Review and Resource Manual

Family Nurse Practitioner

6th Edition

Volume 1

Edited by
Courtney Reinisch, DNP, RN, FNP-BC, DCC
Mary Elizabeth Duffy, DNP, RN, FNP-BC, ACNP-BC, DCC

ANA
AMERICAN NURSES ASSOCIATION

The ANA is the only full-service professional organization representing the interests of the nation's 4.2 million registered nurses through its constituent/state nurses associations and its organizational affiliates. The ANA advances the nursing profession by fostering high standards of nursing practice, promoting the rights of nurses in the workplace, projecting a positive and realistic view of nursing, and by lobbying the Congress and regulatory agencies on health care issues affecting nurses and the public.

American Nurses Association
8403 Colesville Road,
Silver Spring, MD 20910

Library of Congress Control Number: 2024940653

ISBNs
Print Volume 1: 978-1-953985-43-9
Print Volume 2: 978-1-953985-44-6
ePDF: 978-1-953985-45-3
ePub: 978-1-953985-46-0
Mobi: 978-1-953985-47-7
SAN: 851-3481

CONTENTS

VOLUME 1

VOLUME 1

CHAPTER 1

PREPARING FOR THE CERTIFICATION EXAMINATION

Before You Begin Studying

Confirm the eligibility criteria. The eligibility criteria will vary for each exam, but may include things like clinical practice hours, degree and license required, etc. Please check the American Nurses Credentialing Center (ANCC) website for details on the particular eligibility criteria for your exam.

Review the general testing handbook. The general testing handbook can be found on ANCC's website under "Additional Information and Resources (https://www.nursingworld.org/certification/certification-policies/). It provides information on how the exam is scored, policies, etc.

TAKE ADVANTAGE OF ALL OF ANCC'S RESOURCES

1. **Test Content Outline.** The test content outline includes the number of questions for each domain of practice and identifies the areas that are included on the examination.
2. **Test Reference List.** Review the test reference list for review resources. While the list is not all-inclusive, it will act as a guide to help you prepare.
3. **Sample Questions.** In addition to the review questions at the back of this book, you can find sample questions that are similar to those on the actual examination on ANCC's website. For many exams there are also banks of practice questions available from the American Nurses Association's website: https://www.nursingworld.org/continuing-education/ce-subcategories/certification-review/. Make sure to look at practice tests designed for the exam.
4. **Readiness Tests:** Take a practice test in a simulated test environment either at a Prometric Testing Center or via Live Remote Proctoring to increase your comfort with the test environment and procedures. Find more details about Readiness Tests on ANCC's website: https://www.nursingworld.org/certification/readiness-tests/

Develop a personal study plan approximately 3 months before you plan to take your exam. This could include self-study, finding a study buddy or group, taking a review course, taking an online narrated review course, reviewing current textbooks and articles, or other methods. The key is to have a study plan that works for you and follow through on it.

Arrange for special testing accommodations. The American Nurses Credentialing Center and its testing vendor make every effort to reasonably accommodate candidates with documented disabilities as defined by the Americans with Disabilities Act (ADA). If you have a disability as defined under the ADA, you must notify ANCC by submitting a report regarding your request from your physician or a qualified healthcare professional. The information must be on the physician's or other qualified healthcare professional's letterhead, typed, dated, and signed by the healthcare professional. Refer to the General Test Handbook for more details.

Tips for Preparing for the Exam

STEP 1: ASSESS CURRENT KNOWLEDGE

General Content

Examine the table of contents of this book and the test content outline, available at [insert website]

- What content do you need to know?
- How well do you know these subjects?

Take a Review Course

- Taking a review course is an excellent way to assess your knowledge of the content that will be included in the exam.
- If you plan to take a review course, take it well before the exam so you will have plenty of time to master any areas of weakness the course uncovers.
- If some topics in the review course are new to you, concentrate on these in your studies.

STEP 2: DEVELOP YOUR STUDY PLAN

- Write up a formal plan of study.
    - Include topics for study, timetable, resources, and methods of study that work for you.
    - Decide whether you want to organize a study group or work alone.
    - Schedule regular times to study.

- ◇ Avoid cramming; it is counterproductive. Try to schedule your study periods in 1-hour increments.
- ◇ Gather your study resources (general test handbook, Test Content Outline, Test Reference List, Review Manual, sample questions, etc.)

- ♦ You will need to know facts and be able to interpret and analyze this information utilizing critical thinking.

Personalize Your Study Plan

- ♦ How do you learn best? Choose study methods that fit your learning style.
- ♦ Have a specific place with good lighting set aside for studying. Find a place with no distractions. Assemble your study materials.
- ♦ Make sure to focus on the areas you are weakest and reassess periodically

STEP 3: IMPLEMENT YOUR STUDY PLAN

- ♦ Refer to your study plan regularly. Write it up or type it out and put it someplace you will see it regularly. Post it at your desk or even put it into your calendar.
- ♦ Stick to your schedule.
- ♦ Take breaks when you get tired.
- ♦ If you start procrastinating, get help from a friend or reorganize your study plan.
- ♦ It is not necessary to follow your plan rigidly. Adjust as you learn where you need to spend more time.
- ♦ Make sure you reference the Test Reference List and Test Content Outline on ANCC's website for the latest updates and information about the exam.

Pace Your Studying

- ♦ Stop studying for the examination when you start to feel overwhelmed and take a break. If you need to, adjust your study plan:
  - ◇ Break overwhelming tasks into smaller tasks that you know you can do.
  - ◇ Try a new study method.

Work With Others

- Put together a study group.
  - Study groups can provide practice in analyzing cases, interpreting questions, and critical thinking.
  - You can discuss a topic and take turns presenting cases for the group to analyze.
  - Study groups can also provide moral support and help you stay on track.

STEP 4: FINAL PREPARATION

Use practice exams when studying to get accustomed to the exam format and time restrictions. The American Nurses Association has a bank of sample questions available online in many specialty areas.

Practice tests can help you learn to judge the time it should take you to complete the exam and are useful for gaining experience in analyzing questions. However, keep in mind that books of questions may not uncover the gaps in your knowledge that a more systematic content review text like this manual will reveal. If you feel that you don't know enough about a topic, refer to a text from the reference list to learn more. After you feel that you have learned the topic, practice questions are a wonderful tool to help improve your test-taking skills.

Know your test-taking style and be aware of your potential pitfalls. Do you rush through the exam without reading the questions thoroughly? Practice reading the question completely, including all four choices. Choice "a" may sound good at first glance, but "d" is actually correct. Do you get stuck and dwell on a question for a long time? Remember that computer-based exams allow you to mark questions you are unsure about and go back to them later. You should spend about 45 to 60 seconds per question and finish with time to review the questions you marked. There is also no penalty for guessing; you are encouraged to respond to every examination question.

The Night Before the Exam

- Be prepared to get to the exam on time.
  - Know the test site location and how long it takes to get there.
  - Take a "dry run" beforehand to make sure you know how to get to the testing site, if necessary.
- Get a good night's sleep.
- Eat sensibly.

- Avoid alcohol the night before.
- Assemble the required material to be admitted to the exam. Make sure you have the required form of ID. Reference the general test handbook for information about what you'll need.
- Read over the exam room rules. Know what you can and cannot bring with you.

The Day of the Exam

- Get there early. You must arrive to the test center at least 15 minutes before your scheduled appointment time. If you are late, you may not be admitted.
- You will be given a dry erase board, which will be collected at the end of the exam.
- Nothing else is allowed in the exam room. You will be required to put all personal items in a designated area such as a locker.
- Items such as eye-wear, jewelry, etc. are subject to visual inspection
- No water or food will be allowed. You may leave the testing room to use the restroom or get a drink of water, but you will need to sign out according to the instructions that will be explained at the test site. Your testing time will not be increased to accommodate a break.
- Think positively. You have studied hard and are well-prepared.
- Remember your anxiety reduction strategies.

Tips for Dealing with Anxiety

LEADING UP TO THE EXAM:

Everyone experiences anxiety when faced with taking the certification exam.

- Taking a review course or setting up your own study plan will help you feel more confident about taking the exam. There is no substitute for being well-prepared.
- Take practice tests and time yourself to get used to feeling of working on a timer. Remember that the total time for each test is usually 4 hours. Time is not meant to be a factor in the examination.
- Brush up on test-taking skills.
- Practice relaxation techniques. A few minutes of deep breathing, meditation, or even just listening to soothing music can help you calm down and focus.

- Don't put too much stock in what others tell you about their exam experience. Remember that everything they can tell you is based on their memory of a stressful situation; it may not be very accurate. People tend to remember those items with which they are less comfortable; for instance, those with a limited background in women's health may say that the exam was "all women's health." In fact, the test content outline ensures that the exam covers multiple content areas without overemphasizing any one topic.

EXAM DAY ANXIETY:

Test anxiety is a specific type of anxiety. Symptoms include upset stomach, sweaty palms, tachycardia, trouble concentrating, and a feeling of dread. But there are ways to cope with test anxiety.

- Avoid alcohol, excess coffee, caffeine, and any new medications that might sedate you, dull your senses, or make you feel agitated.
- Take a few deep breaths and concentrate on the task at hand.
- Use relaxation techniques such as breathing exercises, progressive muscle relaxation, or imagery and visualization.
- Go into the exam with a strategy in mind. Plan to take water and bathroom breaks at specific intervals and take that opportunity to stretch. Mark questions you're unsure of to come back to them later rather than spending too much time on one question.

INTERNET RESOURCES:

- ANCC website: [insert website]
  - Test Content Outline
  - Test Reference List
  - Sample Questions
  - Readiness Tests
- General Testing and Renewal Handbook: https://www.nursingworld.org/~4aae16/global assets/certification/certification-policies/ancc-generaltestingrenewalrequirements4-1 -2017_final.pdf
- ANA Bookstore: https://www.nursingworld.org/education-events/Books/.
  - ANA Nursing: Scope and Standards of Practice
  - ANA specialty scope and standards

- ◊ Code of Ethics for Nurses
- ◊ Other titles that may be listed on your Test Reference List

- American Nurses Association certification review resources: https://www.nursingworld.org/continuing-education/ce-subcategories/certification-review/
  - ◊ Practice questions
  - ◊ Webinars and review courses
  - ◊ Certification Exam Test-Taking Strategies Web Course

CHAPTER 2

IMPORTANT FACTORS INFLUENCING THE NURSE PRACTITIONER ROLE

Angela Richard-Eaglin, DNP, MSN, FAANP-BC, CNE, FAANP, CDE®

Legal Dimensions of the Role

LEGAL AUTHORITY FOR PRACTICE

State Nurse Practice Acts—Rules and Regulations

Authority for nurse practitioner (NP) practice is found in state legislative statutes and in rules and regulations. The Nurse Practice Act of every state customarily authorizes a board of nursing to establish statutory authority to define who may be called an NP (title protection), what they may do (scope of practice), restrictions on their practice, the requirements an NP must meet to be credentialed within the state as an NP (education, certification, etc.), and disciplinary grounds for infractions. See National Council of State Boards of Nursing's (NCSBN's) website (www. ncsbn .org) for a listing of state nursing board requirements. In many states, legislative acts may specifically require that an NP develop a collaborative practice agreement with a physician that defines general supervision and delegation of authority. Collaborative agreements describe what types of drugs, devices, or diagnostics might be ordered, and define limits related to NP practice.

Statutory law is implemented in regulatory language. The rules and regulations for each state may further define scope of practice, practice requirements, and/or restrictions.

In 1999, the National Council of State Boards of Nursing (NCSBN) began the implementation of an interstate compact for nursing practice to reduce state-to-state discrepancies in nursing requirements for practice. The Advanced Practice Registered Nurse (APRN) Compact addresses the need to promote consistent access to quality advanced practice nursing care within states and across state lines. The Uniform APRN Licensure/Authority to Practice Requirements, developed by NCSBN with APRN stakeholders in 2000, establishes the foundation for this APRN Compact. Like the existing Nurse Licensure Compact for recognition of registered nurse (RN) and licensed practical nurse (LPN) licenses, the APRN Compact gives states the mechanism for mutually recognizing APRN licenses/authority to practice. To be eligible for the APRN Compact, a state must either be a member of the current nurse licensure compact for RNs and LPNs or choose to enter both compacts simultaneously. To see which states participate view the state compact map at www.ncsbn.org/public-files/NLC_Map.pdf.

NURSE PRACTITIONER PROFESSIONAL PRACTICE STANDARDS

Licensure

- Licensure is "[a] process by which an agency of government grants permission to individuals accountable for the practice of a profession to engage in the practice of that profession and prohibits all others from legally doing so" (Committee for the Study of Credentialing in Nursing, 1979; U.S. Department of Health, Education, and Welfare [DHEW], 1971).
- The purpose of licensure is to protect the public by ensuring a minimum level of professional competence. Licensure benefits both the public and the individual nurse because essential qualifications for nursing practice are identified; a determination is made as to whether an individual meets those qualifications; and an objective forum is provided for review of concerns regarding a nurse's practice when needed. Licensure benefits nurses because clear legal authorization for the scope of practice of the profession is established. Licensure also protects the use of titles. Only a licensed nurse is authorized to use certain titles (i.e., registered nurses [RNs], licensed practical/vocational nurses [LPN/VNs], advanced practice registered nurses [APRNs], etc.) or to represent themself as a licensed nurse (NCSBN, 2011).

Certification

- Certification is "[a] process by which a non-governmental agency or association certifies that an individual licensed to practice as a professional has met certain pre-determined standards specified by that profession for specialty practice" (DHEW, 1971).
- The purpose of certification is to assure the public that a person has mastery of a body of knowledge and has acquired the skills necessary to function in a particular specialty. Some certifications are required for entry into practice (e.g., for licensure within a state) and thus have a regulatory function; some certifications denote professional competence and recognize excellence.

Accreditation

- Accreditation is "[t]he process by which a voluntary, non-governmental agency or organization appraises and grants accreditation status to institutions and/or programs or services [that] meet predetermined structure, process and outcome criteria" (DHEW, 1971). The purpose is to ensure that the organization has met specific standards.

Scope of Practice

- *Scope of practice* defines a specific legal scope determined by state statutes, boards of nursing, educational preparation, and common practice within a community.
  - For example, adult nurse practitioners (ANPs) are not legally authorized to care for children. The state might require an NP to have formal educational preparation in pediatrics. There is broad variation from state to state.
- General scope of practice is specified in many published professional documents (e.g., *Scope and Standards of Advanced Practice Registered Nursing*, ANA, 1996). Many organizations have completed role delineation studies that attempt to qualify the core behaviors that all advanced practice nurses (APNs) must possess, as well as the core knowledge and behaviors required of persons in a particular specialty.
  - For example, core knowledge for a pediatric nurse practitioner (PNP) is inherently different from that for a geriatric nurse practitioner (GNP). It is critical that these statements about specific scope and standards exist so that everyone—including nurses—will have access to materials to which they can refer when there are specific questions related to role. This is especially important when the traditional role of nurses is changing or "advancing" at an uneven rate through changes in state law.
  - Because the NP role has expanded into new practice settings, including hospice, acute care hospitals, and home care, it is important that core knowledge and state law protecting NPs in these practice settings also expand, providing the legal authorization and title protection necessary for these practice settings.
- Prescriptive authority is recognized as within the scope of practice for nurse practitioners in all 50 states, although there is major variability from state to state. This variability has created inherent difficulty in collecting data related to NP prescribing practices. The *Nurse Practitioner Journal* publishes a comprehensive update of legislative requirements and recent changes in its January issue each year. Data collected by Nurse Practitioner Alternatives, Inc., since 1996 has documented stability within prescribing patterns by NPs. Data from 2004 documents indicate that the majority of NPs possess their own Drug Enforcement Administration (DEA) numbers (72%), write between 6 and 25 prescriptions in an average clinical day (79%), recommend between 1 and 20 over-the-counter (OTC) preparations in an average clinical day (90%), and manage between 25% and 100% of their patient encounters independently (97%; Nurse Practitioner Alternatives, Inc., 2004).

Standards of Practice

- Standards of practice are authoritative statements by which the quality of practice, service, or education can be judged (e.g., *Scope of Practice for Nurse Practitioners*, American Association of Nurse Practitioners, 2019; *Code of Ethics for Nurses*, ANA, 2015).
- Professional standards focus on the minimum levels of acceptable performance as a way of providing consumers with a means of measuring the quality of care they receive. These standards may be written at the generic level to apply to all nurses (e.g., following standard precautions) as well as to define practice by each specialty.
- The presence of accepted standards of practice may be used to legally describe the standard of care that a provider must meet. These standards may be precise proto cols that must be followed or recommendations for more general guidelines.

The Future of Nurse Practitioner Education and Practice

- In 2020, the National Organization of Nurse Practitioner Faculties (NONPF) released the new and revised Post-baccalaureate Doctor of Nursing Practice (DNP) Program Curriculum and Competency Mapping Templates. As documented by the NONPF, the intent of these documents is to support NONPF's goal to transition all NP programs to the DNP by 2025. These documents can be viewed at https://www.nonpf.org/page/DNPResources?&hhsearchterms=%22practice+and+doctorate+and+entry+and+level+and+competencies%22
- In 2022, as part of a multi-organization collaboration, NONPF (www.nonpf.org), released the *Standards for Quality Nurse Practitioner Education (NTFS)*, 6th edition, A Report of the National Task Force on Quality Nurse Practitioner Education. This consensus-based document provides new standards and revised criteria that facilitate program development, quality, and continuous improvement through assessment, sustainability, and planning. This document can be viewed at https://cdn.ymaws.com/www.nonpf.org/resource/resmgr/2022/ntfs_/ntfs_final.pdf

THE NP ROLE IN UNDERSTANDING AND ADVOCATING FOR PATIENT RIGHTS

Confidentiality

- The patient and family have a right to assume that information given to the health care team will not be disclosed; that is, their information will be kept confidential. This has several dimensions.

- *Verbal information*: Health care providers shall not discuss any information given to them during the health care encounter with anyone not directly involved in a patient's care without the patient's or family's permission (when the family has decision-making permission).
- *Written information*: Confidentiality of the health care encounter is protected under federal statute through the Health Insurance Portability and Accountability Act of 1996 (HIPAA). The Administrative Simplification provisions of HIPAA require the U.S. Department of Health and Human Services to establish national standards for electronic health care transactions and national identifiers for providers, health plans, and employers. The provisions also address the security and privacy of health data. Information may be accessed at http://www.cms.gov/regulations-and-guidance/ hipaa-administrative-simplification/hipaageninfo/thehipaalawandrelated-information.html. The person's right to privacy is to be respected when requesting or responding to a request for a patient's medical record.
- The statute requires that the provider discuss confidentiality issues with patients (parents in the case of a minor), establish consent, and clarify any questions about disclosure of information.
- The provider is required to obtain a signed medical authorization and consent form to release medical records and information.
- Exceptions to guaranteed confidentiality occur when the need for information outweighs the principle of confidentiality. Examples include the following:
  - Release of records to insurance companies
  - Release of records to attorneys involved in litigation
  - Court orders, subpoenas, or summonses
  - Meeting state requirements for mandatory reporting of diseases or conditions
  - In cases of suspected or actual child abuse
  - If a person reveals an intent to harm someone

Informed Consent

- *Informed consent* is the right of all competent adults (age 18 or older) and emancipated minors (age 17 or younger who are married, a parent, or self-sufficiently living away from the family domicile) to accept or reject treatment by a health care provider. (Some states have laws concerning birth control or abortions that apply to patients younger than 18.)
- The clinician has the duty to explain relevant information to patients to assist them in making informed decisions. This information usually includes diagnosis, nature and purpose of proposed treatment or procedure, risks and benefits, prognosis, availability

of alternative methods of treatment and their risks and benefits, and all possibilities of serious harm.

- It must be documented in the medical records that this information has been provided.
- Informed consent does not absolve the NP of allegations of malpractice.

Care of Minors

- In most jurisdictions, persons under the age of 18 cannot receive health care services without permission of a competent parent or legal guardian.
- Exceptions to this rule may be made in some jurisdictions in the case of an emancipated minor, a pregnant minor, or in matters pertaining to sexually transmitted diseases and birth control.

Advance Directives

- When a patient is incapable of making decisions, the person's preferences may be expressed in a written living will or a health care durable power of attorney created when the patient was still competent. Such documents are called *advance directives.*
- *Living wills* are written documents prepared in advance in case of terminal illness or nonreversible loss of consciousness.
- Their provisions go into effect when:
  - The patient has become incompetent,
  - The patient is declared terminally ill, and
  - No further interventions will alter the patient's course to a reasonable degree of medical certainty.

Durable Power of Attorney for Health Care

- People can identify in writing an agent to act on their behalf, should they become mentally incapacitated. The decisions of the designated agent are:
  - Binding,
  - Not limited to the circumstances of terminal illness,
  - Flexible enough to carry out the patient's wishes throughout the course of an illness, and
  - Often accompanied by a durable power of attorney over financial issues.

Ethical Decision-making

- Moral concepts such as advocacy, accountability, loyalty, caring, compassion, and human dignity are the foundations of ethical behavior.
- The ethical behavior of nurses has been defined for professional nursing in an American Nurses Association policy statement (ANA, 2015).
- Ethical behavior incorporates respect for a person's autonomy. Ethical behavior means that a patient must be allowed to make decisions regarding their care to the full extent of their personal capacity to do so.
- Duty to help others (beneficence), avoidance of harmful behavior (nonmaleficence), and fairness are also foundational components of ethical behavior.

Quality Assurance

- *Quality assurance* (QA) is a system designed to evaluate and monitor the quality of patient care and facility management.
- Formal programs provide a framework for systematic, deliberate, and continuous evaluation and monitoring of individual clinical practice.
- Programs promote responsibility and accountability to deliver high-quality care, assist in the evaluation and improvement of the patient's care, and provide for an organized means of problem-solving.
- A good program identifies educational needs, improves the documentation of care, and reduces the clinician's overall exposure to liability.
- Programs identify components of structure, process, and outcomes of care. They also look at organizational effectiveness, efficiency, and client and provider interactions.
    - QA may be implemented through audits, utilization review, peer review, outcome studies, and measurements of patient satisfaction.

Quality & Safety Education for Nurses (QSEN)

- Quality & Safety Education for Nurses (QSEN) was funded by the Robert Wood Johnson Foundation to address the knowledge, skills, and attitudes necessary to ensure the quality and safety of the health care systems in the United States.
- The National Academy of Medicine (NAM), along with numerous professional organizations representing nursing, identified competencies to be used in the education, certification, and continuing education of advanced practice nurses.

- Areas identified that affect advanced practice include:
  - ◇ Patient-centered care focus,
  - ◇ Teamwork and collaboration,
  - ◇ Use of evidence-based practice,
  - ◇ Continuous quality improvement,
  - ◇ Safety to minimize harm to patients and providers, and
  - ◇ Use of informatics and technology.

NURSE PRACTITIONER LEGAL AND FINANCIAL ISSUES

Liability

- NPs should be aware of liability issues or exposure to legal risk, which include
  - ◇ Patients,
  - ◇ procedures, and
  - ◇ Quality of medical records.
- There are methods of risk reduction or management:
  - ◇ Activities or systems have been designed to recognize and intervene to reduce the risk of injury to patients and subsequent claims against health care providers.
  - ◇ Malpractice insurance does not protect clinicians from charges of practicing outside their legal scope of practice. All clinicians carry their own liability insurance coverage to ensure their own legal representation by an attorney to advocate for them.

Malpractice

- Malpractice involves negligent professional acts of persons engaged in professions requiring highly technical or professional skills.
- The plaintiff has the burden of proving the four elements of malpractice.
  - ◇ *Duty*: The clinician does not exercise reasonable care when undertaking and providing treatment to the patient when a patient–clinician relationship exists.
  - ◇ *Breach of duty*: The clinician violates the applicable standard of care in treating the patient's condition.
  - ◇ *Proximate cause*: There is a causal relationship between the breach in the standard of care and the patient's injuries.
  - ◇ *Damages*: There are permanent and substantial damages to the patient because of the malpractice.

- Types of malpractice insurance
  - *Claims-made policy*: Covers a claim only as long as both the incident and the claim take place while the policy is in force.
  - *Occurrence-based policy:* Covers any claim that results from an incident that occurs during the term of the policy, regardless of how long it takes before the claim is made.
  - *Tail coverage*: Additional or supplemental insurance that covers the provider for incidents that occurred during the term of a claims-made policy but are not brought forward until after the policy has expired.

National Practitioner Data Bank (NPDB)

- The Health Care Quality Improvement Act of 1986 established a databank to scrutinize members of the health care profession and list those practitioners who have had malpractice claims asserted against them.
- Currently few NPs are listed in the NPDB, but the number of NPs who have malpractice claims filed against them is increasing as the number of NPs in practice increases.

Reimbursement

- NPs are reimbursed for their services as primary care providers under Medicare, Medicaid, the yes Federal Employees Health Benefits Program, TRICARE (formerly known as CHAMPUS), veterans' and military programs, and federally funded school-based clinics.
- Medicare: People age 65 and over, some disabled people under the age of 65, and people with kidney disease treated with dialysis or transplant are eligible for Medicare.
  - Medicare A: Hospital insurance that requires no premium. Part A covers inpatient care, including hospitals, skilled nursing facilities (not custodial or long- term care), hospice, and eligible home health care services.
  - Medicare B: Outpatient insurance that requires a premium. Patients may decline coverage. Part B covers outpatient services, durable medical equipment, physical and occupational health services, home health care, and eligible preventive care services.
  - Medicare C: Combines Part A and Part B of Medicare.
  - Medicare D: Covers prescription drugs; usually requires a premium. The patient may decline coverage.
  - Medicare E: Offers incentive/reimbursement for providers participating in electronic prescribing.

- Incident to billing: Medicare regulation. Pays 100% of the physician charge to an NP who provides care to patients under specific guidelines (see the Centers for Medicare & Medicaid Services [CMS] website for full guidelines):
  - Services are furnished as an integral, although incidental, part of the physician's care.
  - Physicians must provide the initial service and regular subsequent visits.
  - A physician must be present in the office but not necessarily in the exam room.
  - Services are billed under the physician's provider number at 100% of the physician rate.
- Medicaid
  - Individual states administer and make the rules for Medicaid.
  - States must adhere to CMS rules and regulations when directing the Medicaid program.
  - By federal law, Medicaid will cover services of family and pediatric NPs.
  - If a state has applied to CMS for a Medicaid waiver, it is important that NPs are allowed to be primary care providers.
  - NPs must apply to state Medicaid for Medicaid provider numbers.
  - Full CMS guidelines are available at www.cms.gov
- Private insurance plans may elect to reimburse for NP services even if not mandated to do so by state law. In some states, however, the insurance code may be interpreted rigidly to exclude the reimbursement of NPs.
- Managed care organizations (MCOs) have frequently excluded NPs from being designated as primary care providers carrying their own caseloads. Thus, in many MCOs, the only option for NPs is to be salaried employees. As salaried employees, the NP contributions are often not visible and may be credited to their collaborating physician, giving them a "ghost" provider status. Without a legitimate method to document services provided and revenue generated, the NP can find that job security is often at risk. Many state NP organizations have recently focused legislative activity on enacting state laws allowing NPs to function as primary care providers in both health maintenance organizations (HMOs) and preferred provider organizations (PPOs). These efforts have led to opposition from state medical organizations.
  - There is considerable flux in state and national policy on what services and procedures NPs may bill for and whether they will be paid directly. Incorrect billing places health care providers at risk of fraud and abuse charges, regardless of whether they knowingly violate the law or are simply ignorant of the regulations.
  - NPs must be aware of specific regulations and policies for patient care services. Resources include CMS bulletins, among others (www.cms.hhs.gov/).

◊ Coding and billing practices are the responsibility of the NP provider, and knowledge of the regulations for payors is a requisite competency.

◊ Specific rules and regulations for Medicare and Medicaid can be found at www.cms.hhs.gov

Performance Assessment

- The NPDB and Health Integrity and Protection Data Bank (HIPDB) are maintained by the U.S. Department of Health and Human Services, Health Resources and Services Administration, Bureau of Health Professions, Division of Practitioner Data Banks. Developed because of the Health Care Quality Improvement Act of 1986, the NPDB and HIPDB are flagging systems intended to facilitate a comprehensive review of the professional credentials of health care practitioners, with a goal of improving the quality of health care. The information contained in the NPDB includes a practitioner's licensure, professional society memberships, malpractice payment history, and record of clinical privileges. An NP may perform a self-query by visiting the site at www.npdb-hipdb.com/
- Other programs monitoring and comparing health quality include the Healthcare Effectiveness Data and Information Set (HEDIS), developed by the National Committee on Quality Assurance (NCQA). HEDIS is a set of standardized performance measures designed to ensure that purchasers and consumers have the information they need to reliably compare the performance of managed health care plans (www.ncqa. org).

Health Records

Electronic health record (EHR) systems readily allow access to medical records at a national level for more definitive monitoring of the effectiveness and outcomes of interventions. The data collected assists in determining the most effective clinical interventions and establishing effective guidelines for health care providers.

Centers for Medicare & Medicaid Services and Electronic Health Records

- CMS is promoting the use of EHRs to assist in attaining national health care accuracy and efficiency and better meet established goals.
- The term "meaningfully" is being used for the EHR to assess the efficiency of an electronic system. The 2009 American Recovery and Reinvestment Act delineates three essential components for meaningful use of EHRs for electronic prescribing, exchange of information, and measurement of clinical quality. In 2011, the first of the three stages

was implemented, with the final stage implemented in 2015. The program is voluntary and requires application according to established guidelines. Reimbursement for program participation is based on specific criteria, such as benchmarks for recording accurate vital signs, height, body mass index (BMI), immunizations, and other health care interventions.

- Benefits for the patient include receiving reminders for appointments by email, accessing portions of the medical record to review lab work, and leaving messages for providers. Specifics may be found on the CMS website at https://www.cms.gov/regulations-and-guidance/legislation/ehrincentiveprograms.
- E-scribe: Electronic submission of prescriptions is now common practice, and specific laws regarding e-scribing vary slightly from state to state. Refer to specific state laws for accurate rules regarding the use of e-scribing by means of certified EHR.

Current Trends and Topics in Nurse Practitioner Education and Practice

CONSENSUS MODEL FOR APRN REGULATION: LICENSURE, ACCREDITATION, CERTIFICATION, AND EDUCATION

- Consensus document from more than 40 nursing and advanced practice organizations and the NCSBN APRN Advisory Committee
- Published July 2008
- Provides a national baseline for APRN licensure, accreditation, certification, and education (LACE)
- Defines APRN practice, describes APRN regulatory model, identifies titles to be used, defines specialty, describes emergence of new roles and population foci, and presents strategies for implementation
- Key issues:
  - Goal is standardization of APRN education, licensure, and practice across all states and territories
  - Limits APRN title to four roles: nurse practitioner, nurse anesthetist, nurse midwife, and clinical nurse specialist
  - Identifies six population foci, with potential for more as practice changes
  - Provided for elimination of separate geriatric and adult NP role and certification; replaced with combined ANP-GNP role, education, and certification

FIGURE 2–1.
APRN REGULATORY MODEL

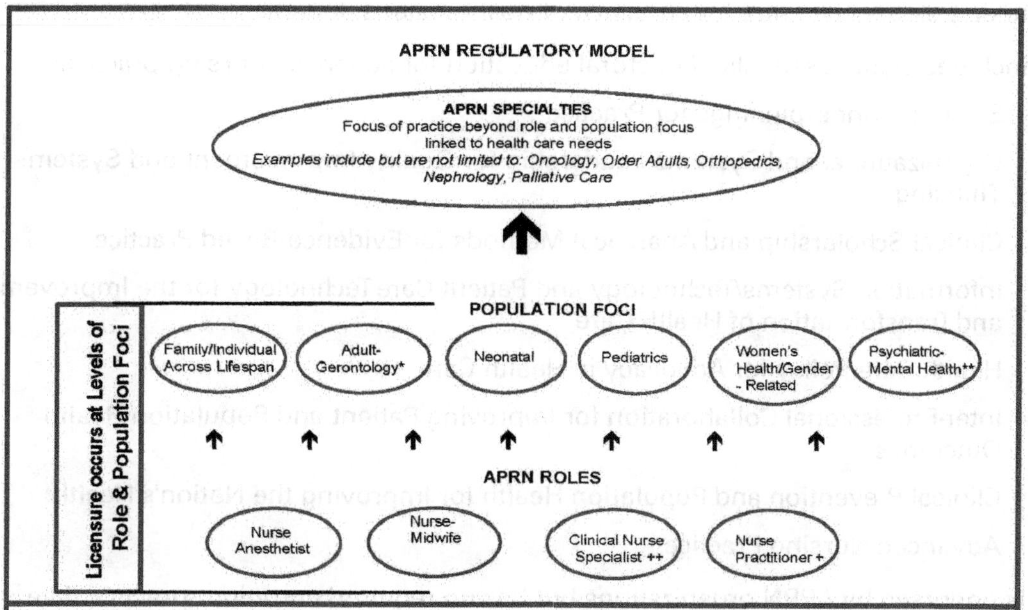

+The certified nurse practitioner (CNP) is prepared with the acute care CNP competencies and/or the primary care CNP competencies. At this point in time the acute care and primary care CNP delineation applies only to the pediatric and adult-gerontology CNP population foci. Scope of practice of the primary care or acute care CNP is **not setting specific** but is based on patient care needs. Programs may prepare individuals across both the primary care and acute care CNP competencies. If programs prepare graduates across both sets of roles, the graduate must be prepared with the consensus-based competencies for both roles and must successfully obtain certification in both the acute and the primary care CNP roles. CNP certification in the acute care or primary care roles must match the educational preparation for CNPs in these roles.

Reprinted from *Consensus Model for APRN Regulation: Licensure, Accreditation, Certification, & Education* (p. 10), by the APRN Consensus Work Group and the National Council of State Boards of Nursing APRN Advisory Committee, 2008. Retrieved from https://www.ncsbn.org/ Consensus_Model_for_APRN_Regulation_July_2008.pdf

DOCTOR OF NURSING PRACTICE (DNP)

- 2004: American Association of Colleges of Nursing (AACN) members approved DNP Position Statement and 2015 target implementation date.
- 2006: *The Essentials of Doctoral Education for Advanced Nursing Practice* was published.
- DNP is the degree associated with practice-focused doctoral nursing education.
- The goal is to prepare graduates for the highest level of nursing practice beyond the initial preparation in the discipline.

- It includes the four current APN roles: clinical nurse specialist, nurse anesthetist, nurse midwife, and nurse practitioner.
- The degree may be entry into practice or post-master's degree.
- It includes eight essentials of doctoral education for advanced nursing practice:
    - Scientific Underpinnings for Practice
    - Organizational and Systems Leadership for Quality Improvement and Systems Thinking
    - Clinical Scholarship and Analytical Methods for Evidence-Based Practice
    - Information Systems/Technology and Patient Care Technology for the Improvement and Transformation of Health Care
    - Health Care Policy for Advocacy in Health Care
    - Inter-Professional Collaboration for Improving Patient and Population Health Outcomes
    - Clinical Prevention and Population Health for Improving the Nation's Health
    - Advanced Nursing Practice
- It is endorsed by APRN organizations but has no required entry-into-practice date established for NPs.

***NONPF committed to moving all entry-level nurse practitioner (NP) education to the DNP degree by 2025 (NONPF, 2018). NONPF developed new and revised the post-baccalaureate DNP Program curriculum and competency mapping templates (NONPF, 2020). More information can be found at the following link: https://www.nonpf.org/page/DNPResources

Practice Environment, Policy, and Advocacy

NAM'S FUTURE OF NURSING 2020–2030

At the request of the Robert Wood Johnson foundation and on behalf of the national academy of medicine, an ad hoc committee conducted a study to develop strategies that improve opportunities for nurses to leverage their expertise to advance health equity and optimize health outcomes for all people.

Future of nursing 2020–2030: charting a path to achieve health equity explores nursing's role in reducing health disparities, promoting equity, keeping costs at a minimum, utilizing technology, and maintaining patient- and family-focused care into 2030. Although the goal is to keep costs at bay, NPS must not do so at the expense of assisting patients to achieve optimal health outcomes. The goal of achieving health equity by eliminating health disparities requires that NPS prioritize the service aspect of health care. Using technology requires advocacy for equitable access to and assistance with literacy. Therefore, the np must promote and develop innovations that support persons and families with ease of access, effective and efficient communication, and high-quality telehealth to monitor health conditions. The report also outlines the critical areas that the nursing professions must bolster to have an impact on the goals of decreasing disparities and advancing health equity. These areas include the nursing workforce, nursing leadership, nursing education, well-being, emergency preparedness and response, and nursing's responsibility regarding individual and structural determinants of health. Nurses work in a broad array of settings, which provide opportunities to improve health through multiple intervention strategies, including the following:

- Advocacy
- Securing resources and making appropriate referrals
- Patient, family, community, and population-focused education
- Team-based/integrative care models
- Active involvement in health policy
- Participation in patient-centered outcomes research

For more information on *the Future of Nursing 2020–2030: Charting a Path to Achieve Health Equity*, visit https://nam.edu/publications/the-future-of-nursing-2020-2030/

NONPF CALLS FOR GREATER RACIAL AND ETHNIC DIVERSITY IN NURSE PRACTITIONER EDUCATION (2018)

In alignment with the mission and vision of NONPF, the organization strives to champion a culture of diversity and inclusivity across all NP education programs and calls upon NP faculty to consider increases in racially and ethnically diverse patient populations, persistence of racial and ethnic disparities in health care delivery, and disparate representation of racially and ethnically diverse groups among NP faculty and within the professional workforce.

ANA POSITION STATEMENT

The Nurse's Role in Addressing Discrimination: Protecting and Promoting Inclusive Strategies in Practice Settings, Policy, and Advocacy states that the ANA seeks to eliminate all forms of discrimination, improving access to and attainment of quality health care, providing inclusive and impartial health care that is devoid of bias, and actively seeking and engaging in opportunities to eradicate disparities. The full ANA statement can be viewed at https://ojin.nursingworld.org/MainMenuCategories/ANAMarketplace/ANAPeriodicals/OJIN/Columns/ANA-Position-Statements/Nurses-Role-in-Addressing-Discrimination.html

AMERICAN ACADEMY OF NURSING (AAN) EQUITY, DIVERSITY, AND INCLUSIVITY STATEMENT

The Academy envisions "Healthy Lives for All People" and their mission is to "Improve health and achieve health equity by impacting policy through nursing leadership, innovation, and science." The Academy is committed to integrating its core values of equity, diversity, and inclusivity as the foundation for developing an anti-racist agenda and the ongoing goal of eliminating all forms of discrimination. "To the Academy, equity is assuring the right conditions for all people to thrive and achieve their full potential. The Academy defines diversity as affirming all the ways in which people differ. Inclusivity, as defined by the Academy, refers to the welcoming and active engagement of all voices within every aspect of the organization and with an intentional emphasis on acknowledging those who experience or have experienced marginalization or disenfranchisement." The full statement can be viewed at https://www.aannet.org/about/about-the-academy/edi

HEALTHY PEOPLE 2030

The *Healthy People 2030* mission is "Building a Healthier Future for All." The 10-year goals focus on improving health and well-being through data-driven objectives in three categories: (1) 10 core objectives, (2) developmental objectives, and (3) research objectives. The core objectives focus on evidence-based interventions to impact high-priority public health issues. The role of the NP in achieving the *Healthy People* goals is to apply the data to surveillance, implement strategic interventions, engage in research, and collaborate in the development of population- and issue-specific intervention strategies. The *Healthy People 2030* goals initiative and Social Determinants of Health (SDOH) can be viewed at **https://health.gov/healthypeople**

NOTABLE CONSIDERATIONS FOR ADVANCING HEALTH EQUITY

Acquisition and Application of Cultural Intelligence

Nurse practitioners across roles have the responsibility of caring for individuals and communities that represent a vast array cultural backgrounds and must be prepared to provide culturally responsible individual- and population-centric care to advance health equity and eliminate health disparities and health care disparities. Critical to achieving these goals, the *Healthy People 2030* goals, and the goals associated with the SDOH is the development of cultural intelligence (CQ). CQ is the skill and ability to function effectively in multicultural situations and environments. CQ can significantly improve cultural literacy and fluency, thereby eliminating barriers, such as personal and institutional biases, that impede the provision of culturally sensitive health care.

The NP has an integral role in promoting and advancing health equity through practice, policy, and advocacy for all people Diversity, equity, inclusion, anti-discrimination, and anti-racism are central to the elimination of health disparities and optimizing health outcomes for all people. There is consensus among professional nursing organizations that supports the responsibility of nurses at all levels of practice to function professionally in concert with the humanitarian ethos, which is predicated on providing care to all humans from the lens of impartiality. The humanitarian principles undergird the code of ethics for nurses, highlighting the values of compassion, service, sympathy, mercy, trust, and respect for human life and dignity.

Providing culturally responsible care requires that the NP be aware that clinical guidelines are meant to *guide* heath care practices and treatment plans, but that to achieve best practices, plans of care must be adapted to meet the individual needs of each person with whom they engage. The NP must engage in culturally responsible and inclusive care, regardless of personal preferences and biases. Consideration and integration of the cultural preferences and practices of each individual and community are crucial in holistically addressing heath care needs, thus creating opportunities to shift the determinants of health toward equitable health care and optimal health outcomes for all individuals and communities.

Bias

Bias is a preference for or aversion to someone that may advantage or disadvantage those at whom the bias is aimed. Bias is a personal, and oftentimes, unsubstantiated judgement, labeling, or stereotyping of someone or something. In health care, bias is a leading cause of health inequity and the subsequent health disparities and adverse health outcomes. Much of the literature addresses the impact of implicit bias on health inequities; however, both implicit and explicit bias may equally negatively impact morbidity and mortality among the most impacted populations. Bias often impacts patient–provider interactions, clinical decision-making, and ultimately, patient and population health. From a geopolitical perspective, bias also affects the distribution of resources, many of which affect the overall health and well-being of individuals on the receiving end of bias and discrimination. Nurse practitioners have the responsibility to be aware of their own personal biases and to recognize and stand against the biased-influenced decisions of others. All NPs must be willing to consistently participate in trainings that facilitate bias-reduction strategies to positively influence health outcomes for all human beings.

Health Disparities

It is important to note that there are two types of disparities that impact health outcomes: health care disparities and health disparities. Health care disparities are systems-based disparities that impact individuals and populations, and health disparities refer to the actual health of people. According to the U.S. Department of Health and Human Services Agency for Healthcare Research and Quality, health care disparities refer to variances in the availability of and access to health care resources, including facilities and services. For more information, visit https://www.ahrq.gov/topics/disparities.html.

The Centers for Disease Control and Prevention (CDC) refers to health disparities as preventable variances in disease burden, injury, violence, and/or opportunities to achieve optimal health that are experienced by socially disadvantaged populations. The CDC acknowledges that "health inequities are directly related to the historical and current unequal distribution of social, political, economic, and environmental resources." Factors such as race/ethnicity, gender, sexual orientation, sex, ability, social and economic status, education level, and geographical location heavily influence health disparities and health care disparities. As determined by the NAM Future of Nursing 2020–2030 Report and the *Healthy People 2030* initiative, intentionally and adequately addressing the SDOH can improve health outcomes through targeted efforts to decrease and eliminate social, economic, and health care disparities. Nurse practitioners have the power and unique opportunities to influence change in these areas. More information can be accessed at https://www.cdc.gov/healthyyouth/disparities/index.htm

Health Literacy

The Health Resources and Services Administration (HRSA) defines health literacy as the ability of an individual to obtain, process, and understand basic health information necessary for making decisions about their health care. It is critical for the NP to know that low health literacy is most prevalent among specific populations, such as older adults, historically underrepresented populations, financially disadvantaged populations, and people from medically underserved populations. However, NPs must not generalize, stereotype, or make assumptions about all individuals or communities who fall within these groups. Cultural intelligence and individualized care must be applied to all people. It is the responsibility of the NP to interview and assess each person to determine individual needs and provide appropriate education. More information on health literacy can be found at https://www.hrsa.gov/about/organization/bureaus/ohe/health-literacy/index.html

Social Determinants of Health

The CDC defines SDOH as "factors that contribute to a person's current state of health." These factors may be biological, socioeconomic, psychosocial, behavioral, or social in nature. Holistic FNP practice incorporates all components into patient care (https://www.cdc.gov/social-determinants/index.htm).

Economic Stability

Goal: Help people earn steady incomes that allow them to meet their health needs.

One in 10 people in the United States live in poverty, making it difficult for many people to afford healthy foods, health care, and adequate housing. One of the foci of *Healthy People 2030* is to help people achieve economic stability. Steady employment decreases the likelihood of living in poverty and increases the likelihood of being healthy. Living with certain disabilities, injuries, and health conditions often limits employment opportunities. NPs play a pivotal role in identifying financial burdens, barriers to access to health care, and barriers to acquisition of health-promoting foods and other resources. It is also within the role of the NP to serve as a liaison and assist in building relationships with social service entities that provide people and communities with needed resources. Other ways that NPs can help to advance the Heathy People 2030 goals is to be aware of and promote existing employment programs, career counseling, and high-quality childcare opportunities, all of which can help more people with job attainment and job security. In addition, many NPs are active in policy engagement, which provides prime opportunities to impact the revision of and/or development of policies aimed at subsidies to help people buy healthy foods, obtain safe housing, increase access to affordable health care, and quality education. Each of these initiatives can reduce poverty and improve health and well-being. More information on the *Economic Stability SDOH* can be viewed at https://health.gov/healthypeople/objectives-and-data/browse-objectives/economic-stability

Education Access and Quality

Goal: Increase educational opportunities and help children and adolescents do well in school.

Higher educational levels increase the likelihood of people being healthier and life expectancy growth. *Healthy People 2030* focuses on ensuring high-quality educational opportunities for children and adolescents and on helping them perform well in school. Stress associated with living in poverty can adversely affect brain development in children and make it more difficult for them to perform well in school.

Of note for NPs is that children from low-income families, children with disabilities, and children who routinely experience forms of social discrimination are more likely to struggle with certain academic subjects, especially math and reading. They are also less likely to graduate from high school or pursue college education. This directly affects their ability to obtain safe jobs with decent wages, and consequently contributes to the development of health problems such as heart disease, diabetes, and depression. In caring for children and adolescents, the NP should be vigilant in screening for and identifying indicators and risk factors related to low-quality education. Beyond identification, the NP serves as an advocate for families experiencing inadequate child and adolescent education and should engage in seeking ways to connect these families with appropriate resources. Interventions that aid children and adolescents with school performance and providing financial resources for college may have long-term health benefits. More information can be found at https://health.gov/healthypeople/objectives-and-data/browse-objectives/education-access-and-quality

Health Care Access and Quality

Goal: Increase access to comprehensive, high-quality health care services.

Many people in the United States do not have health insurance, making it less likely to have a primary care provider, less likely to have consistent health care, and less likely to participate in wellness promotion, all of which adversely impact morbidity and mortality among these individuals. The overall health and well-being of individuals cannot improve without adequate health care, including access (i.e., locations, transportation, health insurance, timeliness, and adequate employment to cover co-pays and prescriptions) and high-quality health care services. The number of individuals who cannot get access to health care as needed and those who are unable to obtain prescription medications when needed has increased over the past several years and is continuing to worsen, according to the *Healthy People 2030* overview on the SDOH. NPs have a moral and professional responsibility to engage in policy and advocacy initiatives aimed at increasing access for affected individuals for significant change in the direction of comprehensive and high-quality health care to occur. Developing innovative interventions that facilitate increased access to health care is essential, and NPs can play a vital role in that. More information on health care access and quality can be found at https://health.gov/healthypeople/objectives-and-data/browse-objectives/health-care-access-and-quality

Neighborhoods and Built Environments

Goal: Create neighborhoods and environments that promote health and safety.

The environment has a major influence on the health and well-being of people and communities. Air and water quality, physical safety (violent vs. non-violent; sidewalks and places to safely access physical activity), number of people interacting within a space (over- or under-populated). Historically underrepresented racial and ethnic minorities and financially disenfranchised people are more likely to live in high-risk places. These factors are key components of a holistic assessment and cannot be overlooked. It is within the purview of the NP to be an active participant in health promotion and safety. *Healthy People 2030* recognizes that improving neighborhoods and built environments can impact health and safety in all the places where people live and interact.

Nurse practitioners should engage in interventions and policy changes at every level of government to aid in health and safety risk reduction, health promotion, and improved quality of life and overall health outcomes. Additional information may be found at https://health.gov/healthypeople/objectives-and-data/browse-objectives/neighborhood-and-built-environment

Social and Community Context

Goal: Increase social and community support.

Opportunities for interpersonal interactions in a variety of places may significantly affect overall health and well-being. In alignment with the focus of *Healthy People 2030* on assisting people with social support needs, NPs should also identify and support this effort through advocacy and active engagement in interventions and innovations, and through interprofessional collaboration with other relevant health care advocates, including other professionals and organizations. More information can be accessed at https://health.gov/healthypeople/objectives-and-data/browse-objectives/social-and-community-context

RESEARCH

- Nurse Practitioners should understand research methods, advocate for ethical and culturally responsible research methods and practices and be able to translate research into practice.
- Research Ethics: The ANA and other organizations provide codes of ethics related to research activities.
- Quantitative vs. Qualitative Research
  - Quantitative research: Research that uses objective measurements to provide numerical and statistical information and data in the form of numbers, percentages, and ratios; may include interventions and treatments
  - Qualitative research: Investigation of a problem using inquiry methods and developing conclusions based on observations, quotes, and themes
- Translational Research
  - Understanding research methodology and bio-statistical data to evaluate, interpret, and implement research findings
  - Identification of evidence-based research and use of critical thinking to implement new research findings and ideas into practice
- FNPs must be prepared to be
  - Lifelong learners: identifying research problems, participating in research affects, and applying research findings
  - Scholars: Providing outcomes research data through various dissemination modes such as publications, speaking engagements, and professional presentations
- Assurance of Safe Practice
- A system to evaluate and monitor the quality of patients' care and facility management.

- Formal programs that provide a framework for continuous, consistent monitoring and evaluation:
  - ◊ Structure, process, and outcomes of care
  - ◊ Client interactions
  - ◊ Clinical competence
  - ◊ Performance assessment
- Knowledge of standards of care and clinical guidelines
- Minimizing clinical errors and complications by using risk-reducing tools such as smart phones and tablets, flow sheets, and electronic resources
- Promoting a safe work environment using principles of QSEN
- Evaluation of clinical outcomes using
  - ◊ Continuous Quality Improvement (CQI)
  - ◊ Peer review
  - ◊ Audit

DISASTER AND EMERGENCY CARE AND PLANNING

Attention is increasingly being paid to preparing RNs to assume emergency roles during a time of mass casualties from either natural disasters or terrorist attacks. The International Nursing Coalition for Mass Casualty Education was established to help nurses to identify the educational competencies for RNs responding to mass casualty incidents. The coalition aspires to improve the ability of all nurses to respond safely and effectively to mass casualty incidents through the identification of existing and emerging roles and responsibilities of nurses, ensuring robustness of education for mass casualty incidents, helping to understand response frameworks, and ensuring collaborative efforts. As outlined in the *NAM Future of Nursing 2020–2030 Report, nurses* are expected to be prepared to respond to emergencies. Information on the objectives and work that has been done toward a uniform curriculum in this area may be obtained at http://www.nursing.vanderbilt. edu/advantage/emergency.html In addition, the Emergency Nurses Association, with endorsement from NONPF, published specialty competencies for the NP who practices in emergency care (Emergency Nurses Association {ENA}, 2008). The 2021 updated competencies from the American Academy of Emergency Nurse Practitioners and the ENA can be found at https://www.ena.org/docs/default-source/education-document-library/enpcompetencies_final.pdf?sfvrsn=f75b4634_0 .

The Centers for Disease Control and Prevention also maintains emergency preparedness resources for health care providers. These can be found at http://emergency.cdc.gov/

COMPLEMENTARY AND INTEGRATIVE HEALTH

There is greater recognition of the use of complementary and integrative modalities. The National Center for Complementary and Integrative Health (NCCIH) is the federal government's lead agency for scientific research on complementary and integrative health (https://nccih.nih.gov). Delivery of holistic, patient-centered, and culturally intelligent care requires NPs to fully engage persons seeking wellness care and those who access care during times of illness in the development and management of treatment plans. The role of the NP in complementary and integrative health is to assess individual levels of health literacy and provide education accordingly. The focus of the plan of care should be on optimal health and well-being, as defined by each individual. Resources for health care providers can be found at https://www.nccih.nih.gov/health/providers.

Definitions (NCCIH)

- NCCIH uses the following terms:
  - "Complementary health approaches" is used when discussing practices and products of nonmainstream origin.
  - "Integrative health" is used when discussing practices that incorporate complementary approaches into mainstream health care.
  - If a practice is nonmainstream and used together with conventional medicine, it is referred to as "complementary."
  - If a practice is nonmainstream and used in place of conventional medicine, it is considered "alternative."

Demographics

- More than 30% of adults and 12% of children use complementary or alternative approaches to health care.
- Many drug–herb interactions have been identified.
- Sixty-eight percent of clinically significant drug–herb reactions are related to five herbs:
  - Kava
  - Garlic
  - Ginkgo biloba
  - St. John's wort
  - Valerian

- The prescription medications most frequently affected:
  - Warfarin
  - Sedative/hypnotics
  - Antidepressants
  - Insulin
  - Oral antidiabetic agents
  - Hepatotoxic medications
  - Oral contraceptives

Role of Nurse Practitioner

Nurse practitioners should be aware of current evidence and resources regarding Complementary and Alternative Medicine (CAM) interventions.

- Maintain objectivity and be supportive about patients' choice to use CAM.
- Proactively ask all patients about the use of and response to CAM:
  - Request that patients bring their supplements (bottles, tubes, containers, packaging, etc.) to visits.
  - Ask about alternative therapies.
  - Document all CAM information and referrals in patient's record.
  - Use caution with women of childbearing age—many herbals are category C.

TABLE 2–1.
NCCIH TYPES OF COMPLEMENTARY HEALTH APPROACHES

APPROACH	EXAMPLES
Natural Products*	Vitamins and minerals, probiotics, herbs (also known as botanicals)
Mind and Body Practices	Acupuncture, relaxation techniques, guided imagery, tai chi, qigong, healing touch, hypnotherapy, movement therapies, yoga, chiropractic, meditation, massage therapy
Other Complementary Health Approaches	Homeopathy, traditional healers, Ayurvedic medicine, naturopathy, traditional Chinese medicine

*Herbal products, probiotics, and vitamins are not approved by the U.S. Food and Drug Administration (FDA) and are considered food supplements.

Source: National Center for Complementary and Integrative Health (NCCIH). Retrieved from https://nccih.nih.gov/health/integrative-health#term

TABLE 2–2.
SELECT DRUG–HERB INTERACTIONS

HERB	DRUG(S)	EFFECT
Garlic	Warfarin	Decreased blood concentrations
Ginkgo biloba	Anticoagulants, aspirin, NSAIDs	Increased risk of bleeding with warfarin
	Thiazide diuretic	Increased blood pressure
	Trazodone	Coma
	Anticonvulsants, TCAs	Decreased seizure threshold
Kava	Benzodiazepines	Additive CNS depression
	Levodopa	Increased "off" periods in patients with Parkinson's Disease
St. John's wort	Warfarin and related anticoagulants, cyclosporin, amitriptyline, digoxin	Decreased blood concentrations
	Piroxicam, tetracyclines	Increased phototoxicity
	Antidepressants, CNS stimulants	Additive effects
	Theophylline	Decreased xanthine levels
Valerian	CNS depressants	Additive CNS depression

Note. NSAIDs = nonsteroidal anti-inflammatory drugs; TCAs = tricyclic antidepressants; CNS = central nervous system.

TABLE 2–3.
COMMON TYPES OF COMPLEMENTARY HEALTH APPROACHES

TEN MOST COMMON COMPLEMENTARY HEALTH APPROACHES IN USE BY ADULTS IN THE UNITED STATES	
17.7%	Natural products
10.9%	Deep breathing
10.1%	Yoga, tai chi, or qi gong
8.4%	Chiropractic or osteopathic manipulation
8.0%	Meditation
6.9%	Massage
3.0%	Special diets
2.2%	Homeopathy
2.1%	Progressive relaxation
1.7%	Guided imagery

Source: *Trends in the use of complementary approaches among adults: United States, 2002–2012.* National health statistics report no. 79, by T. C. Clarke, L. I. Black, B. J. Stussman, P. M. Barnes, and R. L. Nahin, 2015, Hyattsville, MD: National Center for Health Statistics.

CARING FOR PEOPLE WITH DISABILITIES

Definitions

The Americans with Disabilities Act (ADA) is a civil rights law that was enacted in 1990. It prohibits discrimination against individuals with disabilities in all areas of public life, including employment, schools, transportation, and all public and private places that are open to the public. The law ensures that people with disabilities have equal and equitable rights and opportunities as compared to everyone else. The civil rights protections for individuals with disabilities are like those provided to individuals based on race, color, sex, national origin, age, and religion. It guarantees that individuals with disabilities have equal opportunities in public accommodations, employment, transportation, state and local government services, and telecommunications. A person with a disability has a physical or mental impairment that substantially limits one or more major life activities, *or* a record or history of such an impairment, *or* is regarded/perceived by others as having such an impairment. When used in reference to the ADA, the term "disability" is used in a legal rather than medical context. Nurse practitioners should be aware of this distinction. More information about the ADA may be obtained at: https://adata.org/learn-about-ada

- Characteristics of disabilities vary in severity:
  - Very mild (inconvenience)
  - Moderate (interfere with some activities)
  - Severe (need assistance for activities of daily living [ADL] and instrumental ADL)
  - Very severe (need technology for survival)
- Disabilities vary in type:
  - Physical
  - Sensory (vision and hearing)
  - Psychiatric or mental health
  - Cognitive or intellectual
  - Communication
- Disabilities vary in visibility:
  - Not at all visible to others
  - Visible to informed others
  - Visible to all
- Issues for providers
  - Access and care
    - People with disabilities encounter serious barriers to receiving quality health care, preventive care, screening, and reproductive care.

- People with disabilities have received lower quality of care, less aggressive treatment, and are offered few choices. Health care providers are often under-prepared for addressing sexuality, pregnancy, childbearing, and common health problems in people with disabilities. This increases the risk for health inequities, health disparities, and sentinel events.

◊ Barriers to optimal care in people with disabilities include:

- Lack of awareness and knowledge about specific disabilities and of disability in general,
- Lack of CQ regarding interacting with and caring for people living with disabilities,
- Lack of accountability of health care providers for providing culturally responsible and inclusive care for all people,
- Lack of knowledge about the law or disregard for the legal mandates,
- An erroneous assumption is that people with disabilities are dependent on others and incapable of making their own decisions.

◊ Consequences of lack of substandard and non-inclusive care

- Negative encounters, often resulting in people with disabilities avoiding health care providers unless and until necessary
- Inadequate health care, including preventive screening
- Delay in treatment or lack of treatment
- Low level of participation in health-promotion activities
- Poor health status, isolation, and psychological issues

Preventing health disparities using an inclusive excellence approach

Inclusive excellence embodies the principles of cultural intelligence, the humanitarian ethos and principles, and ethical principles as defined in the ANA Code of Ethics for nurses. It embraces diversity, equity, equality, inclusion, belonging, and all the characteristics that make individuals and populations unique. The role of the NP is to adopt and employ supportive strategies that assist in the provision of care in ways that deter discriminatory practices and bias-influenced care, to increase opportunities to advance health equity, and improve population health. Some of those strategies include:

♦ Self-awareness, bias acknowledgement, and mitigation and/or de-activation of bias-influenced decisions

- Cultural intelligence application:
  - ◊ Discuss culture and cultural preferences with each patient.
  - ◊ Do not generalize, stereotype, or make assumptions about people from specific affinity groups, including race, gender identification, sex, nationality, ethnicity, disability, body composition, families, or communities.
- Adopt inclusive language:
  - ◊ Ask about pronouns and use appropriate pronouns.
  - ◊ Ask about gender identification.
- Approach the care of all persons as a partnership, not a dictatorship. People have the right to be active participants in and make the ultimate decisions regarding health care.
- Attend trainings and other educational opportunities related to caring for people from underrepresented, marginalized, and stigmatized populations.
- Provide appropriate and relevant accommodations for all persons who are consumers within the health care system.
- Practice the concept of "nothing about us without us" and the concept that no policy should be decided by a group or representative without participation of members of the affected group.

GENETICS AND GENOMICS

Overview

- Genetics and genomic science are redefining the understanding of the continuum of human health and illness. Recognition of genomics as a central science for health professional knowledge is essential.
- The human genome project was completed in April 2003.
- This science is number one on the list of the 10 most important medical advances in the first decade of the 21st century.
- Care for all people, across the life span, will increasingly require familiarity with genetic and genomic information related to
  - ◊ Prevention, screening, diagnostics, prognostics, selection of treatment, monitoring of treatment effectiveness, referral, and the International HapMap Project (haplotype map).
    - Genetic databank allows exploration of relationships between genetic differences and diseases
    - A global catalog of common human genetic variants

- Contains a description of each variant, identifies where it occurs in human DNA, and describes variation and distribution within and across populations
- Links genetic markers with human traits (e.g., celiac disease) and/or presence or absence of disease

Definition

- ♦ *Genetics:* The study of individual genes and their impact on relatively rare single gene disorders
- ♦ *Genomics:* The study of all the genes in the human genome together, including their interactions with one another, the environment, and the influence of psychosocial and cultural factors

Role of the FNP

- ♦ Understand the relationship of genetics and genomics to health, prevention, screening, diagnostics, prognostics, selection of treatment, and monitoring of treatment effectiveness
- ♦ Facilitate access to genetic specialists
- ♦ Develop a family history
  - ◊ Complete detailed family history, including genetic and environmental risk factors
  - ◊ Use these mnemonics to identify "red flag" issues:
    - SCREEN
      - Some concern
      - Reproduction
      - Early disease, death, or disability
      - Ethnicity
      - Nongenetic
    - Family GENES
      - Family: multiple affected siblings or persons in multiple generations
      - G: groups of congenital anomalies
      - E: extreme or exceptional presentation of common conditions
      - N: neurodevelopmental delay or degeneration
      - E: extreme or exceptional pathology
      - S: surprising laboratory values

- Pharmacogenomics
  - Drug metabolism is orchestrated by complex interactions among dozens of different genes.
  - There is the potential for safer drugs, more effective prescribing, more accurate dosing, targeted vaccines, and reduced cost (e.g., warfarin).
- Lifestyle
  - Lifestyle risk factors are known to affect overall health (sedentary lifestyle, obesity).
  - Biologic processes are complex and poorly understood.
  - Findings in telomere studies identify some impact of lifestyle on the life of the gene.
  - Further genetic research may identify susceptibility factors.
- Genetic counseling and screening
  - Multidisciplinary health care team provides counseling and screening
  - Considerations for genetic counseling and/or screening:
    - Those who have or are concerned that they might have an inherited disorder or birth defect
    - Women who are pregnant or planning to be at age 35 or older
    - Couples who already have a child with an inherited disorder, undiagnosed disease, or birth defect
    - Couples whose infants have a genetic disease diagnosed by routine newborn screening
    - Women who have had three or more miscarriages or babies who died in infancy
    - People concerned that their jobs, lifestyles, or medical histories may pose a risk to the outcome of pregnancy (common causes of concern include exposure to radiation, medications, illegal drugs, chemicals, or infections)
    - Couples who would like testing or more information about genetic conditions that occur frequently in their ethnic groups
    - Couples who are first cousins or other close blood relatives
    - Pregnant women whose ultrasound examinations or blood testing indicate that their pregnancies may be at increased risk for certain complications or birth defects
- Prenatal testing
  - Began in 1970s with alphafetoprotein testing
  - Quad screen with ultrasound can identify approximately 90% of trisomy 21 cases.
  - Markers help identify high-risk pregnancies such as preeclampsia, fetal growth restriction, fetal demise, and placental abnormalities

- Gene therapy
  - This is a technique for correcting defective genes responsible for disease development. All therapies require "carrier molecule" or vector to carry therapeutic gene to patient's target cells; the most common vector is a genetically adapted virus.
  - Several approaches:
    - Most common: normal gene inserted into a nonspecific location within the genome to replace a nonfunctional gene
    - Abnormal gene could be switched with normal gene through homologous recombination
    - Abnormal gene repaired through selective reverse mutation that returns a gene to its normal function
    - Gene regulation (the degree to which a gene is turned on or off) could be altered
  - The U.S. Food and Drug Administration (FDA) has not yet approved any human gene therapy product for sale; all are still experimental.
  - Ethical questions and opinions about gene therapy abound.
- NPs need to become increasingly familiar with pharmacogenomics and the most recent indications for medication prescribing.

END-OF-LIFE CARE

All patients are entitled to counsel regarding end-of-life care to ensure that patients have input and can involve their families with their care at the end of life. Advance care directives ensure that the patient's desires are known and followed when the patient is no longer able to communicate. Nurse practitioners play a unique role in this care delivery process in both inpatient and outpatient settings.

- Palliative care is comprehensive and coordinated, using all resources available within the community, with no exclusions regarding curative therapy.
- Hospice care is more focused on keeping patients comfortable at the end of life and generally does not include treatment intended to be curative.

Palliative care

- Comprehensive care for short- or long-term illnesses, including incurable conditions
- Multidisciplinary approach
- Includes pain and symptom management

- Addresses social, psychological, and spiritual needs as well as physical (including pain management)
  - Information available from the Hospice and Palliative Nurses Association (www .hpna.org/) and the Center to Advance Palliative Care (www. getpalliativecare.org)

Hospice care

- Available when all curative treatment options are exhausted or refused
- Multidisciplinary approach
- Focuses on pain control and comfort measures
- Stresses quality of life
- Provides family support
  - Exclusions regarding therapeutic interventions delineated before patient enters hospice care

DIRECT-TO-CONSUMER ADVERTISING

Patients frequently present to the office already having formed their diagnosis and requesting specific treatments. NPs must become knowledgeable about the newest products on the market and how they are marketed to consumers to appropriately counsel and treat patients. NPs critically read clinical studies and make evidence-based decisions about the appropriateness of medications and therapies based on individual patient presentation.

TELEHEALTH

With rapidly expanding technology, the use of telecommunications in health care delivery is ever- changing. Telehealth in part includes "use of information and technologies that are emerging, as well as the ability to move the caregiver and information to where the patient is rather than moving the patient to centralized places to deliver health services and information." (Huston, 2013)

Areas to be included in these advances:

- High-quality video conferencing between provider and patient
- Medical records
- Surgical robots
- Remote monitoring of implanted medical devices such as pacemakers, defibrillators, and some pain medication delivery systems

Since the release of the IOM report *To Err is Human: Building A Safer Health System* (1999), increased attention has been paid to changes all health care providers should make to reduce medical errors. In response, The Joint Commission (formerly known as JCAHO, or The Joint Commission on Accreditation of Healthcare Organizations, www.jointcommission.org/) has issued a list of abbreviations that should not be used in health care. In addition, the Institute for Safe Medication Practices has published a list of dangerous abbreviations related to medication use that it recommends should be explicitly prohibited (http://www.ismp.org/). The list of banned abbreviations includes many symbols traditionally used in patient charts and in written prescriptions.

THERAPEUTIC COMMUNICATION

Overview

- *Therapeutic communication* is a transaction between the sender and the receiver. Both parties participate simultaneously.
- In the transactional model, both participants perceive each other, listen to each other, and simultaneously engage in the process of creating meaning in a relationship, focusing on the patient's issues.
- Both patient and provider bring unintended bias to the exchange influencing the intended message and its interpretation.
- Interactions must be viewed in the context and intersectionality of identities of both the patient and the provider:
  - Values, attitudes, and beliefs
  - Gender
  - Age or developmental level
  - Cultural influences
  - Religious of spiritual affiliations
  - Social status
  - Economic/financial status
  - The environment
- Requirements for therapeutic relationships:
  - Authenticity
  - Rapport
  - Trust
  - Respect

- ◊ Honesty
- ◊ Empathy
- ◊ Consistency

- ♦ Therapeutic communication involves actively listening and observing, both verbal and nonverbal cues.
  - ◊ Nonverbal
    - Body language (i.e., body movement, eye contact, eye movements, posture)
    - Affect and demeanor
  - ◊ Verbal
    - Giving broad openings—offering general leads
    - Using silence—accepting
    - Giving recognition—restating
    - Reflecting—focusing
    - Exploring—seeking clarification and validation
- ♦ Nonverbal behaviors to promote active listening:
  - ◊ **S**—Sit squarely facing the patient
  - ◊ **O**—Observe an open posture
  - ◊ **L**—Lean forward, toward the patient
  - ◊ **E**—Establish eye contact
  - ◊ **R**—Relax

Therapeutic Boundaries

- ♦ Effective communication is a core skill in primary care.
  - ◊ The therapeutic relationship is a planned, goal-directed, and contractual relationship between the provider and the patient for the purpose of providing care to the patient to meet his or her physical, emotional, and spiritual health care needs.
  - ◊ Therapeutic relationships occur along a dynamic continuum.
  - ◊ The provider is accountable and takes responsibility for setting and maintaining the boundaries of a therapeutic relationship, regardless of the client's actions or requests.
  - ◊ Professional boundaries identify the parameters of the therapeutic relationship.
  - ◊ Establishing, maintaining, and communicating professional boundaries to the patient is imperative to the therapeutic relationship. Boundary crossing is a

conscious or unconscious decision by the provider that deviates from established ethical and professional boundaries, including these examples:

- Accepting gifts
- Self-disclosure by the provider
- Embarking on a social relationship with a patient
- Sexual misconduct
- Exploiting the therapeutic relationship for the emotional, financial, sexual, or personal advantage or benefit of the provider

Teaching Strategies/Group Dynamics/Literacy

Patient education is a matter of quality, safety, and is essential to successful clinical interventions. It should occur at each clinical visit. Busy clinical settings should not hinder patient education, as NPs are responsible and accountable for providing education as part of a holistic model of care. Literacy levels differ considerably within the clinical setting. The average literacy level for patients is estimated to be at the fifth grade, and inadequate functional health literacy may be as high as 80% in some clinical settings. Health care expenses escalate considerably in the lower-literacy populations. The NP must not allow literacy levels to induce bias and does not excuse the responsibility of providing adequate health education to all patients, regardless of literacy level.

- Teaching strategies include using written patient education materials in the preferred primary language, and multimedia approaches such as audio and video that are specific to the literacy level of the patient. Best practices require the NP to move beyond just giving the materials to the patient or care supporter, but to read through or discuss the materials to ensure understanding by offering a space for questions and explanations.
- Group dynamics may alter the efficacy of group teaching and require considerable time on the part of the clinician. This should not deter the NP from this responsibility.
- Improving patient education using multimedia computer programs and touch screens is rapidly becoming a more feasible option, followed by one-on-one interaction with the instructor and/or smaller group interaction. The role of the NP is to ensure that people who are provided these materials receive explicit instructions on use of the technology and the health care information provided in this format.

PROFESSIONAL ORGANIZATIONS

- Participation in professional organizations is critical in affecting advancement of the nursing and nurse practitioner profession. Through active participation in professional organizations, NPs have a voice in NP education, health policy, NP autonomy, including independent practice, and governance. There is power in numbers, and all NPs should be involved and active in their professional organizations at the national, state, and local levels to broadly influence academia, health care systems, and clinical practice.

- State organizations work diligently to monitor and affect laws and regulations affecting NP practice and health policy. In addition, these associations provide peer-networking and continuing education opportunities. Many state NP organizations have local chapters.
- National organizations
  - American Association of Nurse Practitioners (AANP): the American Academy of Nurse Practitioners and the American College of Nurse Practitioners joined to create the largest full-service national professional membership organization for NPs of all specialties in 2013 (www.aanp.org). The mission of AANP is to lead NPs in transforming patient-centered health care with a vision of "providing high-quality health care for all by the patient's provider of choice" (AANP, 2013).
  - The National Organization of Nurse Practitioner Faculties (NONPF) is an organization of nurse practitioner educators who are instrumental in setting standards for nurse practitioner education. NONPF has developed core competencies describing the domains of practice with critical behaviors that should be exhibited by all entry-level NPs.

Theory and Principles of Family-Focused Care

The traditional family nurse practitioner (FNP) provides primary and secondary preventive care to persons across the life span living alone or in nuclear or extended family networks. Today's family consists of individuals who identify themselves as family members, not limited by walls, genetics, or legally defined relationships. Friedman (2002) defines family as "two or more persons who are joined together by bonds of sharing and emotional closeness and who identify themselves as being part of the family" (p. 9).

Family members may live together or within proximity in a common community and participate together in educational, social, and religious experiences. Families may form as an outgrowth of kinship bonds with others in the community or because of culturally specific extended family networks. Family forms are varied—the FNP will interact with many different family forms such as the gay and lesbian family, the single-parent family, the extended family, adoptive or stepparent families.

Family-focused care is the specialized role of the FNP, who acknowledge that the family process is an interaction among members that serves to promote mental and physical health, prevent disease, and restore health in times of illness. FNPs provide a comprehensive psychosocial approach to caring for people that fosters health-promoting lifestyles among family members. The FNP interacts across the interdependent roles of individual, family, and community to act as advocate, case manager, coordinator, counselor, and expert provider of care.

The FNP assesses family structure and dynamics to help people maximize their health, given the realities of their personal and family health histories, psychosocial histories, genetic makeups, cultural and religious values, traditions, and social and economic contexts. FNPs teach family members to recognize the influences of their family health patterns and risks, use family members as resources for knowledge and support during periods of health, maintain psychosocial ties with their family of origin, and assume functions that help optimize health in family members by using resources in the community.

The FNP role is interpreted as a unique NP role. It is not, as some would suggest, an adult NP plus pediatric NP plus geriatric NP role, but it requires mastery of a unique constellation of knowledge and tasks involving the care of an individual within a family context. The FNP is not expected to have the depth of knowledge of NPs practicing in the specialty areas but is expected to know something about many different diseases and processes affecting the person throughout the life span. As such, the FNP works closely with physician colleagues in the diagnosis and development of the initial treatment regimen and is prepared to refer to specialists.

FAMILY THEORY—ASSESSMENT AND INTERVENTION

In general, family theory serves as a basis for assessing and coming to understand the structure, development, and function of families through the process of family assessment. Authors such as Friedman (2002), Kaakinen et al. (2015), and Wright and Leahey (2012) have developed family assessment tools. Family theory is grounded in general systems theory, including structural functional theory, family systems theory (Bowen), family development theory (Duvall, 1977), child development theory (Erikson; 1959 Havighurst, 1952), and other social science theories, including communication, stress, and interactional theory.

THEORETICAL BASIS FOR FAMILY THEORY—GENERAL SYSTEMS THEORY

General systems theory provides a framework that explains the dynamic structure and function of the family within the context of a unified whole. The family performs activities reflected by the actions of interacting parts or subsystems. Any *system* is defined as "a bounded set of interrelated elements exhibiting coherent behavior as a trait" (Constantine, 1986, p. 67). Families are considered systems because they are made up of interrelated elements or objectives, exhibit coherent behaviors, have regular interactions, and are interdependent.

These are the major principles of systems theory adapted from Friedman (2002), Kaakinen et al. (2015), and Wright and Leahey (2012):

- Each system has its own characteristics, and the whole is greater than the sum of the parts, rather than just the sum of the characteristics of individual parts of a system.

- All parts of the system are dependent on one another, even though each part has its own role within the system.
- Families are organized in a way that enables the interdependence and interactivity of their members.
- Each family system has mechanisms for the exchange of information within the system and between the system and the broader environment.
- Boundaries that are open, closed, or operate at random exist within family systems.
- Family systems change over time as both individuals and the whole respond to change in the internal and external environments. With change, families become more complex, reflecting adaptation and differentiation of their members.
- Change occurs through feedback processes that allow for circular interaction within the family system, rather than a linear cause-and-effect pattern.
- A change affecting one part of a family manifests itself as change in the whole family system.
- Families strive for homeostasis or a predictable steady state that reflects a balance between change and stability.

The value of systems theory lies in understanding that families are composed of interacting parts in constant interaction with one another and the larger environment, and that change in one part of the family is reflected in change in the family. As families expand, grow, and experience stress and illness, their ability to be changed and yet maintain homeostasis reflects the health and coping strategies of the family to adapt. Families with poor coping strategies may resist change or be unable to restore homeostasis after change. Stress and illness may trigger dysfunctional coping patterns or disequilibrium. Families with closed boundaries may resist help from outside resources during periods of disequilibrium.

STRUCTURAL FUNCTIONAL THEORY

- Families are social systems that form interdependent and independent relationships referred to as *subsystems* both within and outside of the family. Structure describes relationships within families, such as the husband–wife subsystem, parent–child subsystem, sister–brother subsystem, and so on.
- Internal family subsystems function as a microcosm of society, reflecting the larger sphere of human needs. Rank order within families is a component of structure, such as the ordering of children by birth in the family or by age if they are adopted or stepchildren.

- Function includes the tasks that families carry out to provide members with safety, reproduction, education, parenting, sexual expression, economic security, transfer of cultural traditions and inheritance, social support, play, relaxation, and health promotion opportunities.
- Supra-systems form outside the family and reflect functional needs not met within the family. Relationships with teachers, schools, religious and civic organizations, the health care system, and friends are examples of supra-systems that meet needs not fulfilled by interactions within the family system. Multiple relationships are formed through supra-systems that reflect family values, beliefs, and emotional boundaries. By developing an ecomap, the FNP can visualize the relationships of family members with systems outside the family system (Wright & Leahey, 2012).
- These are the principles of structural functional theory adapted from Friedman (2002), Hanson et al. (2005), and Wright and Leahey (2012):
  - Families are social systems with instrumental and expressive functions that include activities of daily living, communication, social support, role acquisition, values, beliefs, problem-solving, and relationships.
  - In optimally functioning families, members take on predictable roles that meet the instrumental and expressive needs of their members.
  - Families are composed of small numbers with characteristics of small-group behavior.
  - Families are social systems that carry out functions necessary to meet the need for orderly transfer of wealth, procreation, and education of members of society.
  - People adopt norms, values, and cultural traditions that are learned as part of the process of family socialization.
  - Disease or ill health can interfere with the family's ability to carry out its internal functions and meet the responsibilities it has formed in relationships with systems outside the family. Families with multiple unmet needs may experience guilt, stress, dysfunction, and poor coping strategies during periods of stress and illness.

FAMILY DEVELOPMENTAL THEORY

- Developmental theory explains human growth and development according to theorists such as Erikson, Piaget, and Havighurst. Duvall (1977) and Duvall and Miller (1985) further applied the concept of development to the sociological study of family. The model outlines the eight consecutive stages in the family life cycle, offers a predictive overview of the activities that occur in families over time, and serves as a basis for anticipatory guidance when assessing and teaching families.

- According to Duvall (1977), families pass through eight chronological stages; as in child development theory, success in one task sets the stage for success in subsequent tasks. Failure in one task leads to frustration or delays in subsequent tasks or stages in the family life cycle. These stages are supported by Duvall's model and adapted from Friedman (2002):
  - Beginning family
  - Childbearing family (oldest child up to 30 months of age)
  - Family with preschool children (oldest child 2½ to 5 years of age)
  - Family with school-aged children (oldest child 6 to 12 years of age)
  - Family with adolescents (oldest child 13 to 20 years of age)
  - Launching center family (grown children leaving the home)
  - Family with middle-aged parents (empty nest, up to time of retirement)
  - Family with old age and retirement
- Underlying assumptions (adapted from Friedman, 2002; and Hanson et al., 2005)
  - Families change over time because of the influence of environmental conditions.
  - Developmental tasks are the aims, although they are not completed at one time and may overlap with other developmental tasks.
  - Families demonstrate different forms of membership across developmental stages that perform age-related functions.
  - Families bring with them an experience of their pasts as well as current circumstances.
  - Families share common developmental processes with other families.
  - Families express developmental milestones in a variety of ways.

COMMUNICATION THEORY

As described by Friedman (2002), Hanson et al. (2005), and Wright and Leahey (2012):

- Communication theory emphasizes the interaction of people that includes both verbal and nonverbal communication among members of a family.
- Communication functions include emotional support, shared information, and instruction.
- The content of messages is time-bound and must be appreciated within the context of the sender.

- Communication that lacks clarity may lead to family dysfunction or poor coping strategies.
- Communication conveys values and beliefs between members and the external environment.
- Communication with clarity and congruence promotes positive behavior within the family.

CASE STUDIES

CASE 1

A family nurse practitioner (FNP) has worked part time in a college health center since graduating 3 earlier. The FNP has accepted a position in a family practice setting. In addition to providing family practice care, the responsibilities include covering the prenatal clinic 1 day a week. The collaborating physician has agreed to provide direct supervision during the first 6 to 8 weeks of employment and will be present in the clinic while the FNP is seeing patients.

1. Is the FNP legally authorized to provide care to prenatal women? To children?
2. Should the FNP accept this assignment? Why or why not?
3. What standards of care should be followed in providing care to prenatal patients?

CASE 2

A 16-year-old presents in the clinic for sexually transmitted disease (STD) testing. The patient does not have a parent or legal guardian present.

1. What are the legal issues presented in this case?
2. What ethical principles should guide decision-making regarding this case?

CASE 3

The RN approaches the NP to give a brief report on the next patient who is waiting to be examined. The RN whispers the following to the NP "The name on the chart is Jessie, but I'm not sure if *'it's'* a boy or girl. *It* looks like a boy because of the facial hair, but the hairstyle looks like a girl and the nails are done."

1. What should the NP's response be to the RN?
2. What are some best practices/strategies for ensuring that the patient receives high-quality care without the influence or bias?
3. What ethical principles should guide interactions with the RN, NP, and with the patient?

CASE STUDIES DISCUSSION

CASE 1

1. Is the FNP legally authorized to provide care to prenatal women? To children?

   If certification has been maintained as a family nurse practitioner, there is legal authorization to provide care in this setting.

2. Should the FNP accept this assignment? Why or why not?

   The FNP is legally authorized and can accept this assignment because adequate supervision will be provided during this training period, and the collaborating physician has also agreed to be present for support while the FNP is seeing patients.

3. What standards of care should the FNP follow in providing care to prenatal patients?

   Standards of care are developed by professional organizations such as the American Nurses Association, which has created the Standards for Advanced Practice Nursing, and the American Association of Colleges of Nursing (AACN) and the National Organization of Nurse Practitioner Faculties (NONPF), which have created population-focused Nurse Practitioner Primary Care Competencies. The NP should use established guidelines and standards of practice that guide safe and appropriate care for prenatal patients.

CASE 2

1. What are the legal issues presented in this case?

   The main legal issue is the provision of care to minors without the consent of a parent or legal guardian. In the case of sexually transmitted infections, a minor's legal right to provide informed consent to receive STD and/or HIV services without the consent, knowledge, or involvement of a parent or guardian varies by state. It is the responsibility of the NP to be familiar with the laws of the state where the services are being provided.

2. What ethical principles should guide decision-making regarding this case?

   The ethical principles of service, mercy, empathy, compassion, trust, and beneficence are a few examples that may guide decision-making. Decisions should also be guided by the ANA Code of Ethics, NP scope of practice standards, and HIPAA laws.

CASE 3

1. What should the NP's response be to the nurse?

   The NP should use this situation as an opportunity to have a non-aggressive, but assertive, conversation with the RN about respect for human life and dignity, that is, not referring to a person as "it," to briefly educate the RN about the importance of using inclusive language. In addition, the NP should remind the RN that the best course of action for maintaining effective, therapeutic communication, best practices, and inclusive excellence is to explicitly ask the person about their gender identification and what their pronoun preferences.

2. What are some best practices/strategies for ensuring that the patient receives high-quality care without the influence of bias?

   - Self-assessment/awareness/acknowledgment regarding personal biases toward transgender people
   - Obtain upstander training and apply it in situations where bias and actual discrimination or potential for discrimination is apparent
   - Work to develop a high level of cultural intelligence
   - Provide inclusive, patient-centered care

3. What ethical principles should guide interactions with the RN, NP, and the patient?

   - The ethical principles of service, mercy, empathy, compassion, trust, and beneficence are a few examples that may guide decision-making.

REFERENCES

Alligood, M. R. (2018). *Nursing theorists and their work* (7th ed.). Philadelphia: Elsevier-Health Sciences Division.

American Academy of Emergency Nurse Practitioners & Emergency Nurses Association (2021). *Emergency nurse practitioner competencies.* https://www.ena.org/docs/default-source/education-document-library/enpcompetencies_final.pdf?sfvrsn=f75b4634_0

American Academy of Nursing. (2021). *Equity, diversity, and inclusivity statement.* Retrieved from https://www.aannet.org/about/about-the-academy/edi

American Association of Colleges of Nursing. (2021). *The essentials: Core competencies for professional nursing education.* Retrieved from https://www.aacnnursing.org/Portals/42/AcademicNursing/pdf/Essentials-2021.pdf

American Association of Colleges of Nursing. (2018). *Fact sheet: The doctor of nursing practice (DNP).* Retrieved from https://www.aacnnursing.org/News-Information/Fact-Sheets/DNP-Fact-Sheet

American Nurses Association. (2015). *Nursing: Scope and standards of practice* (3rd ed.). Silver Spring, MD: Nursesbooks.org.

American Nurses Association. (2015). *Code of ethics for nurses with interpretive statements.* Silver Spring, MD: Nursesbooks.org.

American Psychological Association. (n.d.). Psychology & aging: Addressing the needs of older adults. Washington, DC: APA. Retrieved from https://www.apa.org/pi/aging/resources/guides/aging.pdf

American Recovery and Reinvestment Act (ARRA) of 2009. (2009). Pub. L. No. 111-5, 123 Stat. 115, 516. Retrieved from http://www.govtrack.us/congress/bills/111/hr1

Americans with Disabilities Act of 1990. Retrieved from https://adata.org/learn-about-ada

ANA Ethics Advisory Board (June 7, 2019) "ANA Position Statement: The Nurse's Role in Addressing Discrimination: Protecting and Promoting Inclusive Strategies in Practice Settings, Policy, and Advocacy" *OJIN: The Online Journal of Issues in Nursing, 24*(3). https://doi.org/10.3912/OJIN.Vol24No03PoSCol01

Ang, S., Rockstuhl, T., Ta, M.L. Cultural Intelligence and Competencies. (2015). *International Encyclopedia of the Social & Behavioral Sciences, 5,* 433–439. dx.doi.org/10.1016/B978-0-08-097086-8.25050-2

APRN Consensus Work Group & the National Council of State Boards of Nursing APRN Advisory Committee. (2008). *Consensus model for APRN regulation: Licensure, accreditation, certification, & education.* Retrieved from http://www.aacn.nche.edu/education-resources/aprnrport.pdf

Berger, K. S. (2017). *The developing person through the life span* (10th ed.). NewYork: Worth.

Bernard, V. (2015). The humanitarian ethos in action. *International Review of the Red Cross, 97*(897–898), 7–18. doi:10.1017/S1816383115000831

Buppert, C. (2014). *Nurse practitioners' business practice and legal guide* (5th ed.). Sudbury, MA: Jones & Bartlett.

Buppert, C. (2018). *Nurse practitioners' business practice and legal guide* (6th ed.). Sudbury, MA: Jones & Bartlett.

Butts, J. B., & Rich, K. L. (2013). *Nursing ethics across the curriculum and into practice* (3rd ed.). Sudbury, MA: Jones & Bartlett.

Centers for Disease Control and Prevention. (2019). Public health genomics. Retrieved from https://www.cdc.gov/genomics/default.htm

Centers for Disease Control and Prevention. (2021). State laws that enable a minor to provide informed consent to receive HIV and STD Services. Retrieved from https://www.cdc.gov/hiv/policies/law/states/minors.html

Clarke T. C., Black, L. I., Stussman, B. J., Barnes, P. M., & Nahin, R. L. (2015). *Trends in the use of complementary health approaches among adults: United States, 2002–2012.* National health statistics reports, no 79. Hyattsville, MD: National Center for Health Statistics.

Committee for the Study of Credentialing in Nursing. (1979). *Credentialing in nursing: A new approach.* Kansas City, MO: American Nurses Association.

Constantine, L. (1986). *Family paradigms: The practice of theory in family therapy.* NewYork: Guilford Press.

Duvall, E. M. (1977). *Marriage and family development* (5th ed.). Philadelphia: Lippincott.

Duvall, E. M., & Miller, B. C. (1985). *Marriage and family development* (6th ed.). Philadelphia: Lippincott.

Edmunds, M. W., & Mayhew, M. S. (2013). *Pharmacology for primary care providers* (4th ed.). St. Louis, MO: Mosby.

Facchiano, L., & Snyder, C. H. (2012). Evidence-based practice for the busy nurse practitioner: Part one: Relevance to clinical practice and clinical inquiry process. *Journal of the American Academy of Nurse Practitioners, 24,* 579–586.

Federation of State Medical Boards of the United States. (1988). *Non-physician duties and scope of practice* (Position Statement 210.003, July). Dallas, TX: Author.

Ford, L. C. (1992). Advanced nursing practice: Future of the nurse practitioner. In L. H. Aiken & C. M. Fagin (Eds.), *Charting nursing's future: Agenda for the 1990s.* Philadelphia: Lippincott.

Friedman, M. (2002). *Family nursing: Research, theory, and practice* (5th ed.). Upper Saddle River, NJ: Prentice Hall.

Geisler, C., Cheung, C., Steinhagen, S. J., Neubeck, P., & Brueggeman, A. D. (2015). Nurse practitioner knowledge, use, and referral of complementary/alternative therapies. *JAANP, 27*(7), 380–388.

Giger, J. N. (2013). *Transcultural nursing* (6th ed.). St Louis, MO: Mosby.

Glanz, K., Rimer, B. K., & Viswanath, K. (Eds.). (2015). *Health behavior and health education: Theory, research, and practice* (4th ed.). Hoboken, NJ: John Wiley & Sons.

Gopal, D. P., Chetty, U., O'Donnell, P., Gajria, C., & Blackadder-Weinstein, J. (2021). Implicit bias in healthcare: Clinical practice, research and decision making. *Future Healthcare Journal, 8*(1), 40–48. https://doi.org/10.7861/fhj.2020-0233

Gray, B., & Orrock, P. (2014). Investigation into factors influencing roles, relationships, and referrals in integrative medicine. *Journal of Alternative and Complementary Medicine, 20*(5), 342–346.

Health Insurance Portability and Accountability Act of 1996 (HIPAA). Pub. L. 104–191.

HealthIT.gov. (2015). EHR incentives & certification. Retrieved from http://www.healthit.gov/providers-professionals/meaningful-use-definition-objectives

Health Resources and Services Administration. (2019). Health literacy. Retrieved from https://www.hrsa.gov/about/organization/bureaus/ohe/health-literacy/index.html

Huston, C. (2013) The impact of emerging technology on nursing care: Warp speed ahead. *OJIN: The Online Journal of Issues in Nursing, 18*(2), Manuscript 1. DOI: 10.3912/OJIN.Vol18No02Man01

Institute of Medicine. (2012). *The role of telehealth in an evolving health care environment: Workshop summary*. Washington, DC: National Academies Press. Available from http://iom.nationalacademies.org/reports/2012/the-role-of-telehealth-in-an-evolving-health-care-environ-ment.aspx

Institute for the Future. (2003). *Health & health care 2010: The forecast, the challenge*. Hoboken, NJ: John Wiley & Sons.

Institute of Medicine. (1999). *To err is human: Building a safer health system.* Available from http://nationalacademies.org/hmd/reports/1999/to-err-is-human-building-a-safer-health-sys-tem.aspx

Institute of Medicine. (2010). *The future of nursing: Leading change, advancing health.* Available from http://nationalacademies.org/hmd/reports/2010/the-future-of-nursing-leading-change-advancing-health.aspx

International Council of Nurses. (2000). *ICN position statement: Prevention of disability and the care of people with disabilities.* Retrieved from http://www.icn.ch/images/stories/docu-ments/publications/position_statements/A16_prevention_disability_care.pdf

Kirschner, K. L., & Curry, R. H. (2009). Patients with disabilities. *JAMA, 302*(12), 1334–1335.

Josen, A. R., Winslade, W. J., & Siegler, M. (2015). *Clinical ethics: A practical approach to ethical decisions in clinical medicine* (8th ed.). Columbus, OH: McGraw-Hill.

Mason, D. J., Leavitt, J. K., & Chaffee, M. W. (2015). *Policy & politics in nursing and health care* (7th ed.). Philadelphia: Elsevier.

Mullen, F., Politzer, R. M., Lewis, C. T., Bastacky, S., Rodak, J. Jr., & Harmon, R. G. (1992). The National Practitioner Data Bank: Report from the first year. *JAMA, 268,* 73–79.

Murray, R. B., Zentner, J. P., & Yakimo, R. (2009). *Health promotion strategies through the life span* (8th ed.). Upper Saddle River, NJ: Prentice Hall.

Nahin, R. L., Stussman, B. J., & Herman, P. M. (2015). Out-of-pocket expenditures on complementary health approaches associated with painful health conditions in a nationally representative adult sample. *Journal of Pain, 16*(11), 1147–1162.

National Academy of Medicine. (2021). The future of nursing: Charting a path to achieve equity. Retrieved from https://nam.edu/publications/the-future-of-nursing-2020-2030/

National Center for Complementary and Integrative Health. (2022). *Resources for health care providers.* Retrieved from https://www.nccih.nih.gov/health/providers

National Council of State Boards of Nursing. (1993). *Regulation of advanced nursing practice* (National Council Position Paper, 1993). Chicago, IL: Author.

National Council of State Boards of Nursing. (2011). *What you need to know about nursing licensure and boards of nursing.* Retrieved from https://www.ncsbn.org/Nursing_Licensure.pdf

National Council of State Boards of Nursing. (2007). *A nurse's guide to the importance of appropriate professional boundaries.* Chicago: Author. Retrieved from https://www.ncsbn.org/ProfessionalBoundaries_Complete.pdf

National Hospice and Palliative Care Organization. (2015). Hospice and palliative care. Retrieved from http://www.nhpco.org/about/hospice-care

National Institutes of Health: National Center for Complementary and Integrative Health. (2011). *Children and the use of complementary health approaches.* Retrieved from https://nccih.nih.gov/health/children#key

National Institutes of Health: National Center for Complementary and Integrative Health. (2015). Complementary, alternative, or integrative health: What's in a name? Retrieved from https://nccih.nih.gov/health/integrative-health

National Institutes of Health: Office of Dietary Supplements. (n.d.). Dietary supplement fact sheets. Retrieved from http://ods.od.nih.gov/

Ogungbe, O., Mitra, A.K., & Roberts, J.K. (2019). A systematic review of implicit bias in health care: A call for intersectionality. IMC Journal of Medical Science, 18(1), 19.

Papero, D.V., & Kerr, M. E. *Bowen family systems.* Upper Saddle River, NJ: Allyn & Bacon.

Pearson, L. J. (2015). *The Pearson Report.* Burlington, MA: Jones & Bartlett.

Pohl, J. M., Nath, R., Zheng, K., Rachman, F., Gans, D. N., & Tanner, C. (2013). Use of a comprehensive patient safety tool in primary care practices. *Journal of the American Academy of Nurse Practitioners, 25*(8), 415–418.

Quinlan, E., & Robertson, S. (2013). The communicative power of nurse practitioners in multidisciplinary primary healthcare teams. *Journal of the American Academy of Nurse Practitioners, 25,* 91–102.

Robert Wood Johnson Foundation. (2010). *Quality and safety education for nurses.* Retrieved from http://qsen.org/about-qsen/

Saba, V. K., & McCormick, K. A. (2015). *Essentials of nursing informatics* (6th ed.). New York, NY: McGraw-Hill.

Sand-Jecklin, K., Murray, B., Summers, B., & Watson, J. (2010). Educating nursing students about health literacy: From the classroom to the patient bedside. *Online Journal of Issues in Nursing, 15*(3). Retrieved from http://www.medscape.com/viewarticle/729395

Tsai, H. H., Lin, H. W., Pickard, A. S., Tsail, H. Y., & Mahady, G. B. (2012). Evaluation of documented drug interactions and contraindications associated with herbs and dietary supplements: A systematic literature review. *International Journal of Clinical Practice, 66*(11), 1056–1078.

U.S. Department of Health and Human Services. (n.d.). *National practitioner data bank.* Retrieved from http://www.npdb-hipdb.hrsa.gov/

U.S. Department of Health and Human Services. (2003). *OCR privacy brief: Summary of the HIPAA privacy rule.* Washington, DC: U.S. Dept. of Health & Human Services Office for Civil Rights.

U.S. Department of Health and Human Services. (2010). *Healthy People 2020* (3rd ed.). McLean, VA: International Medical Publishing Inc.

U.S. Department of Health and Human Services. (2014). *Healthy People 2020 leading health indicators progress update.* McLean, VA: International Medical Publishing Inc.

U.S. Department of Health, Education and Welfare. (1971). *Report on licensure and related health personnel credentials* (DHEW Pub. No. (HSM) 72–11). Washington, DC: Author.

U.S. Food and Drug Administration: U.S. Department of Health and Human Services. (2015). *Questions and answers on dietary supplements.* Retrieved from http://www.fda.gov/Food/DietarySupplements/UsingDietarySupplements/ucm480069.htm

U.S. Office of Technology Assessment. (1986). *Nurse practitioners, physician's assistants and certified nurse midwives: A policy analysis.* Washington, DC: U.S. Government Printing Office.

Villaseñor, S., & Piscotty, R. J. (2015). The current state of e-prescribing: Implications for advanced practice registered nurses. *AANP.* Online preview 5-5-2015. Retrieved from http://onlinelibrary.wiley.com/doi/10.1002/2327-6924.12263/full

Wright, L. M., & Leahey, M. (2012). *Nurses and families: A guide to family assessment and intervention* (6th ed.). Philadelphia, PA: F. A. Davis.

CHAPTER 3

HEALTH CARE ISSUES

Laura Reed, DNP, FNP
Michael A. Carter, DNSc, DNP, FNP, GNP, FAAN, DCC

General Approach

- All countries throughout the world have financial limits on their abilities to support health care systems.
- The United States spends about 50% more per person than any other country in the world (Tikkanen, R., & Abrams, M. K., 2020).
- Health care access and health disparities in the United States continue even after passage and modifications of the Patient Protection and Affordable Care Act.
- There are 7447 primary care Health Professional Shortage Areas (HPSAs) representing the underserved with limited access to care.
- The leading causes of infant mortality in the United States are congenital malformations, disorders of short gestation and low birth weight, injuries, sudden infant death syndrome, and maternal pregnancy complications.
- A resurgence of previously controlled infections and the emergence of newer infections, coupled with antibiotic resistance and an increasingly global environment, make infectious disease a persistent threat to people at either end of the age spectrum.
- Current health care trends support greater emphasis on disease prevention, risk reduction, health promotion, and chronic disease management rather than exclusive disease management.
- There is increased emphasis on evidence-based practice (the use of current and best evidence to make decisions about care) and early translation of the best evidence into practice to improve health care quality and outcomes of care.
- There is increasing health care complexity through technological advances, particularly in health care information systems.

RED FLAGS

- *Health disparities*: "A type of health difference that is closely linked with social, economic, and/or environmental disadvantage." (U.S. Department of Health and Human Services, 2020)
- *Access*: the availability (or lack thereof) of health care services to all
- *Medically underserved community*: a setting with a shortage of primary care, dental, and/or mental health services
- *Vulnerability*: open to physical, emotional, and/or socioeconomic harm
- *Disadvantaged*: inhibited from knowledge, skills, and abilities to participate in the health care system as a provider and/or a receiver of health care because of economic, social, ethnic, or racial background, and/or physical or mental impairment
- *Underrepresented minorities*: racial and ethnic populations whose representation among the health professions is lower than their proportion of the general population
- *Social determinants of health*: defined by the World Health Organization as "conditions in which people are born, grow, live, work, and age, and the wider set of forces and systems shaping the conditions of daily life" (WHO, 2015)

THE PATIENT PROTECTION AND AFFORDABLE CARE ACT

- Patient Protection and Affordable Care Act (ACA) became law in 2010 (U.S. Department of Health and Human Services, n.d.).
- In 2020, 8.6% of U.S. citizens (28.0 million) did not have health insurance at any point during the year (https://www.census.gov/library/publications/2021/demo/p60–274.html)
- The ACA ended preexisting condition exclusions, keeps adults younger than 26 years of age on their parents' plan, and ended lifetime limits.
- The ACA requires insurers to offer preventive care with no copayment.

NATIONAL PREVENTION STRATEGY

The National Prevention Strategy (Centers for Disease Control and Prevention, n.d.) presents evidence-based recommendations designed to reduce the burden of the most-common preventable causes of disease and death. The aim of this initiative is to guide the nation in the most effective and achievable ways to improve health and well-being. The strategic directions include healthy and safe community environments, clinical and community preventive services, empowered people, and the elimination of health disparities. Here are the priority areas:

- Tobacco-free living
- Preventing drug abuse and excessive alcohol use
- Healthy eating
- Active living
- Injury- and violence-free living
- Reproductive and sexual health
- Mental and emotional well-being

Model Epidemiologic Principles

DEFINITION

- The study of how disease is distributed in populations
- Includes factors that influence this distribution (Gordis, 2014)

NATURAL HISTORY OF DISEASE

The course of disease is one of development, expression, and progression in a person over time. Several stages appear to be universally descriptive:

- Stage of susceptibility (pre-pathological)
- Stage of pre-symptomatic disease (subclinical)
- Stage of clinical disease
- Stage of disability (or death)

PREVENTION OF DISEASE

The goal is to intervene as early as possible to prevent disease or disability.

Primary Prevention

- Interventions at the stage of susceptibility, directed at preventing disease from occurring
- Education, exercise, nutrition, water fluoridation, immunizations, food-handling regulations, pollution control

Secondary Prevention

- Interventions at the subclinical stage, directed at early detection of the illness or problem to reduce the progress and severity of the disease
- Genetic testing in newborns, lead screening, vision and hearing screening, smoking cessation programs, cholesterol screening, and mammography

Tertiary Prevention

- Interventions at the clinical stage of disease, directed at treatment and rehabilitation of the illness to prevent or minimize progression of the disease or its sequelae, such as disability
- Use of inhaled steroids in the management of asthma and penicillin prophylaxis in patients with sickle cell anemia

ETIOLOGY

The cause or the web of causation of a disease or problem:

- Any factors (direct or indirect) that increase the likelihood of disease
- Prevalence rates describe the number of persons who have a condition in the population at a specific time divided by the number of people in the population.
- Incidence rates describe the number of new cases that occur during a specified time in a group at risk. (See Table 3–1, which identifies the leading causes of death per age group.)

RISK FACTORS

- Age, sex, social, cultural, familial, racial/ethnic, genetic, occupation, and lifestyle history represent potential sources of problems and diseases that may be difficult or impossible to alter.
- Risk-reduction programs may be established to decrease the vulnerability of persons to certain problems by modifying some risks.

TABLE 3–1.
LEADING CAUSES OF DEATH BY AGE GROUP

AGE	CAUSE OF DEATH
Under 1 year	Congenital anomalies
	Short gestation
	Sudden infant death syndrome (SIDS)
	Unintentional injuries
	Maternal complications
	Placenta, cord, or membranes
	Bacterial sepsis
	Respiratory distress
	Circulatory system disease
	Neonatal hemorrhage
1–4 years	Unintentional injuries
	Congenital anomalies
	Homicide
	Malignant neoplasms
	Heart disease
	Influenza and pneumonia
	Cerebrovascular
	Perinatal period
	Septicemia
	Benign neoplasms
5–9 years	Unintentional injuries
	Malignant neoplasms
	Congenital anomalies
	Homicide
	Heart disease
	Influenza and pneumonia
	Chronic lower respiratory disease
	Cerebrovascular disease
	Benign neoplasms
	Suicide

Continued

TABLE 3–1.
(CONTINUED)

AGE	CAUSE OF DEATH
10–14 years	Unintentional injuries
	Suicide
	Malignant neoplasms
	Homicide
	Congenital anomalies
	Heart disease
	Chronic lower respiratory disease
	Diabetes mellitus
	Influenza and pneumonia
	Cerebrovascular
15–24 years	Unintentional injuries
	Homicide
	Suicide
	Malignant neoplasms
	Heart disease
	COVID-19
	Congenital anomalies
	Diabetes mellitus
	Chronic lower respiratory disease
	Complicated pregnancy
25–34 years	Unintentional injuries
	Suicide
	Homicide
	Heart disease
	Malignant neoplasms
	COVID-19
	Liver disease
	Diabetes mellitus
	Cerebrovascular disease
	Complicated pregnancy

Continued

TABLE 3–1.
(CONTINUED)

AGE	CAUSE OF DEATH
35–44 years	Unintentional injuries
	Heart disease
	Malignant neoplasms
	Suicide
	COVID-19
	Liver disease
	Homicide
	Diabetes mellitus
	Cerebrovascular disease
	Influenza and pneumonia
45–54 years	Malignant neoplasms
	Heart disease
	Unintentional injuries
	COVID-19
	Liver disease
	Diabetes mellitus
	Suicide
	Cerebrovascular disease
	Chronic lower respiratory disease
	Homicide
55–64 years	Malignant neoplasms
	Heart disease
	COVID-19
	Unintentional injuries
	Chronic lower respiratory disease
	Diabetes mellitus
	Liver disease
	Cerebrovascular disease
	Suicide
	Influenza and pneumonia

Continued

TABLE 3–1.
(CONTINUED)

AGE	CAUSE OF DEATH
65 years and older	Heart disease
	Malignant neoplasms
	COVID-19
	Cerebrovascular disease
	Alzheimer's disease
	Chronic lower respiratory disease
	Diabetes mellitus
	Unintentional injuries
	Nephritis
	Influenza and pneumonia

Adapted from "10 Leading Causes of Death by Age Group, United States—2020," by Centers for Disease Control and Prevention, 2020. https://wisqars.cdc.gov/data/lcd/home

COMMUNICABLE OR INFECTIOUS DISEASES

Illnesses caused by organisms that attack and invade vulnerable persons

- Involve identification of causative agents,
- Rely on microbiology principles to understand the life cycle of organism,
- Focus on intervention at vulnerable phases in the course of disease or life cycle of organism, and
- Use selected infectious disease definitions (Box 3–1).

Reservoirs of Infection

- Cases and carriers
- Animal carriers (lower vertebrate animals)
- Invertebrate hosts (insects)
- Inanimate objects: Some infectious agents are free living in the environment, multiplying on inanimate objects (such as *Salmonella* in food, *Legionella* in pools of water, and *Histoplasma* in oil).

BOX 3–1.
INFECTIOUS DISEASE DEFINITIONS

General Definitions

- *Infection*: Colonization and multiplication of an organism in the host, typically producing an immune response but no signs or symptoms.
- *Disease*: Stage when an infection produces signs and/or symptoms (including pathologic changes). Certain organisms (such as influenza virus) are capable of infection with or without producing disease; other organisms (such as measles virus) always produce disease in susceptible persons. Disease may vary in severity.
- *Colonization*: The organism invades the host at a particular site, multiplies, and acts as a parasite but does not produce infection, immune response, or disease.
- *Carrier state*: Persistence of an organism in a host; this stage may follow infection, disease, or colonization and may be infectious to others.

Agent (Organism) Properties

- *Infectivity*: Ability of an organism to invade and multiply in a susceptible host. Varicella is highly infective, rhinovirus is intermediate, and tubercle bacilli are of low infectivity.
- *Pathogenicity*: Ability of an organism to produce disease. Rabies, rhinovirus, and varicella are highly pathogenic; adenovirus and rubella are intermediate; and tubercle bacillus is low.
- *Virulence*: Severity of disease that an organism can produce, measured by criteria such as number of days in bed or the frequency of serious sequelae including death (fatality rate). Rabies virus is highly virulent (nearly 100% fatality rate); poliovirus is moderately virulent; and varicella and rhinovirus are of low virulence (almost zero fatality rate).
- *Immunogenicity*: Ability to produce a lasting and effective immunity. Rhinovirus, which primarily acts locally, results in a poor systemic immune response. Systemic viral infections such as measles produce lasting immunity.

Continued

BOX 3–1. (CONTINUED)

Agent–Host Relations

- *Latent infection*: The organism is not shedding or obtainable (likely hidden in host cells).
- *Patent infection:* The organism is shedding and/or obtainable from such areas as feces, urine, blood, or respiratory tract. Certain infections may remain permanently patent (some cases of hepatitis B) or be intermittently patent (herpes virus), or, after being latent for a long time, may reactivate and produce disease (tuberculosis and herpes zoster).
- *Period of communicability*: The time when sufficient numbers of organisms are shed to cause transmission; usually concurrent with disease but not always.
- *Incubation period*: The time from exposure to the onset of disease.

Mechanisms of Transmission of Infection

- Direct: through touching, kissing, sexual intercourse, childbearing, breastfeeding, transfusions
- Indirect: through air, vector (insects, animals), vehicle (food, water, towels)

Control Measures

- Measures directed against the reservoir: isolation, quarantine, insect spraying
- Measures that interrupt the transmission of organisms: water purification, milk pasteurization, barrier protection during sexual intercourse
- Measures that reduce host susceptibility: immunization, appropriate use of antibiotics, improved nutrition

Concepts of Epidemic vs. Endemic Infections

- *Generation time:* interval between receipt of infection and the maximal communicability of the host; applied to both subclinical and clinical infections (incubation period applies only to clinical cases); used to describe and analyze the spread of infectious diseases (i.e., common vehicle, single-exposure epidemic, determined by the incubation or generation time)

- *Herd immunity:* resistance of a group to invasion and spread of an infectious agent because a large portion of the group is immune; decreases the likelihood of an epidemic in an area
- *Endemic*: a disease or infectious agent that is usually present in a population
- *Epidemic:* occurrence of disease in excess of what is normally expected in a population
- *Morbidity:* occurrence of illness in a population
- *Mortality:* occurrence of death in a population

Human Development

DEFINITION

- Most development is patterned and orderly, with both a purpose and a direction.
- Development is continuous throughout life, although the degree of change in many areas decreases after adolescence.
- Development may occur simultaneously in several areas, such as physical and social, but the rate of change in each area varies.
- The pace of development varies among persons.
- Physical and mental stress during periods of critical developmental change, such as puberty, may make a person particularly susceptible to outside stressors.
- Anticipatory guidance is an important component of patient and family education throughout the life span.

INFANT AND CHILD DEVELOPMENT

- Assessment of growth is determined by routine monitoring of height, weight, head circumference (until age 2), dental development, and appearance of secondary sex characteristics.
- Adequacy of growth is determined by comparison with normal growth parameters (see Tables 3–2 through 3–5) and/or plotting the measurements of height, weight, and head circumference on a standard National Center for Health Statistics (NCHS) (2010) growth chart.

TABLE 3–2.
NORMAL GROWTH PARAMETERS FOR HEIGHT AND WEIGHT

AGE	WEIGHT*	HEIGHT*
Newborn	95% of newborns weigh 5–10 lbs. Approximately 5%–10% of body weight is lost in the first few days; then birth weight is regained in 7–10 days.	95% of newborns are between 18 and 22 in. long.
Birth–6 months	Weekly gain 140–200 g (5–7 ounces). Birth weight doubles by 6 months.	Monthly gain is 2.5 cm (1 in.).
Older than 6–12 months	Weekly gain 85–140 g (3–5 ounces); triples by age 1 year 50% by age 1 year.	Monthly gain is 1.25 cm (0.5 in.). Birthweight length increases by approximately 50% by age 1.
Toddlers	Yearly gain 2–3 kg (4½–6½ lbs).	Growth is approximately 12 cm (5 in.) between ages 1 and 2 years and 6–8 cm (2½–3½ in.) between ages 2 and 3 years. Approximately 50% of adult height is reached by age 2 years.
School age	Yearly gain approximately 2–3 kg (4½–6½ lbs).	Growth is approximately 5–6 cm (2–2½ in.) per year. Birth length doubles by age 4 years and triples by age 13 years.
Puberty—girls (10–14 years)	Weight gain 15–55 lbs (mean 38 lbs).	Growth is approximately 5–25 cm (2–10 in.); 95% of adult height is achieved by menarche (skeletal age of 13 years).
Puberty—boys (11–16 years)	Weight gain 15–65 lbs (mean 52 lbs).	Growth is approximately 10–30 cm (4–12 in.); 95% of adult height is achieved by skeletal age of 15 years.

*These measurements are averages.

Adapted from "CDC Growth Charts," by National Center for Health Statistics, 2010. Retrieved from http://www.cdc.gov/growthcharts/

- There are two periods of rapid growth: infancy and adolescence; in-between, growth is steady but slower.
- The growth of most body tissues parallels physical growth, which is most rapid in the first 2 years; lymph tissue growth is rapid in the preschool and early school-age years; growth of reproductive organs remains slow until puberty.

Patterns of Development

- The sequence of development is basically the same in all children, but the rate varies.
- Attainment of developmental landmarks in one area does not always run parallel to another area of development.
- Development is dependent on maturation of the nervous system.
- Generalized activity precedes specific movements. (A young infant kicks and waves arms with excitement, whereas an older infant reaches out and grasps.)
- Development occurs in a cephalocaudal direction (head control develops before walking) and a proximal-to-distal direction (shoulders before fingers).
- Certain primitive reflexes must be lost before the corresponding voluntary movement is acquired. (Grasp reflex lost before deliberately grasping objects can occur.)

Tooth Eruption

- Deciduous teeth usually begin at 6 months of age with the central incisors and move laterally.
- All 20 deciduous teeth are usually in place by 2½ to 3 years of age.
- Delayed dentition is considered when no teeth have erupted by 13 months of age.
- Shedding of deciduous teeth begins at about 6 years of age and continues through age 12.
- Eruption of the first permanent teeth occurs with the first molars, at about age 6 years.
- Eruption of all 32 permanent teeth may not be complete until ages 17 to 21, with third molars.

Developmental Landmarks and Milestones

- Development is typically assessed in four areas: gross motor, fine motor, language, and social skills.
- The purpose is to identify children in need of further assessment and determine if a developmental disability exists.
- All states are required to have a system to identify and treat developmental disabilities in children ages 3 to 5 years; most states have voluntarily extended this age range.

Interpreting Results

- Attainment of milestones is in ranges.
- A significant finding in any developmental assessment is the loss of developmental milestones previously achieved or lack of key milestones by a certain age (see Table 3–3).
- Language and fine motor skills are sensitive indicators of intellectual development.
- Early attainment of gross motor skills is not a significant indicator of advanced intellectual development but does usually preclude the diagnosis of intellectual disability. Developmental warning signs can be found in Table 3–4.
- No child is intellectually disabled if delayed in one area but normal in all others.

ADOLESCENT PUBERTAL CHANGES

Boys

- Average age at onset is 10.5 to 16 years.
- Precocious puberty is the development of secondary sex characteristics before age 9 and is often associated with a pathological etiology in boys.
- Delayed puberty is lack of changes by age 14 years.
- First change is testicular enlargement, followed by pubic hair development at the base of the penis (adrenarche); testicular size larger than 2 to 2.5 cm indicates puberty has begun.
- Penile growth occurs approximately 6 to 12 months after testicular enlargement; penis grows from a prepubertal size of 3.5 to 5.5 cm to an adult length of 12 cm (7.5 to 15.5 cm).
- Growth spurt begins about 1 year after the first testicular changes (average age 12.5 years), peaks after 1.5 years, and lasts 2 to 4 years.
- Accompanying changes, such as axillary and facial hair and deepening voice, occur later in puberty.

TABLE 3–3.
DEVELOPMENTAL MILESTONES

TASKS	AVERAGE AGE (RANGE)*
GROSS MOTOR SKILLS	
Moves head from side to side	2 weeks
Lifts shoulders while prone	2 months
Moves both arms and both legs	2 months
Rolls over	4 months (2–6 months)
Head control (no bobbing)	4 months
Pushes up with straight arms when on tummy	6 months
Sits alone	6 months (5–9 months)
Crawls (reciprocal)	9 months (8–11 months)
Cruises	9 months (8–13 months)
Pulls to stand	12 months
Walks alone	12 months (9–15 months)
Drinks from cup without lid as it is held	12 months
Runs, walks upstairs holding rail	18 months (14–21 months)
Throws ball overhand	19–20 months (16–24 months)
Pedals tricycle	28 months (21–36 months)
Balances on one foot	28–30 months (22–38 months)
Jumps off ground with both feet	30 months
Unbuttons some buttons	4 years
Hops on one foot	4 years (3–4½ years)
Tandem walk	5 years (3½–5 years)
Skips	5 years
FINE MOTOR SKILLS	
Unfists	3–4 months
Holds objects placed in hand	3–4 months (2½–5 months)
Reaches for objects	4 months (3–5 months)
Transfers objects	6 months (4½–7 months)
Ulnar raking	6 months (5–7 months)
Looks for objects when dropped out of sight	9 months
Inferior pincer	9–10 months

Continued

TABLE 3–3. (CONTINUED)

TASKS	AVERAGE AGE (RANGE)*
Mature pincer	11–12 months
Deliberate throw	12–13 months
Spontaneous scribble	14–16 months (12–16 months)
Tower of 2	15 months (12½–20 months)
Tower of 4	18 months (16–20 months)
Tower of 6	24 months (17–30 months)
Imitates line	24 months (19–30 months)
Tower of 10	36 months
Copies circle	36 months (2½–3½ years)
Uses scissors	3 years
Copies square	4 years (4–5 years)
Draws 3-part figure	4 years (3½–5 years)
Copies triangle	5 years
Draws 6-part figure	5½ years (4½–6 years)
LANGUAGE (RECEPTIVE AND EXPRESSIVE)	
Localizes sound	4–9 months
Babbling vowels	5–6 months
Babbling consonants	6–7 months
"Dada"/"mama"—nonspecific	9–10 months
"Dada"/"mama"—specific	10–12 months
13 words	11–13 months
Follows one-step command	11–15 months
10–15 words, 25% intelligible	15–18 months
Points to named pictures when asked "show me"	18–24 months
Approximately 100-word vocabulary by 2nd birthday; says "me" and "mine" Uses 2- to 3-word phrases. (As a rule, the number of words in a sentence equals the child's age [2 by age 2, 3 by age 3])	2 years
Approximately 50-word vocabulary; 2-word combinations with 1 action word	30 months
Follows 2-step commands without gesture	30 months

Continued

TABLE 3–3.
(CONTINUED)

TASKS	AVERAGE AGE (RANGE)*
Few possessives ("my ball") and progressives (the—ing: "I playing")	30 months
Concept of "I" questions	30 months
Knows few colors, pronouns, plurals, full name, age, approximately 250-word vocabulary, 3–4 word sentences (75% intelligible)	36 months
Asks who, what, when, where, or why questions	3 years
Says first name when asked	3 years
Counts to 4, can say a nursery rhyme, asks and answers why, how, when, knows opposite analogies, and uses past tense	4 years+
Uses complex sentences, understands meanings of words, counts to 10, has fluent speech, uses future tense	5 years
Answers simple questions about a book or story after read or told	5 years
SOCIAL, INTERACTIVE, VISION	
Regards face	0–1 month
Smiles responsively when approached, talked to, smiled at	2 months
Calms down when spoken to/picked up	2 months
Chuckles (not a full laugh) when you try to make laugh	2 months
Attempts to keep attention with eye contact, movement, or making sounds	4 months
Hand regard	4–5 months
Smiles at mirror image	5 months
Plays peek-a-boo	9 months
Recognizes familiar people	6 months
Laughs	6 months
Shows facial expressions	9 months
Plays pat-a-cake	12 months
Waves goodbye	10 months (7–14 months)
Indicates wants	12 months (10–14 months)
Imitates housework	15 months (13–18 months)

Continued

TABLE 3–3. (CONTINUED)

TASKS	AVERAGE AGE (RANGE)*
Shows liked object	15 months
Shows affection with hugging	15 months
Claps when excited	15 months
Puts out hands to be washed and dried	18 months
Puts on clothing	18 months
Notices when others are upset/hurt	24 months
Verbalizes "Look at me" to show what they can do	30 months
Follows simple routines when told	30 months
Notices other children and joins play	3 years
Likes to be a "helper"	4 years
Does simple chores at home	5 years

*Ages will vary with different tests.

Adapted from Zubler, J. M., Wiggins, L. D., Macias, M. M., Whitaker, T. M., Shaw, J. S., Squires, J. K., . . . & Lipkin, P. H. (2022). Evidence-informed milestones for developmental surveillance tools. *Pediatrics, 149*(3).

Girls

- Average age at onset is 11 years, with a range of 8 to 13 years.
- Precocious puberty is the onset of changes before 8 years of age or menarche before age 10 years.
- Delayed puberty is no breast development by age 13 years or no menses by 15 to 16 years.
- First pubertal change is usually breast budding under the areola and pubertal fine hair over the mons pubis (adrenarche or pubarche).
- Menarche occurs at an average age of 12.5 years (range 10 to 15 years).

TABLE 3–4.
DEVELOPMENTAL WARNING SIGNS

6 weeks	Absence of auditory alertness Lack of visual fixation (focusing) Excessive head lag on pulling-to-sitting position
6 months	Persistence of hand regard Failure to follow 180 degrees (for both near and far objects) Persistent fisting Preference of one hand
10 months	Absence of babble No smiling or social responsiveness Absence of weight-bearing while hand held Failure to sit without support
18 months	No spontaneous vocalizations No single words No pincer grasp Inability to stand without support
2 years	No recognizable words No walking

Health Maintenance

Current factors support greater emphasis on health promotion and disease prevention.

Healthy People 2030 (U.S. Department of Health and Human Services, n.d.):

- A set of goals and objectives based on annual targets to guide the nation's health promotion and prevention effofrts
- National objectives that emphasize disease prevention and define leading health indicators necessary to measure health; as a group, reflect major health concerns in United States in the 21st century
- Emphasizes social determinants of health and promotion of health across all stages of life and use of technology, such as interactive websites, as the main vehicle of dissemination of evidence-based resources for implementation

- Leading health indicators selected based on their ability to motivate action, availability of data to measure progress, and importance as public health issues. They include:
  - Increase the proportion of people with health insurance
  - Increase the use of oral health care system
  - Reduce severe maternal complications identified during delivery hospitalizations
  - Reduce the number of days people are exposed to unhealthy air
  - Reduce the rate of acute hepatitis
  - Reduce the proportion of people 21 years of age or over who engaged in binge drinking in the past month
  - Reduce the number of diabetes cases diagnosed yearly
  - Reduce the proportion of children and adolescents with lifetime tooth decay
  - Reduce current tobacco use in adolescents
  - Reduce the rate of hospital admissions for urinary tract infections among older adults
  - Increase knowledge of HIV status
  - Reduce suicide rate
  - Reduce *Clostridium difficile* (C. Diff.) infections that people get in the hospital
  - Increase the proportion of adults with diabetes who have a yearly eye exam
  - Increase past-year attempts to quit smoking in adults
  - Reduce the rate of hospital admissions for pneumonia among older adults
  - Reduce congenital syphilis
  - Reduce pelvic inflammatory disease in female adolescents and young women
  - Reduce the syphilis rate in men who have sex with men
  - Reduce current cigarette smoking in adults
  - Increase the proportion of people with a usual primary care provider
  - Increase the proportion of sexually active female adolescents and young women who get screened for chlamydia
  - Increase the proportion of people who no longer have hepatitis C
  - Increase the proportion of people who know they have chronic hepatitis B
  - Reduce maternal deaths
  - Reduce drug overdose deaths
  - Increase employment in working-age people
  - Reduce the rate of hepatitis A
  - Reduce household food insecurity and hunger

◇ Increase the proportion of fourth graders with reading skills at or above the proficient level
◇ Increase the proportion of people who get the flu vaccine every year
◇ Reduce the proportion of children and adolescents with obesity
◇ Increase the rate of acute hepatitis B
◇ Increase the proportion of adults who do enough aerobic and muscle-strengthening activity
◇ Reduce the rate of infant deaths
◇ Increase the proportion of adults who get screened for colorectal cancer
◇ Increase the control of high blood pressure in adults
◇ Reduce homicides
◇ Reduce consumption of added sugars by people 2 years of age or older

Health Maintenance Practice

LIFESTYLE/HEALTH BEHAVIORS

Routine counseling and chemoprophylaxis in primary prevention may prevent certain conditions (see Table 3–5). Specific health behaviors that are amenable to intervention can be found in Table 3–6.

Exercise

- Recommendation is 30 minutes of moderate physical activity on most days of the week; does not have to be continuous
- Recommendation is as important for children as for adults

Child and Adolescent Pre-Participation Sports Assessment

- Children and adolescents participating in sports should have a pre-participation evaluation (PPE). Almost all states require medical clearance before sports participation, although no standardization of PPEs exists, and evaluations may vary. The American Academy of Pediatrics and the American Association of Sports Medicine Physicians each have developed guidelines.
- The PPE should involve parents for athletes younger than 18 years of age.

TABLE 3–5. CHEMOPROPHYLAXIS FOR DISEASE PREVENTION

CONDITION	RATIONALE	RECOMMENDATIONS
PREVENTING PRIMARY DISEASE		
Neural tube defects	Disorders of the cranium, spine, and nervous system that occur when the neural tube fails to close. Folic acid supplementation has resulted in more than 50% reduction in these birth defects. The average North American diet includes less than half of the recommended dietary intake of folic acid.	All women of childbearing years, whether pregnant or not, should take 0.4 mg daily of folic acid either alone or as part of a multivitamin supplement. The dose is increased with pregnancy.
Hemorrhagic disease of the newborn	Newborn gut lacks the bacteria necessary to synthesize vitamin K, which is used for coagulation.	Vitamin K (phytonadione), 1 mg, is administered once immediately after birth.
Ophthalmia neonatorum	Primary purpose is the prevention of gonococcal and chlamydial conjunctivitis in the neonate. Silver nitrate is not effective against *Chlamydia*.	Instilled immediately postpartum: a single application of 0.5% erythromycin ophthalmic ointment, or 1% tetracycline ophthalmic ointment
Group B *Streptococcus* (GBS) (prevention in the newborn)	In the early 1970s, GBS was a primary cause of neonatal sepsis and meningitis. Prevention strategies began to screen women for GBS and provide antibiotic prophylaxis for women who were positive or had specific risk factors.	Screen pregnant women for GBS in one of two ways: ♦ Obtain vaginal and rectal cultures at 35–37 weeks of gestation. ♦ If no culture results are available, the decision for chemoprophylaxis is based on the presence of one or more risk factors: delivery at 37 weeks of gestation or less, membranes ruptured for more than 18 hours, intrapartum fever of 38° C or higher, or mother had a previous infant with GBS disease or had GBS bacteriuria herself.

Continued

TABLE 3–5.
(CONTINUED)

CONDITION	RATIONALE	RECOMMENDATIONS
		Whichever screening method is used, the treatment is the same: IV penicillin G, 5 million units, followed by 2–5 million units every 4 hours until delivery. Treatment is most effective if at least two doses of penicillin are given.
Dental caries	Reduction of dental caries can be accomplished with fluoride and sealants. Excess fluoride will cause fluorosis (mottling of the teeth).	Dose of fluoride is dependent on fluoride concentration in the water and age of the child. Sealants are plastic coverings applied by the dentist for secondary molars.
DISEASE PREVENTION IN HIGH-RISK PEOPLE		
Respiratory syncytial virus (RSV)	RSV is responsible for the majority of lower respiratory tract infections in children. RSV is a paramyxovirus that produces fusion of human cells in tissue. RSV attacks the upper and lower respiratory tracts, often causing life-threatening pneumonia and bronchiolitis. Bronchiolitis may begin as a mild upper respiratory tract infection that progresses to difficulty breathing with a cough and wheeze. RSV causes potentially life-threatening airway obstruction.	Employ shared decision making to recommend a single dose of RSV vaccine for adults ages 60 and older, (CDC, 2024). Treatment is focused on symptom relief. Airway management with bronchodilators, hydration, and antivirals may be used to manage RSV.

Continued

TABLE 3–5. (CONTINUED)

CONDITION	RATIONALE	RECOMMENDATIONS
Infective endocarditis (IE) or subacute bacterial endocarditis (SBE)	SBE prophylaxis with antibiotics is recommended for people with specific cardiac conditions who are undergoing procedures that may induce a transient bacteremia. *High-risk conditions* include prosthetic valves, most congenital heart malformations, rheumatic heart disease, hypertrophic cardiomyopathy, mitral valve prolapse with regurgitation, and previous bacterial endocarditis. *High-risk procedures* include most types of dental work (tooth extractions, cleaning, and surgery) and operations within the oropharynx, gastrointestinal, and genitourinary tract. Failures may occur even with adherence to recommendations.	Recommended prophylaxis: oral amoxicillin, 50 mg/kg (maximum 2 grams) 1 hour prior to the procedure. If allergic to penicillin, use cephalexin (50 mg/kg, maximum 2 grams) or azithromycin or clarithromycin (15 mg/kg, maximum 500 mg). Post-procedural antibiotics are no longer recommended.
Streptococcus pneumoniae (pneumococcal disease)	Extended (possibly lifelong) antibiotic prophylaxis is recommended for those persons at risk for developing fulminant pneumococcal disease, particularly patients with sickle-cell disease and asplenia. Pneumococcal vaccine may change these recommendations, but currently antibiotics are recommended even if vaccine is given.	Penicillin G or V Younger than 5 years of age, 125 mg twice a day 5 years of age and older, 250 mg twice a day

Continued

TABLE 3–5. (CONTINUED)

CONDITION	RATIONALE	RECOMMENDATIONS
PREVENT RECURRENCES OF DISEASE		
Acute rheumatic fever (ARF)	Continuous antibiotics effective against group A streptococcus are provided for persons who have a documented history of ARF to prevent recurrences. Antibiotic prophylaxis should begin as soon as the diagnosis of ARF is made and continue through life.	Benzathine penicillin IM every 4 weeks or daily oral antibiotics: ♦ Penicillin V, 125–250 mg twice a day, or ♦ Erythromycin 250 mg twice a day, or ♦ Sulfadiazine 60 pounds and over, 1 g daily; less than 60 pounds, 0.5 g daily
Urinary tract infections (UTIs)	Children (infants to adolescents) with recurrent UTIs (more than 2 to 3 episodes) may be candidates for antibiotic prophylaxis to prevent recurrences.	Daily antibiotic therapy, usually with nitrofurantoin or trimethoprim- sulfamethoxazole, is given for various lengths of time: ♦ Children with normal urinary tracts are usually treated until infection-free for 6–12 months. ♦ Children with vesicoureteral reflux are treated until the reflux resolves. ♦ Children with urinary tract abnormalities are often on long-term therapy.
PREVENT DISEASE AFTER EXPOSURE		
Meningitis (*Neisseria meningitidis* or *Haemophilus influenzae*)	Antibiotic prophylaxis is recommended for household members and child-care contacts of infected person.	Administer rifampin within 24 hours of identifying the person at 10 mg/kg every 12 hours × 2 days (four doses) for *Neisseria*; for *Haemophilus*, use a 4-day regimen.

Continued

TABLE 3–5. (CONTINUED)

CONDITION	RATIONALE	RECOMMENDATIONS
Pertussis	Household contacts of infected person should receive antibiotic prophylaxis.	Administer erythromycin estolate (some experts use azithromycin) at 40–50 mg/kg/day (maximum 2 grams/day) for 14 days.
Sexually transmitted diseases	Symptomatic or asymptomatic persons exposed to partners with chlamydia, gonorrhea, or syphilis are treated with appropriate antibiotics.	Same treatment regimen is used for the infected and the exposed person.

https://www.aafp.org/dam/AAFP/documents/patient_care/clinical_recommendations/cps-recommendations.pdf.

- The goal of the PPE is to identify those who may need conditioning or rehabilitation, need further evaluation for clearance, or should be excluded from participation. Particular attention should be directed at the cardiopulmonary and musculoskeletal systems.
- Sports physicals should not replace the routine physical exam but may include preventive health care teaching on topics such as the use of supplemental aids and prevention of injuries.
- Results of the PPE may allow for full participation (the majority), temporary deferral (due to illness or injury), partial deferral (i.e., no contact or collision sports), the recommendation for an appropriate sport for certain conditions, and/or exclusion.

Exercise Recommendations for Adults

- Focus on fundamental fitness and not sport-specific skills
- Goal: Sustain target heart rate for 30 minutes for maximum cardiopulmonary conditioning
  - Subtract the patient's age from 220
  - Multiple result by 0.8 for target heart rate
  - A 40-year-old patient's target heart rate is 144 bpm

TABLE 3–6.
SPECIFIC HEALTH BEHAVIORS AMENABLE TO INTERVENTION

FACTOR	STRENGTH OF EVIDENCE	BENEFIT	AGE FOR WHICH RECOMMENDED	RECOMMENDATION
Exercise	Good evidence	Many, including preventing cardiac disease, death	All ages	Individualize
Nutrition	Simple, focused intervention can be effective	Help with many chronic conditions	No upper limit	Counseling about adequate diet
Calcium	Good evidence in high-risk patients	Reduce risk of osteoporosis	Postmenopausal women	1000–1500 mg/day for women; no recommendation for men
Cholesterol	Diet not shown sufficient to reduce cholesterol level; normal levels protect young to middle-aged men	Reduce hyperlipidemia, atherosclerotic cardiovascular disease (ASCD)	No support for screening and treatment over age 75	Total cholesterol under 200, low-density lipoprotein (LDL) depends on risk factors
Weight loss	Well-documented in adults up to 65	Reduce risk factor for atherosclerotic coronary disease	Not studied in older adults	Maintain ideal body weight
Stop smoking	Strongest recommendation, simple interventions can have 5%–10% quit rate	Reduce risk for cardiovascular, pulmonary, gastrointestinal diseases and malignancies	Quitting at any time improves pulmonary function and decreases risk of myocardial infarction (MI) and death	Ask about and encourage cessation at each visit
Alcohol	Cessation difficult to achieve in alcoholics	Reduce risk for falls and confusion in the older adults	No age limit to improve safety	Ask about, counsel to use in moderation

Continued

TABLE 3–6.
(CONTINUED)

FACTOR	STRENGTH OF EVIDENCE	BENEFIT	AGE FOR WHICH RECOMMENDED	RECOMMENDATION
Drugs	Well documented	Reduce many risks of polypharmacy: adverse reactions, drug interactions, death in the older adults	Never too late	Check medications at each visit; ask about over-the-counter and herbal remedies; use only medications that are medically necessary
Safety, injury/abuse prevention	Few data on prevention effectiveness	Reduce risk of falls, sixth leading cause of death	Different focus in older adults	Home safety evaluation
Aspirin	Evidence in middle-aged men; few studies in older adults, look promising	Primary and secondary prevention of cardiovascular and cerebrovascular disease	Recommended for men over 40 or 50	Low dose: 81 mg/day for cardiovascular health
Estrogen	Well-documented; weigh risks (such as increased risk of breast cancer) vs. benefits	Reduce risk of osteoporosis	Postmenopausal women with no contraindications	Progestin reduces risk of endometrial cancer, increases risk of breast cancer
IMMUNIZATION				
Influenza	Well-documented incidence, severity of influenza	Reduce	65+ years	Annually
Pneumonia	60% efficacy *Streptococcus pneumoniae* infection	Prevent	65+ years	Once, may repeat in 5 years
Tetanus	Well-proven	Prevent tetanus	No age limit	Every 10 years

- Before prescribing an exercise program for any patient, conduct a history and physical examination and evaluate:
  - Fatigue, shortness of breath, chest pain
  - Risk factors for thromboembolic disease
  - Excessive bruising
  - Cardiac murmurs, clicks, hums
  - Carotid bruits
  - Other physical indicators of undiagnosed vascular disease
  - Current medications
- Decrease intensity or components of the exercise program if the patient
  - Is unable to talk while exercising,
  - Is fatigued for more than 1 hour after finishing, or
  - Develops swelling or pain.
- Increase intensity and/or time as patient develops tolerance

General Nutrition

- Goal: maintain or achieve ideal body weight and supply all essential body nutrients to maintain or regain health
- Normal growth requires appropriate intake of protein, fat, carbohydrates, water, vitamins, minerals, and trace elements.
- Recommended dietary allowances (RDAs) are estimates of safe and adequate amounts of nutrients recommended to be consumed daily to maintain health. The RDA is the amount of nutrient needed to meet the known nutrient requirements of approximately 97% of the population.
- U.S. Department of Agriculture (USDA; n.d.) MyPlate suggests:
  - Make half your plate of fruits and vegetables
  - Switch to fat-free or low-fat (1%) milk
  - Make at least half your grains whole
  - Compare sodium, sugars, and saturated fats in foods and choose the foods with lower numbers

Infant/Childhood/Adolescent Nutrition

Diet planning

- Energy requirements can be determined using charts or the calculations in Table 3–7.
- Adolescents who have completed their growth and wish to lose weight will need to reduce calorie intake by 500 calories per day for each pound they wish to lose each week.
- No more than 2 pounds should be lost per week.
- Weight loss is not recommended for growing children (except under special circumstances and with close supervision).
- For children older than 2 years, 55% to 60% of calories should come from carbohydrates, 10% to 15% from protein, and no more than 30% from fat (with saturated fat 10% or less), and less than 300 mg of cholesterol per day.
- Fat and cholesterol should not be restricted in the first 2 years of life.
- Recommended fiber intake is 0.5 g/kg/day, to a maximum of 35 g/day.

Recommended Nutritional Supplements

- Vitamin K, 1 mg IM, given at birth to all newborns to prevent hemorrhagic disease
- Vitamin D, 200 units/day, recommended for all breastfed infants until they are ingesting a minimum of 500 mL/day of vitamin D–fortified formula or milk
- Ferrous sulfate, 2–3 mg/kg/day (max 15 mg/day), recommended for breastfed pre-term infants by 2 months old

TABLE 3–7.
DETERMINING ENERGY REQUIREMENTS

AGE	AVERAGE KCAL/KG/DAY
0–6 months	110–120
7–12 months	90–105
1–10 years	80
Adolescence	30–55

Example: 9-month-old infant weighing 8 kg requires approximately 800 calories/day (8 kg × 100 kcal/kg/day = 800)

- Iron-fortified cereals starting by 6 months of age in all infants to replace iron stores, which are depleted by the time the infant doubles birth weight at approximately age 4 to 5 months
- Fluoride supplements to reduce susceptibility to dental caries
- No fluoride supplements before 6 months of age and where water fluoride content is higher than 0.6 ppm, to avoid fluorosis (excessive mottling of the teeth; see Table 3–8)

Infant Nutrition

- Breast milk and/or formulas are sufficient to meet the nutrient needs of infants up to 4 to 6 months of age (exceptions noted above); see Table 3–9.
- Advantages of breast milk: nutritionally balanced, contains antibodies and macrophages, allergic reactions are rare, savings on time and money
- Possible disadvantages: milk supply may be insufficient, mechanical difficulties such as inverted nipples may occur, medications and infectious organisms may pass to infant, nutritional deficiencies in the mother may affect infant
- All U.S. Food and Drug Administration (FDA)–approved infant formulas meet minimum nutrient standards and are
- 20 calories/ounce except for those specifically labeled as higher in calories (e.g., Enfamil 24 calories/ounce).
- Evaporated milk formula not recommended, although it may be used in extenuating circumstances (e.g., unable to breastfeed and/or cannot afford formula). It is made by mixing one can of evaporated milk (13 ounces) with 19½ ounces of water and 3 tablespoons of corn syrup. These infants must also receive a multivitamin with iron; dosage varies with age.

TABLE 3–8.
RECOMMENDED FLUORIDE DOSES WHEN WATER HAS 0.3–0.6 PPM

AGE	BELOW 0.3 PPM	0.3–0.6 PPM
6 months–3 years	0.25 mg	0
3–6 years	0.5 mg	0.25 mg
6–11 years	1.0 mg	0.5 mg

TABLE 3–9.
INFANT FORMULAS

	COW'S MILK–BASED	SOY PROTEIN ISOLATE	PROTEIN HYDROLYSATES
Examples	Enfamil, Similac, Good Start	Isomil, ProSobee	Nutramigen, Pregestimil, Alimentum
Composition comments	Casein/whey ratio varies with manufacturer Lactose is usual carbohydrate (CHO) source; lactose-free formulas using corn syrup and/or fructose now widely available Available in iron- fortified and low-iron preparations; low-iron formulas not recommended	CHO—sucrose and/or glucose Methionine added to all soy formulas to correct deficiencies All are iron fortified	Partially hydrolyzed protein that results in peptides that do not elicit an immunologic response Most are lactose free
Uses	Routine use in well infants	Infants with lactose intolerance Infants with cow's milk protein sensitivity (approximately 20% of infants allergic to cow's milk also allergic to soy)	Infants with cow's milk and soy sensitivity
Contraindications	Milk protein sensitivity Lactose intolerance Galactosemia	Soy protein allergy Preterm infants—CHO, protein, mineral absorption of soy formulas in preterm infants is not adequately documented and American Academy of Pediatrics (2004) does not recommend their use; soy formulas specifically developed for preterm infants available Infants with renal disease	None reported

Food Introduction

- Guidelines have been directed more by tradition than by science.
- May be introduced when infant is able to sit with support and has good neuromuscular control of head and neck, typically around 4 to 6 months of age
- Tradition has held that cereals are a good place to begin; use a spoon and avoid adding to bottle.
- Start with single-ingredient foods and add one new food at a time, with up to 4 to 7 days between foods to identify intolerances.

Food/Formula Cautions

- No low-iron formula use
- No cow's milk in the first year of life
- No honey before age 1 year because of possible development of infantile botulism
- Avoid foods high in salt or sugar, such as canned or processed foods; RDA for sodium for infants is 17.6 mg/kg/day.
- Avoid foods that are easily choked on, such as grapes, popcorn, hot dogs, raisins, nuts, candy, and peanut butter.
- Home preparation of foods such as spinach, beets, carrots, or collard greens may have enough nitrates to cause methemoglobinemia and are therefore not recommended in infancy.
- Foods considered highly allergenic—such as eggs, wheat, seafood, and nuts—have traditionally been withheld in the first year of life to avoid a possible allergic reaction, but the validity of this practice is uncertain.

Adult Nutrition

- Calculate body mass index (BMI) to determine overweight and obesity: weight in pounds ÷ height in inches^2) × 703. BMI of 25 or higher is considered overweight according to the Centers for Disease Control and Prevention (CDC), Assessing Your Weight (n.d.).
- An online BMI calculator can be found at www.cdc.gov/nccdphp/dnpa/bmi/adult_ BMI /english_bmi_calculator/bmi_calculator.htm
  - ◊ Normal weight: BMI 18.5–24.9
  - ◊ Overweight: BMI 25–29.9

- ◊ Class I obesity: BMI 30–34.9
- ◊ Class II obesity: BMI 35–39.9
- ◊ Class III obesity: BMI 40 or higher

Losing Weight

- In establishing realistic weight goals, calculate the relationship of current weight compared to ideal body weight:
- Determine ideal body weight (IBW)
- Divide IBW by current body weight
- Multiply by 100
- Subtract 100
- Result gives percent over or under ideal body weight

Diet Planning

- Determine caloric needs by adding basal calories (IBW × 10) and activity calories (IBW × 3) for sedentary people, IBW × 5 for moderately active people, or IBW × 10 for people involved in strenuous activity.
- Example: IBW = 120 lbs for a sedentary person
- 120 × 10 = 1,200 basal calories; 120 × 3 = 360
- 1200 + 360 = 1,560 total calories needed per day
- People who wish to lose weight will need to reduce calorie intake by 500 calories per day for each pound they wish to lose each week.
- Diets should limit fat to 30% or less of total calories, carbohydrates to 55% to 60% of calories, and the rest of calories from protein.

Geriatric Nutrition

- Goal: Supply all essential body nutrients to maintain or regain health
- Maintain, gain, or lose weight if necessary
- Adequate calcium intake: 1,000–1,500 mg a day

- Adequate vitamin D intake: 800 IU a day but consider higher deficiency levels in home-bound
- Frail older adults at risk for malnutrition—low albumin levels

Safety

CHILDHOOD INJURIES

- Injury is the number one cause of death among children ages 16 and younger
- Motor vehicle accidents, suffocation, drowning, poisoning, fires, and falls are some of the most common ways children are hurt or killed
- Many injuries are preventable (see Table 3–10)

INJURY PREVENTION IN ADULTS/GERIATRICS

- Home safety evaluation for fall prevention
    - Bathrooms are the site of most falls
    - Throw rugs are dangerous
        - Use contrast lighting to reduce hazards
        - Sufficient lighting is needed both inside and outside the home
        - Safe and appropriate assistive devices are important
- Driving evaluations for safety
    - Driving is essential for independence, making patients reluctant to give it up
    - Driving can be impaired due to dementia, impaired vision, slowed reflexes, or musculoskeletal disorders.
    - Seat belts are necessary for safety.
- Smoke and carbon monoxide detectors
- Safety locks on firearms
- Tips for environmental safety can be found in Table 3–11.

TABLE 3–10.
INJURY AND PREVENTION

TYPE OF INJURY	EPIDEMIOLOGY	PREVENTION
Motor vehicle accident (MVA)	MVAs account for about half of all unintentional injury deaths; infants and adolescents usually injured as occupants, school-age children predominantly injured as pedestrians.	Use of child restraints and seat belts is the most effective way to prevent occupant injuries. There are four basic types of restraints: 1. Infant/toddler (birth to 2 years): Place semi-inclined and backward facing in the back seat. 2. Toddler/preschool: Convertible seats and forward-facing seats with harnesses as long as possible up to the weight or height limit by the manufacturer. 3. School-aged: Belt positioning booster seat. Place preferably in the back seat. An infant or toddler car seat fits if the child's ears are below the top of the seat's back and shoulders are below the seat strap slots. 4. Older children: Use lap and shoulder belts. All children younger than 13 years should be restrained in rear seats. A shoulder strap should not be used if it goes across the face or throat. Child should be in booster seat to keep shoulder strap in proper place. See https://www.healthychildren.org/English/safety-prevention/on-the-go/Pages/Car-Safety-Seats-Information-for- Families.aspx Car seat adaptations are available for premature infants and patients in casts, on ventilators, or with special medical conditions such as spina bifida.

Continued

TABLE 3–10. (CONTINUED)

TYPE OF INJURY	EPIDEMIOLOGY	PREVENTION
Drowning	Drowning is the second leading cause of accidental death for children 1 to 4. Poor supervision plays a key role in drowning of young children and infants. Adolescent drowning is often associated with alcohol use. Approximately 75% of drowning occurs in bodies of water that are part of the person's home, particularly bathtubs and pools. Infants can drown in inches of water and in unusual ways, such as in pails of water and toilet bowls. Approximately one-third of all survivors of drowning will suffer irreversible brain injury.	Supervision is the key to prevention: 1. Leave no children unattended in or near water and observe closely. 2. Keep the bathroom door closed. 3. Empty all pails of water. 4. Keep swimming pools completely fenced with a locking gate. 5. Make life jackets a must. 6. Teach children to swim and to behave safely around water, such as using life preservers. Infant swim lessons are not recommended because of the risk of water intoxication.
Fire and burns	More than 300 children between the ages of 0 and 19 are treated in emergency rooms daily for burn-related injuries. More than 1 million burn injuries occur per year and as many as 30,000 people younger than 15 in are hospitalized yearly for burns. Approximately 75% of all burns are scalds that occur in the kitchen. Bathtub water can cause burns if hotter than 120° F. Skin damage rarely occurs at temperatures below 110° F, but a full-thickness burn can occur in 1 second in water 160° F. Approximately 85% of all deaths from fire are due to smoke inhalation during house fires.	Keep smoke alarms on each floor of the house and check the batteries every month. (All three types—photoelectric, and ionization and combination of both—are effective.) Keep pot handles turned inward on the stove. Keep an ABC-rated fire extinguisher the kitchen. Do not allow children to sit in adults' laps when they are drinking hot liquids. Teach children fire escape route and rules, and practice escapes. Keep temperature at 120°F

Continued

TABLE 3–10. (CONTINUED)

TYPE OF INJURY	EPIDEMIOLOGY	PREVENTION
Asphyxiation	This type of injury accounts for approximately 40% of all choking unintentional deaths in children younger than 1 year of age. Food items commonly choked on are hot dogs, candy, nuts, grapes, raisins, and raw vegetables. Nonfood items that children choke on include balloons, undersized infant pacifiers, small toys with small parts Asphyxiation occurs from situations such as hanging from drapery cords or bibs tied around neck; crib strangulations (head entrapment); toy chest lids falling on a child's head and neck; or when the nose and mouth are covered in a soft pillow, beanbag, or waterbed.	Do not feed small, round, hard foods to children less than 2 to 3 years of age. Do not allow children to run with food. Keep small objects out of the reach of children; evaluate all toys for safety. No balloons before age 3 years and then monitor. Encourage parents to learn the Heimlich maneuver. Tie up all cords. Use bibs with Velcro balls and jacks, coins, pop-tops, instead of ties. Use cribs with slat and safety pins spacing 2 3/8 in. or less. Do not place infants on any soft or enveloping surfaces.

Adapted from *Guide to clinical preventive services,* by Agency on Healthcare Research and Quality. (2014). Washington, DC: Department of Health and Human Services. Retrieved from http://www.ahrq.gov/professionals/clinicians-providers/guidelines-recommendations/guide/index.html

ASSESSMENT FOR VIOLENCE AND ABUSE

- Clinicians should ask about and watch for signs of physical abuse during encounters with patients.
- Patients will often admit to problems, but only if they are asked.
  - Know and use state laws in determining requirements for reporting suspected abuse.
  - Learn state requirements for a sexual assault examination.

TABLE 3–11.
PREVENTION OF ENVIRONMENT-RELATED HEALTH PROBLEMS

SAFETY HAZARD	RISK	RECOMMENDATIONS
Secondhand smoke	Increased risk of respiratory problems and cancer	No smoking in the home, car, or around children
Carbon monoxide exposure	Ranges from chronic flu-like symptoms to death	Use acceptable carbon monoxide detector in home; properly use and maintain fuel-burning devices
Radon	Increased risk of cancer	Test home for radon with a home test kit; if level exceeds 4 pCi/L, identify and seal basement leaks
Lead	Lead poisoning—neurological damage, anemia	Do not use lead-containing utensils for cooking or eating. Renovations done with proper precautions. Employment in high-risk places/occupations—use precautions

Adapted from *Guide to clinical preventive services,* by Agency on Healthcare Research and Quality. (2014). Washington, DC: Department of Health and Human Services. Retrieved from http://www.ahrq.gov/professionals/clinicians-providers/guidelines-recommendations/guide/ index.html

Geriatric Abuse and Neglect

- Risk factors include age over 84; social isolation; lack of support; cognitive impairment; and physical, emotional, and financial dependency.

STRESS

- Stress is the emotional and physical response to an increase in the environmental demands beyond the resources of a person to cope with those demands.
- Small amounts of stress may add excitement and variety and increase the quality of life. Large amounts of stress may be overwhelming and lead to disease.
- The goal is to find the right balance of stress in life.
- People often seem to have vulnerability to stress in one system (e.g., hypertension, ulcer, mental problems).

Management

Stress may be managed through various techniques:

- Avoid unnecessary change during stressful times.
- Manage time by keeping to predetermined goals and priorities.
- Avoid stressful triggers (people, activities, etc.) when possible.
- Create habits or routines to decrease stress.
- Develop alternative activities or friendships that increase pleasure.
- Physical exercise often decreases stress.
- Participate in religious, motivational, or service projects that increase self-esteem or change focus to helping others.
- Use biofeedback, tension-relaxation exercise, yoga, or imagery to control stress reactions.

Interpersonal Support

- High-quality interactions with others help persons maintain or regain health (Pender, 1996).
- Types of supporting behaviors (Friedman, 1998)
  - Instrumental support gives direct assistance and service.
  - Informational support uses advice, suggestions, and information in solving problems.
- Emotional support comes when love, care, empathy, and trust are provided through relationships.
  - Appraisal support uses feedback and affirmation to help people evaluate themselves.

Stressors in the Older Adult

- A common myth about the older adults is that they do not tolerate change.
- The older adults do face major life changes, especially losses—death of spouse and/or friends, having to move, retiring, or losing jobs, the ability to do many activities, etc.; these changes cause major stress in the older adults.

DEPENDENCY

- A common personality tendency that, in its extreme form, causes a person to rely on other people or activities, such as eating food, drinking alcohol, having sex, gambling, or other activity, to try to satisfy an emotional hunger
- Action begun voluntarily but, through repetition, becomes involuntary
- Becomes addiction when there is loss of control (compulsivity), continuation despite adverse consequences, and obsession or preoccupation with the activity
- Treatment may be complex and require long-term therapy.

PHARMACOLOGY IN THE GERIATRIC POPULATION

- Polypharmacy of five or more drugs at one time is a common problem with potential drug interactions.
- Age-related changes increase risk of drug toxicities.
  - Absorption is slower, with delayed onset
  - Distribution in tissues affected by a change in the fat-to-muscle ratio
  - Metabolism slowed, increasing toxicity by drugs metabolized by the cytochrome P450 system
  - Excretion through the kidneys may be decreased due to reduced renal function
- Drug toxicities are more common and more serious in the older adults.
  - Use lower doses and titrate up slowly.
  - Monitor over-the-counter drug use closely.

Health Maintenance

CHILD HEALTH SUPERVISION

- The general health of children can be improved significantly through the effective use of health care supervision (e.g., disease prevention, early detection, and intervention of disorders, providing anticipatory guidance).
- Health supervision should be done at regularly scheduled well visits and should include obtaining a history and physical exam; vital signs; assessment of growth and development; obtaining age-appropriate screening tests; and counseling about nutrition, safety, and other topics.

- Recommended ages for well visits are at 2 weeks; 2, 4, 6, 9, 12, 15, 18, and 24 months; yearly from ages 3 to 6 years; every other year from ages 6 to 11 years; and yearly during adolescence.
- Additional visits may be needed for children outside the recommended well visit schedule, for example: sports physicals, and presurgical clearance or evaluation.

PEDIATRIC HEALTH SCREENING

- Purpose: early detection of treatable conditions (see Table 3–12)
- Not all abnormal results are identified on screening tests, so continual monitoring of the patient's condition and repeat testing may be necessary.
- Use of screening tests will change as the incidence of disease changes (e.g., lead testing) and as technology improves (e.g., newborn hearing tests).
- Screening tests may be recommended primarily for high-risk groups (e.g., lead, cholesterol) at certain ages; others are universal tests for all children (anemia).

ADULT/GERIATRIC HEALTH SCREENING AND SUPERVISION

- Routine periodic health supervision visits have not been established for adults.
- Routine screening recommendations are established by the U.S. Preventive Services Task Force and are updated for asymptomatic persons, based on evidence supporting the effectiveness of preventive measures (see Table 3–13).
- Various specialty groups, such as the American Cancer Society, National Cancer Institute, American College of Obstetricians and Gynecologists (ACOG), and American Academy of Family Physicians, also make recommendations, and these may not agree with the U.S. Preventive Services Task Force.
- Clinicians should be prepared to clearly identify and document the basis for their preventive practices because there is not always agreement among the recommending bodies.

GERIATRIC ASSESSMENT

Nonspecific presentation of illness

- The older adults often present with vague complaints or deterioration in functional independence as an early subtle sign of illness.

TABLE 3–12. PEDIATRIC SCREENING RECOMMENDATIONS

SCREENING TESTS	AGES FOR SCREENING	TESTING AND INTERPRETATION
Neonatal, metabolic, and genetic screening (PKU test)	All full-term infants before discharge and in 1–2 weeks	All states screen for phenylketonuria (PKU) and hypothyroidism; most screen for galactosemia. Other tests are determined on a state-by-state basis and may include sickle-cell disease, maple syrup urine disease, homocystinuria, congenital toxoplasmosis, adrenal hyperplasia, and cystic fibrosis. All positive screening results require immediate confirmation and/or referral.
Hearing	All newborns	Newborns to be screened appropriately for hearing impairment.
Hearing	3, 4, 5, 10, 12, 15, and 18 years of age	Audiometric screening: Minimal screening evaluation should be 20 dB HL with frequencies of 1, 2, and 4 kHz. Any unheard frequency is a failure, and the child should be retested at a later date. Failure again requires a referral.
Anemia	Hemoglobin and hematocrit for asymptomatic children 6–12 months who are at increased risk of iron-deficiency anemia	Hemoglobin is sensitive for iron-deficiency screening anemia but not mild-deficiency states.
Lead screening	Selectively obtain blood lead levels (BLLs) in children at 9–12 months and possibly again at 2 years. BLLs above10 μg/dL require retesting and possible further evaluation and treatment, depending on the level.	1. Screen children who live in at-risk communities for elevated BLLs, areas where 27% or higher of housing was built before 1950 and in populations in which the percentage of 1- and 2-year-olds with elevated BLLs is 12% or higher. (Such information is provided by state health officials.) 2. In all other communities, screen children who live in or regularly visit homes/facilities built before 1950, or 1978 if renovated in the past 6 months, or who have siblings/playmates with elevated BLLs.

Continued

TABLE 3–12. (CONTINUED)

SCREENING TESTS	AGES FOR SCREENING	TESTING AND INTERPRETATION
		3. Screen all children where community and home information is unknown. 4. Any child may be screened if other risk factors for lead exposure exist, such as cultural practices (use of lead pottery or lead-containing folk medicines), parent occupation, adoption from countries where lead poisoning is prevalent, or where elevated BLLs may be contributing to a problem such as developmental delay.
Tuberculin (TB) skin test	Annual testing, with Mantoux purified protein derivative (PPD) skin test for children at high risk. For children with no risk factors who live in high-prevalence regions or who lack a clear history, do periodic testing at ages 1, 4–6, and 11–16 years of age (suggested; can be any age). Interferon-Gamma Release Assays (IGRA) blood test may be used in place of skin test.	Children at high risk include those who: 1. Have contacts with infected adults 2. Have clinical or x-ray findings suggestive ofTB 3. Are immunosuppressed (HIV) 4. Have chronic illness (diabetes, renal disease) 5. Come from high-prevalence countries (or their parents did) 6. Have or had frequent exposure to high-risk adults: HIV positive, homeless, drug abuser, poor health, nursing home resident, malnutrition, or migrant worker. Induration considered positive if: Larger than 5 mm: risk factors 1–3 (see above) Larger than 10 mm: risk factors 4–6, or any child younger than 4 years old Larger than 15 mm: all others

Continued

TABLE 3–12. (CONTINUED)

SCREENING TESTS	AGES FOR SCREENING	TESTING AND INTERPRETATION
Vision screening	Obtain visual acuity (V/A) and binocular vision by age 3–5 years.	Test V/A with the Snellen chart standardized at 20 feet. Use a Tumbling E or Lea chart (uses symbols—apple, circle, square, and house) if letters cannot be recognized. A failed test is V/A 20/40 or greater in either eye, or if there is a two-line discrepancy between the eyes (e.g., 20/20 in one eye and 20/40 in another). All children should be tested once for color blindness. Make referrals for all failures.

Adapted from *Guide to clinical preventive services,* by Agency on Healthcare Research and Quality. (2014). Washington, DC: Department of Health and Human Services. Retrieved from http://www.ahrq.gov/professionals/clinicians-providers/guidelines-recommendations/guide/index.html

- This generally occurs in the absence of classical (typical) symptoms and signs of disease.
- Acutely ill older adults often present with
  - Confusion or delirium,
  - Increased difficulty performing activities of daily living (ADLs),
  - Incontinence, or
  - Falls.

Functional Assessment

- Assessment tools provide standardized data to follow trends and evaluate response to treatment.
- Cognitive and functional assessments are the keystone to providing geriatric care.
- Many assessment tools are available.

TABLE 3–13. ADULT/GERIATRIC SCREENING RECOMMENDATIONS

PROBLEM OR ISSUE	GENERALLY ACCEPTED RECOMMENDATIONS
Asymptomatic heart disease	Do not screen asymptomatic adults at low risk for coronary heart disease
Breast masses	Screen women 50–74 years every 2 years with mammography. Diagnostic exam if positive or with mass.
Cervical cancer	The USPSTF recommends screening for cervical cancer every 3 years with cervical cytology alone in women aged 21 to 29 years. For women aged 30 to 65 years, the USPSTF recommends screening every 3 years with cervical cytology alone, every 5 years with high-risk human papillomavirus (hrHPV) testing alone, or every 5 years with hrHPV testing in combination with cytology (cotesting).
Colon cancer	Screen ages 45–75 with High-sensitivity guaiac fecal occult blood test (HSgFOBT) or fecal immunochemical test (FIT) every year Stool DNA-FIT every 1 to 3 years Computed tomography colonography every 5 years Flexible sigmoidoscopy every 5 years Flexible sigmoidoscopy every 10 years + annual FIT Colonoscopy screening every 10 years Selectively screen adults aged 76 to 85 years for colorectal cancer. https://www.uspreventiveservicestaskforce.org/uspstf/recommendation/colorectal-cancer-screening
Vision	Screen visual acuity with Snellen testing and refer people at high risk for glaucoma to eye specialists.
Dental/oral	Yearly exam and counseling
Hearing	Assess hearing through physical exam and refer as needed.
Hyperlipidemia	Men older than 34 and women older than 44 who are at increased risk for coronary heart disease. Screening for others has lower-level evidence.
Hypertension	Blood pressure screening every 2 years in normotensive patients older than 21
Menopause	Counsel all perimenopausal and postmenopausal women about the potential risks and benefits of hormone replacement.

Continued

TABLE 3–13. (CONTINUED)

PROBLEM OR ISSUE	GENERALLY ACCEPTED RECOMMENDATIONS
Osteoporosis	Counsel all women about the risks and benefits of hormone replacement therapy, dietary calcium, vitamin D, weight-bearing exercise, and smoking cessation. Bone density measurement for women age 65 and older, earlier in women at increased risk. Optimal intervals not established.
Prostate cancer	No recommended routine screening for prostate cancer such as digital rectal examinations, prostate-specific antigen (PSA), or transrectal ultrasound. Potential harm is greater than benefit.
Testicular cancer	No evidence supports routine screening of asymptomatic men.
Hypothyroidism	Evidence does not recommend screening with thyroid stimulating hormone (TSH) in asymptomatic persons.
Skin cancer	Counsel about minimizing exposure to ultraviolet radiation. Screening not recommended for general population.
Dementia, functional	Not recommended in asymptomatic persons
Sexually transmitted	Offer high-intensity counseling for adults at increased risk for sexually transmitted disease (STDs).

Adapted from *Guide to clinical preventive services,* by Agency on Healthcare Research and Quality. (2014). Washington, DC: Department of Health and Human Services. Retrieved from http://www.ahrq.gov/professionals/clinicians-providers/guidelines-recommendations/guide/index.html. https://www.ahrq.gov/prevention/guidelines/index.html

Normal Changes of Aging

- What is normal becomes less uniform as patients age.
- Normal changes usually mean less functional reserve.
- It is often difficult to differentiate among normal aging, chronic disease, medication effect, and disuse.

IMMUNIZATION

- Recommended for various age groups to prevent the spread of disease and to reduce the mortality and morbidity related to diseases that are responsive to vaccines

- Immunization schedules change from time to time, so the advanced practice nurse must review updated schedules annually, as well as stay apprised of schedule and vaccine changes for all age groups. This information is located on the Centers for Disease Control and Prevention's Vaccine and Immunization website (http://www.cdc.gov/vaccines/schedules/hcp/index.html).
- Most children are immunized by the time they enter school, but many remain unimmunized until that time, leaving them at unnecessary risk for infections or considered risks to other children.
- Many adults are inadequately immunized from lack of immunization as children, failure to get boosters, or have not received newly recommended immunizations for adults.
- Some categories of workers may require additional immunizations such as food handlers, those working with animals, and travelers.
- Older adults are the largest age group acquiring tetanus.

Immunization Guidelines

- All states require children entering school and licensed day care to have vaccines. To check individual state laws, refer to the Immunization Action Coalition (http://immunize.org/laws/index.htm).
- The immunization schedule must be modified when immunization has not begun in early infancy or was interrupted. Previously given vaccines do not need to be repeated.
- The child is considered not immunized if the vaccine status is unknown.
- Preterm infants should be immunized with regular doses according to postnatal chronological age.
- Adverse effects: Common to almost all the vaccines are local injection-site reactions such as pain, tenderness, and erythema that are mild and transient, and mild to moderate fevers and myalgias for 24 to 48 hours.
- General contraindications to vaccinations include hypersensitivity reactions (urticaria, shock, wheezing) and prior encephalopathy within 7 days of pertussis vaccine; undefined illnesses where administering vaccines may confuse the diagnosis; and prior severe reactions where administering the vaccine would be more harmful than withholding.
- Not contraindications: minor illnesses, family history of seizure disorders, sudden infant death syndrome, presence of a pregnant woman in the household

- There is no contraindication to simultaneous administration of routine vaccines.
- Informed consent from parent/guardian prior to vaccination with information provided regarding the disease to be prevented, risks and benefits of the vaccine, and potential adverse effects
- Additional vaccines may be indicated or recommended for specific illnesses and/or disorders, travel, geographical area, and/or special circumstances. Adult vaccines are listed in Table 3–14.
- Free vaccines are available through the Vaccines for Children program for uninsured and Medicaid-eligible children and Native American and Alaska Native children.

OTHER DISEASE-PREVENTION PROGRAMS

Back to Sleep Program

- For the prevention of SIDS, the most common cause of death in children under 1 year of age
- Risk factors for SIDS: sleep position, exposure to cigarette smoke, low birth weight, and prematurity; highest incidence in Black people and Native Americans, and lowest in Asian people
- Recommends positioning infants on the back or side for sleeping. Incidence of SIDS has decreased dramatically with these sleeping positions.

Smoking Cessation

- More than 40% of U.S. children are exposed to environmental tobacco smoke in their own homes.
- Teenage smokers experience a decrease in physical fitness and lung function and, later, an increase in the risk of lung cancer and heart disease.
- Encourage cessation of smoking first without pharmacologic interventions; if unsuccessful, may educate regarding the products available for assistance.

TABLE 3–14.
IMMUNIZATION GUIDELINES FOR ADULTS

TYPE OF IMMUNIZATION	RECOMMENDATIONS FOR ADULTS
COVID-19	Detailed information can be found in CDC's Interim Clinical Considerations for Use of COVID-19 Vaccines Currently Approved or Authorized in the United States (see www.cdc.gov/vaccines/covid-19/clinical-considerations/covid-19- vaccines-us.html)
Hepatitis A	Two doses if another risk factor is present (medical, occupation, or lifestyle indication)
Hepatitis B	All people 12–25 years with no history of infection or previous immunization; high-risk adults
Human papillomavirus (HPV)	Women through age 26 years, men through age 21 years; men who have sex with men and men who have compromised immune systems including HIV through age 26
Influenza	Pregnant women; annually for all adults 50+ years of age; others if at high risk or household contacts of those at high risk. Healthy, ages 2–49, and nonpregnant women, can receive either intranasally administered live, attenuated influenza vaccine (LAIV), (FluMist), or IIV. Annually for health care workers, particularly those who care for severely immunocompromised people (i.e., those who require care in a protected environment); should receive IIV rather than LAIV. (CDC, 2023).
Measles, mumps, and rubella (MMR)	Administer one or two doses to anyone 18 years of age and older born after 1957 with no documented proof of immunity. Contraindicated in pregnancy or immunocompromising conditions
Meningococcal	First year college students living in dormitories and travelers to endemic areas with no history of prior infections; anyone whose spleen was damaged or removed
Pneumococcal polysaccharide (PPSV23)	Once at 65+; one or two doses age18 and older if at high risk and repeat if injection was more than 5 years ago
Pneumococcal 13-valent conjugate (PCV13)	One dose for adults age 18 and older with another risk factor present
Rubella screen or immunization	Women of childbearing age

Continued

TABLE 3–14. (CONTINUED)

TYPE OF IMMUNIZATION	RECOMMENDATIONS FOR ADULTS
Tetanus, diphtheria, pertussis (Tdap/DTaP/Td)	Substitute one-time dose of Tdap for Td booster, and then booster every 10 years; booster at 5 years for wound management. Administer one dose of Tdap vaccine to pregnant women during each pregnancy (preferred during 27–36 weeks of gestation), regardless of number of years since prior Td or Tdap vaccination.
Varicella	Administer two doses in adults with no history of varicella or previous vaccination. Contraindicated in pregnancy and immunocompromising conditions.
Zoster	Once at 60+ for all adults with history of chicken pox infection

Please visit http://www.cdc.gov/vaccines/schedules/hcp/imz/adult.html for the latest vaccination guidelines as the recommendations change frequently.

Adapted from *Immunization schedules,* by Centers for Disease Control and Prevention. (2022). Retrieved from http://www.cdc.gov/vaccines/schedules/hcp/index.html

https://www.cdc.gov/vaccines/covid-19/downloads/COVID-19-immunization-schedule-ages-6months-older.pdf

CDC's interim clinical considerations for use of COVID-19 vaccines can be found at www.cdc.gov/vaccines/covid-19/clinical-considerations/covid-19-vaccines-us.html.

Other Health Care Considerations

CULTURAL INFLUENCES

- The health care provider who is sensitive to issues surrounding health care and the traditional health beliefs of the patient can provide more comprehensive health care.
- Family structure and values have an impact on the health encounter.
- Ethnicity is based on the race, tribe, or nation with which a person identifies and influences the person's beliefs and behaviors.

ENVIRONMENTAL FACTORS

- General circumstances such as climate, altitude, and temperature affect all people in a region and cannot be modified unless the person relocates.

- Other factors such as air pollution, water fluoridation and contamination, crime, poverty, and transportation are examples of factors that might be manipulated to have a positive effect on the community.

EVIDENCE-BASED MEDICINE

- The trend today is to base decisions on evidence from randomized controlled research trials when possible but at times evidence with less confidence is used. Many sources of recommendations are available through U.S. government–sponsored websites like CDC, National Institutes of Health (NIH), and AHRQ.
- There are conflicting guidelines among various organizations, and these must be reconciled by the practitioner.

CLINICAL GUIDELINES

- Standards of practice are devised from research by experts in the field to guide and standardize practice across the nation. Nurse practitioners should know how to analyze clinical guidelines to determine those that are written by objective scholars and are without organizational, professional, or pharmaceutical bias. (See the National Guideline Clearinghouse at www.guideline.gov.)
- Factors to consider in evaluating guidelines include source of guideline; appropriateness of methodology used to develop guideline such as randomized trials; use of expert opinion/clinical experience in decision-making; public policy considerations; feasibility issues; use of peer preview; and congruence with other practice guidelines, timeliness, and funding source.

CASE STUDIES

CASE 1

Emily, 2 months old, has been brought by her parents to the clinic for her well baby exam. Her gestation and birth history are unremarkable. She was born at 39 weeks with a birth weight of 7 pounds, 8 ounces (3.4 kg) and length of 20.5 inches. She is breastfed on demand, about every 3 to 4 hours. She has not had any immunizations.

1. What vaccines will Emily need today?
2. What developmental milestones would you assess for in a 2-month-old?
3. There is no fluoride in the tap water at her home. When should you start Emily on fluoride? How much will you give her each day?
4. Emily's mother is thinking about discontinuing breastfeeding and starting infant formula. What information should you provide to her that might encourage her to continue to breastfeed?

CASE 2

Travis, a 4½-year-old, comes to the clinic for a school physical. His last checkup was at 3 years of age. He is 40 pounds and 39 inches. His immunization records indicate he has had four DTaP, three IPV, one MMR, two hepatitis B, and three Hib vaccine shots.

1. What vaccines would he need today?
2. What anticipatory guidance and safety issues would you discuss with Travis and his parents?

CASE 3

Josh, Travis's 14-year-old brother, needs a pre-participation sports physical. Josh weighs 225 pounds and is 5 feet, 8 inches tall.

1. What would be the focus of your assessment examination?
2. What counseling does Josh need?
3. What immunizations might Josh need?

CASE 4

You have been asked to set up a health fair for a large computer company. The company would like to focus on employees, their families, and retired workers. You research the company and find out that equal numbers of employees with young children, single employees, and retired employees plan to attend the health fair.

1. What primary prevention topics would you address for parents of young children?
2. What secondary prevention topics would you address for adults ages 18 to 50?
3. What secondary prevention topics would you address for adults 50 and older?
4. How would you educate the participants about stress management?

CASE 5

Jose M. is a 65-year-old man who has scheduled his "Welcome to Medicare" exam with you. He has recently moved to this community to be closer to his children and is new to your practice.

He is particularly interested in remaining healthy and wants to do what is appropriate in screening and prevention.

1. What are the age- and gender-specific screening tests that you would recommend?
2. What vaccines would you recommend?
3. What specific counseling would you recommend?

CASE 6

Ms. J. is a 45-year-old Black woman who has been told she has type 2 diabetes mellitus and that she should attempt to reduce her weight. She is 68 inches tall and weighs 237 pounds.

1. What is her BMI? What is a desired BMI for her?
2. She reports that she has seen Internet advertisements for weight-loss programs that guarantee she will lose 5 pounds in the first week and that some people have lost over 100 pounds on this plan. She asks for your advice on enrolling on this plan. What is your recommendation?

CASE 7

Cynthia is a 48-year-old transgender woman who is seeing you today in the clinic for an annual wellness exam. The name on her chart is "Richard Smith" and she prefers the pronouns she/her. She is in a long-term monogamous relationship with a cisgender man. She has no past medical or surgical history and tells you she does not trust medical providers. When asked about medication use, she does admit to using injectable estrogen that she orders off the Internet.

1. What screening and prevention tests would you recommend today?
2. What immunizations would you recommend today?
3. What counseling would you provide today for this patient?

CASE STUDIES DISCUSSION

CASE 1

1. What vaccines will Emily need today?

   DTaP, IPV, HBV, Hib, PCV, and rotavirus

2. What developmental milestones would you assess for in a 2-month-old?

   Begins to smile at people, coos, makes gurgling sounds; begins to follow things with eyes; can hold head up

3. There is no fluoride in the tap water at her home. When should you start Emily on fluoride? How much will you give her each day?

   Begin at older than 6 months with 0.25 mg per day. Patients from 6 months to 3 years of age should receive fluoride concentration of 0.25 mg per day (NIH, 2002).

4. Emily's mother is thinking about discontinuing breastfeeding and starting infant formula. What information should you provide to her that might encourage her to continue to breastfeed?

   Ask why she is considering the change. Breastmilk is nutritionally balanced and contains antibodies and macrophages, which are important to immunity and wound healing.

   Allergic reactions are rare. Breastfeeding may save money.

CASE 2

1. What vaccines would he need today?

   DTaP, IPV, MMR, hepatitis B, and varicella; depending on time of year, add influenza and give hepatitis A, if not given

2. What anticipatory guidance and safety issues would you discuss with Travis and his parents?

   Recreational sports protection gear (helmets, pads); swimming safety; automobile (street safety, seatbelts); knows his address, phone number, how to call 911; smoke alarms in the house; access to/storage of guns in the home

CASE 3

1. **What would be the focus of your assessment examination?**

   History, immunization status, vital signs, pubertal development, musculoskeletal, and cardiopulmonary systems

2. **What counseling does Josh need?**

   Weight management (his BMI is 34.2), safety (seatbelts, recreational protective gear)

3. **What immunizations might Josh need?**

   Ensure that he completed the seriesTdap, HBV, varicella, MMR, IPV, MCV, and HAV. Tdap and MCV if he did not have at age 11 to 13 years. HPV series to begin at age 11.

CASE 4

1. **What primary prevention topics would you address for parents of young children?**

   Nutrition, iron intake, fluoride, safety (car seats, falls, poisonings, drowning), immunizations, sunscreen, access/storage gun safety

2. **What secondary prevention topics would you address for adults ages 18 to 49?**

   Exercise, weight management, stop smoking, influenza prevention, mammography, Pap smears

3. **What secondary prevention topics would you address for adults 50 and older?**

   Mammography, Pap smears, colon screening, avoid UV radiation

4. **How would you educate the participants about stress management?**

   Large amounts of stress can lead to disease. Discuss stress management techniques (relaxation, imagery, time management). Seek out support. Recognize sources of stress for the geriatric clients—loss.

CASE 5

1. **What are the age- and gender-specific screening tests that you would recommend?**

   Some form of colon screening, lipid screening, blood pressure

2. **What vaccines would you recommend?**

   Flu every year,Tdap booster every 10 years, zoster, PCV13, PCV23. HAV and HBV series if he has not had these. Others depend on his medical history.

3. What specific counseling would you recommend?

   Depends on his risk factors; general counseling for exercise, balanced diet, avoiding ultraviolet radiation, STDs if at risk

CASE 6

1. What is her BMI? What is a desired BMI for her?

   Her BMI is 36. A desired BMI is between 18.5 and 25.

2. She reports that she has seen Internet advertisements for weight-loss programs that guarantee she will lose 5 pounds in the first week and that some people have lost over 100 pounds on this plan. She asks for your advice on enrolling on this plan. What is your recommendation?

   Plans that propose more than 1 or 2 pounds of weight loss per week are difficult to sustain. Advertised programs are often expensive and may not consider the needs of people with diabetes. She will need to lose over 70 pounds to reach her desired BMI, and this may take a year or more to achieve and sustain.

CASE 7

1. What are screening and prevention tests will you recommend today?

   Anal cancer screening, depression/anxiety screening; diet/exercise; alcohol/tobacco use; cardiovascular screening such as blood pressure and lipid screening; and prostate, testicular, and colon cancer screening

2. What immunizations would you recommend today?

   Influenza vaccine annually, Td/Tdap Booster every 10 years, HBV and HAV series if not already completed

3. What counseling would you provide today for this patient?

   You should discuss sexual health and complete a sexual risk assessment annually and as indicated at future visits, diet /exercise, smoking cessation if applicable, STD testing if at risk

REFERENCES

Agency on Healthcare Research and Quality. (2014). *Guide to clinical preventive services.* Washington, DC: Department of Health and Human Services https://www.ahrq.gov/sites/default/files/wysiwyg/professionals/clinicians-providers/guidelines-recommendations/guide/cpsguide.pdf

Berul, C. (2000). Cardiac evaluation of the young athlete. *Pediatric Annals, 29*(3), 163.

California Health Care Almanac. (2022). *Health care costs 101: Slow growth persists.* https://www.chcf.org/publication/2022-edition-health-care-costs-101/

Celentano, D., & Szklo, M. (2019). *Gordis epidemiology* (6th ed.). Philadelphia, PA: Elsevier.

Centers for Disease Control and Prevention. (n.d.). Assessing your weight. http:// www.cdc.gov/healthyweight/assessing/index.html

Centers for Disease Control and Prevention. (n.d.). National prevention strategy: America's plan for better health and wellness. Retrieved from http://www.cdc.gov/features/preventionstrategy/

Centers for Disease Control and Prevention. (2020). 10 leading causes of death by age group, United States—2020. https://www.cdc.gov/injury/wisqars/leadingcauses.html

Centers for Disease Control and Prevention. (2022). Immunization schedules. http://www.cdc.gov/vaccines/schedules/hcp/index.html

Centers for Disease Control and Prevention. (2023). Prevention and Control of Seasonal Influenza with Vaccines: Recommendations of the Advisory Committee on Immunization Practices (ACIP)—United States, 2023–24. https://www.cdc.gov/flu/professionals/acip/summary/summary-recommendations.htm#recommend

Center for Disease Control and Prevention (2024). Vaccines and preventable diseases: Respiratory syncytial virus (RSV) immunizations. https://www.cdc.gov/vaccines/vpd/rsv/index.html

Friedman, M. (2003). *Family nursing: Research, theory, and practice* (5th ed.). Norwalk, CT: Appleton & Lange.

Galan, N. (2018). The Affordable Care Act: An update. *Medical News Today.* Retrieved from https://www.medicalnewstoday.com/articles/247287.php

Gordis, L. (2018). *Epidemiology* (6th ed.). Philadelphia: Elsevier.

Harvard Countway Library (2022) LGBTQIA+ Health: Practice Guidelines. Retrieved from https://guides.library.harvard.edu/c.php?g=721845&p=5145849

Hockenberry, M. J., & Wilson, D. (2014). *Wong's nursing care of infants and children* (10th ed.). St. Louis, MO: Elsevier.

Immunization Action Coalition. (n.d.). State mandates on immunization and vaccine-preventable diseases. http://www.immunize.org/laws/

James, P., Oparil, S., Carter, B., Cushman, W., Dennison-Himmelfarb, C., Handler, J., . . . Ortiz, E. (2014). 2014 evidence-based guideline for the management of high blood pressure in adults. *Journal of the American Medical Association, 311*(5), 507–520.

Jarvis, C. (2015). *Physical examination and health assessment* (7th ed.). St. Louis, MO: Elsevier.

Marcdante, K. J., & Kliegman, R. M. (2014). *Nelson essentials of pediatrics* (7th ed.). Philadelphia, PA: Elsevier.

National Center for Health Statistics. (2010). CDC growth charts: United States. http://www.cdc.gov/nchs/data/ad/ad314.pdf

National Center for Health Statistics. (2013). Health expenditures. http://www. cdc.gov/nchs/fastats/health-expenditures.htm

National Institute of Health. (2002).The use of fluoride in infants and children. *Pediatrics & child health, 7*(8), 569–582. https://doi.org/10.1093/pch/7.8.569

National Institute on Aging. (2008). Health disparities toolbox. http://www.nia.nih. gov/about/features/links-minority-research-training-fall-2008

Pender, N., Murdaugh, C., & Parsons, M. A. (2014). *Health promotion in nursing practice* (7th ed.). Upper Saddle River, NJ: Prentice Hall.

Tanner, J. M. (1962). *Growth of adolescents* (2nd ed.). Oxford, England: Blackwell Scientific.

Tikkanen, R., & Abrams, M. K. (2020). *U.S. Health care from a global perspective, 2019: Higher spending, worse outcomes.* https://www.commonwealthfund.org/publications/issue-briefs/2020/jan/us-health-care-global-perspective-2019

U.S. Census Bureau. (2021) Health insurance coverage in the United States: 2020.

U.S. Department of Agriculture. (n.d.). MyPlate and historical food pyramid resources. https://www.myplate.gov/

U.S. Department of Health & Human Services. (n.d.). Affordable Care Act. https://www.hhs.gov/answers/health-insurance-reform/what-is-the-affordable-care-act/index.html

U.S. Department of Health and Human Services, Office of Disease Prevention and Health Promotion. (n.d.). *Healthy people 2030.* Retrieved from https://health.gov/healthypeople

World Health Organization. (2015). What are social determinants of health? http:// www.who.int/social_determinants/sdh_definition/en/ https://www.who.int/health-topics/social-determinants-of-health#tab=tab_1

Zubler, J. M., Wiggins, L. D., Macias, M. M., Whitaker, T. M., Shaw, J. S., Squires, J. K., . . . & Lipkin, P. H. (2022). Evidence-informed milestones for developmental surveillance tools. *Pediatrics, 149*(3). [e2021052138]. https://doi.org/10.1542/peds.2021-052138

CHAPTER 4

INFECTIOUS DISEASES

Elizabeth Istorico RN, FNP-BC

General Approach

- Making the correct diagnosis of infectious disease in the family setting requires familiarity with the infectious organisms *commonly* seen in each age group.
- Mild illness is common in children, particularly upper respiratory infections in infants and toddlers.
- A fever is a temperature greater than 38°C (100.4°F) rectal, 37.5°C (99.5°F) oral, and 37°C (98.6°F) axillary. The normal temperature varies throughout the circadian rhythm, being lowest in the early morning and higher in the afternoon.
- Transmission of infection is influenced by the type of organism, its mode of transmission, its viability in the environment, the number of organisms present in the environment, the resistance of the potential host to the organism, and the frequency of the asymptomatic or carrier state.
- Antibiotic resistance is a growing concern. All providers need to ensure appropriate prescribing to prevent increasing resistance in communities and populations.
- Vaccine refusal by parents and some communities has resulted in increases in incidences of some illnesses such as measles. In 2019 there were 1282 cases of measles in 31 states. From year-to-year, measles cases average from fewer than 100 to a couple of hundred. This is a key reminder of how quickly measles can spread in the unvaccinated (CDC, 2019b). See Centers for Disease Control and Prevention (CDC) April 2019 report on the increase in measles cases in the United States: https://www.cdc.gov/mmwr/volumes/68/wr/mm6817e1.htm.
- Evolving diseases that are now drug resistant (such as gonorrhea and tuberculosis) add to the concern.

ASSESSMENT

- Obtain a thorough history of the symptoms of the present illness, as well as possible contacts.
- Factors indicating possible bacterial infection include loss of appetite, dehydration, high fever, chills, significant weakness, and/or malaise.
- Perform a physical examination, evaluating for signs of infection, including vital signs; skin (noting rash); eyes (noting conjunctival erythema or discharge); ears, nose, and throat (noting erythema and drainage); neck (noting nuchal rigidity, adenopathy); lungs (noting dull, diminished, or adventitious breath sounds); heart (noting murmurs or rubs); abdomen (noting tenderness, change in bowel sounds, organomegaly); and musculoskeletal (noting tenderness, warmth, edema, and erythema).
- A neurological exam, including mental status evaluation, may be needed to exclude central nervous system (CNS) infection or complication.
- Rapid testing for strep, mono, flu, and other available on-site testing may be used as an initial screen to determine the best approach and course of treatment.
- Obtain a culture to determine causative organism(s) before treatment to prevent false-negative results.
- Sensitivity testing helps clarify the most appropriate antibiotic(s) to use.

MANAGEMENT

- Assess for allergies to medications and clarify type of reaction to previous antibiotic use.
- Be aware of drug-resistance patterns in the community.
- Avoid treating a viral illness with an antibiotic "just in case" or because the patient or parent insists on one. Improvement with antibiotics usually occurs in 2 to 3 days for most infections. Beyond this time frame, consider reassessing the patient and treatment plan.
- It is important to educate the patient and document the criteria for reevaluation if the patient is not improving.
- Adequate hydration is important in the treatment of infectious illnesses, especially in children.
- Ninety percent of respiratory infections are viral.
- To avoid the risk of a patient developing Reye's syndrome, do not prescribe or administer aspirin, or products containing aspirin, for viral infections to patients younger than 19 years of age.

- Due to a decreased immune response, older adults have an increased risk of secondary bacterial infections.
- If the patient is pregnant, use antibiotics in pregnancy category B; be aware that most antibiotics pass into breast milk.
- Know local health department guidelines for reporting communicable diseases.
- Seek referrals to infectious disease specialists earlier rather than later during unknown or unusual infection.
- Be alert to endemic diseases.
- Be alert to diseases that may be a result of international travel or bioterrorism.

RED FLAGS

- The very young and very old are at special risk for severe infections, as are those with compromised immune systems, such as people with a history of splenectomy or concomitant illness such as diabetes.
- The social determinants of health are the economic and social conditions that influence individual and group differences in health status. According to the Centers for Disease Control and Prevention (CDC) it is "life-enhancing resources, such as food supply, housing, economic and social relationships, transportation, education, and health care, whose distribution across populations effectively determines length and quality of life" (CDC, 2022c).
- Recognize the unique physiologic and psychological responses of older patients to infectious disease and therapy.
- Public health measures such as social distancing and masking have their psychological challenges with children as well as adults.
- A fever with listlessness or flaccidity requires an aggressive evaluation, no matter the patient's age.
- Bacteremia and sepsis may present with fever or hypothermia, chills, tachycardia, tachypnea, hypotension, or altered mental status; mortality is nearly 50% in septic shock.
- Consult or refer to a specialist if the illness does not respond to initial therapy or the presentation is unusual; hospitalization may be necessary if the patient is unable to take oral medication or maintain hydration or has a severe infection requiring intravenous antibiotics.
- Know and recognize common diagnostic features of certain illnesses, such as Koplik spots in measles (rubeola), subcutaneous nodules in rheumatic fever, and so on.

- Educate the patient and caregiver, document recommendations, and follow-up with the patient and caregiver when an infection is not resolving as expected.

PEDIATRIC ISSUES

- Any infant with fever who is younger than 4 weeks of age, or 1 to 3 months of age with fever and no focal sign of infection, may require admission with a workup, including urine and blood cultures, lumbar puncture, and chest X-ray.
- Frequent (up to 10) viral illnesses, especially upper respiratory illnesses, per year are common in infants and toddlers.
- To avert the risk of Reye's syndrome, the family nurse practitioner should educate the caregivers of patients between newborn and 19 years of age and educate adolescents to avoid over-the-counter medications and other products that contain salicylates and other related compounds.
- Transmission of infections in older infants and toddlers is mainly through droplet secretions on hands and sharing toys in group settings.
- Children are contagious long before they are symptomatic. Although it is important to exclude sick children from group settings and contact with other children, parents and day care workers need to understand that this will not necessarily reduce the spread of infection to others.
- Good handwashing is the single most effective tool in the prevention of illness.
- Washing toys may prevent the spread of illness.

Childcare Exclusion List

- Providers should seek state and local department of health guidance for the most up-to-date childcare exclusion guidelines.
- This list applies to:
  - All children in out-of-home childcare
  - All students in 3-, 4-, and 5-year-old classrooms, and kindergarten
  - Medically fragile students in 1st through 12th grades—those students with special health care needs and/or developmental delays that require close assistance with feeding or personal hygiene activities. (The parents, in concert with the child's school, will determine whether a child is considered medically fragile.)

Varicella

Children with chickenpox may return to day care or school with a parent note once all the sores and blisters are dried or scabbed over, or, if there are no scabs, until no new sores appear.

Coronavirus Infectious Disease 2019 (COVID-19)

Exclude students or staff with a positive polymerase chain reaction (PCR). Consult cdc.gov and local or state health department for current exclusion and masking guidelines. Guidance will vary based on population, for example: school aged children or persons living in long term care settings. Criteria to return: 10 days after symptoms started and 24 hours since the last fever without using fever-reducing medication and symptoms improved.

Diarrhea

For *most kinds* of diarrhea (defined as three or more loose stools in 24 hours), students in 1st through 5th grades should stay home until diarrhea stops, or until a health care provider clears the child to return to school.The child can return with a parent note when the diarrhea has stopped. Older children in 6th through 12th grades with diarrhea do not have to stay home, unless they are spreading illness in the school setting or have diarrhea with blood or mucus.

- Students of any age must have a medical clearance to return to school after having diarrhea that contains blood or mucus.
- Students who can use the restroom or whose stools are contained in diaper-type underwear do not have to be excluded if the diarrhea is known to be from a noncontagious condition, or if it continues after the child completes antibiotics for a diarrhea-causing illness.
- A medically fragile child or child who needs help with toileting may be excluded for fewer than three episodes of diarrhea if his or her condition makes it hard for caretakers to maintain sanitary conditions in the classroom.

Diarrhea from Campylobacter, Escherichia coli, Giardia, Norovirus, Rotavirus, Salmonella, or Shigella

Students of any age are excluded for one of these infections. A child may return to school with a medical note for the following conditions:

- *Campylobacter, norovirus, rotavirus, Shigella, and most types of Salmonella:* after diarrhea stops
- *E. coli:* For the most severe type of *E. coli,* students of any age must be out of school until the diarrhea stops and two lab tests taken 24 hours apart test negative for *E. coli* O157:H7, which causes bloody diarrhea.

- *Giardia:* once diarrhea stops, or child has taken antibiotics for at least 24 hours
- *Salmonella enterica* typhi (typhoid fever): after 24 hours without diarrhea and three negative lab tests, if a doctor clears the child to return
- *Shigella:* after 5 days of antibiotics or a negative lab test

Fever by Itself

- Infants 4 months old and younger: Keep them home for rectal temperature of 101°F or higher.
- Children over 4 months old: Keep the child home for a fever with a temperature of 101°F or higher by mouth, 100°F or higher if taken under the arm (axillary), or 102°F or higher if taken in the rectum.
- Children can return with a parent note when the fever has resolved.

Fever with Rash, Behavior Change, or Other Symptoms

A child should be taken to a health care provider or clinic for any fever if he or she also has signs of severe illness such as a rash, change in behavior, earache, vomiting, confusion, sore throat, or irritability. A medical note is required to return.

Flu/Influenza or Influenza-Like Illness (ILI)

A student with ILI or the flu will be excluded for a temperature of 100°F with cough and/or sore throat until they are fever-free for at least 24 hours without any fever medications.

Rubella/German Measles/3-Day Measles

Keep a child at home until 7 days after rash starts. The child may return with a medical note.

Head Lice

Children with crawling lice or nits (eggs) one-fourth inch or closer to the scalp may be sent home at the end of the day if head-to-head contact with other children can be avoided. Otherwise, they may be excluded immediately. A child may return with a parent note after his or her first treatment with a school-approved lice-removal product, if there are no active lice crawling on the child's head. The school or center should check the child 7 days after treatment for any newly hatched crawling lice. If any are present, the child will have to be re-treated for lice to return to school or childcare.

Hepatitis A/Yellow Jaundice

Children with acute hepatitis A may return with a medical note 1 week after the start of the jaundice.

Hib disease (Haemophilus influenzae type b)

Students with proven Hib disease need to be out of school until at least 24 hours after they complete their antibiotics. A medical note is required to return.

Impetigo

A child who has dry, honey-colored, crusty sores that cannot be covered should be sent home at the end of the school day until 24 hours after starting antibiotics.

If the sores are weepy, oozing, or wet, or cannot be covered and kept dry, the child will be sent home immediately. The child may return after 24 hours of antibiotics if the sores have stopped oozing and are starting to get smaller. A medical note is needed to return to school.

Rubeola/Measles/Red Measles/10-Day Measles

Children with measles can return with a medical note 4 days after the rash begins if they have no fever and feel well enough to participate in regular school activities.

Meningitis

A student with signs of meningitis (high fever, rash, stiff neck) must remain out of school until a health care provider says that the student may return.

Mononucleosis (Mono)

A child's health care provider will decide when a child is well enough to go back to childcare or school after having mono. No contact sports, heavy lifting, or strenuous activity for the first 2 to 3 weeks and for as long as splenomegaly persists (extend to 8 weeks).

Mumps

Children with mumps can return with a medical note 5 days after the beginning of swelling.

Conjunctivitis/Pinkeye

Children whose eyes are red or pink, and who have eye pain and reddened eyelids, with white or yellow eye discharge or eyelids matted after sleep, should not be in school until they have been examined and treated. A medical note is required to return.

Rash

A student who has a rapidly spreading rash or a rash with fever or behavior change should be excluded from school immediately. A medical note is required to return.

Tinea Corporis/Ringworm

Children with ringworm of the scalp must remain out of school until they have begun treatment with a prescription oral antifungal medication.The child may return with a medical note. Children with ringworm of the body may return with a parent's note once they have begun oral or topical antifungal treatment, unless the affected area can be completely covered by clothing the entire time that the child is at school or in childcare.

Scabies

Children with scabies should be out of school until treatment/medication has been applied. A medical note is required to return.

Herpes Zoster/Shingles

Children who have shingles lesions/sores/blisters that cannot be covered should be kept at home.They may return with a parent note once the lesions are dried/scabbed.

Sores Inside the Mouth

Children with sores inside the mouth who also drool should stay home until their health care providers say that the sores are not contagious. A medical note is needed to return to school.

Staph or Strep Skin Infections (Including Methicillin-resistant Staphylococcus aureus [MRSA])

A child with a draining sore, boil, or abscess that cannot be covered, or with sores that ooze through and soak dressings, should remain home. The child may return once the draining stops, or if the drainage (oozing) can be contained in the dressing, so that no one else comes into contact with the drainage.

Streptococcal Pharyngitis/Strep Throat

A child with strep throat can return to school with a medical note 24 hours after starting antibiotics if there is no fever.

Sty (or Stye)

A child with a draining/oozing sty/stye should remain home until the draining stops.

Tuberculosis (TB)

A child with TB should be kept home until the health care provider treating the TB writes a medical note that says the child is no longer contagious.

Vomiting

A child who has vomited two or more times in 24 hours should stay home until the vomiting stops.

Pertussis/Whooping Cough

A child with whooping cough can return to school with a medical note after completing 5 days of prescribed antibiotics, unless directed otherwise by the local health department or the school nurse.

For more information, go to http://www.scdhec.gov/health/childteenhealth/schoolexclusion/

Viral Infections

FIFTH DISEASE (ERYTHEMA INFECTIOSUM)

Description

- A mild, self-limiting viral disease characterized by erythematous and macular rash first appearing on the cheeks and ears, leading to a "slapped cheek" appearance

Etiology

- Caused by human parvovirus B19
- Transmitted via droplet, most often through contact with infected saliva, nasal secretions, and sputum, and sometimes blood
- Communicable before onset of symptoms; not infectious after onset of rash
- Incubation period 4 to 14 days, up to 21 days; rash and joint symptoms occur 2 to 3 weeks after acquiring the infection

Incidence and Demographics

- Cases often occur as part of community outbreaks during late winter and early spring; may also occur sporadically.
- Spread to household contacts is common.

Risk Factors

- Institutional-style day care setting
- School age
- Adults without immunity
- Contact with saliva, nasal secretions, and sputum of infected persons

Prevention and Screening

- May reduce transmission through rigorous handwashing and careful handling of used facial tissues.

Assessment

History

- Prodrome is usually absent; if present, it includes mild fever, malaise, headache, mild pruritus, and myalgia; occurs 7 to 10 days before rash.
- Rash, beginning on face and ears, with circumoral pallor, leading to slapped cheek appearance; progressing to erythematous, maculopapular, "lacy" (often pruritic) rash beginning on the trunk and moving to arms, buttocks, and thighs
- Arthralgia and arthritis may also be present; more common in infected adults, especially women.

Physical Exam

- Fever is low grade if present.
- Note characteristic appearance of rash on face and body (see Fifth Disease description section above).
- Rash fluctuates in intensity with environmental changes up to weeks and months after appearance; may increase or reappear following sunlight exposure, warm bath, or vigorous play.
- No lymphadenopathy or focal signs of infection
- May also see evidence of arthralgia and arthritis, more common in infected adults, especially women

Diagnostic Studies

- None usually performed in uncomplicated cases
- White blood cell (WBC) count usually normal; anemia with decreased reticulocyte count is possible
- Detection of parvovirus B19–specific immunoglobulin (Ig) M antibody is possible to confirm diagnosis in complicated cases (persist for 2 to 4 months); IgM is usually detectable 3 days after infection; IgG antibody usually detectable 7 days after infection; positive IgG antibody in the absence of IgM antibody indicates previous infection and immunity
- Pregnant women exposed to fifth disease in first trimester should be serologically tested for IgM and IgG antibodies; if susceptibility or a positive infection, weekly fetal ultrasounds are indicated for 4 to 8 weeks after exposure or 2 to 4 weeks after infection to detect fetal hydrops

Differential Diagnosis

- Undifferentiated viral syndrome before appearance of rash
- Other viral infections with rash

Management

Nonpharmacologic Treatment

- Symptomatic
- Isolation not indicated, but the infected individual should avoid contact with pregnant women and immunocompromised patients

Pharmacologic Treatment

- Acetaminophen or ibuprofen for fever, myalgia, or arthralgia in patients younger than 19 years of age
- Antipruritic medication, if necessary
- Intravenous immunoglobulin for chronic infection in immunocompromised patients
- If evidence of fetal hydrops, fetal transfusion may be considered

How Long to Treat

- Until symptoms resolve

Special Considerations

- Infections during pregnancy may cause fetal hydrops and death, although risk is relatively low.
- The highest risk is if the mother is exposed during the first 20 weeks of pregnancy.
- Parvovirus B19–infected fetuses may be treated with intrauterine blood transfusions.
- Persons with sickle-cell disease or other chronic anemia are at risk for developing severe anemia, if infected.
- Immunocompromised people are at risk of serious illness, if infected.

- Aspirin and aspirin-containing products should not be administered to anyone younger than 19 years of age for a viral illness to avoid risk of developing Reye's syndrome.

When to Consult, Refer, Hospitalize

- Refer to hematologist for complications—aplastic crisis, chronic anemia

Follow-Up

- Unnecessary in low-risk patients
- Closely with immunocompromised patients or those experiencing aplastic crisis

Complications

- Aplastic crisis, chronic anemia
- Arthritis, arthralgia in adults

HERPANGINA

Description

- Acute viral illness causing fever, ulcerative mouth lesions, cough, coryza, pharyngitis

Etiology

- Enterovirus (Coxsackievirus A and B)
- Transmitted by fecal–oral and oral–oral route
- Incubation 3 to 6 days

Incidence and Demographics

- Seen more frequently in temperate climates (summer and fall)
- Affects primarily children, day care through school age

Risk Factors

- More frequent in congregate settings, day care, and school.

Prevention and Screening

- Good handwashing

Assessment

History

- The prodrome of fever is as high as 106°F, pharyngitis, malaise, headache, backache, anorexia, drooling, vomiting, diarrhea

Physical Exam

- 1–2 mm vesicles and ulcers on the anterior tonsillar pillars, soft palate, uvula, tonsils, pharyngeal wall, and posterior buccal surfaces

Diagnostic Studies

- Throat culture to exclude streptococcal pharyngitis

Differential Diagnosis

- Herpes simplex gingivostomatitis
- Aphthous stomatitis
- Hand, foot, and mouth disease
- Vincent's angina
- Streptococcal pharyngitis

Management

Nonpharmacologic Treatment

- Symptomatic—rest and fluids

Pharmacologic Treatment

- Acetaminophen or ibuprofen for fever and discomfort in patients younger than 19 years of age
- Variety of suspension—viscous lidocaine 2%, diphenhydramine, and either Maalox or Kaopectate—can be applied to lesions to relieve discomfort

How Long to Treat

- Until symptoms resolve

Special Considerations

- None

When to Consult, Refer, Hospitalize

- Consult if symptoms persist for longer than 2 weeks or if child is unable to drink or eat.

Follow-Up

- None usually needed

Expected Course

- Resolves in 3 to 5 days

Complications

- Rarely myocarditis, meningitis, or encephalitis

HUMAN IMMUNODEFICIENCY VIRUS (HIV) INFECTION AND ACQUIRED IMMUNODEFICIENCY SYNDROME (AIDS)

Description

- HIV: Viral infection with the human retrovirus that destroys cells with critical immune system functions. HIV-1 can infect all cells expressing the T4 (CD4+) antigen, which serves as a receptor for HIV; once in the cell, it replicates and causes cell fusion or death. The virus depends on reverse transcriptase for replication, and because the CD4+ lymphocyte directs many other cells in the immune network, infection of the CD4+ lymphocyte allows for disorder of virtually all body systems.
- AIDS: Disease characterized by opportunistic infections; or HIV+ persons with CD4 cell counts less than 200 cells/μL or a CD4 percentage less than 14%.

Etiology

- Viral transmission—HIV usually transmitted through sexual intercourse; IV drug use; transfusions of blood or blood products; needle stick or mucous membrane exposure in health care workers; injections with unsterilized, used needles such as acupuncture, tattooing, or medical injection; perinatal; breastfeeding (mother to child)
- Seroconversion takes an average of 3 weeks from initial infection.
- Median time from infection with HIV to AIDS in persons who are not on antiretroviral treatment is estimated to be 10 years.
- Stages of HIV disease include acute HIV infection (acute retroviral syndrome), early infection, asymptomatic chronic infection, symptomatic HIV infection, and AIDS or advanced HIV infection.

Incidence and Demographics

- At the end of 2019, an estimated 1,189,700 people ages 13 or older had HIV in the United States including 158,500 people whose infection had not been diagnosed (CDC, 2022b).
- The rate of HIV diagnosis in African Americans remains higher than in any other ethnic group: 42% (15,305) of the 36,801 new HIV diagnoses in the United States and dependent areas in 2019 (CDC, 2022b).
- The highest new HIV infection incidence in 2019 was in the 25–34 age group (CDC, 2022b).
- Men who have sex with men (MSM) are more severely affected by HIV than any other group in the United States. Of the 34,800 estimated new HIV infections in the United States in 2019, 70% were in gay and bisexual men (CDC, 2022b).

Risk Factors

- Unprotected anal, oral, or vaginal sex with multiple partners
- Unprotected sex with HIV-positive person or IV drug user
- IV drug use or needle-stick exposure
- Blood transfusion outside United States, or in United States 1977–1985
- Unprotected sex with person with recent or history of sexually transmitted diseases (STDs)
- Personal diagnosis of STD
- Children born to HIV+women
- People sustaining occupational exposure to blood or bodily fluids
- Incarceration—high rates in prison populations who take infection back to community upon release

Prevention and Screening

- Incorporate and promote HIV testing as part of routine primary care, per CDC (2022b) and U.S. Preventive Services Task Force (USPSTF, 2019) recommendations.
- Promote sexual abstinence or decrease the number of sexual partners; reduce unsafe sexual behavior; encourage condom use.
- Treat STDs.
- Evaluate and offer HIV preexposure prophylaxis (PrEP), if appropriate.
- Prevent/treat IV drug use. Counsel regarding not sharing injection drug-using equipment.
- Test plasma, organ, and tissue donors for HIV.
- Provide health care workers with postexposure antiretroviral prophylaxis treatment.
- Counsel HIV+mothers about the risks of transmission of HIV to their infants associated with breastfeeding.
- Screen all pregnant women.
- Give antiretroviral treatment (ART) to HIV+women during pregnancy and labor; newborns should receive ART after delivery to prevent perinatal transmission.
- Refer to http://aidsinfo.nih.gov/contentfiles/perinatalgl.pdf for current guidelines

Assessment

History

- Index of suspicion is raised by obtaining a complete history of symptoms, risk factors, and personal medical history, although the patient may remain asymptomatic for years.
- Complaints causing parents to seek care for their children are generalized lymphadenopathy, failure to thrive, recurrent or persistent thrush, recurrent infections.
- Adolescents may present with sexually transmitted infections, persistent vaginal candidiasis, or persistent "colds."
- Adults may present with a variety of complaints at any stage of HIV.

Physical Exam

- A complete physical exam is necessary.
- An infant born to an infected mother may not be developing to expected milestones for 1 year or more.
- An infant/child may show failure to gain weight (failure to thrive), generalized lymphadenopathy, hepatosplenomegaly, recurrent or persistent thrush, recurrent or chronic parotitis, recurrent infections, or infections that fail to respond to treatment; *Pneumocystis jirovecii (pneumocystis pneumonia [PCP])* infection may be first manifestation.
- Adolescents and adults may show a wide variety of physical findings related to STDs: serious infections, malignancies, and cardiac and neurologic dysfunction.
- Hairy leukoplakia of the tongue and Kaposi sarcoma (KS) are highly linked to HIV infection.

Diagnosis by Stage of HIV

- Acute HIV infection: time from exposure to onset of symptoms usually 2 to 4 weeks
- Typical symptoms include fever (96%), adenopathy (74%), pharyngitis (70%), rash (erythematous maculopapular; 70%), myalgia or arthralgia (54%), diarrhea (32%), headache (32%), nausea and vomiting (27%), hepatosplenomegaly (14%), and thrush (12%).
- Early and asymptomatic infection: clinically asymptomatic or in some cases persistent generalized lymphadenopathy
- Symptomatic HIV infection: conditions more common and more severe in HIV infection but are not AIDS-indicator conditions

  - ◊ Examples: thrush, oral hairy leukoplakia, peripheral neuropathy, cervical dysplasia, constitutional symptoms (fever, weight loss), recurrent herpes zoster, idiopathic thrombocytopenic purpura, and listeriosis

- ♦ AIDS (CDC definition): HIV+ persons with CD4 cell counts less than 200 cells/µL, a CD4 percentage less than 14%, or a variety of conditions such as candidiasis of esophagus, trachea, bronchi, or lungs; invasive cervical cancer; recurrent bacterial pneumonia; Kaposi's sarcoma; pneumocystis pneumonia; wasting syndrome due to HIV; and others

For Diagnosis in Infants and Children

Infants younger than 18 months

- ♦ Positive results on at least one specimen (excluding cord blood) using one or more HIV virologic (non-antibody) tests:
  - ◊ HIV-1 nucleic acid (DNA or RNA detection)
  - ◊ HIV-1 p24 antigen test, including neutralization assay in a child older than 1 month of age
  - ◊ HIV isolation (viral culture)
  - ◊ HIV nucleotide sequence (genotype)
- ♦ Presumptive diagnosis for children younger than 18 months: may be based on positive results of HIV virologic tests on one serum specimen and no subsequent negative tests or diagnosis of HIV infection based on laboratory criteria and documented in the medical record by health care provider or presence of AIDS-defining conditions as defined by the CDC
- ♦ Children younger than 18 months born to an HIV-infected mother categorized as "not infected with HIV" if child does not meet the criteria for infection and has at least two negative HIV antibody screening tests from separate specimens at 6 months of age or older or at least two negative HIV virologic tests from separate specimens at 1 month to 4 months of age *and* no other laboratory or clinical evidence of HIV infection (definitive criteria)
- ♦ Presumptive criteria for children younger than 18 months born to HIV-infected mother categorized as "not infected with HIV" if child does not meet definitive criteria but has one negative HIV antibody test at 6 months of age or older and no positive HIV virologic tests *or* has one negative HIV virologic test performed at 4 months of age or older and no positive virologic tests *or* one positive HIV virologic test with at least two subsequent negative virologic tests, at least one of which is at 4 months of age older or negative HIV antibody results, at least one of which is at 6 months of age or older *and* no other laboratory or clinical evidence of infection *or* designation by health care

provider to be "not infected" and health care provider has noted testing results in medical record *and* no other laboratory or clinical evidence of HIV infection is noted

- Children 18 months and younger born to HIV+ mothers and not meeting above criteria for HIV infection or "not infected with HIV" categorized as having perinatal exposure
- Children older than 18 months and adolescents diagnosed as having HIV infection if have positive screening test for HIV antibody and positive result on a confirmatory test *or* positive result of HIV virologic test *or* diagnosis of HIV infection based on laboratory tests and recorded in medical record by healthcare provider *or* presence of AIDS-defining conditions.

Diagnostic Studies

- Fourth generation HIV antigen/antibody test
- Negative fourth generation antigen/antibody test: does not guarantee person is HIV uninfected; window of time from infection to reactive test can be delayed by several weeks; retesting is recommended 4 to 12 weeks from last high-risk exposure
- If acute HIV infection suspected, HIV viral load testing should be ordered
    - CD4 count: used to assess degree of immune suppression.
    - HIV viral load: used to monitor response to ART; used in conjunction with antigen/antibody test to confirm acute HIV infection
    - Maternal antibodies: may remain present for up to 15 months so antibody tests are unreliable in infants

Differential Diagnosis

- Cancer
- Endocrine diseases
- Malabsorption syndromes
- Candidiasis
- Tuberculosis
- Other infections
- Hepatic disease
- Lymphoma
- Enterocolitis

- Endocarditis
- Renal disease

Management

Nonpharmacologic Treatment

- Counsel regarding prevention of transmission through use of condoms, cleaning up blood spills, and not sharing razor blades or needles.
- Stress that patients must adhere to a drug regimen if it is to be helpful.
- Encourage a healthy lifestyle: balanced diet, smoking cessation, substance abuse cessation, decreased stress, and adequate sleep.
- Discuss protection from contagious disease: washing hands after contact with soil; avoiding cleaning litter box (toxoplasmosis) or rough play with kittens (cat scratch disease); maintaining food safety.
- Health maintenance referral: dental exam every 6 months, ophthalmology examination at diagnosis and annually; when CD4+ count is less than 50 cells/μL, refer to ophthalmologist or optometrist trained in cytomegalovirus (CMV) retinitis for screening
- Tests to determine concomitant diseases, immunity status; Mantoux tuberculin skin test (purified protein derivative; PPD) or Interferon Gamma Release Assay (IGRA), rapid plasma reagin (RPR) or Treponemal-specific assay, cervical Pap smear every 6 to 12 months, hepatitis B surface antigen (HBsAg), hepatitis C antibody, toxoplasmosis IgG, cytomegalovirus IgG, varicella IgG, chest X-ray
- Baseline labs before drug therapy: HIV viral load, CD4+ count, HIV genotype, metabolic panel, liver function, renal profile, complete blood count (CBC) with differential and platelets, fasting lipids, fasting glucose or hemoglobin A1c (HbA1c), urinalysis, pregnancy testing

Immunizations: annual inactivated influenza vaccine

- Persons with immune compromise can be considered for vaccination outside of routine administration schedule (CDC, 2023)
- Pneumococcal vaccine (PCV13 and PPV23)
- Consider hepatitis B virus (HBV); Hep B is a three-dose schedule unless evidence of immunity) and *H. influenzae* b (Hib) vaccines
- Consider meningococcal vaccines if indicated

- Tetanus-diphtheria (Td) vaccine should be given if the patient has not been vaccinated within the last 5 years.
- Substitute one-time dose of tetanus-diphtheria and acellular pertussis (TDaP) at time of next booster; then Td every 10 years.
- If the patient has not received the primary series of Td, the patient should begin the primary series of three doses of Td with the first two doses administered 4 weeks apart and the third dose administered 6 to 12 months later.
- A dose of TDaP can be substituted for any of the three doses of Td.
- Give inactivated polio, hepatitis A vaccine (HepA is a two-dose schedule unless serologic evidence of previous disease), and HepB vaccine (unless evidence of immunity) for protection to all HIV positive persons.
- Varicella zoster and measles, mumps, and rubella (MMR) vaccine for asymptomatic patients with CD4 counts greater than 200 cells/μL and no evidence of immunity or significant exposure.
- Human papillomavirus virus (HPV) vaccine recommended for those who have not received the three-dose series and who meet the recommended age requirements. The second dose should be given 2 months after the first and the third dose given 6 months later.
- Avoid live vaccines for any patient who is severely immunocompromised (CD4 counts less than 200 cells/μL): MMR, varicella zoster, bacilli Calmette-Guerin (BCG), live attenuated influenza vaccine (LAIV, FluMist). MMR, and varicella zoster are also contraindicated in pregnant women.

Pharmacologic Treatment

- Antiretroviral treatment should be offered to all patients, regardless of CD4+ count or viral load.
- The Panel on Antiretroviral Guidelines for Adults and Adolescents classifies the following regimens as Recommended Initial Regimens for Most People with HIV (in alphabetical order) (clinical.info.hiv.gov):
    - Bictegravir/tenofovir/lamivudine/emtricitabine (AI; see Table 4.1: Rating of Evidence and Recommendations)
    - Dolutegravir/abacavir/lamivudine—only for individuals who are HLA-B*5701 negative and without chronic HBV co-infection (AI)
    - Dolutegravir plus (emtricitabine or lamivudine) plus (tenofovir alafenamide [TAF] or tenofovir disoproxil fumarate [TDF]) (AI)

TABLE 4.1
RATING OF EVIDENCE AND RECOMMENDATIONS

RATING OF EVIDENCE	RATING OF RECOMMENDATIONS		
	A = STRONG	B = MODERATE	C = OPTIONAL
I = Data from randomized controlled trials	AI	BI	CI
II = Data from well-designed nonrandomized trials, observational cohort studies with long-term clinical outcomes, relative bioavailability/bioequivalence studies	AII	BII	CII
III = Expert opinion	AIII	BIII	CIII

https://clinicalinfo.hiv.gov/en/guidelines/adult-and-adolescent-arv/what-start-initial-combination-regimens-antiretroviral-naive?view=full

- ◊ Doluetgarvir/lamivudine (AI)—except for individuals with HIV RNA above 500,000 copies/mL, HBV co-infection, or when ART is to be started before the results of HIV genotype *resistance testing for reverse transcriptase or HBV testing are available.*

- ♦ Selection of a regimen should be individualized on the basis of virologic efficacy, toxicity, pill burden, dosing frequency, drug–drug interaction potential, resistance testing results, and comorbid conditions.
- ♦ Based on individual patient characteristics and needs; in some instances an alternative regimen may actually be a preferred regimen for a patient.
  - ◊ Initiate *P. jirovecii* if CD4+ count is less than 200 cells/µL and Mycobacterium avium prophylaxis if CD4+ count is less than 50 cells/µL.
  - ◊ Treat concurrent infections of disseminated tuberculosis and/or viral hepatitis

Pre-exposure Prophylaxis (PrEP)

- ♦ For people who do not have HIV but are at risk of getting HIV
- ♦ Three HIV medications are approved by the U.S. Food and Drug Administration (FDA) for use as PrEP
  - ◊ Emtricitabine/tenofovir disoproxil (Truvada*)
  - ◊ Emtricitabine/tenofovir alafenamide (Descovy*)

* Note—PrEP is most effective when taken consistently each day

- ◇ Cabotegravir (CAB) intramuscular (IM) injection given every 2 months for sexually active men, women, and transgender persons with indications for PrEP use; recently FDA approved.

When to Consult, Refer, Hospitalize

- ♦ Every HIV-infected infant, child, adolescent, pregnant woman, and older adult should be referred to and followed by an HIV specialist knowledgeable for that age group.
- ♦ Refer HIV patients to appropriate support groups.
  - ◇ All 50 states; Washington, DC; and U.S. territories require reporting AIDS cases to local health authorities.

Special Considerations

- ♦ Always maintain patient confidentiality.
- ♦ In older HIV patients, it is important to differentiate between geriatric conditions and HIV symptoms (such as dementia) and be aware of potential drug interactions.

Follow-Up

- ♦ See U.S. Department of Health & Human Services publications for guidelines on HIV primary care, ART recommendations, and opportunistic infection prevention and treatment. ART treatment guidelines are updated at least annually. (ClinicalInfoHIV.gov, n.d.)
- ♦ Assess for mental health issues and social isolation.

HEALTH CARE WORKER EXPOSURES TO BLOOD AND OTHER BODY FLUIDS THAT MAY CONTAIN HIV

Description

- ♦ Exposure may place a health care worker (e.g., an employee, student, contractor, attending clinician, public safety worker, volunteer) at risk for HIV infection and, therefore, requires consideration for postexposure prophylaxis (PEP).
- ♦ Exposure is a percutaneous injury; contact with mucous membrane or non-intact skin; contact with intact skin when the duration of contact is prolonged (i.e., several minutes or more) or involves an extensive area with blood, tissue, or other body fluids; or any direct contact with concentrated HIV in a research laboratory or production facility.

Etiology

- Fluids with known risk of HIV transmission: blood, bloody fluids, semen, vaginal fluids, concentrated HIV materials in research labs
- Fluids with suspected risk of HIV transmission: pleural fluid, cerebrospinal fluid, peritoneal fluid, synovial fluid, pericardial fluid, amniotic fluid
- Materials with doubtful risk of HIV transmission: feces, vomitus, urine, saliva, sweat, tears (unless bloody)

Risk Factors

- Device visibly contaminated with patient's blood; procedure that involved a needle placed directly in a vein or artery, or deep injury
- After percutaneous exposure to HIV-infected blood—approximately 0.3%; mucous membrane exposure—0.09%; skin exposure lower risk
- Contact with blood or other body fluids from patients in health care or laboratory setting

Prevention and Screening

- Health care workers should always follow CDC recommendations for universal or standard precautions.
- Wear gloves when contact with blood or bodily fluids is possible.
- Use "personal protective equipment" (masks, goggles, gowns) when engaging in procedures that involve blood or bodily fluids.
- Prevent needle injuries, use puncture-proof containers, use "safety" needles, and refrain from recapping or post-use manipulation of needles.

Assessment

History

- Evaluate exposure: type of fluid, type of exposure (needle gauge, depth of needlestick, visible blood, mucous membrane), and duration of exposure.
- Evaluate exposure-source person: prior HIV testing results, history of possible HIV exposures, and risk for HIV (IV drug use, sexual contact, acute HIV syndrome).

- If source person is HIV positive, document current HIV RNA levels (viral load), CD4 levels, and current or previous ART and compliance.

Physical Exam

- Assess site or wound, anxiety level of health care worker.

Diagnostic Studies

- Source person: If HIV serologic status is unknown, request HIV antibody after incident, provide pretest counseling and consent form; also test for HBV and HCV.
- If consent cannot be obtained, follow local and state laws.
- If source person is HIV seronegative, no testing of worker is needed.
- Exposed health care workers: Offer HIV antibody testing for baseline evaluation with worker consent.
- Test health care workers for hepatitis B immune status.
- Pregnancy testing should be offered to all women of childbearing age.
- Maintaining confidentiality of test results and documentation is critical.

Management

Nonpharmacologic Treatment

Immediately following exposure:

- Skin: Wash thoroughly with soap and water.
- Eyes: Irrigate immediately with saline or water. Tilt head back, hold eyelid open, pour water or saline over eye, and pull eyelid up and down to cleanse entire area. If wearing contact lenses, do not remove lenses while irrigating eye. After flushing the affected eye, remove contact lenses and clean thoroughly.
- Mouth or nose: Use clean water rinse/flush.
- Consider and discuss the risks and benefits of postexposure prophylaxis, based on type of fluid, source risk, and type of exposure.
- Counsel exposed worker to follow measures to prevent secondary transmission, especially the first 6 to 12 weeks: practice sexual abstinence or use condoms; refrain

from donating blood, plasma, organs, tissue, or semen; and refrain from breastfeeding if applicable.

Pharmacologic Treatment

- Tetanus diphtheria (Td) vaccine should be given if the patient has not been vaccinated within the last 5 years.
  - Patients 65 years or older who have never received TDaP should receive a dose of TDaP instead of Td.
  - If the patient has completed the primary series of three doses Td, a dose of TDaP vaccine should be substituted for Td as a booster.
  - If the patient has not received the primary series of Td, the patient should begin the primary series of three doses of Td with the first two doses administered 4 weeks apart and the third dose administered 6 to 12 months later.
  - A dose of TDaP can be substituted for any of the three doses of Td.
    - Hepatitis B vaccine series (if not already vaccinated and no evidence of immunity)
    - Hepatitis B immune globulin (if source antigen positive or high risk for hepatitis B and health care worker not immune)
    - After evaluation/assessment of HIV infection risk, determine need for postexposure prophylaxis
    - Current guidelines recommend the use of a tenofovir + emtricitabine with raltegravir as the standard regimen. Consultation with an HIV expert may be required if the source patient has extensive HIV treatment history.

How Long to Treat

- PEP should be provided for 28 days.

Special Considerations

- Pregnant women
  - Consider short- or long-term effects on fetus and newborn when offering PEP.
  - Counsel regarding potential risk for HIV transmission based on type of exposure, stage of pregnancy (first trimester = period of maximal organogenesis and risk for teratogenesis), and safety of drug combinations.

- Breastfeeding: Consider temporary discontinuation of antiretroviral therapy.
- Resistance of the source virus to antiretroviral drugs; if resistance known or suspected, consultation with an HIV expert is recommended

When to Consult, Refer, Hospitalize

- Consult with HIV expert; refer to current U.S. Department of Health and Human Services guidelines.
- The Clinician Consultation Center, (888) 488–4911, provides clinician-to-clinician guidance for PEP, non-occupational post-exposure prophylaxis (nPEP).

Follow-Up

- Advise exposed health care workers to seek medical evaluation for any acute illness occurring during the follow-up period; illness characterized by fever, rash, myalgia, fatigue, malaise, or lymphadenopathy may indicate acute HIV infection.
- Health care providers with high-risk exposure or exposed to HIV+ source: HIV testing with a fourth generation assay at 6 weeks and 4 months after exposure

Complications

- HIV seroconversion
- Side effects from ART such as nausea/vomiting, nephrolithiasis, hemolytic anemia, hyperglycemia, or worker unable to finish medication
- All FDA-approved HIV PEP medications are associated with hepatotoxicity.

INFECTIOUS MONONUCLEOSIS

Description

- Acute viral illness with fever, fatigue, pharyngitis, and adenopathy; some risk of complications

Etiology

- Epstein-Barr virus (EBV), a gamma herpesvirus, is the causative organism.
- The transmission is commonly via the oropharyngeal route (saliva); blood, semen, and cervical secretions are less-common routes.
- Communicability: Respiratory tract viral shedding can occur for months after infection.
- Incubation is 30 to 50 days, making it difficult to pinpoint exact date of exposure.
- Transmission of the virus to others is possible for 3 months or longer.

Incidence and Demographics

- Common in high school and college age (no sexual predisposition)
- Not seasonal or cyclical

Risk Factors

- Living in group settings

Prevention and Screening

- Handwashing
- Avoid sharing eating or drinking utensils.
- Avoid close personal contact (kissing, sexual contact).

Assessment

History

- Fatigue, fever, swollen lymph nodes, sore throat occur in most people.
  - Fever (rarely exceeding 102°F) lasts about 10 days; fatigue may linger for several weeks.
  - Malaise, myalgia, and headache (50%) also frequently occur.

Physical Exam

- Lymphadenopathy may be significant and include posterior cervical and occipital nodes; lasts 1 to 4 weeks.
- Exudative pharyngitis (50%) often confused with streptococcal pharyngitis; tonsillar ulceration (20%).
- Petechiae of palate and eyelid edema may occur; body rash occurs in a few cases.
- Skin rash (maculopapular, pruritic, copper-colored or tan) in one-third of patients thought to be due to those with infectious mononucleosis who are prescribed amoxicillin.
- Hepatomegaly or particularly splenomegaly may occur in about 40% of people; this is a late finding and lasts about 4 weeks.
- Jaundice is rare with less than 5% of patients having this symptom.

Diagnostic Studies

- Monospot is the usual screening test—rapid, nonspecific test for heterophile antibody agglutination (85% sensitive and 94% specific); should not be used beyond 1 month; 25% false negative within first week of symptoms
- CBC with differential shows lymphocytosis (greater than 50%) with 10% atypical; elevated white blood cell count (10,000–20,000 μg/L)
- Abnormal liver function tests: aminotransferases alanine transaminase (ALT), aspartate transaminase (AST) and gamma-glutamyl transferase (GGT) levels elevated in 80% to 90% of cases; may need to follow in severe infection
- Consider throat culture to exclude group A streptococcal infection.
- Consider EBV antibody titer (viral capsid antigen, early antigen) if diagnosis is in doubt, especially in older patients or early in the disease state.

Differential Diagnosis

- Other viral syndromes: rubella, adenovirus, toxoplasmosis, cytomegalovirus
- Serum sickness
- Leukemia
- Hepatitis
- Group A streptococcal or viral pharyngitis

Management

Nonpharmacologic Treatment

- Symptomatic, no isolation required (see Prevention and Screening)
- Warm saltwater gargles for pharyngitis
- No contact sports, heavy lifting, strenuous activity for first 2 to 3 weeks and while splenomegaly persists (extend to 8 weeks).
- Realistic schedule of rest, including bed rest
- Increased fluid intake

Pharmacologic Treatment

- Give acetaminophen or ibuprofen for fever and discomfort in patients younger than 19 years of age.
- Do not prescribe ampicillin or amoxicillin unless comorbid streptococcal pharyngitis exists; if needed, treatment may cause rash.
- Steroids may be given to treat pharyngitis that leads to airway obstruction or hematologic complications (5- to 7-day taper).

Special Considerations

- Patients with recent EBV infection should not donate blood.

When to Consult, Refer, Hospitalize

- Refer to hematologist, neurologist, hepatologist, etc., early if any complications suspected.
- Hospitalization may be necessary for complications.

Follow-Up

- Based on clinical course; no follow-up may be necessary if fever and symptoms resolve after 10 days; do if jaundice, hepatosplenomegaly, or complications develop

Expected Course

- Duration variable, 3 to 4 weeks
- If symptoms persist after 6 months, further evaluation should take place.

Complications

- Tend to occur in young or older patients
- CNS disorders such as aseptic meningitis, encephalitis, seizures, Guillain-Barré syndrome, optic neuritis, coma, transverse myelitis, Bell's palsy
- Hematologic complications such as hemolytic anemia, aplastic anemia, thrombocytopenia, hemolytic uremic syndrome
- Other rare complications: upper airway obstruction (1% to 5%), splenic rupture (0.5% to 1%), myocarditis, pericarditis, pleural effusion, pneumonitis, hepatitis, erythema multiform, nephrotic syndrome, uveitis, mono-arthritis
- Chronic fatigue is the most reported sequelae, occurring in up to 7% of adolescents at 12 months.

INFLUENZA

Description

- Acute viral illness that occurs in epidemics, usually in the fall and winter

Etiology

- It is caused by an orthomyxovirus that appears in antigenic types A and B.
- Frequent mutations produce new strains each flu season; H1N1, prime example

Incidence and Demographics

- Very common
- Frequently leads to pneumonia in older adults, contributing to fifth leading cause of death in that population; young children also commonly affected

Risk Factors

- Close contact with infected people
- Nursing home residents
- Older adult patients residing with children
- Pregnant women
- Persons with chronic pulmonary, cardiovascular, renal, hepatic, hematological, metabolic, neurologic, or immunosuppressive disorders

Prevention and Screening

- Handwashing
- Influenza vaccine provides immunity to 85% (live vaccine) and 71% (inactivated vaccine) of those inoculated; however, many host factors may individually affect immunity.
- Protection begins about 2 weeks after vaccination and lasts several months.
- Vaccination recommended universally for everyone older than 6 months of age.
- No influenza vaccines are approved for children younger than 6 months, although pregnant and lactating women are highly targeted to receive influenza vaccine to protect their infants.
- Consider high-dose (four times the dose of traditional vaccine) vaccine in those age 65 and older.
- Administer antiviral medication such as oseltamivir, 75 mg orally, once a day for 5 days and zanamivir, two 5-mg inhalations, once a day for 5 days after exposure in influenza A or B.
- Live attenuated influenza vaccine (LAIV), FluMist (a flu vaccine nasal spray), may be used in all healthy people between 2 years and 49 years of age without a history of asthma or wheezing; it is *not* to be administered to pregnant women, children and adolescents on aspirin therapy, persons with history of Guillain-Barré syndrome, or people with allergy to chicken eggs or nasal spray components.

Assessment

History

- Acute onset
- Malaise
- Headache
- Nausea
- Muscle aching
- Nasal stuffiness

Physical Exam

- Fever, chills
- Mild pharyngeal injection
- Conjunctival redness

Diagnostic Studies

- CBC: leukopenia common
- Nasal or throat swab for identifying influenza antigen

Differential Diagnosis

- Rhinovirus
- Bronchitis
- Pneumonia
- Respiratory syncytial virus (RSV)
- Coronavirus disease 2019 (COVID-19)
- Other acute febrile illnesses

Management

Nonpharmacologic Treatment

- Rest
- Encourage fluids

Pharmacologic Treatment

- Analgesics
- Cough suppressant (*Note:* Over-the-counter cough formulations are not recommended for children younger than 2 years of age.)
- Antiviral medication must be started within 2 days of symptom onset to be effective.
- Oseltamivir (Tamiflu), 75 mg orally twice a day; or zanamivir (Relenza), two 5-mg inhalations twice a day for 5 days, for influenza A or B

When to Consult, Refer, Hospitalize

- Refer all very young and older adults to an infectious disease specialist.

Follow-Up

Expected Course

- Usual duration is 1 to 7 days
- Often a longer and more severe course in older adults

Complications

- ◊ Pneumonia
- ◊ Death

MEASLES (RUBEOLA)

Description

- Acute viral disease with fever (temperature higher than 101°F)
- Erythematous
- maculopapular rash
- cough
- coryza
- conjunctivitis
- characteristic rash of oral mucous membranes known as Kolpik's spots

Etiology

- Measles virus (RNA virus, paramyxovirus family)
- Transmitted by direct contact with infectious droplets, or less commonly by airborne spread; highly contagious
- Incubation period 7 to 21 days
- Communicable 1 to 2 days before symptoms begin: 3 to 5 days before rash to 4 days after rash onset

Incidence and Demographics

- Greater than 99% reduction in the reported incidence of measles since vaccination began in 1963
- Most new cases are secondary to importation from other countries.
- In 2014, the United States experienced a record number of measles cases, the highest number since measles was declared eliminated.

Risk Factors

- Lack of immunization; up to 5% of cases secondary to vaccine failure

Prevention and Screening

- Vaccine, usually given as MMR (measles, mumps, rubella) subcutaneous per routine schedule with first dose at 12 to 15 months, booster at 4 to 6 years of age

Assessment

History

- Prodrome of fever higher than 101°F, malaise; cough, coryza, and/or conjunctivitis—the three C's of measles

Physical Exam

- Red, maculopapular rash beginning on face and neck; progressing slowly down trunk and extremities (cephalocaudal) between the second and fourth days and lasting 5 to 7 days
- Rash begins as discrete lesions and then becomes confluent and salmon-colored (morbilliform rash); lesions initially blanch with pressure
- When fever subsides, rash fades to faint brown stain; skin may desquamate
- Kolpik's spots are tiny, bluish-white spots on an erythematous base, clustered on the buccal mucosa near the molars, and are pathognomonic for measles. They appear 1 to 2 days before onset of rash and may last up to 12 to 15 days.

Diagnostic Studies

- Acute (when rash appears) and convalescent (2 to 4 weeks) antibody titers
- Serum IgM antibodies peak 10 days after onset of rash; disappear after 20 to 60 days
- Measles virus detected from nasopharyngeal secretions, conjunctiva, blood, urine

Differential Diagnosis

- Rubella
- Scarlet fever
- Roseola

Management

Nonpharmacologic Treatment

- Symptomatic: rest and fluids
- Isolation for 4 days after appearance of rash
- Avoid bright lights (photosensitivity)

Pharmacologic Treatment

- Give acetaminophen or ibuprofen for fever and discomfort (no aspirin-containing products in patients younger than 19 years of age).
- Consider vitamin A (200,000 IU orally if older than age 1 year; 100,000 IU orally for infants 6- to 12-months-old) in children at high risk for complications such as pneumonia (e.g., immunodeficiency, malabsorption, malnutrition); repeat in 24 hours and in 4 weeks if any ophthalmologic evidence of vitamin A deficiency.
- Give to all children in communities with vitamin A deficiency, particularly in developing countries.
- Live measles vaccine given within 72 hours of exposure may provide protection in some cases.
- Immune globulin may be given within 6 days of exposure; do not give with live vaccine. Susceptible household contacts should receive immune globulin because identification of the index case usually occurs after 72 hours (American Academy of Pediatrics [AAP], 2021).
- Immune globulin dosing: 0.25 mL/kg body weight, IM; immunocompromised children should receive 0.5 mL/kg body weight; maximum dose 15 mL

Special Considerations

- Do not prescribe or administer aspirin or aspirin-related products for a viral infection or syndrome because of the risk of Reye's syndrome in patients younger than 19 years of age.
- Children between 6 and 11 months traveling outside the United States should be administered monovalent measles vaccine, or MMR if unavailable, before traveling, if possible. The dose administered before 12 months of age should not count toward the MMR series (CDC, 2019).

- Children 12 months of age and older traveling outside the United States should receive two doses of MMR at least 28 days apart before departing (CDC, 2019).

When to Consult, Refer, Hospitalize

- No reason to refer in uncomplicated cases

Follow-Up

- Daily during acute phase, 3 to 4 days after onset of rash; more often if indicated (high-risk person, infant, presence of complications)

Expected Course

- Recovery within 3 to 4 days after onset of rash, resolves in 10 days

Complications

- Otitis media, bronchopneumonia, laryngotracheobronchitis, diarrhea, acute encephalitis (1 in 1,000 cases)
- subacute sclerosing panencephalitis (SSPE) is very rare and may develop years after measles infection

MUMPS (PAROTITIS)

Description

- Acute viral disease affecting salivary glands, primarily parotid gland

Etiology

- Caused by a paramyxovirus
- Transmitted via respiratory route (direct contact)
- Communicable 1 to 2 days before 5 days after onset of parotid swelling
- Incubation period 16 to 18 days, but cases may occur 12 to 25 days after exposure

Incidence and Demographics

- Fewer than 1,000 cases per year; dramatic decline since implementation of vaccination
- Most reported cases in children 5 to 14 years of age; declining since introduction of second MMR vaccine in early childhood
- May see outbreaks in immunized populations; however, most cases of parotitis in immunized children not due to mumps

Risk Factors

- Unimmunized people

Prevention and Screening

- Primary prevention through vaccination; vaccine, usually given as MMR subcutaneous per routine schedule with first dose at 12 to 15 months, booster at 4 to 6 years of age; postexposure vaccination not effective
- Exclusion from school or day care until 9 days from onset of parotid gland swelling
- During outbreaks, exclusion of unimmunized children from school or day care for 26 days after onset of parotid gland swelling of the last person with mumps in affected school or day care

Assessment

History

- Fever, malaise, pain in or behind ear during chewing or swallowing
- "Classic" symptom is extreme pain when ingesting tart or sour substances

Physical Exam

- Tender, swollen parotid glands, typically covering angle of jaw; may also see submaxillary and sublingual gland involvement; parotid glands may not be involved; approximately one-third of mumps cases do not have clinically apparent salivary gland swelling.
- Tenderness persists 1 to 3 days; swelling persists 7 to 10 days

- Openings of ducts of involved salivary glands may be red and swollen.
- Fever may be normal, slight, or high (up to 104°F).

Diagnostic Studies

- WBC count may show leukopenia and lymphocytosis.
- Isolation of mumps virus in cell culture, best collected from saliva
- Rise in serum IgG titers or positive mumps IgM antibody test
- Serum amylase level increased in approximately 90% of patients with parotitis not specific to mumps. Helpful in differentiating parotitis from cervical adenopathy.

Differential Diagnosis

- Parotitis from other causes, including infectious, tumor, or parotid duct obstruction
- Tooth infection or abscess
- Cervical adenitis

Management

Nonpharmacologic Treatment

- Supportive—encourage fluids, bed rest, warm or cold compresses to swollen areas (whichever is more soothing).
- Avoid tart, sour, acidic food and drink, and mucous membrane irritants such as peppermint.
- Wash mouth with fat-free broth or saline solution.
- Isolate until swelling is gone.

Pharmacologic Treatment

- Give acetaminophen or ibuprofen for fever and discomfort (no aspirin-containing products in patients younger than 19 years of age).

When to Consult, Refer, Hospitalize

- Refer to specialist with any suggestion of complications.
- Mumps must be reported to the CDC.

Special Considerations

- International travelers are at risk for exposure to mumps. Immunization is recommended if a person is unsure of his or her immunity status. Evidence of presumptive immunity includes documentation of health care provider–diagnosed disease, laboratory evidence of immunity, documentation of administration of two doses of live mumps vaccine, or birth date before 1957 (CDC's Health Information for International Travel, 2018; the Yellow Book).
- Non-U.S. citizens traveling to the United States must be fully vaccinated with accepted COVID-19 vaccine and a negative viral test no more than 1 day before boarding flight
- U.S. citizen, U.S. national, and lawful permanent resident need a negative viral COVID test no more than 1 day before traveling to the United States.

Follow-Up

Expected Course

- Up to 10 days

Complications

- Meningitis—symptomatic in approximately 10% of patients
- Other CNS involvement, including cerebellar ataxia
- Orchitis common in infection after puberty, but sterility rare
- Rare: arthritis, thyroiditis, mastitis, glomerulonephritis, oophoritis, pancreatitis, myocarditis, transverse myelitis, thrombocytopenia, paresis of the facial nerve, hearing impairment

ROSEOLA

Description

- Acute viral disease of infants and young children characterized by significant fever for 7 to 10 days; when resolved, followed by faint, erythematous, maculopapular rash lasting hours to days

Etiology

- It is caused by the human herpes virus 6 (HHV-6).
- HHV-6 is a common cause of febrile illness in infants and young children, with or without rash.
- Roseola-like illnesses may be caused by a variety of different viruses, such as Coxsackieviruses, echoviruses, adenoviruses, and parainfluenza virus.
- Transmission is by droplet and fecal–oral route.
- Incubation period is 9 to 10 days.

Incidence and Demographics

- Affects children ages 3 months to 4 years; peak age 6 to 24 months

Risk Factors

- Institutional-style day care setting

Prevention and Screening

- Prevention difficult; should institute droplet and secretion precautions in institutionalized patients
- Remove from day care until afebrile
- No risk of spread after fever resolves, even if rash still present

Assessment

History

- Sudden onset of fever (may be sustained or spiking); temperature may be as high as 106°F; fever is what usually prompts parents to seek medical attention; lasts 3 to 7 days
- Cough, sore throat; faint rash that appears when the temperature begins to decrease

Physical Exam

- Presence of fever (temperature up to 106°F)
- Faint blanching, erythematous, maculopapular rash beginning on day 4 (lasts 1 to 2 days)
- May have lymphadenopathy (suboccipital, posterior cervical, postauricular), mild pharyngitis

Diagnostic Studies

- None indicated; if CBC performed, may see leukopenia and lymphocytosis

Differential Diagnosis

- Other viral, febrile illnesses with rash
- Drug reaction rash

Management

Nonpharmacologic Treatment

- Supportive—encourage fluids in febrile phase

Pharmacologic Treatment

- Acetaminophen or ibuprofen for fever and discomfort in patients younger than 19 years of age

How Long to Treat

- While symptomatic

Special Considerations

- None

When to Consult, Refer, Hospitalize

- No reason to refer in uncomplicated cases

Follow-Up

Expected Course

- Mild, self-limiting

Complications

- Seizures (probably associated with high fever as opposed to viral invasion of cerebrospinal fluid [CSF] or cerebral structures), aseptic meningitis, encephalitis, thrombocytopenia purpura

GERMAN MEASLES (RUBELLA)

Description

- Mild viral disease with low-grade fever and generalized erythematous, maculopapular rash; generalized lymphadenopathy, most commonly suboccipital, postauricular, cervical; high risk if contracted during pregnancy

Etiology

- Rubella virus is an RNA virus of *Togaviridae* family
- Transmitted by direct or droplet contact with nasopharyngeal secretions

- Incubation period 14 to 23 days
- Communicable a few days before rash onset and for 5 to 7 days after rash appears
- Infants with congenital rubella may shed virus for 1 year or more

Incidence and Demographics

- Incidence has declined by 99% since onset of vaccination; most cases now occur in young non-immunized or inadequately immunized adults (outbreaks in colleges or occupational settings).

Risk Factors

- Non-immunized or inadequately immunized young adults

Prevention and Screening

- Administer live attenuated vaccine, usually in the form of MMR, to non-immunized persons, especially women of childbearing age. Vaccine is usually given as MMR subcutaneous per routine schedule with first dose at 12 to 15 months and a booster at 4 to 6 years of age.
- Active immunization after exposure will not prevent infection; initiation of passive immunity with immune globulin is not helpful.
- Women of childbearing age should be tested for rubella antibody titer and, if titer is low, should receive vaccine; avoid pregnancy for at least 28 days after vaccination.

Assessment

History

- History of cough, coryza, malaise, fever, headache, and possibly arthralgia

Physical Exam

- Maculopapular rash, beginning on face and spreading rapidly to trunk; second day, rash begins to disappear in same pattern; usually resolves by third day
- Fever, lymphadenopathy (suboccipital, postauricular, cervical), conjunctivitis, pharyngitis

Diagnostic Studies

- Virus can be detected on nasal smear.
- Acute (7 to 10 days) and convalescent (2 to 3 weeks) serum titers (fourfold rise or more)
- Determine immune status—latex agglutination immunoassay

Differential Diagnosis

- Other viral diseases characterized by fever and rash

Management

- Symptomatic—rest and fluids
- Isolation if in an institution
- Stay home from work or school for 7 days after onset of rash.

Special Considerations

- Maternal infection is associated with a high incidence of congenital anomalies and/or fetal demise.
- Follow droplet precautions when caring for infants with congenital rubella until three or more successive negative nasopharyngeal and urine cultures are obtained.
- Be sure patients are immune to rubella before taking a cruise; outbreaks of rubella have been reported on cruise ships.

When to Consult, Refer, Hospitalize

- No reason to refer in uncomplicated cases
- Must be reported to the CDC

Follow-Up

Expected Course

- Usually acute, self-limiting illness
- Arthritis and/or neuritis may occur in young children; more common in older children and adults.

Complications

- Congenital rubella is associated with congenital anomalies and/or fetal demise.
- Rare complications of postnatal acquired rubella include encephalitis and thrombocytopenia.

CHICKENPOX (VARICELLA ZOSTER)

Description

- Usually, mild acute viral disease characterized by fever and generalized, pruritic, vesicular rash

Etiology

- Caused by varicella zoster virus (herpes virus family)
- Highly contagious; transmitted by airborne respiratory secretions from infected people
- Rarely spread through contact with fluid from vesicles
- Can be caused by contact with patients with herpes zoster (shingles) in susceptible persons
- Communicable 1 to 2 days before rash until vesicles are crusted, approximately 5 days after onset of rash
- Incubation period usually 14 to 16 days but may be 10 to 21 days

Incidence and Demographics

- Seen in all ages; most frequent in young schoolchildren, children attending day care

Risk Factors

- Unimmunized person

Prevention and Screening

- Vaccination is the best form of prevention. Health care providers may refer to the *Centers for Disease Control and Prevention Recommended Immunization Schedule for Adults Aged 19 Years and Older—United States* (CDC, 2022).
- Isolate infected people.
- Children should not return to school or day care and adults should not return to work until all lesions are crusted over.

Assessment

History

- Headache, mild fever, malaise

Physical Exam

- Rash in various stages; progresses from macules to papules to vesicles on erythematous base within 6 hours after onset
- Vesicles crust in 4 to 6 days.
- Some medical authors note vesicles appearing first on scalp and mucous membranes; others report vesicles appearing first on the trunk and back simultaneously with mucous membranes, and then spreading to scalp and extremities.
- Vesicles may be seen in the conjunctivae, mouth, throat, esophagus, trachea, rectum, and vagina; little scarring occurs.
- Vesicles rarely appear on the palms and soles.
- Pruritus is present in areas of crusted vesicles.
- Vesicles usually appear in three crops on three successive days.

Diagnostic Studies

- In some cases, serologies IgM/IgG or varicella zoster virus PCR
- May see leukopenia
- May see WBC elevation with secondary infection
- May perform acute and convalescent titers
- Can be detected in vesicular scrapings during the first 3 to 4 days of the eruption

Differential Diagnosis

- Herpes simplex virus
- Papular urticaria
- Multiple insect bites
- Allergic skin reaction
- Scabies
- Smallpox
- Other viral fever and rash diseases
- Impetigo

Management

Nonpharmacologic Treatment

- For pruritus: calamine or Cetaphil lotion; baths with baking soda or oatmeal

Pharmacologic Treatment

- May administer varicella vaccine to exposed, susceptible children within 72 hours (up to 120 hours) after varicella exposure; may prevent or modify the disease
- Acetaminophen or ibuprofen for fever and discomfort for persons younger than 19 years of age
- Antipruritic medication such as diphenhydramine 5 mg/kg/day, divided every 6 hours.

- Consider oral acyclovir (Zovirax) or other antiviral medication for people at high risk of severe infection (older than age 12, chronic disease, immunocompromised, long-term salicylate therapy) if initiated within 24 hours of onset of rash.
- Administer varicella zoster immune globulin (VZIg) within 72 to 96 hours after exposure in immunocompromised children.

Special Considerations

- Varicella zoster virus remains latent in nerve roots and may emerge later in life as herpes zoster (shingles).
- Do not prescribe or administer aspirin or aspirin-related products to persons younger than 19 years of age because of associated risk of Reye's syndrome.
- Because of increased risk of severe disease and complications in children older than 12, adolescents without reliable history of disease should be immunized.

When to Consult, Refer, Hospitalize

- No reason to refer in uncomplicated cases

Follow-Up

- Return to day care, school, or work only after all lesions are crusted.

Complications

- Secondary, bacterial infection of skin (impetigo)
- Scarring—may be a cosmetic concern
- Encephalitis, nephritis, hepatitis, glomerulonephritis
- Reye's syndrome
- Thrombocytopenia
- Pneumonia

WEST NILE VIRUS (WNV)

Description

- Viral infection causing febrile illness, headache, fatigue, rash, arthritis, myalgia, weakness, lymphadenopathy, and meningoencephalitis

Etiology

- WNV is caused by the arbovirus of family *Flaviviridae*. The transmission cycle is spread by infected mosquitoes to birds and from infected birds to feeding mosquitoes.
- Human infection is primarily from the bite of an infected mosquito.
- Domestic animals, including horses, are sometimes infected by bites of infected mosquitoes; however, there is no documentation of spread of the disease from animal to animal or animal to human.
- Although rare, infection can be spread through blood transfusions, organ transplantation, and prenatal transmission.

Incidence and Demographics

- Reported in Asia, Africa, Europe, and United States
- In 2021, 49 states within the United States reported cases of WNV (CDC, 2022).
- Incubation period 5 to 15 days
- Mild illness in 20% of infected people, lasting 3 to 6 days
- As of 2022, a total of 2,695 cases of WNV disease have been reported to the CDC. Of these, 1,855 (69%) were classified as neuroinvasive disease (such as meningitis or encephalitis) and 840 (31%) were classified as non-neuroinvasive disease. (CDC, 2023)
- Adults 60 years of age or older at greatest risk for serious illness
- Mortality 5%; most deaths in older adults

Risk Factors

- Outdoor activities when mosquito activity is high
- Outdoor occupation

- Blood transfusion and organ transplant
- Older adults

Prevention and Screening

- Avoid mosquito bites: Minimize outdoor activity, wear protective clothing, and protect home and yard from breeding mosquitoes by draining standing water and maintaining window screens.
- When outdoors, apply insect repellent containing diethyltoluamide (DEET) (up to 50% strength), picaridin, or oil of lemon eucalyptus; permethrin is also recommended for use on clothing, shoes, and other gear.
    - *Pediatric note:* Oil of lemon eucalyptus products should not be used on children younger than 3 years of age. AAP does not recommend the use of DEET on infants younger than 2 months.
- Apply repellent to clothing and exposed skin, avoiding eyes and mouth; do not apply to skin under clothing—efficacy of repellent is affected by concentration, perspiration, and getting wet. Reapply repellent as needed.
- Communities can control vectors by public health spraying against mosquitoes.
- Wear gloves when disposing of dead birds.
- Report dead birds to local health department.
- Screen blood donations for WNV using nucleic acid-amplification test.

Assessment

History

- Determine exposure to mosquitoes.
- Check for history of blood transfusion or organ transplantation.

Physical Exam

- Nondescript fever with maculopapular or morbilliform rash on neck, trunk, arms, and legs
- Arthritis, myalgia, generalized weakness, and lymphadenopathy
- Meningitis: fever, headache, and nuchal rigidity

- Encephalitis: fever, headache, and altered mental status ranging from confusion to coma, with or without additional signs of brain dysfunction (paresis, flaccid paralysis, ataxia, sensory deficits, optic neuritis, seizures, and abnormal reflexes)

Diagnostic Studies

- CSF with IgM antibody for WNV is confirmative; CSF with pleocytosis (increased number of lymphocytes)
- WNV antibody in serum is presumptive of recent infection in patients with acute CNS infection; greater than a fourfold increase in antibody titers 2 to 4 weeks apart is confirmative
- Pleocytosis: increased number of lymphocytes in CSF

Differential Diagnosis

- California encephalitis
- Eastern equine encephalitis
- Western equine encephalitis
- Powassan encephalitis
- St. Louis encephalitis
- Colorado tick fever
- Dengue fever

Management and Treatment

Nonpharmacologic Treatment

- Supportive care
- Monitor for complications

Pharmacologic Treatment

- Appropriate treatment of complications

How Long to Treat

- Continue supportive care until improvement.

Special Considerations

- See CDC website: http://www.cdc.gov/ncidod/dvbid/westnile/index.htm/

When to Consult, Refer, Hospitalize

- Report WNV encephalitis cases to the state health department.
- Immediately refer patients to an infectious disease specialist.
- Patients with deteriorating mental status should be referred immediately to a health care provider for hospitalization.
- WNV must be reported to the CDC.

Follow-Up

- The majority have very minor illness and recovery without complications.

Complications

- Central nervous system abnormalities
- Death

Bacterial And Other Infections

LYME DISEASE

Description

- Tick-borne infection from a spirochete transmitted via deer tick bite, often begins with rash (erythema migrans), and progresses to headaches, arthritis, and neurologic sequelae; up to 20% of patients have complications; most do not have permanent sequelae

Etiology

- Caused by the spirochete *Borrelia burgdorferi;* the most common vector-borne disease in the United States.
- Transmitted to humans by *Ixodes scapularis* tick (deer tick); not transmitted by larger dog tick
- Size of tick 2–9 mm
- Painless bite; ticks usually drop off unnoticed in 2 to 4 days; must be embedded longer than 24 hours to transmit disease
- Incubation period from bite to appearance of erythema migrans 3 to 31 days; usually 7 to 14 days

Incidence and Demographics

- Ninety percent of cases are diagnosed in the Mid-Atlantic, Northeastern, and North Central areas of the United States.
- Preliminary results from three different evaluation methods suggest that the number of people diagnosed with Lyme disease each year in the United States is around 300,000.
- Patients with Lyme disease are most likely to have illness onset in June, July, or August and less likely to have illness onset from December through March (CDC, 2022).

Risk Factors

- Live in endemic region
- Spend time outdoors for recreation or occupation
- Exposed skin
- No use of repellents
- Thirty percent to 50% of cases in children and adolescents; reported cases of Lyme disease are most common among boys 5 to 9 years of age

Prevention and Screening

- *Reduce exposed skin*: Wear light-colored clothing to see ticks; wear long pants and long sleeves; tuck shirts into pants, tuck pants into socks. When outdoors, apply insect repellent containing DEET (up to 50% strength), picaridin, or oil of lemon eucalyptus; permethrin is also recommended for use on clothing, shoes, and other gear.

  - ◊ *Pediatric note*: Oil of lemon eucalyptus products should not be used on children younger than 3 years of age. The AAP does not recommend the use of DEET on infants younger than 2 months.

- ♦ Apply repellent to clothing and exposed skin, avoiding eyes and mouth. Do not apply to skin under clothing: efficacy of repellent is affected by concentration, perspiration, and getting wet. Reapply repellent as needed.
- ♦ Walk in the middle of a path; avoid walking near tree branches, bushes, or grass; inspect skin, hair, and scalp after spending a day outside; examine clothing before coming into the house.
- ♦ Examine pets for ticks regularly.
- ♦ The Lyme disease vaccine was withdrawn from the market in 2002 by the manufacturer because of low sales and is no longer commercially available.
- ♦ Prophylactic antibiotics are not routinely used following tick bites.
- ♦ Factors to take into consideration include:
  - ◊ Was the tick on the person for 24 hours before being removed or falling off?
  - ◊ Has it been at least 3 days since the person removed the tick or it fell off?
  - ◊ Is Lyme disease common in the location where the person was exposed to the tick?

Assessment

History

- ♦ Most unable to identify tick bite, but have history of possible exposure

Physical Exam

- ♦ Complete physical exam
- ♦ Characteristic rash (target lesion); may find tick or tick remnant in Stage 1 Lyme disease (see Table 4–2 for descriptions of each stage of disease)
- ♦ Signs of cranial nerve palsies, meningeal signs, pericarditis, mono-arthritis in Stage 2 Lyme disease
- ♦ May see recurrent tendonitis, bursitis, synovitis late in disease; memory loss; motor or sensory deficits; iritis, optic neuritis, and other eye manifestations

TABLE 4–2.
STAGES OF LYME DISEASE

STAGE	SYMPTOMS
Stage 1: Early localized disease	♦ Flu-like symptoms of fever, chills, myalgia, arthralgia, headache may develop 3–30 days post tick bite. ♦ 50%–90% of patients develop distinctive rash termed erythema migrans within about 1 week of tick bite: begins as red macule or papule, expands rapidly over several days to annular, erythematous patch with central clearing, larger than 5 cm to as large as 30 cm ♦ Resolves in 3–4 weeks without treatment; usually in area of tick bite but may occur anywhere
Stage 2: Early disseminated spirodisease (weeks to months postexposure)	♦ Begins roughly 3–5 weeks after initial infection, as disease spreads ♦ Wide variety of symptoms, most notably persistent fatigue ♦ Migratory arthralgia common ♦ Cranial nerve palsies (especially facial nerve) common ♦ Meningitis, conjunctivitis may occur; carditis with heart block rare ♦ Most common manifestation is multiple erythema migrans lesions, usually smaller than initial lesion
Stage 3: Late disease (months years later)	♦ Months to years after initial infection, a recurrent polyarticular arthritis affecting large joints (knees) may develop ♦ Central and peripheral nervous system affected, may develop subacute encephalopathy, distal paresthesias ♦ Memory, mood, sleep problems may be noted ♦ Cardiac involvement

Diagnostic Studies

- Lyme disease is primarily a clinical diagnosis; serology has uncertain sensitivity but is used to confirm the presence of specific antibodies to *B. burgdorferi* in serum (see Table 4–3).
- Step 1: Enzyme-linked immunosorbent assay (ELISA) method is preferred: more sensitive and specific. If positive, proceed to Step 2.
- Step 2: Western blot assay can detect both IgM and IgG and is used as a confirmatory test.
- Serologic tests are not necessary if patient has classic presentation of exposure to endemic area and erythema migrans; test results are often negative early in disease course.

TABLE 4–3.
LABORATORY FINDINGS IN LYME DISEASE

SERUM TEST	EARLY FINDINGS	MIDCOURSE	LATE FINDINGS
	2–4 weeks after erythema migrans	6–8 weeks	4–6 months
IgM	Appears	Peaks	Declines to low levels
IgG	Negative	Appears	Peaks; remains elevated but at lower level

- For late disease, patient must have specific symptoms and objective signs before testing.
- Patients with Lyme disease may not have elevated titers during the first several weeks of illness (false-negative test result).
- Do not test patients with nonspecific symptoms for Lyme disease as there is a relatively high incidence of false positives in the general population.

Differential Diagnosis

- Rocky Mountain spotted fever
- Rheumatic fever
- Viral disease
- Fibromyalgia
- Other forms of arthritis

Management and Treatment

Nonpharmacologic Treatment

- Hydrate patients; keep skin well lubricated.
- Remove tick using firm tension and fine tweezers. Clean site. Do not squeeze or puncture the tick. If the tick head or other parts are not removed, clean with antimicrobial as removing head can cause tissue damage and has no effect on risk of Lyme disease.

Pharmacologic Treatment

- Adults
  - Early disease: doxycycline, 100 mg twice a day orally for 14 to 21 days
  - Late disease: same as early disease but 21 to 28 days
  - Persistent or recurrent arthritis, carditis, meningitis, or encephalitis:
    - Ceftriaxone (Rocephin), 2 g once daily or 1 g twice daily IV or IM for 14 to 21 days

      or
    - Penicillin G IV, 20 million units in four divided doses
- Pediatric
  - Early disease: younger than 8 years of age, amoxicillin 25–50 mg/kg/day orally divided into two doses daily, not to exceed 2 g/day for 14 to 21 days
  - Early disease: 8 years of age or older, doxycycline 100 mg twice a day orally for 14 to 21 days
  - Late disease: same as early disease except extend treatment for 21 to 28 days
  - Persistent or recurrent arthritis, carditis, meningitis, or encephalitis:
    - Ceftriaxone (Rocephin) 75–100 mg/kg once daily, not to exceed 2 g/day for 14 to 21 days

      or
    - Penicillin G IV, 300,000 U/kg/day in four divided doses not to exceed 20 million U/day

How Long to Treat

- 14 to 21 days for early disease and 21 to 28 days for late disease
- 30 to 60 days for meningitis or encephalitis

Special Considerations

- Amoxicillin is recommended for children and for pregnant and lactating women.

When to Consult, Refer, Hospitalize

- Refer to infectious disease specialist and/or to other specialist as soon as diagnosis is suspected. Monitor for central nervous system or cardiac involvement, uncertain diagnosis, or failure to respond to oral medication.

- Consult if IV therapy is required.
- Lyme disease must be reported to the CDC (CDC, 2019c).

Follow-Up

Expected Course

- Most respond promptly; complete resolution of symptoms in 4 weeks
- Long-term outcome not clear. In one study, many had residual symptoms; however, treatment is often delayed, or patients undertreated

Complications

- Recurrent arthritis, chronic neurologic symptoms, congestive heart failure, cardiomyopathy

PERTUSSIS

Description

- An upper respiratory illness characterized by a progressive cough lasting longer than 2 weeks with one of the following symptoms: spasms of coughing, inspiratory "whoop," or post-tussive vomiting; or in infants younger than 1 year, apnea with or without cyanosis

Etiology

- *Bordetella pertussis*
- Transmission is respiratory
- Incubation 6 to 20 days
- Communicable until 5 days after treatment initiated

Incidence and Demographics

- Following the introduction of the pertussis vaccines in the 1940s when cases frequently were greater than 100,000 per year, incidence declined dramatically to less than 10,000 by 1965. In the 1980s, pertussis reports began increasing, and by 2019, more than 18,000 cases were reported nationwide. (https://www.cdc.gov/pertussis/surv-reporting/cases-by-year.html)

Risk Factors

- Lack of immunization

Prevention and Screening

- See CDC immunization schedule for pertussis vaccine for children and adults (https://www.cdc.gov/vaccines/schedules/index.html).

Assessment

History

- Catarrhal stage: mild upper respiratory symptoms with cough, nasal congestion, rhinorrhea, sneezing, low grade fever, and mild conjunctival injection (most contagious stage); indistinguishable from the common cold
- Paroxysmal stage: severe bursts of cough with inspiratory whoop followed by vomiting; fever absent or low grade (less than 101°F); cough is forceful, rapid, staccato sequence; child unable to breath between coughing attacks, which are often accompanied by emesis; face may become reddened or have petechiae; cough is worse at night

Physical Exam

- Depending on stage, patient may appear tired; apnea may occur in young infants.
- Obtain vital signs; check eyes, ears, nose, throat, lymph, respiratory, and cardiac exam to exclude other illnesses.

Diagnostic Studies

- PCR swab of nasal cavity or nasopharyngeal cultures in the catarrhal stage or IgA testing for *B. pertussis* to confirm diagnosis
- CBC will show leukocytosis.

Differential Diagnosis

- Bronchiolitis
- Bronchitis
- Pneumonia
- Other viral and bacterial upper respiratory infections
- Cystic fibrosis
- Foreign body

Management and Treatment

Nonpharmacologic Treatment

- Symptomatic—rest and fluids
- Admission for infants younger than 6 months of age

Pharmacologic Treatment

- Erythromycin, 40–50 mg/kg/day, in four divided doses *or*
- Trimethoprim/sulfamethoxazole (Bactrim), 8mg/kg/day (trimethoprim component) given twice a day
- Beta-2 agonists to control paroxysmal cough
- Corticosteroids for severely ill patients

How Long to Treat

- 14 days

Special Considerations

- Give antibiotics early; they are not effective late in the course of illness except to deal with complications.
- Antibiotics do not significantly shorten the disease but do reduce transmission.

- The CDC recommends antibiotic treatment for everyone in proximity to a person with pertussis illness regardless of age.
- Do not use cough suppressants.

When to Consult, Refer, Hospitalize

- Consult for infants younger than 6 months and others who present with potentially severe disease; they often require hospitalization for supportive care.
- Pertussis must be reported to the CDC.

Follow-Up

- Follow via telephone contact; discourage clinic visits.

Expected Course

- May be 10 weeks in uncomplicated cases

Complications

- Pneumonia
- Seizures
- Encephalopathy
- Death

RHEUMATIC FEVER (RF)

Description

- Serious inflammatory systemic immune process occurring 1 week to 6 months after group A beta-hemolytic streptococcal pharyngitis

Etiology

- Anti-streptococcal antibodies cross-react with human cardiac myocytes, cartilage, and thalamic and subthalamic nuclei of the CNS, causing carditis, arthritis, and chorea.
- Heredity may play a role, causing a particular immune response to strep.

Incidence and Demographics

- Frequency and severity have decreased due to better treatment of pharyngitis.
- RF remains an important cause of cardiac death in 5- to 25-year-olds.
- Many older patients have valvular disease caused by rheumatic fever.

Risk Factors

- Immigrants to the United States
- Genetic predisposition
- Ages 5 to 15
- More common in girls and Black people
- Living in the Midwest or Intermountain West in the mid- to late 1980s

Prevention and Screening

- Timely antibiotic treatment of group A beta-hemolytic streptococcal upper respiratory infection

Assessment

History

- May have history of recent sore throat
- Presents with gradual onset of fever, malaise, and joint pain (classically migratory pain and possible inflammation of large joints; disappears in 3 to 4 weeks)
- Fatigue, irritability, abdominal pain, epistaxis (rare)

Physical Exam

- Heart murmurs indicating mitral valve 75%, aortic valve 30%, tricuspid or pulmonic less than 5% involvement; occur within 2 weeks; may be permanent
- Pericarditis, myocarditis; may last 6 weeks to 6 months
- Subcutaneous nodules (painless, freely movable over extensor surfaces of elbows, knees, and wrists)
- Neurologic: facial grimaces and tics and chorea (purposeless, involuntary, rapid movements of trunk and/or extremities) are late findings
- Rash is rare; presents with erythematous, macular lesions with rounded or serpiginous margins and pale centers; transient and migratory, and occurs mainly on trunk and proximal extremities
- Guidelines for diagnosis—Jones criteria
  - Required: evidence of a preceding streptococcal infection such as elevated or increasing antistreptolysin O titer or other streptococcal antibodies, positive rapid antigen detection test (RADT) or throat culture for group A streptococcus, or recent scarlet fever
  - Also required: two major symptoms or one major and two minor symptoms (see Table 4–4)

Diagnostic Studies

- Current strep throat: RADT or throat culture; may or may not be positive
- Preceding strep infection: streptococcal antibody titers—obtain acute and convalescent serum titers (2 to 4 weeks)

TABLE 4–4.
JONES CRITERIA FOR RHEUMATIC FEVER

MAJOR SYMPTOMS	MINOR SYMPTOMS
Carditis (common) Polyarthritis (common) Chorea (uncommon) Erythema marginatum (uncommon) Subcutaneous nodules (uncommon)	Clinical: fever (temperature, 101°F –102°F), arthralgia, previous rheumatic fever (RF) or preexisting rheumatic heart disease Laboratory: acute phase reaction (leukocytosis, elevated erythrocyte sedimentation rate [ESR], abnormal C-reactive protein or prolonged PR interval or other electrocardiographic changes)

- To confirm diagnosis and evaluate severity of illness:
  - Erythrocyte sedimentation rate (ESR) elevation
  - C-reactive protein elevation
  - Prolonged PR interval on electrocardiography (ECG)

Differential Diagnosis

- Rheumatoid arthritis
- Systemic lupus erythematosus
- Lyme disease

Management and Treatment

Nonpharmacologic Treatment

- Strict bed rest (this is debated among professionals) until C-reactive protein level has been normal for 2 weeks, and ESR and temperature normal

Pharmacologic Treatment

- Depends on specific symptoms and severity of disease; refer to specialist
- Pain—codeine rather than nonsteroidal anti-inflammatory drugs (NSAIDs)
- Carditis—inotropic agents, diuretics, vasodilators, and corticosteroids as indicated
- Chorea treated with sedatives and benzodiazepines

How Long to Treat

- Bed rest until temperature, lab results, pulse rate (less than 100/min in adults), and ECG return to normal
- Antibiotics as per specialist recommendation

Special Considerations

- Educate patient regarding meticulous oral hygiene to prevent bacterial seeding.
- Educate patient to notify health care providers about cardiac condition before any procedure.
- Treat patients who have a history of rheumatic fever prophylactically to prevent recurrence (secondary prevention). The usual antibiotic is penicillin. These patients should take a full course of antibiotics followed by a continuous prophylactic dose for 10 years if the patient had carditis; 5 years if patient did not have carditis.
- Prophylaxis before procedures that may cause bacteremia is important indefinitely (see Table 4–5).
- Patients who should receive prophylaxis:
    - High-risk
- Prosthetic valve; previous bacterial endocarditis; complex, cyanotic congenital heart disease; surgically constructed systemic pulmonary shunts or conduits
    - Medium or moderate risk
- Patients with acute rheumatic fever (ARF) who have acquired valvular dysfunction but *not* patients with previous ARF without valvular dysfunction
- Patients with uncorrected cardiac congenital defects, hypertrophic cardiomyopathy, mitral regurgitation, mitral valve prolapse with murmur, and possibly men 45 years and older with mitral valve prolapse without murmur

TABLE 4–5.
RHEUMATIC FEVER PROPHAXIS GUIDELINES

Primary Prophylaxis: Treat *Streptococcus pyogenes* pharyngitis	Benzathine Pen G, 1.2 million units IM	Penicillin for 10 days prevents rheumatic fever even when started 7–9 days after onset of illness Alternative Pen VK, 250 mg orally twice a day, sulfadiazine 1 g, orally once a day, or erythromycin 250 mg, orally twice a day
Secondary Prophylaxis (previous documented rheumatic fever)	Benzathine Pen G, 1.2 million units, IIM every q3—4 weeks	Duration: No carditis: 5 years or until the age of 21, whichever is longer; carditis without residual heart disease: 10 years since last attack; carditis with residual valve disease: 10 years since last attack or until age 40, whichever is longer.

Adapted from Gilbert, D. N., Moellering, R. C., & M. A. Sande. (2022). *The Sanford Guide to Antimicrobial Therapy* (52nd ed.). Hyde Park, VT: Antimicrobial Therapy, Inc.

When to Consult, Refer, Hospitalize

- Refer to rheumatologist and/or cardiologist for all suspected cases.
- Hospitalize for acute carditis and/or chorea.

Follow-Up

- Usually by cardiologist to monitor C-reactive protein; reevaluate every 4 to 6 weeks when patients present for prophylaxis

Expected Course

- Initial episodes may last months in children and weeks in adults.

Complications

- Recurrent ARF secondary to streptococcal reinfection
- Cardiomegaly, heart failure, pericarditis, mitral regurgitation, aortic insufficiency
- Death in 1% to 2%
- American Heart Association (AHA) dental prophylaxis guidelines (2021) refer to most updated guidelines: https://www.heart.org/-/media/files/health-topics/infective-endocarditis/infective-endocarditis-wallet-card.pdf

ROCKY MOUNTAIN SPOTTED FEVER (RMSF)

Description

- Moderate systemic febrile illness with rash caused by vasculitis of small vessels; systemic symptoms including fever, characteristic rash; risk of severe complications and death

Etiology

- *Rickettsia rickettsii* transmitted by bite of infected tick
- Tick must attach and feed for 4 to 6 hours to transmit infection

- No person-to-person transmission; disease confers immunity
- Incubation 2 to 14 days

Incidence and Demographics

- More than 50% of cases in South Atlantic region, predominantly in southeastern and central states; also, upper Rocky Mountain states, Canada, Mexico, and South and Central America
- The number of cases has risen in the last two decades from 495 cases in 2000 to a peak of 6,258 in 2017 (CDC, 2019).
- People 40 years of age and older account for the highest number of cases; however, children younger than 10 represent the highest number of reported deaths.

Risk Factors

- Exposure to tick bites; camping or yardwork; exposed skin due to short pants, sleeves; no repellent

Prevention and Screening

- Avoid tick bites (see Lyme disease).

Assessment

History

- Triad: headache, fever, rash (and history of tick bite, although not all present at time of initial assessment)
- Presents with sudden onset of fever (temperature higher than 104°F) in nearly 100% of patients
- Severe headache unrelieved by analgesics; myalgia (particularly in calf and thigh)
- Rash: small, flat, pink, non-pruritic on wrists, forearms, and ankles, and then spread to trunk (sometimes palms and soles), turning purple and petechial

- Malaise, anorexia, nausea and vomiting, abdominal pain, lymphadenopathy, cough, and confusion are possible
- History of possible tick bite or exposure

Physical Exam

- Characteristic maculopapular rash usually appears before the sixth day of illness; spreads from wrists and ankles to trunk, neck, and face.
- If untreated, rash becomes petechial in about 4 days, and progresses to purpuric and coalesced.
- Moderate to high fever; conjunctival injection
- Splenomegaly in approximately 50% of patients

Diagnostic Studies

- Titers: acute and convalescent sera (fourfold increase in antibody titer) may not rise for 10 to 14 days
- Routine blood work may show nonspecific changes, identify complications: CBC with differential (thrombocytopenia, variable WBC count, mild anemia), prothrombin time (PT) and partial thromboplastin time (PTT; prolonged), blood urea nitrogen (BUN) and creatinine (elevated in renal insufficiency), electrolytes (mild hyponatremia), and elevated liver function tests (LFTs)

Differential Diagnosis

- Systemic viral infection
- Bacterial sepsis
- Meningitis
- Meningococcemia
- Lyme disease
- Rubella
- Scarlet fever
- Mononucleosis

- Rheumatic fever
- Drug reaction
- Erythema multiforme
- Ehrlichiosis

Management

Nonpharmacologic Treatment

- Rest and fluids
- Isolation not indicated

Pharmacologic Treatment

- **Important to treat promptly**; treatment before day 5 of illness in children affords the highest likelihood of good outcome
- Doxycycline is the treatment of choice in adults who are not pregnant and children of all ages unless they are hypersensitive to tetracyclines
- Adults
  - ◊ Doxycycline, 100 mg twice a day after loading dose of 200 mg once
  - ◊ If patient is sensitive to tetracyclines, use:
- Amoxicillin, 500 mg three times a day *or*
- Cefuroxime (Ceftin), 500 mg twice a day
- Late stage: ceftriaxone (Rocephin), 2 g IV once a day
- Pediatric
  - ◊ Less than 45 kg: doxycycline, 2–4mg/kg/day orally in two divided doses
  - ◊ More than 45 kg: doxycycline, 100 mg orally twice a day
- Pregnant women
  - ◊ Chloramphenicol (Chloromycetin), 500 mg every 6 hours

How Long to Treat

- 5 to 10 days or until afebrile 2 to 5 days

Special Considerations

- Educate patient on the tick associated with RMSF and ways to avoid the infection.

When to Consult, Refer, Hospitalize

- Consult with infectious disease specialist as soon as possible for potential hospitalization, any signs of complications.
- Rocky Mountain spotted fever must be reported to the CDC.

Follow-Up

- See patient for follow-up every 2 to 3 days if not hospitalized until symptoms resolved.

Expected Course

- Follow-up 1 to 2 days after initial visit; advise patients to return at first sign of complications.
- Most cases resolve without complication if treated promptly; infection can persist for 3 weeks.
- Refer for tertiary care as soon as complications develop or if patient has a petechial rash on first visit.

Complications

- CNS, cardiac, pulmonary, gastrointestinal, and renal involvement; disseminated intravascular coagulation, shock, death

SCARLET FEVER

Description

- Acute infectious disease usually associated with streptococcal pharyngitis and characterized by a vascular response to bacterial exotoxin

Etiology

- Toxin produced by group A hemolytic streptococcus (GAS) and occasionally produced by certain strains of staphylococci.
- Strep toxin usually has a pharyngeal source.
- Strep or staph infections from wounds or burns is a rare source.
- Transmitted by direct projection of large droplets or physical transfer of respiratory secretions
- Incubation 3 to 5 days
- Communicable during incubation and clinical illness, 10 days; no longer communicable after 24 hours of antibiotic

Incidence and Demographics

- Usually occurs in children 6 to 12 years, but also occurs in adults

Risk Factors

- Outside-the-home day care setting
- School-age children

Prevention and Screening

- Early identification of GAS by RADT or throat culture and removal from school or childcare for 24 hours after initiation of antibiotics
- Good handwashing
- Household contact screening for GAS or prophylactic treatment not effective

Assessment

History

- Prodrome: 1 to 2 days of fever, sore throat, headache; abdominal pain and vomiting may be present
- Rash appears in 1 to 5 days.

Physical Exam

- Initial pharyngitis is beefy red with or without exudate; white coating on tongue on days 1–2 that sheds by days 4–5 (shiny red with prominent papillae)
- Rash presents as fine eruptions on an erythematous bases, texture of sandpaper, blanches with pressure, initially on chest and axilla, and spreads to abdomen and extremities
- Red streaks in skin folds of axillae and antecubital fossa (Pastia's lines)
- Flushed face with circumoral pallor
- Rash becomes generalized; desquamation begins on face after 7 to 10 days

Diagnostic Studies

- Rapid antigen test or throat culture for strep
- Antistreptolysin O titer to confirm recent infection with group A streptococcus (not useful in management of acute streptococcal pharyngitis)

Differential Diagnosis

- Viral syndromes
- Mononucleosis
- Drug reaction

Management

Nonpharmacologic Treatment

- Rest and fluids

Pharmacologic Treatment

- Prompt therapy imperative to prevent rheumatic fever and other complications
- Penicillin V (Pen VEE K), 500 mg twice a day; erythromycin, 250 mg every 6 hours; or cefadroxil (Duricef), 500 mg twice a day
- For staphylococcal scarlet fever, dicloxacillin

How Long to Treat

- 10 days

Special Considerations

- Recurrence of GAS pharyngitis may be treated with prophylactic penicillin during times of increased risk of infection (spring, late fall, and winter)

When to Consult, Refer, Hospitalize

- Chronic GAS pharyngitis
- Evidence of pneumonia, bacteremia, shock, or other severe complications

Follow-Up

- Repeat throat culture indicated for patients at risk for rheumatic fever

Expected Course

- Improvement should be seen 2 to 3 days after starting antibiotic.

Complications

- Otitis media, sinusitis, bacteremia, rheumatic fever, glomerulonephritis
- Risk is reduced with prompt diagnosis and treatment.

Illnesses of Unknown Origin

FEVER WITHOUT LOCALIZING SIGNS

Description

- Fever (temperature 38.4°C [101.1°F] or higher) at least once in 24 hours with no source of infection or cause for hyperthermia; also known as fever without focus. For children with fever longer than 10 days, the term "fever of unknown origin" (FUO) is used; some experts suggest that fever should be present for 3 weeks as an outpatient or 1 week as an inpatient before the term FUO is applied.

- In many cases, no diagnosis can be established, and fever abates spontaneously.
- In up to 25% of cases in which fever persists, cause of fever remains unclear, even after thorough evaluation.

Etiology

- The principal causes of FUO are rheumatologic disease, infection, and neoplasm; drug fever is uncommon.
- Most FUOs result from atypical presentations of common diseases.

Incidence and Demographics

- Fever without localizing signs or symptoms, usually of acute onset and present for less than 1 week, is a common diagnostic dilemma in children younger than 36 months of age.
- An infectious agent, usually viral, is identified in 70% of infants younger than 3 months of age with fever.

Risk Factors

- Independent of age, fever with petechiae with or without localizing signs indicates high risk of life-threatening bacterial infections such as bacteremia, sepsis, and meningitis.

Prevention and Screening

- Have routine wellness exams.
- Avoid infected people.
- Seek medical attention if fever does not resolve with rest, fluids, and antipyretics within 24 hours of onset.

Assessment

History

- Note onset of fever, degree, duration, diurnal variation.
- Changes in environment, foods, and/or lifestyle changes around time of fever onset, particularly history of exposure to animals (domestic and wild), travel history
- Uncommon dietary habits or pica, tick bites, ethnic background, family history of disease
- Recent sick contacts (health care workers or day care)
- Medications and transfusions
- Number of school days missed
- Family stresses
- Review systems; particularly note intermittent rashes, arthralgia, weight loss, behavior changes

Physical Exam

- May be entirely normal or demonstrate mild findings such as clear rhinorrhea
- Absence of sweating: may indicate familial dysautonomia

Diagnostic Studies

- CBC with differential and platelets: Blood, urine, and CSF cultures should be obtained, as indicated.
- Consider ESR, chest X-ray, andTB skin testing.
- The course of action and diagnostic studies performed should be individualized based on presentation and child's age.

Differential Diagnosis

- Inflammatory disease
- Viral illness
- Bacterial infections

- Neoplasm
- Abscess
- Familial dysautonomia
- Hypothalamic dysfunction
- Drug fever

Management

Nonpharmacologic Treatment

- Maintain hydration, good nutrition, adequate sleep.
- Treat symptomatically.

Pharmacologic Treatment

- See Box 4–1.

Special Considerations

- Do not prescribe or administer aspirin or aspirin-related products to patients younger than 19 years of age.

When to Consult, Refer, Hospitalize

- All HIV-infected infants, children, adolescents, pregnant women, and adults presenting with FUO should be referred to and followed by an HIV specialist with knowledge of that age group/circumstance.

Follow-Up

- If not hospitalized, follow-up in 1 to 3 days, depending on age of child, degree of fever; occasionally, the source of infection will become identifiable in time.
- If blood or CSF cultures are positive and a child is not hospitalized, admit and treat with IV antibiotics.

BOX 4–1. GUIDELINES FOR MANAGEMENT OF FEVER

Infants Younger than 1 Month of Age

- Infants may acquire community pathogens; also, at risk for late-onset neonatal bacterial diseases and perinatally acquired herpes simplex virus infection
- CBC, blood culture, urine culture; consider lumbar puncture and culture
- Always treated aggressively in hospital; maintain on prophylactic antibiotics for 3 days pending culture results. Some practitioners hospitalize infants younger than 3 months of age if no focus of infection found on physical exam in office.

Infants Between 1 and 3 Months of Age

- Serious bacterial disease occurs in 10%–15%, including bacteremia in 5%, of febrile infants younger than 3 months old.
- Infants who appear generally well, have been previously healthy, have no focus for infection, total WBC count 5,000–15,000 cells/mm^3, absolute band count lower than1,500 cells/mm^3, and normal urinalysis are unlikely to have a serious bacterial infection. The negative predictive value of these criteria for serious bacterial infection is greater than 98%, and greater than 99% for bacteremia.
- CBC, blood culture, urine culture; consider lumbar puncture
- Usually treated aggressively with 24-hour hospital observation and prophylactic antibiotics
- If CBC is within normal limits and adequate follow-up assured, consider treatment with IM ceftriaxone pending culture results.

Children older than 3 Months of Age/Adults

- Low-grade fever: Give antipyretics and observe.
- Acetaminophen, 15 mg/kg/dose no more than every 4 hours and no more than five doses in 24 hours
- Ibuprofen, 10 mg/kg/dose if older than 6 months old; no more than every 6 hours and no more than four doses in 24 hours
- Fever (temperature higher than 102°F), obtain a CBC. If WBC is higher than 15,000/mm^3, obtain a blood culture and administer IM ceftriaxone. Obtain urine culture in boys younger than 6 months and girls younger than 2 years; some providers obtain urine cultures in all children with high fever and no focus of infection found on exam.

Complications

- Children with FUO have a better prognosis than do adults, depending on the primary disease process, which is usually an atypical presentation of a common childhood illness.

KAWASAKI DISEASE

Description

- Acute, self-limiting, multisystem vascular illness with rash and fever; also known as mucocutaneous lymph node syndrome
- Leading cause of acquired heart disease in children in the United States

Etiology

- Unknown; most likely infectious

Incidence and Demographics

- Eighty percent of cases in children younger than 5 years old (peak age 18 to 24 months); 5% of cases in children older than 10 years of age; rare in children older than age 15
- 1.5:1 male-to-female ratio
- Recurrence low
- No clear genetic pattern, although the incidence is lowest among White Americans and highest among Americans of Asian and Pacific Island descent
- Epidemics in the United States seem to occur during the winter and spring in 2- to 3-year intervals.
- No person-to-person spread, although siblings seem to be affected at higher rate.

Risk Factors

- Unknown

Prevention and Screening

- Unknown

Assessment

History

- May report recent history of cold, cough, or ear infection
- Persistent fever, red mouth and lips, and swollen hands with rash

Physical Exam

- Erythematous mouth and pharynx with "strawberry tongue" and red, swollen, and cracked lips
- Bulbar conjunctivitis without exudate
- Cervical lymphadenopathy—usually unilateral, involves at least one node swollen to greater than or equal to 1.5 cm diameter
- Polymorphous, generalized, erythematous rash
- Induration of hands and feet
- Periungual and groin desquamation may occur.

Diagnostic Criteria

- Persistent fever plus four of the five criteria in Box 4–2 *or*
- Persistent fever plus three of the criteria in Box 4–2 and evidence of coronary artery abnormalities
- Infants—may have atypical Kawasaki disease; irritability, abdominal pain, diarrhea, vomiting may be apparent with coronary artery disease

Diagnostic Studies

- None available; nonspecific tests include ESR, platelet counts, serum C-reactive protein

BOX 4–2.
DIAGNOSTIC CRITERIA FOR KAWASAKI DISEASE

Persistent fever for more than 5 days without an identifiable source, presence of four of five other clinical criteria, and unresponsive to antibiotics; diagnosis can be made if fever and only three criteria are met along with documented coronary artery disease

1. Mucous membrane involvement (erythematous mouth, pharynx; strawberry tongue; dry, fissured lips)
2. Non-purulent bilateral conjunctivitis
3. Polymorphous, erythematous, generalized rash
4. Cervical lymphadenopathy involving at least one node ≥1.5 cm in diameter
5. Polymorphous exanthema

**Adapted from *Red Book 2021*, American Academy of Pediatrics: Elk Grove Village, IL.

- CBC with differential: WBC count usually elevated with left shift (increased band forms); thrombocytosis develops in second week
- ECG and echocardiogram indicated to assess presence of cardiac or coronary artery disease

Differential Diagnosis

- Rickettsial diseases
- Rubella
- Rubeola
- Scarlet fever
- Rheumatic fever
- Epstein-Barr virus
- Drug reaction (Stevens-Johnson syndrome)
- Lyme disease
- Juvenile rheumatoid arthritis
- Scalded skin syndrome
- Toxic shock syndrome

Management

Nonpharmacologic Treatment

- Supportive: rest, fluids, protection of skin (lubrication, good hygiene)
- No tart or acidic beverages
- Bland diet (secondary to mouth ulceration)

Pharmacologic Treatment

- High-dose aspirin as anti-inflammatory (80–100 mg/kg/day four times a day); dose reduced after acute phase to prevent coronary thrombosis; if coronary artery abnormalities present, continue low-dose aspirin therapy (3–5 mg/kg) indefinitely
- High-dose intravenous immune globulin (IVIG) therapy (2 g/kg as single dose)—initiate as soon as possible; efficacy questionable if initiated after 10th day of illness
- Initiation of aspirin and IVIG within 10 days of fever onset—substantially reduces the prevalence of coronary artery dilation and aneurysms
- Hold measles and varicella immunizations for 11 months after IVIG therapy; if at high risk for measles exposure, may immunize and repeat immunization after 11 months

Special Considerations

- Aspirin therapy in patients younger than 19 years of age should be monitored closely due to risk of Reye's syndrome.

When to Consult, Refer, Hospitalize

- All suspected cases of Kawasaki disease are managed in a hospital.
- Refer all suspected cases to a cardiologist.

Follow-Up

- Long-term management depending on degree of cardiac involvement; echocardiogram in 6 to 8 weeks

Expected Course

- Without treatment, fever resolves in 12 days: other symptoms resolve 6 to 8 weeks after onset
- Myocardial infarction and sudden death may occur months to years later.

Complications

- Bacterial superinfection (desquamating skin)
- Coronary aneurysms
- Pericardial effusion
- Myocarditis
- Myocardial infarction
- Arthritis and arthralgia
- Jaundice, liver, and gallbladder problems
- Aseptic meningitis

SEVERE ACUTE RESPIRATORY SYNDROME CORONAVIRUS 2 (SARS-COV-2)

The first reported case of SARS-COV-2 infection was in China in 2019 and became a global pandemic. As of April 2022, more than 503 million cases of coronavirus disease 2019 (COVID-19) have been reported globally, including more than 6.2 million deaths. (https://covid19.nih.gov/)

Diagnostic Studies (EUA—emergency use authorization)

- Reverse-transcription polymerase chain reaction (RT-PCR) is the gold standard for detecting current SARS-CoV-2 infection
- Antigen-based diagnostic tests (detect viral antigens) are less sensitive but highly specific. Advantages are their low cost, rapid turnaround time, and use for home testing.
- Serology or antibody tests can detect recent or prior SARS-CoV-2 infection

Vaccines

The most effective way to prevent SARS-CoV-2 infection

- mRNA vaccines
    - Pfizer-BioNTech
    - Moderna
- Adenovector vaccine
    - Johnson & Johnson/Janssen (because of the risk of serious adverse events associated with this vaccine, the Pfizer and Moderna vaccines are preferable)

Treatment

- Post-exposure prophylaxis
    - Monoclonal antibodies have emergency use authorization (EUA)
    - Antivirals (EUA)
        - Ritonavir-boosted nirmatrelvir (Paxlovid) oral
        - Remdesivir intravenous; inpatient use only

INFECTIONS FROM BIOWEAPONS (BW)

Description

Biological agents with bioweapon potential are characterized as Category A agents. These agents can be easily disseminated or transmitted from person to person, cause high mortality with potential for major public health impact, and require prompt action. Numerous viruses, several bacteria, and toxins may be used as weapons, but those that are known to have been weaponized, have effective dispersal methods, and be environmentally stable include anthrax, botulism, plague, smallpox, tularemia, and viral hemorrhagic fevers (Ebola, Marburg, Lassa, dengue, yellow fever, and others).

Etiology

- Naturally occurring organisms that have been altered to increase lethality

Incidence and Demographics

- Smallpox is no longer found in a wild form; all other potential bio-agents occur naturally.
- Inhalation anthrax is rare, although dermatologic infection is still found fairly
- often in farm workers.
- Large-scale outbreaks of botulism have never occurred.

Risk Factors

- Any population can be at risk, although bioweapons attacks are more likely to occur in densely populated, urban areas or at large, crowded events, such as sporting events.

Prevention and Screening

- Primary care providers must maintain an elevated level of suspicion.
- Family nurse practitioners must be aware of the modes of transmission, incubation periods, and communicable periods of these diseases; an excellent source of information is the CDC Emergency Preparedness and Response website: http://emergency.cdc.gov/

Assessment

History

- Symptoms for most agents may initially mimic those of common viral illnesses and include fever, fatigue, malaise, muscle aches, headache, cough, vomiting, diarrhea, rashes.
- For most agents, symptoms will quickly increase in intensity and severity.
- The first indication of an unannounced biologic attack is likely to be an unusual increase in number of people seeking care.

Physical Exam

- Ill-appearing patient, often out of proportion to degree of illness prevalent in the community

Diagnostic Studies

- Blood cultures, CBC, electrolytes
- Other studies dictated by clinical picture

Differential Diagnosis

- Common wild viral agents (fifth disease, coxsackievirus, varicella)
- Other potential biological agents

Management

Nonpharmacologic Treatment

- Rapidly isolate patient and contacts.
- Refer to infectious disease specialists.
- Rapidly notify public health authorities.
- Psychological and mental health problems brought on by the event will require significant expertise.

Pharmacologic Treatment

- See Table 4–6.
- Empiric therapy may be indicated if large numbers of people present with a nonspecific febrile illness in a limited time frame and location under credible threat of attack. Empiric therapy is ciprofloxacin or doxycycline orally or intravenously at routine recommended doses.

Special Considerations

- Appropriate management of postexposure prophylaxis and its complications will be critical in containing spread of infection.

TABLE 4–6.
POTENTIAL BIOWEAPONS AGENTS

BIOLOGICAL AGENT	TRANSMISSION/ INCUBATION	CLINICAL PRESENTATION	DIAGNOSIS	MANAGEMENT
Anthrax (*Bacillus anthracis*): Gram-positive, spore- forming aerobic rod that causes cutaneous or pulmonary infection	Inhalation of aerosolized spores; person-to person transmission does not occur Incubation up to 6 weeks	Biphasic, with initial prodrome of nonspecific febrile flulike illness. May be followed by brief period of improvement, and then rapid onset of high fever and severe respiratory distress Shock, death within 24–36 hours.	Chest X-ray shows mediastinal widening; Gram-positive bacilli on unspun peripheral blood smear	Ciprofloxacin or doxycycline for 60 days; standard contact precautions Prophylaxis should be offered with the same agents. A vaccine is available, but supply is limited. Raxibacumab is a new drug containing antibodies that neutralize anthrax toxins
Cutaneous anthrax does not have bioweapon (BW) potential.	1–7 days	Skin blisters	History, clinical, wound culture	7- to 10-day antibiotic course
Botulism: Caused by neurotoxin produced by *Clostridium botulinum*, a spore- forming, obligate anaerobe found in soil. Botulinum toxin is the most lethal natural poison known	Toxin can be aerosolized; sources of entry include wounds and gastrointestinal (GI) and respiratory tracts. It can also be dispensed in food. There is no person-to-person transmission. Incubation 12–36 hours.	Symmetric cranial neuropathies (e.g., drooping eyelids, weakened jaw clench, difficulty swallowing, speaking), blurred vision or diplopia, symmetric descending weakness in a proximal-to-distal pattern, respiratory dysfunction	Routine laboratory tests usually unremarkable. Definitive diagnostic testing for botulism available only at the CDC; diagnosis is primarily clinical.	Supportive care, including ventilator support. Passive immunization with equine antitoxin

Continued

TABLE 4–6.
(CONTINUED)

BIOLOGICAL AGENT	TRANSMISSION/ INCUBATION	CLINICAL PRESENTATION	DIAGNOSIS	MANAGEMENT
Plague (*Yersinia pestis*): Non-motile bacillus	Bubonic: transmitted by bites from infected fleas of rodents; most common type is pneumonic: inhalation of respiratory droplets from a human or animal with respiratory plague; may be aerosolized Secondary cases would occur from contact with infected persons. A BW attack most likely to produce pneumonic plague. Incubation 2–4 days	Bubonic: enlarged, painful, regional lymph nodes (buboes), fever, chills, headache, malaise, GI symptoms, and prostration Pneumonic: fever, weakness, and rapidly developing pneumonia with shortness of breath, chest pain, cough, and sometimes bloody or watery sputum Can be fatal without treatment.	Clinical diagnosis important as treatment must begin in fewer than 24 hours. Large numbers of patients with severe pneumonia, particularly if accompanied by hemoptysis, must trigger prompt presumptive treatment and isolation. Prophylaxis of close contacts	Streptomycin, gentamicin, tetracycline, or chloramphenicol begun within 24 hours greatly improves prognosis; isolation and supportive care necessary Prophylactic therapy begun within 7 days is very effective in preventing infection. Vaccine under investigation.
Smallpox: Caused by a DNA virus genus orthopoxvirus	Person-to-person transmission; spread by inhalation of air droplets or aerosols. Smallpox virus is specific for humans; animal infection does not occur. Weaponized smallpox can be spread by aerosol or by bombs or missiles.	High fever, malaise, severe aching pains, prostration Later, a papular rash develops over the face and spreads to the extremities; soon becomes vesicular and later, pustular. Rash is most dense on face.	Patients are most contagious from time of onset of rash until scabs form. Initial diagnosis must occur at a military facility. After confirmation of community disease, subsequent diagnoses made on basis of clinical presentation.	No known effective antiviral agents Treatment is supportive. All potentially infected persons should be hospitalized in their homes.

	Secondary infection would occur from direct person-to-person spread, via both droplet and infected fomites (clothing, bedding). Incubation 12–14 days.			In event of widespread outbreak, specific hospitals would be designated for treatment of smallpox patients. Widespread vaccination would be indicated; smallpox vaccine is effective only if administered within 4 days of exposure. Vaccine is available, although supply is government controlled.
Tularemia (*Francisella tularensis*): Gram-negative coccobacillus. Type A most virulent and likely to be weaponized. Very small amount (10–50 organisms) can produce disease.	Naturally occurring in temperate areas of North America, Europe, and Asia. F. tularensis can be used as a biological weapon as an aerosol, with infection occurring secondary to inhalation, skin, or mucous membrane contact, or GI exposure from contaminated soil, water, food, or animals. Person-to-person transmission is not known to occur.	Presentation dependent on route of administration. Inhalation most likely Symptoms include abrupt onset of fever with progression to pneumonia and respiratory disease, hilar lymphadenopathy, and pleuritis. Inhalation can also cause sepsis without respiratory symptoms; this syndrome has a high fatality rate	No means of rapid testing is widely available. Diagnosis is initially clinical. *F. tularensis* may be identified by culture done in biological safety level (BSL) 3 labs.	Streptomycin IM or gentamicin IV for infection Ciprofloxacin or doxycycline at usual doses recommended for mass casualties or postexposure Vaccine is not widely available and immunity is incomplete.

Continued

TABLE 4–6.
(CONTINUED)

BIOLOGICAL AGENT	TRANSMISSION/ INCUBATION	CLINICAL PRESENTATION	DIAGNOSIS	MANAGEMENT
	Incubation 1–4 days, depending on virulence of strain, site, and size of inoculums.			
Viral Hemorrhagic Fevers (VHFs): A group of illnesses caused by several distinct RNA viruses (*Arenaviridae, Bunyaviridae, Filoviridae, Flaviviridae*), including Ebola hemorrhagic fever*, Marburg virus, Lassa fever, and hantavirus pulmonary syndrome (HPS)	Humans are not the natural reservoir of these viruses and are infected when they encounter secretions of infected hosts. Ebola, for example, is spread through direct contact with the blood or body fluids of a person who is sick with Ebola virus disease (EVD) or objects contaminated with the virus.	Specific signs and symptoms vary by the type of VHF; initial signs and symptoms include marked fever, fatigue, dizziness, muscle aches, loss of strength, and exhaustion. Patients often show signs of bleeding under the skin, in internal organs, or from body orifices (mouth, eyes, ears, etc.).	High index of suspicion; detailed travel history important Lab findings supportive of infection vary; typically, leukopenia, thrombocytopenia occur Immunoglobulin (Ig) M antibody by enzyme-linked immunosorbent assays (ELISA) during the acute illness	There is no cure or established drug treatment for VHFs, although ribavirin has been tried with Lassa fever and recent drug therapy has advanced for EVD. Therapy is supportive and barrier isolation techniques should be initiated, including guidance by the CDC

	However, humans can transmit some viruses to one another, after the accidental transmission from the host. Naturally occurring human cases occur sporadically. Incubation is dependent on virus.	Full-blown VHF evolves to shock and generalized bleeding from the mucous membranes.	Diagnosis by viral cultivation requires 3–10 days and can be done only at BSL 4 labs (CDC, military facilities).	for donning and doffing personal protective equipment (PPE) for health care workers (HCWs). Vaccines are newly available for EVD.

*Ebola virus disease (EVD) is a rare, but deadly, disease that was not diagnosed in the United States until 2014. Four (non-weaponized) cases were confirmed, including three health care workers who were exposed while caring for EVD patients in the United States and in the African nation of Guinea. Although the risk of exposure in the United States is minimal, thorough assessment and identification of persons who have traveled to parts of the world where EVD is prevalent are imperative to prevent the spread of the disease, as is strict adherence to infection-control guidelines specific to EVD.

Adapted from Bell B. P., Damon I. K., Jernigan D. B., et al. "Overview, Control Strategies, and Lessons Learned in the CDC Response to the 2014–2016 Ebola Epidemic." *Morbidity and Mortality Weekly Report.* 2016;65(3):4–11.

When to Consult, Refer, Hospitalize

- Anthrax, botulism, hantavirus, plague, and tularemia must be reported to the CDC.

Follow-Up

Complications

- Dependent on agent
- Most potential agents have high lethality—30% to 100%.

TRANSMISSION-BASED PRECAUTIONS

Contact Precautions

These are used in addition to standard precautions when caring for patients with known or suspected diseases that are spread by direct or indirect contact. These include methicillin-resistant *Staphylococcus aureus* (MRSA), vancomycin-resistant *Enterococcus* (VRE), and *Clostridium difficile*. Contact precautions include gloving and gowning when in contact with the patient, objects, and surfaces within the patient's environment. All reusable items should be cleaned and disinfected according to organizational policy, and disposable items should be thrown away immediately after use.

Droplet Precautions

These require the use of a surgical mask in addition to standard precautions when within 3 feet (6 feet for smallpox) of a patient known to have or suspected of having a disease spread by droplets. These include influenza, pertussis, SARS, and meningococcal disease. Health care workers (HCWs) should observe droplet precautions when examining a patient with respiratory symptoms, especially if the patient has a fever. These precautions should remain in effect until it is determined that the symptoms are not caused by an infection that requires droplet precautions.

Airborne Precautions

These are used in addition to standard precautions when in contact with patients with known or suspected diseases spread by fine particles transmitted by air currents, such as tuberculosis, measles, and severe acute respiratory syndrome (SARS). HCPs must wear a National Institute for

Occupational Safety and Health (NIOSH)–certified, fit-tested N95 respirator just before entry into an area shared with a patient suspected or known to have one of these diseases. If eye protection is needed, wear goggles or a face shield during all contact with the patient, not only if you predict splashes or sprays.

DONNING AND DOFFING PERSONAL PROTECTIVE EQUIPMENT (PPE)

All HCWs involved in the care of EVD patients must have training in the proper use of PPE. No skin should be exposed while working in the PPE. A trained observer must supervise every step of the PPE donning/doffing procedure to ensure that the established protocol has been followed.

Donning PPE

- The gown should fully cover the torso from the neck to the knees, the arms to the wrists, and wrap around the back. It should be tied at the neck and waist.
- Nonsterile gloves should cover the wrist of the gown. They should be put on after the gown.
- The mask's ties should be secured at the back of the head and at the neck. The flexible noseband should be fitted to the bridge of the nose. The mask should fit snugly to the face and extend below the chin.
- The goggles and face shield should be adjusted to fit the face.
- After the PPE is in place, work from clean to dirty and limit the surfaces touched. Keep hands away from face. The equipment should be changed if torn or heavily contaminated.
- Perform hand hygiene before and after putting on PPE.

Doffing PPE

- Remove all PPE before leaving the patient room or anteroom. Remember the outside of all equipment is considered contaminated.
- To remove gloves, grasp the outside of one glove in the palm of the opposite hand and peel off. Hold the removed glove in the gloved hand, while sliding fingers of the ungloved hand under the remaining glove at the wrist and peeling off.
- To remove goggles and face shield, handle by the clean headband or earpieces.

- Remove the gown by unfastening the neck and waist ties and peeling it from each shoulder toward the same hand, turning the gown inside out. Hold the removed gown away from the body, roll it into a bundle, and discard.
- Without touching the front of the mask, remove the mask by grasping the ties.
- Perform hand hygiene.

Tropical/Global Diseases

See Table 4–7.

TABLE 4–7.
TROPICAL/GLOBAL DISEASES

DISEASE	TRANSMISSION METHOD	INFECTED COUNTRIES	SEVERITY/SYMPTOMS	TREATMENT/PREVENTION
Chagas Disease (American trypanoso-miasis)	Parasite transmitted by infected reduviid bugs	South and Central America; now more than 300,000 cases in the United States	Skin lesion, fever, anorexia, lymphadenopathy, hepatosplenomegaly, carditis; later—dementia, heart failure, weight loss	Benznidazole and nifurtimox Prevention: avoid buildings made of mud, adobe, and thatch
Chikungunya	Vector-borne virus (arbovirus) spreads via the *Aedes aegypti* and *Aedes albopictus* mosquitoes	Certain regions of Africa, Asia, Europe; spreading to Caribbean and Central America, with 232 cases now reported in the United States.	Fever, malaise, polyarthralgia, headache, myalgia, rash, lymphopenia; rarely fatal	NSAIDs, hydration, rest Antiviral agents, monoclonal antibody treatments, and several vaccines are in various stages of development
Cholera	Bacterial infection transmitted in contaminated food or water	Developing countries with poor sanitation; more common in warm months	Perfuse, watery diarrhea, abdominal pain, vomiting lasting 1–3 days; can be fatal with profound dehydration	Tetracycline, oral rehydration Prevention: risk generally considered low to travelers and vaccine not available in United States
Dengue fever	Vector-borne virus (arbovirus) spreads via the *A. aegypti*	Any tropical or subtropical country, greater risk in cities	High fever, severe headache, vomiting, backache, eye pain, myalgia, arthralgia, rash for 2–7 days; rarely hemorrhagic	Acetaminophen, hydration, blood transfusions Prevention: protection against daytime mosquitoes
Japanese encephalitis	Several different viruses carried by mosquitoes	Worldwide, although high-risk areas include China, Korea, India, SE Asia	Headache, stiff neck, confusion, irritability, fever, weakness, dizziness, tremors, seizures, paralysis, lethargy, delirium, coma, death	Treatment: symptomatic only Prevention: Vaccine (Je-Vax) recommended only for rural area in high-risk Asian countries for travel more than 30 days.

Continued

TABLE 4–7.
(CONTINUED)

DISEASE	TRANSMISSION METHOD	INFECTED COUNTRIES	SEVERITY/SYMPTOMS	TREATMENT/PREVENTION
Leptospirosis	Exposure to the urine of animals by swimming or bathing in contaminated fresh water	Subtropical and tropical countries pose highest risk	High fever, severe headache, diarrhea, eye inflammation, internal bleeding, liver and kidney failure	Treatment: antibiotics as early as possible Prevention: Avoid fresh water activities in high-risk countries
Malaria	Parasite transmitted by *Anopheles* mosquitoes	Found in every tropical and subtropical country in the world	Flu-like with possible nausea and vomiting, jaundice; fatal without prompt treatment Typically presents within 10–30 days of exposure but can occur up to 1 year	Treatment and prevention: mefloquine (Larium), atovaquone/proguanil (Malarone), or doxycycline Minimize mosquito exposure
Plague	Bacteria carried by rodents and transmitted by fleas	Africa, SE Asia, parts of South America and the United States; risk in rural, mountainous areas	Lymphadenopathy, fever, chills, headache, malaise, fatigue, and GI symptoms; can be fatal without treatment	Streptomycin antibiotics, sulfonamides for children Prevention: insect repellents, avoid handling animals, consider preventive antibiotics Vaccine pending
Polio	Viral infection transmitted in contaminated water or food	Most developing countries in Africa, Asia, Central America, India, the Middle East, and Eastern Europe	Flu-like symptoms, fever, headache, stiff neck and back, myalgia; leading to paralysis. Can be fatal.	Treatment is symptomatic. Prevention: Universal immunization with vaccine is required in infancy. Booster necessary for adults traveling to endemic areas. Inactivated polio vaccine is used.

Rabies	Virus transmitted from exposure to saliva from an infected animal	Worldwide except Antarctica	Disease is nearly always fatal once symptoms develop.	Treatment: rabies human rabies immune globulin (HRIG) after bite(s), vaccine, if not previously vaccinated (previously vaccinated only require booster vaccine); immediately clean wound thoroughly with soap and water Prevention: vaccine is available; does not eliminate need for treatment after exposure
Severe acute respiratory Syndrome (SARS)	Coronavirus spread by infected droplets from coughing or sneezing	First identified in China in 2003; not currently active	High fever, cough, dyspnea, atypical pneumonia, acute respiratory distress	Supportive care Prevention: hand hygiene, avoid contact with SARS patients
Severe acute respiratory syndrome 2 (SARS-2)	Coronavirus spread by infected droplets	First identified in China in December 2019	Range of clinical manifestations from no symptoms to critical illness. Fever, cough, sore throat, malaise, headache, muscle aches, nausea, vomiting, diarrhea, loss of taste/smell to shortness of breath, hypoxia, respiratory failure, septic shock, multiple organ dysfunction	Supportive care Vaccines Monoclonal antibodies Oral/IV antivirals

Continued

TABLE 4–7.
(CONTINUED)

DISEASE	TRANSMISSION METHOD	INFECTED COUNTRIES	SEVERITY/SYMPTOMS	TREATMENT/PREVENTION
Typhoid fever	Bacterial infection with *Salmonella typhi* in contaminated food and water	Any region where food or water is contaminated; common after natural disasters in urban areas of poor countries	Flu-like symptoms, fever, diarrhea, and/or constipation; untreated, can last up to 4 weeks and is fatal in 10% of cases; patients can remain infectious after resolution of symptoms	Antibiotics essential; ciprofloxacin is antibiotic of choice, oral rehydration. Prevention: vaccination recommended for travelers to high-risk countries more than 4 weeks; bottled water only
Yellow fever	Arbovirus transmitted by mosquito	African countries near the equator and in tropical parts of South America	Flu-like symptoms, headache, fatigue, fever, nausea, vomiting, constipation, jaundice, hemorrhagic fever; fatal in 23% of severe cases	Supportive care; lifetime immunity after illness Prevention: vaccination prior to traveling to endemic areas; required for entry into certain countries. Live vaccine contraindicated in pregnancy, infants, lactation, immunocompromised.

CASE STUDIES

CASE 1

An 18-year-old male first year college student complains of losing weight and fatigue for 1 month. He states he is chronically tired, cannot get enough sleep, and feels feverish, but he does not have a thermometer in his dorm room. He has occasional aching joints. Of note is a cold a few weeks ago with a sore throat. He went to the university clinic at that time, had a rapid strep test done, and was told it was negative. He is concerned because he has missed more than eight classes this month.

Past Medical History: Usually healthy. Few occasional colds. Was told he had a heart murmur but not sure if he still does. Chickenpox at age 8. No past surgeries or hospitalizations; not sure of his immunization status. No current medications, no known drug allergies (NKDA).

1. Should you be concerned about measles, mumps, rubella, polio, diphtheria, or pertussis because he does not know if his immunizations are up to date?
2. What other history is needed?

Exam: No lymphadenopathy, pharynx pink without exudate, systolic murmur best heard over the second intercostal space, no joint swelling or tenderness, no rash or skin lesions

3. What is your differential diagnosis?
4. What initial diagnostic and management plan is appropriate?

CASE 2

A 6-year-old boy whose parents both are quite worried because his "hands are swollen, and his eyes are red." Has had a low-grade fever for over 1 week; highest 101°F. He also had a runny nose so mother thought he had a cold. Yesterday, his eyes were red, but they did not notice anything about the hands. Today, his eyes are very red, his lips are red and swollen, and hands are swollen and beginning to peel.

Past Medical History: No childhood illnesses; occasional colds; one or two ear infections as a baby.

Bilateral hernia repair at age 9 months. Immunizations up to date.

1. What are you looking for in a physical exam?
2. What do you suspect from this child's presentation?
3. What is your management plan?

CASE 3

A 14-month-old female infant whose father states, "She had a high fever a few days ago. Now she has a rash." She visited the practice 4 days ago for persistent fever of 2-day history. Fever as high as 104°F. Diagnosed with viral syndrome and sent home with instructions for fever management and to push fluids. Now returns, afebrile, but has a light red rash on her chest and back. Appetite poor, drinking liquids. Her face was flushed when she had the fever, but now her face is pale.

Past Medical History: History of recurrent otitis media; four episodes in 9 months. Immunizations up to date. No current medications.

1. What other history is needed?
2. What screening tests should be done?
3. What is the likely diagnosis and what management is appropriate?

CASE STUDIES DISCUSSION

CASE 1

1. Should you be concerned about measles, mumps, rubella, polio, diphtheria, or pertussis because he does not know if his immunizations are up to date?

   No, it is unlikely that he has missed these immunizations because they would have been required upon entrance to college.

2. What other history is needed?

   Health of his roommates, dorm-mates, and friends; any rash, specific joint pain and swelling; how much weight has he lost; has he had any night sweats or cough; tick bite or outdoor exposure; and his sexual orientation and partner history (how many, use of sexually transmitted infection (STI) protection, any symptoms of STIs in partners), history and symptoms of STIs, any swollen glands, other associated symptoms

3. What is your differential diagnosis?

   Rheumatic fever, mononucleosis (unlikely with no lymphadenopathy), Lyme disease (dependent on history of exposure), HIV primary infection (unlikely without additional symptoms), viral illness (unusual to last this long and be unaccompanied by rash)

4. What initial diagnostic and management plan is appropriate?

   Aortic murmur is significant and rheumatic fever should be highly suspected. Immediate referral to cardiologist is essential with initiation of penicillin treatment. Initial diagnostic testing would include CBC, ESR, C-reactive protein, streptococcal antibody titer, ECG, and two-dimensional (2D) echocardiography.

CASE 2

1. What are you looking for in a physical exam?

   Fever, cervical lymphadenopathy, rash, skin desquamation in groin; eye, ear, nose, throat exam for signs of local infection; cardiac exam for signs of pericarditis, myocarditis; neurologic exam for signs of meningitis; abdominal exam for hepatosplenomegaly; musculoskeletal exam for arthritis; skin for rash

2. What do you suspect from this child's presentation?

   Kawasaki disease

3. What is your management plan?

   Immediate referral to pediatric cardiologist

CASE 3

1. What other history is needed?

   Her contact with other children and if any of them have been ill; does she seem to have a sore throat; how is she eating, sleeping; activity level

2. What screening tests should be done?

   If sore throat is present, a throat swab and a CBC with differential will rule out group A beta-hemolytic streptococcal infection.

3. What is the likely diagnosis and what management is appropriate?

   Given the history of high fevers that relented on the onset of rash on day 4, it is likely to be roseola. Expected physical examination findings would be a blanching erythematous maculopapular rash and may have adenopathy. Rule out otitis media. Continue supportive management.

REFERENCES

American Academy of Pediatrics. (2021). *Red Book 2021: Report of the Committee on Infectious Diseases* (29th ed.). Elk Grove Village, IL: Author.

American Hearth Association. (2021). *Prevention of infective endocarditis.* https://www.heart.org/-/media/files/health-topics/infective-endocarditis/infective-endocarditis-wallet-card.pdf

Burns, C., Dunn, A., Brady, M., Starr, N., & Blosser, C. (2019). *Pediatric primary care* (7th ed.). St. Louis, MO: Saunders.

Centers for Disease Control and Prevention. (2017). *Blood-borne infectious diseases: HIV/AIDS, hepatitis B, hepatitis C management and treatment guidelines.* http://www.cdc.gov/niosh/topics/bbp/

Centers for Disease Control and Prevention. (2018). *Preparation and planning for bioterrorism emergencies.* http://emergency.cdc.gov/bioterrorism/prep.asp

Centers for Disease Control and Prevention. (2019a). *Parvovirus B19 (fifth disease).* http://www.cdc.gov/parvovirusb19/fifth-disease.html

Centers for Disease Control and Prevention. (2019b). Increase in Measles Cases—United States, January 1-April 26, 2019. *MMWR: Morbidity and Mortality Weekly Report 68*(17), 402–404. https://www.cdc.gov/mmwr/volumes/68/wr/mm6817e1.htm.

Centers for Disease Control and Prevention. (2019c). *Reported cases of Lyme disease by year, United States.* http://www.cdc.gov/lyme/stats/chartstables/casesbyyear.html

Centers for Disease Control and Prevention, Division of Global Migration and Quarantine. (2019). *Protection against mosquitoes, ticks, fleas and other insects and arthropods.* http://www.cdc.gov/travel/yellowBookCh3-InsectsArthropods.aspx

Centers for Disease Control and Prevention, Division of Global Migration and Quarantine. (2021). *Lyme disease.* Retrieved from http://wwwn.cdc.gov/travel/yellowBookCh4-LymeDisease.aspx

Centers for Disease Control and Prevention. (2021). *West Nile virus update: United States.* www.cdc.gov/ncidod/dvbid/westnile/index.htm

Centers for Disease Control and Prevention. (2022a). *Recommended immunization schedule for adults aged 19 years and older—United States, 2013.* http://www.cdc.gov/vaccines/adults/index.html

Centers for Disease Control and Prevention. (2022b). *HIV by group.* http://www.cdc.gov/hiv/group/index.html.

Centers for Disease Control and Prevention. (2022c). *Social Determinants of Health at CDC.* https://www.cdc.gov/about/sdoh/index.html.

Centers for Disease Control and Prevention. (2023). *Recommendations & guidelines of the ACIP: Altered Immunocompetence: General best practice guidelines for immunization.* https://www.cdc.gov/vaccines/hcp/acip-recs/general-recs/immunocompetence.html

ClinicalInfoHIV.gov. (n.d.). *Clinical Guidelines.* https://clinicalinfo.hiv.gov/en/guidelines

Gilbert, D., Chambers, H. F., Eliopolis, G., Chambers, H., & Saag, M. (2022). *The Sanford guide to antimicrobial therapy* (52nd ed.). Sperryville, VA: Antimicrobial Therapy, Inc.

Goroll, A., & Mulley, A. (2020). *Primary care medicine: Office evaluation and management of the adult patient* (8th ed.). Wolters Kluwer Health

National Institutes of Health. (2022). *Recommendations for use of antiretroviral drugs in pregnant HIV-1-infected women for maternal health and interventions to reduce perinatal HIV transmission in the United States.* Retrieved from http://aidsinfo.nih.gov/guidelines

South Carolina Department of Health and Environmental Control Bureau of Disease Control. (2022). *Childcare exclusion list.* http://www.scdhec.gov/health/childteenhealth/schoolexclusion/

CHAPTER 5

COMMON PROBLEMS OF THE SKIN

Aaron M. Sebach, PHD, DNP, MBA, AGACNP-BC, FNP-BC, NP-C, CP-C, CEN, CPEN, CGNC, CLNC, CNE, CNECL, SFHM

General Approach

- Dermatologic complaints may be indicative of a dermatologic disorder or a symptom of a systemic problem.
- Dermatologic disorders can have a profound impact on a patient's self-image. Incorporate psychological assessments for patients with dermatologic disorders and address the assessments in the treatment plan.
- Utilize proper terminology to describe dermatologic lesions (Tables 5–1 and 5–2).
- The most important part of a dermatologic assessment is a thorough history.
- Physical examinations are best performed in a well-lit room with a penlight for illumination and shadowing (to determine if a lesion is raised), a Wood's lamp for fluorescing certain types of lesions, a magnifying lens or dermatoscope, glass slides for diascopy (to determine blanching) and skin scrapings, potassium hydroxide (KOH) solution (to illuminate hyphae), 5% acetic acid for aceto-whitening (to illuminate human papilloma virus lesions), mineral oil for suspected scabies, Giemsa or Wright stains (to assess blood morphology), and a microscope.
- Physical examinations should include appearance of the patient (comfortable, agitated, toxic) and vital signs. Toxic patients should be immediately referred to an emergency department.

DERMATOLOGIC SIGNS TO BE ASSESSED AND DOCUMENTED

- Distribution of lesion (generalized or localized, central or peripheral, symmetric or asymmetric, predilection for certain body areas such as extensor or flexor surfaces and intertriginous areas, sun-exposed or pressure areas)

TABLE 5–1. MORPHOLOGIC DEFINITIONS FOR PRIMARY SKIN LESIONS

TERM	DEFINITION AND EXAMPLE	SIZE
Macule	Flat, non-palpable, colored lesion (e.g., freckle)	Up to 5 mm
Patch	Flat, non-palpable, colored lesion (e.g., port-wine stain)	Up to 10 mm
Papule	Solid, elevated, circumscribed lesion (e.g., nevus)	Up to 10 mm
Nodule	Solid, elevated, circumscribed lesion extending into the dermis or subcutaneous tissue (e.g., lipoma, cyst)	0.5–1.2 cm
Vesicle	Fluid-filled, elevated, circumscribed lesion (e.g., herpes simplex)	Up to 5 mm
Cyst	Encapsulated, fluid-filled mass (e.g., epidermoid cyst)	Variable
Bullae	Fluid-filled, elevated, circumscribed lesion (e.g., second-degree burn, bullous pemphigoid)	Larger than 10 mm
Pustule	Pus-filled, elevated, circumscribed lesion (e.g., acne)	Up to 5 mm
Wheal	Elevated, pruritic, plaques caused by local dermal edema (e.g., hives, urticaria)	0.5 to 10 cm diameter
Tumor	Solid, elevated mass	Variable

TABLE 5–2. MORPHOLOGIC DEFINITIONS FOR SECONDARY SKIN LESIONS

LESION	DEFINITION	EXAMPLE
Scale	Dried accumulations of epithelium	Psoriasis
Crust	Dried serum, blood, or pus	Impetigo
Ulcer	Sharply defined, deep erosion	Decubitus ulcer
Scar	Fibrosis that replaces normal skin after injury	Keloid
Lichenification	Induration and thickening of skin resulting from chronic scratching or rubbing	Eczema
Fissure	Linear split through dermis and epidermis	Cheilitis

- Arrangement of lesions (discrete, confluent, scattered, linear, zosteriform, polycyclic, grouped, patchy, accurate, reticular, scarlatiniform)
- Shape or configuration of the primary lesion (annular, oval, nummular, iris, pedunculated, verrucous, umbilicated, gyrate, serpiginous)
- Color of lesions (erythematous, violaceous, hypomelanotic, depigmented, flesh colored, hypermelanotic, variegated)

- Borders or margins of lesions (well-demarcated or ill-defined)
  - Palpable qualities (soft, firm, mobile, fixed, hard, fluctuant, tender, hot/warm/cool, smooth, rough, indurated)
  - Measured dimensions (diameter, width, length, elevation, depression)
  - Descriptive terms (lichenified, atrophied, sclerosed, pigmented, friable, hyperkeratotic, weeping, crusted, mobile or nonmobile, hypertrophic/keloidal, excoriated)
  - Morphology of primary and secondary lesions (see Tables 5–1 and 5–2)
  - Associated symptoms involving hair, vision, nails, mucous membranes, lymphatic system, hepatosplenomegaly, and/or neurologic changes

CHANGES ASSOCIATED WITH AGING

Should be identified and recognized as normal, such as dermatoheliosis or photoaging of the skin evidenced by wrinkles and drying, pigment changes, pseudo scars, senile purpura, solar lentigines, alopecia, seborrheic keratoses (benign epithelial growths that occur with aging and become darkened in color; have a warty, greasy surface; and are raised papules or plaques, 1–3 cm, with a characteristic "stuck on" appearance; no treatment necessary unless skin cancer cannot be ruled out, then biopsy and excise)

HEALTH MAINTENANCE AND SCREENING GUIDELINES

- Skin cancer is the most common cancer in the United States.
- Sun exposure, especially early in life, has been identified as a risk factor for skin cancer.
- Primary prevention involves counseling patients to avoid sun exposure and to protect themselves with appropriate sunscreen and clothing.
- Secondary prevention involves screening for skin lesions with premalignant or malignant characteristics during routine health exams and referring patients at increased risk for melanoma to specialists.
- Tertiary prevention involves removal of precancerous lesions, such as suspicious moles and actinic keratoses. Actinic (solar) keratoses are due to sun exposure and may be precursors to squamous cell carcinoma. Lesions are single or multiple, discrete, flat, or slightly raised, dry, scaly, and brownish or reddish up to 1.5 cm in size. Biopsies are indicated if the lesions are inflamed or indurated. Techniques for lesion removal include liquid nitrogen, curettage, laser ablation, photodynamic therapy, or fluorouracil cream application.

USE OF TOPICAL STEROIDS

- Topical steroids should be prescribed at the lowest dosage and for the shortest duration.
- Table 5–3 reflects topical steroids by potency.
- Fluorinated steroids result in tissue thinning when used long term. Avoid using on the face and genital region.

RED FLAGS

- *Anaphylaxis* may evolve rapidly from a variety of exposures, including drugs, exercise, food, insect stings, and latex; rapidly evolving symptoms may include hives, pruritus, flushing, shortness of breath, wheezing, tachycardia, difficulty swallowing, nausea, vomiting, abdominal cramping, and possible shock. Epinephrine and other emergency measures for anaphylactic reactions include:
  - Dose of epinephrine 1:1,000 (aqueous) 0.01 mL/kg per dose administered subcutaneously.
  - Epinephrine dose infants/children: 0.01 mg/kg, max 0. 3 mg/dose; adults: 0.1–0.5 mg, max dose 1 mg

TABLE 5–3.
COMMON TOPICAL STEROIDS (RANKED BY POTENCY, HIGHEST TO LOWEST)

POTENCY	EXAMPLE
Very High	Augmented betamethasone dipropionate 0.05% (Diprolene), clobetasol propionate 0.05% (Clobex, Olux), desoximetasone 0.25% (Topicort), halobetasol propionate 0.05% (Lexette, Ultravate), halobetasol propionate 0.01% (Bryhali, Duobrii)
High	Amcinonide 0.1%, clobetasol propionate 0.025% (Impoyz), fluocinonide 0.05%, halcinonide 0.1% (Halog), mometasone furoate 0.1%, triamcinolone acetonide 0.5%
Medium	Betamethasone dipropionate 0.05% (Sernivo), betamethasone valerate 0.12% (Luxiq), clocortolone pivalate 0.1% (Cloderm), flurandrenolide 0.05% (Cordran), fluticasone propionate 0.05% (Cutivate), triamcinolone acetonide 0.2% (Kenalog)
Lower Medium	Hydrocortisone butyrate 0.1% (Locoid), hydrocortisone probutate 0.1% (Pandel), prednicarbate 0.1%, triamcinolone acetonide 0.025%
Low	Alclometasone dipropionate 0.05%, desonide 0.05% (DesOwen, Verdeso), fluocinolone acetonide 0.01% (Capex, Synalar)
Lowest	Hydrocortisone acetate 2.5% (Analpram HC, Pramosone), hydrocortisone 1% (Epifoam, Proctofoam HC), hydrocortisone Base 2.5% (Texacort), Hydrocortisone 1%

◇ If life-threatening systemic anaphylaxis occurs, call 911 and emergency transport; give epinephrine as above; start IV, oxygen, and inhaled albuterol (Proventil) nebulizer if bronchospasm is severe.

♦ *Necrotizing fasciitis* is a rapidly progressing deep infection of the subcutaneous tissue that presents as an area or rapidly enlarging erythematous, edematous plaque with a central area of necrosis, pain out of proportion to the degree of cellulitis, fever, and crepitation. It is caused by beta-hemolytic *Streptococcus* and/or *Staphylococcus*. Urgent hospitalization for surgical debridement and IV antibiotics is essential to avoid excessive tissue loss or rapid multi-system failure.

♦ *Malignant melanoma* has five cardinal signs: asymmetry; border is irregular, often scalloped, and poorly defined; color is variable from within the lesion; diameter is large (greater than 6.0 mm); and elevation is almost always present with subtle or obvious surface distortion. It is best assessed by side-lighting of the lesion.

Allergy

CONTACT DERMATITIS

Description

♦ Cutaneous reaction to an external agent—either irritant or allergen (e.g., metal, plants, chemicals, or food substances)

Etiology

♦ Eighty percent of cases are due to universal irritants (soap, detergents, or organic solvents). Irritant contact dermatitis is due to direct toxicity of the skin (e.g., from detergent) without prior sensitization.

♦ Allergic contact dermatitis is a hypersensitivity reaction due to previous immune sensitization (e.g., poison ivy, oak, antimicrobials, adhesive tape, latex).

Incidence and Demographics

♦ Less common in African Americans due to greater compaction of the stratum corneum resulting in an improved barrier function.

♦ More common in females than males due to social and environmental factors.

- Common in all ages; age has no influence on sensitization.
- Occupational sensitization a common cause of disability in industry.

Risk Factors

- Exposure to irritant or allergen.
- Prior sensitization to allergen.
- Atopic dermatitis is associated with an increased risk of irritant contact dermatitis due to a compromised skin barrier.

Prevention and Screening

- Protective clothing in the presence of potential exposure.
- Avoidance of known irritants/allergens.

Assessment

History

- Pruritic rash in unnatural pattern on exposed skin with associated burning sensation
- Known exposure to irritant or allergen
- Acute onset affecting the hands and face as well as sun-exposed skin
- May include systemic symptoms of toxicity if extensive involvement

Physical Exam

- Morphology: erythematous papules, vesicles, or bullae on an inflamed background; scaling, erythema, edema; thickened skin and weepy; local area warm and swollen
- Location/distribution: exposed skin surfaces in unnatural pattern, mimicking possible path of irritant
- Irritant or allergen may be obvious by location of the rash
- Metal allergy: most common offender is nickel in jewelry and clothing
  - ◊ Distribution: neck, wrists, waist, strap line, ear lobes
  - ◊ Generally mild and chronic with scaling, pigmentation changes, and pruritus

- Plant dermatitis
  - Distribution and arrangement are often linear
  - Most caused by poison ivy, poison oak, and poison sumac
  - Secondary signs: weeping, scaling, edema, crusting, and excoriation

Diagnostic Studies

- Primarily a clinical diagnosis
- Patch testing may be warranted for severe or recurrent episodes with unclear etiology

Differential Diagnosis

- Atopic dermatitis
- Nummular eczema
- Impetigo
- Scabies
- Psoriasis

Management

Nonpharmacologic Treatment

- Remove offending irritant or allergen.
- Wash potentially contacted clothing.
- Bathe in tepid water with soap to wash allergen/irritant off skin.
- Use cool compresses with astringent (Domeboro or Burow's solution), pramoxine-containing emollient (Sarna or CeraVe Itch Relief) or colloidal oatmeal suspension (Aveeno) to treat pruritus.

Pharmacologic Treatment

- Oral antihistamines (diphenhydramine, hydroxyzine, loratadine, or cetirizine) should be used for pruritus (dose all pharmacologic interventions by weight in pediatric patients) with best time for administration before sleep because of sedating side effects.

- Topical antihistamines not currently recommended
- Topical corticosteroids may be considered based on the severity and location of the dermatitis
    - High- to mid-potency corticosteroids can be used on thicker skinned areas (e.g., scalp, torso)
    - Low-potency corticosteroids can be used on thinner skinned areas (e.g., neck)
- Systemic steroids may be considered for severe or extensive involvement
    - Prednisone: Begin at 60 mg in adults and taper over 2 to 3 weeks, depending upon the severity of symptoms.
    - Methylprednisolone dose pack is inadequate
- Oral antibiotics should be utilized for infected lesions
- Ultraviolet A (UVA)-Ultraviolet B (UVB) or Psoralen ultraviolet A (PUVA) treatments

How Long to Treat

- Length of treatment determined by extent of involvement and response; often 1 to 2 weeks

Special Considerations

- Steroids should be avoided in pregnancy unless clinically warranted.
- Distribution of symptoms may help determine causative agent.

When to Consult, Refer, Hospitalize

- Consult with/refer to an allergist for patch testing if indicated.
- Hospitalization should be considered for toxic or unstable patients (infants, older adults).

Follow-Up

Expected Course

- The course is usually dictated by irritant or allergen and extent of involvement.
- Metal allergies tend to be low-level and chronic, with possible lichenification and hyperpigmentation.

Complications

- Toxicity and secondary infection

URTICARIA

Description

- Dermis and subcutaneous tissue reaction to various stimuli characterized by erythematous wheals that appear on any part of the body
- Lesions may be round, oval, or form rings or arcs; pruritic; and pale
- Acute urticaria—hives, or wheals, appear abruptly and may last 24 to 36 hours
- Chronic urticaria—lesions persist for longer than 6 weeks
- Spontaneous urticaria: no identifiable causative factor
- Inducible urticaria: specific identifiable causative factor
- May occur with angioedema or with generalized anaphylaxis

Etiology

- May be allergic or nonallergic, immune globulin E (IgE)–mediated or non-IgE–mediated hypersensitivity resulting in a release of chemical mediators (histamine, prostaglandins, serotonin, kinins) from cutaneous mast cells leading to increased vascular permeability
- Fluid extravasates from small blood vessels causing typical lesions
- Many and varied causes—include foods, medicines, inhalants, infectious agents, physical factors (heat, cold, exercise, sunlight)

Incidence and Demographics

- Experienced by up to 20% of population at some point
- Can occur at any age, although is more common in children and adolescents
- Acute urticaria is most common.
- Chronic urticaria can significantly affect quality of life.

Risk Factors

- History of allergies, asthma, atopic diseases

Prevention and Screening

- Allergen avoidance
- Sunscreen or protective clothing if solar urticaria

Assessment

History

- Complete review of recent exposure to possible causative factors (e.g., medications, foods, injections, infections, inhalations, animals)
- Family or personal history of previous episodes of urticaria, atopic disease
- Exposure to sun, cold, stress, water, exercise
- Extent of pruritus
- Assess for lip and hand swelling, shortness of breath, or signs of a more generalized reaction.

Physical Exam

- Mildly erythematous, blanching, flat-topped lesions with pale centers
- Lesions 2 mm to 20 cm in diameter, scattered or coalesced, generalized or localized distribution
- May appear and fade within 24 hours; may reappear later
- A linear distribution may suggest dermographism, reflecting urticaria induced by scratching
- Heat may intensify lesions
- Evaluate mucous membranes and airway
- Evaluate lungs for wheezing and blood pressure for hypotension

Diagnostic Studies

- If fever, assess for infectious underlying cause and perform appropriate diagnostic tests as needed (e.g., chest X-ray, urinalysis, complete blood count [CBC])
- If urticarial vasculitis is suspected, biopsy for hematoxylin and eosin and direct immunofluorescence is recommended to confirm the diagnosis.
- No routine diagnostic testing in acute spontaneous urticaria
- Chronic spontaneous urticaria may consider CBC, erythrocyte sedimentation rate (ESR), and/or C-reactive protein (CRP) based on identification of underlying cause

Differential Diagnosis

- Erythema multiforme
- Contact dermatitis
- Juvenile rheumatoid arthritis
- Mastocytosis
- Pityriasis
- Viral exanthem
- Arthropod bites

Management

Nonpharmacologic Treatment

- Avoid suspected offending agent.
- Avoid aspirin, alcohol, and nonsteroidal anti-inflammatory drugs.

Pharmacologic Treatment

- Oral antihistamines such as diphenhydramine (Benadryl) 5 mg/kg/day in four divided doses or hydroxyzine 2 mg/kg/day in three to four divided doses
- Topical steroids are not useful; systemic steroids should be used for severe or extensive reactions.

  - ◊ Dose of epinephrine 1:1,000 (aqueous) 0.01 mL/kg per dose administered subcutaneously.
  - ◊ Epinephrine dose infants/children: 0.01 mg/kg, max 0. 3 mg/dose; adults: 0.1–0.5 mg, max dose 1 mg
  - ◊ If life-threatening systemic anaphylaxis occurs, call 911 and emergency transport; give epinephrine as above; start IV, oxygen, and inhaled albuterol (Proventil) nebulizer if bronchospasm is severe.
- Prescribe an epinephrine auto-injector (EpiPen) for anaphylaxis treatment and for prophylaxis following bee stings for patients with an allergy.
- First-line therapy: second-generation H1 antihistamines (sgAHs)
- Consider a second antihistamine at night if symptoms are not well controlled.
- Leukotriene receptor agonists (e.g., montelukast, 10 mg daily) are effective as adjunct agents.
- First-generation antihistamines are not recommended because of sedation and safety considerations.

How Long to Treat

- Until symptoms resolve

Special Considerations

- Angioedema and anaphylaxis occur by the same mechanism as urticaria.
- Angioedema occurs in up to 50% of children with urticaria and usually involves the face, hands, and feet.
  - ◊ Anaphylaxis may evolve rapidly with hives, accompanied by airway edema, pruritus, flushing, wheezing, tachycardia, difficulty swallowing, nausea, vomiting, abdominal cramping, and possible shock.
  - ◊ A precise cause of urticaria is often not identified.

When to Consult, Refer, Hospitalize

- Refer to an allergist or immunologist if symptoms persistent for more than 6 weeks.
- Immediately transfer to emergency facility for anaphylaxis with emergency care en route.

Follow-Up

Expected Course

- The course is usually dictated by irritant or allergen and extent of involvement.

Complications

- Angioedema, anaphylaxis, or secondary site infection due to scratching

Eczematous Conditions

ATOPIC DERMATITIS

Description

- Chronic skin condition characterized by inflammation and intense itching along a typical pattern of distribution (e.g., extensor surfaces); the presentation frequently varies according to the age and race of the patient; pruritus is the most characteristic finding
- Scratch-itch-scratch cycle perpetuates and exacerbates the problem.
- Infantile atopic dermatitis lasts from birth to 2 years of age; facial involvement may be worse with teething; extensor surface involvement is often due to crawling.
- Childhood atopic dermatitis lasts from 2 years of age to puberty; affected areas are less vascular; flexor surfaces are commonly affected.
- Adult atopic dermatitis occurs following puberty and presents with thickened and lichenified plaques.

Etiology

- IgE-mediated inherited dermatitis that involves abnormality in the cell-mediated immune system
- Often a manifestation of multisystem atopy, which includes asthma, allergic rhinitis, and atopic dermatitis known as the atopic triad
- Filaggrin gene mutations increase the risk of atopic dermatitis.
- Environmental factors can trigger exacerbations (e.g., food allergens such as cow's milk, skin infections, irritants).

Incidence and Demographics

- Predominantly presents in childhood, with approximately 50% of patients diagnosed by 6 months and then approximately 75% diagnosed by age 5
- Those affected often have a family history of atopic problems such as an inherited IgE-mediated hypersensitivity
- White individuals are commonly affected, followed by African Americans.
- Males and females are affected equally.
- More common in those living in urban areas
- Seventy-five percent to 85% of those with atopic dermatitis will develop allergic rhinitis; 50% will develop asthma.

Risk Factors

- Family history of atopic problems such as an inherited IgE-mediated hypersensitivity; family history of filaggrin gene mutation
- History of asthma or allergic rhinitis
- Dry environment; repetitive skin abrasions
- Emotional stress; hormonal factors (pregnancy, menses, thyroid); infections

Prevention and Screening

- Environmental controls
- Coping skills
- Management of pruritus

Assessment

History

- Pruritic rash in classic distribution
  - Family history of atopic problems such as an inherited IgE-mediated hypersensitivity; family history of filaggrin gene mutation
  - History of asthma or allergic rhinitis

Physical Exam

- Morphology: initially poorly defined erythematous patches, papules, or patches, with or without scales; develops into red, weeping, crusted patches; eventually become lichenified
- Distribution: extensor and exposed surfaces in infants
- Flexor folds: antecubital and popliteal fossae; wrists, neck, and forehead of older children and adults; upper trunk
- In children, assess for allergic shiners—Dennie-Morgan lines around the eyes reflecting blood vessel congestion
- Associated findings: lichenification, excoriations, fissures and erosions, periorbital hyperpigmentation, rhinitis and/or asthma, dermatographism, keratosis pilaris, ichthyosis vulgaris, and cataracts in up to 10% of patients
- African Americans may lose pigmentation in lichenified areas.

Diagnostic Studies

- Mainly a clinical diagnosis
- IgE level
- Patch testing
- Skin biopsy
- Bacterial cultures to rule out *Staphylococcus aureus;* viral cultures to rule out herpes simplex virus

Differential Diagnosis

- Seborrheic dermatitis
- Nummular eczema
- Psoriasis
- Dermatophytosis
- Scabies
- Contact dermatitis

Management

Nonpharmacologic Treatment

- Acute weeping lesions: humidify environment; decrease use of hot water, soap, and abrasive clothing
- Take long, soaking baths in warm water for short periods of time—pat dry; do not use abrasive towels/rubbing; avoid water that is too hot.
- Liberal use of emollients and/or lubricating lotions after bathing. Emollients and humectants improve the barrier function of the skin, reduce pruritis and pain, reduce dryness, and rehydrate the skin
- Oatmeal baths for pruritus
- Relaxation techniques and behavior modification may be helpful in severe cases.
- Stress management techniques are useful to control flare-ups.
- UV phototherapy is often effective due to its immunosuppressive and anti-inflammatory effects; not recommended for use in children.

Pharmacologic Treatment

- Utilize a stepwise treatment approach.
- Topical corticosteroids are the mainstay of treatment. Potency is determined based on clinical response. Use twice a day and sparingly. Use for the shortest amount of time necessary.
- Topical calcineurin inhibitors: pimecrolimus (Elidel) or tacrolimus may be used as monotherapy or in combination with a topical corticosteroid.
- Crisaborole 2% ointment (Eucrisa): non-steroidal option to treat atopic dermatitis for patients with mild/moderate atopic dermatitis. Approved for children who are at least 3 months of age
- Dupixent (dupilumab injection) is a biologic approved for the treatment adults and children 6 months of age and older with moderate to severe atopic dermatitis that is not controlled with current treatment modalities
- Montelukast (Singulair): may use in children older than 2 years and in adults. There is a black box waring for psychiatric side effects such as depression, aggression, sleep disturbances, and suicidal ideation.
- Systemic steroids (prednisone) are sometimes warranted in severe flare-ups; begin at 60 mg and taper down over 2 to 4 weeks

- May need oral antibiotics for secondarily infected lesions
- UVA-UVB and PUVA treatments for recalcitrant cases
- JAK inhibitors—three Janus kinase (JAK) inhibitors are U.S. Food and Drug Administration (FDA) approved disease-modifying antirheumatic drugs (DMARDs). They reduce the overworking of the immune system to treat inflammatory conditions.
    - Abrocitinib (Cibinqo): oral treatment for adults with recalcitrant atopic dermatitis
    - Ruxolitinib (Opzelura): a short-term topical treatment for patients 12 and older for mild to moderate atopic dermatitis
    - Upadacitinib (Rinvoq): oral treatment for patients 12 and older for moderate to severe atopic dermatitis

How Long to Treat

- Prednisone treatment should be limited to a 2-week tapered course.
- Topical preparations are used intermittently as symptoms warrant.
- Treat acute flares until controlled while maintaining and then continuing nonpharmacologic treatment; may require occlusive dressings at night for 2 to 6 weeks.

Special Considerations

- Repeated courses of oral corticosteroids are not recommended and are associated with adverse systemic effects including weight gain, adrenal suppression, and glucose intolerance.
- Systemic steroids are usually contraindicated in pregnancy and lactation.
- Geriatric patients are predisposed to atrophic skin and steroids exacerbate atrophy; therefore, use topical steroids of lower potency.
- *Nummular eczema* is a chronic, pruritic, inflammatory dermatitis in coin-shaped 4–5 cm plaques; usually found on anterior aspects of the lower legs but may also appear on the trunk, hands, and fingers; pruritus is often intense.
    - Secondary skin changes include exudative crusting, scaling, excoriation, lichenification, and post-inflammatory hyperpigmentation.
    - Treatment is the same as for atopic dermatitis.
- *Dyshidrotic eczema* is an acute, chronic, or recurrent dermatosis of palms, fingers, and/or soles characterized by a sudden onset of deep pruritic rash on hands and feet, which may last for weeks.

  - ◇ Initially presents with clear vesicles in clusters on the palms and soles; later scaling, lichenification, and painful fissures
  - ◇ Pruritus is treated with wet dressings of Domeboro solution, oatmeal, high-potency corticosteroid cream twice a day, and oral antihistamines

When to Consult, Refer, Hospitalize

- Refer patients with suboptimal response to the treatment plan above or for PUVA or UVA-UVB treatment.
- Refer those requiring topical calcineurin inhibitors.

Follow-Up

- Every 2 weeks until well controlled

Expected course

- Chronic condition with subacute phases and acute flares
- Usually more symptomatic during winter months

Complications

- Secondary infection, cellulitis, or both
- Skin atrophy, striae from overuse of topical steroids

SEBORRHEIC DERMATITIS

Description

- Chronic, recurrent, and often pruritic inflammatory disease of the skin where sebaceous glands are most active (nasolabial folds, scalp, skin folds)
- Variable course; seldom resolves completely
- Can coexist with rosacea

Etiology

- Unknown definitive etiology; may have a hormonal component
- Proliferation of *Malassezia furfur* species is hypothesized

Incidence and Demographics

- Incidence of 1% to 3% of the population affected, males more than females
- Highest prevalence is infancy (first 3 months of life)
- Increased incidence in immunocompromised patients, particularly those with Parkinson's disease

Risk Factors

- Family history
- HIV infection
- Zinc or niacin deficiency
- Parkinson's disease

Prevention

- Daily cleansing of the skin with soap, water, and clean wash cloth

Screening

- None

Assessment

History

- Gradual onset of greasy, scaly rash on the face (glabella and nasolabial fold) and scalp
- May be associated with *slight* pruritus

- Greasy white skin flakes on clothing and in hair
- Facial mask use

Physical Exam

- Usually see a fine, dry, white, or yellow scale on an erythematous base, or
- Dull red plaques with thick, white, or yellow, scaly, greasy lesions
- Morphology: yellow/red, greasy, moist, sharply marginated lesions; 5–20 mm scaling macules and papules; hypopigmentation may be present in dark-skinned children
- Distribution: scalp, eyebrow, eyelids, nasolabial folds, cheek, behind ears, intertriginous areas
- Secondary signs: possible inflammatory base, sticky crusting (more common on ears), fissures (more common at ear attachments to the scalp)

Diagnostic Studies

- Diagnosis is clinical.

Differential Diagnosis

- Psoriasis
- Impetigo
- Actinic keratosis
- Dermatophytosis
- Atopic dermatitis
- Rosacea
- Systemic lupus erythematous

Management

Nonpharmacologic Treatment

- For infants: anti-seborrheic shampoo three times per week; leave on for 5 minutes before rinsing. For difficult infant scales, apply warm mineral or baby oil for 10 minutes before shampooing.

- Adolescents: Avoid cold creams and moisturizers, which may block sebaceous glands.
- Remove scaling of eyelashes with baby shampoo.

Pharmacologic Treatment

- Shampoo frequently with selenium sulfide (Selsun or Exsel), tar (Polytar, T/Gel, or Tegrin), or pyrithione zinc (Head & Shoulders) shampoos.
- Salicylic acid (T/Sal) may be helpful in removing crusts.
- Oral itraconazole or ketoconazole daily for 2 weeks is indicated for widespread disease in adults
- Topical corticosteroids can be used with potency based on the severity and location
- Use hydrocortisone lotion for resistant areas, and/or ketoconazole (Nizoral) cream

How Long to Treat

- Chronic condition requires initial therapy until symptoms resolve, followed by maintenance therapy of ketoconazole shampoo, lotions, and/or topical steroids

Special Considerations

- Systemic steroids are contraindicated in pregnancy and lactation unless clinically warranted.

When to Consult, Refer, Hospitalize

- Consult or refer for unresponsive cases.

Follow-Up

- Visits every 1 to 2 months during the maintenance phase to monitor for signs of skin atrophy

Expected Course

- Chronic condition requiring initial treatment phase and maintenance therapy

Complications

- Secondary infection
- Skin atrophy, striae from chronic topical steroids

Acne

ACNE VULGARIS AND NODULOCYSTIC ACNE

Description

- A polymorphic disorder of the pilosebaceous unit characterized by inflammation and a variety of lesions ranging from comedones to inflamed cysts on the face, upper torso, and back
    - Acne vulgaris consists of open and closed comedones, inflamed papules, and pustules.
    - Nodulocystic acne or acne conglobata consists of cysts, abscesses, and sinus tracts.
    - Acne fulminans is the most severe form and features suppuration of lesions; may have concurrent systemic symptoms such as fever and arthritis.

Etiology

Factors usually involved:

- Inflammation and immune response
- Sebaceous gland hyperplasia and excess sebum production
- Abnormal follicular differentiation
- Colonization with bacteria (e.g., *Propionibacterium*)
- Genetics
- Mechanical factors such as trauma, cosmetics, oral medications (e.g., corticosteroids, oral contraceptives, and lithium), and mechanical occlusion (e.g., helmets, padding, and other sports equipment)

Incidence and Demographics

- Most common skin condition; present in 80% to 85% of all adolescents because of increased androgen production
- Males are affected more than females; light-skinned people are more affected than darker-skinned people.
- Flares in perimenopausal women may occur because of elevated unopposed adrenal androgens.

Risk Factors

- Elevated circulating androgen hormones as described above
- Use of follicle-blocking cosmetics and hair spray
- Oral contraceptives with high progestin components; anticonvulsants; systemic or topical steroid use
- Genetic predisposition, male

Prevention and Screening

- Good daily skin hygiene, avoidance of follicle-blocking cosmetics that are oil-free and labeled as non-comedogenic

Assessment

History

- Onset associated with puberty or with excess androgen
- May include a history of oil-based cosmetic use and/or harsh scrubbing

Physical Exam

- Mild to moderate acne, or acne vulgaris
  - Presence of comedones, inflamed papules, pustules and cysts on the face, upper torso, and back
- Open comedones, or "blackheads" (follicular orifice is dilated)

- Closed comedones, or "whiteheads" (plug in the sebaceous duct enlarges)
  - Inflamed papules and pustules result from the proliferation of *Propionibacterium acnes*
- Severe acne or nodulocystic acne
  - Cysts and nodulocystic lesions develop as plug enlarges; may result in sinus tracts forming under the skin; inflamed cysts develop as abscesses
  - Possible presence of scarring from healed lesions

Diagnostic Studies

- Diagnosed clinically
- CBC and blood cultures may be indicated if the patient has acne fulminans and appears toxic
- Bacterial culture may be indicated to rule out folliculitis

Differential Diagnosis

- Rosacea
- Abscess
- Cutaneous manifestations of systemic lupus erythematosus (SLE)
- Furunculosis
- Tinea barbae
- Folliculitis
- Syringoma
- Milia

Management

Nonpharmacologic Treatment

- Gentle washing twice a day with mild soap such as Dove, Basis, or Neutrogena, or other non-comedogenic cleanser
- Avoid oil-based cosmetics and hairsprays, which can plug follicles.
- Avoid picking or squeezing lesions, as this may lead to scarring and hyperpigmentation.

Pharmacologic Treatment

- Mild Acne
  - No inflammation—topical retinoid (e.g., tretinoin 0.1%) and topical benzoyl peroxide
  - With inflammation—topical retinoid (e.g., tretinoin 0.1%) and topical antibiotic (e.g., clindamycin 1% foam, erythromycin 2% gel). Can use topical benzoyl peroxide as monotherapy or topical dapsone 7.5% as monotherapy
- Moderate Acne
  - No inflammation—topical retinoid (e.g., tretinoin 0.1%), topical dapsone 7.5%, topical benzoyl peroxide
  - With inflammation—topical retinoid (e.g., tretinoin 0.1%) and oral antibiotic (e.g., tetracycline 500 mg orally twice a day for 2 months; minocycline, 100 mg orally twice a day for 2 months).
- Severe Acne
  - Systemic isotretinoin 0.5–1 mg/kg/day in two divided doses. **(Women of childbearing age must be strongly counseled to use reliable contraception for 1 month before, during, and for 1 month following the use of the medication.)**
- Hormone Related
  - Oral contraceptives
  - Spironolactone 25 to 200 mg daily for 3 to 6 months. Only prescribe to women 25 and older. Monitor CBC, serum potassium, and blood pressure monthly.

How Long to Treat

- Treatment is long term and may continue for years. Topical agents should be started individually or with a combined keratolytic and antibiotic (e.g., Benzamycin gel) once a day and increased to twice a day after 1 to 2 weeks to avoid excessive drying.
- Start oral antibiotics twice to three times a day and taper over time to once a day after improvement is achieved.
- Systemic isotretinoin should be used for 15 to 20 weeks; treatment may restart after a 2-month drug holiday.

Special Considerations

- Advise patients that minimal response is expected in the first 4 to 6 weeks of therapy, and optimal response may take several months on the various regimens.
- Patients should be started on a single agent, with additional agents added as needed.

- Because topical treatments can be drying, start slow (once a day with one agent) and increase to twice a day, adding second and third agents one at a time.
- Sex: Women with polycystic ovaries or other hyperandrogenism and women with late-onset acne may benefit from the use of oral contraceptives with low androgenic activity.
- Race: Darker-skinned people are more likely to develop post-inflammatory hyperpigmentation. Azelaic acid cream possesses hypopigmentation properties and may be useful in limiting post-inflammatory hyperpigmentation.
- Most anti-acne drugs (topical and oral) cause photosensitivity reactions; sun exposure should be limited, and liberal use of oil-free sunscreen gel is advised.
- Pregnancy and lactation: Isotretinoin (Accutane) is a teratogen and must be avoided. **Women of childbearing age must be strongly counseled to use reliable contraception for 1 month before, during, and for 1 month following the use of the medication.** Use of the IPLEDGE (REMS) program is required with two approved forms of birth control for patients of childbearing potential due to the known teratogenic side effects of isotretinoin. Monthly negative pregnancy tests are required during the treatment course and 2 months after discontinuation of isotretinoin
- Laboratory monitoring for patients taking Isotretinoin (Accutane) includes lipid panel, CBC, liver function tests (LFTs), and glucose.

When to Consult, Refer, Hospitalize

- Referral to a dermatologist is appropriate if a suboptimal response is achieved after adequate trial on two or three of the above drugs and if isotretinoin is being considered.
- Dermatology should ideally prescribe Isotretinoin (Accutane).

Follow-Up

- Initial follow-up every 2 months until a stable regimen is established with successful control

Expected Course

- Long-term management often necessary for several years.

Complications

- Excess drying of the skin from topical agents
- Potentially severe side effects with Isotretinoin (Accutane), such as pseudotumor cerebri (increased risk with tetracycline), pancreatitis, hepatotoxicity, corneal opacities, blood dyscrasias, premature epiphyseal closure. Pregnancy category X.

ACNE ROSACEA

Description

- Chronic acneiform inflammation of the central third of the face characterized by redness and flushing
  - Does not involve comedones—the classic lesion of acne vulgaris
  - Characterized by episodes of remission and recurrence

Etiology

- Cutaneous vascular disorder of unknown etiology with the increased reaction of capillaries to triggers (e.g., spicy foods, exercise, stress, heat, sun exposure)
- Sebaceous gland hyperplasia
- Ocular manifestations such as conjunctivitis, blepharitis, and episcleritis occur

Incidence and Demographics

- More common in women than men and in those with fair skin
- Onset is between 30 and 50 years of age
- Rhinophyma is seen almost exclusively in men over the age of 40.

Risk Factors

- Fair skin (Fitzpatrick skin type I or II)
- Family history of rosacea
- Female sex

- Emotional stress
- Excessive alcohol, emotional stress, sunlight, and temperature extremes are triggers.
- Excessive alcohol consumption associated with flares

Prevention and Screening

- None

Assessment

History

- History of abnormal flushing of the central portion of the face after drinking hot or alcoholic beverages or eating spicy foods

Physical Exam

- Two millimeter to 3 mm papular and pustular discrete and clustered lesions on the central portion of the face on an erythematous base; rosy coloration of nose, chin, cheeks; no comedones
- Dilatation of the superficial capillaries causes flushing and eventually leads to telangiectasia.
- Ocular symptoms such as blepharitis or keratitis may be associated.
- Chronic symptoms can lead to lymphatic changes causing cellulitis.
- Irreversible hypertrophy of the nose (rhinophyma) is a result of chronic inflammation and is seen almost exclusively in men over age 40.

Diagnostic Studies

- None
- Diagnosis is clical

Differential Diagnosis

- Acne vulgaris
- Butterfly rash of SLE
- Cellulitis
- Mastocytosis
- Folliculitis
- Seborrheic dermatitis
- Contact dermatitis

Management

Nonpharmacologic Treatment

- Includes avoidance of triggers that cause facial flushing such as hot beverages, alcohol, spicy foods, exposure to sun and wind, emotional stress, and certain medications such as niacin

Pharmacologic Treatment

- Topical metronidazole (Metrogel) 0.75%, erythromycin 2%, or clindamycin (CleocinT) gel twice a day
- Tetracycline 250 mg orally two to three times a day
- Doxycycline (Vibramycin) 100 mg orally twice a day
- Doxycycline (Oracea) 40 mg orally daily. Controlled release anti-inflammatory dosing of doxycycline.
- Minocycline (Minocin) 50–100 mg orally twice a day
- Erythromycin 250 mg orally two to three times a day
- 1% Ivermectin in a Cetaphil base (Soolantra cream) daily

How Long to Treat

- Long-term initially at two to three times a day. dosing, tapering down to once a day maintenance dosing

- If there is no improvement with the above regimens, a trial of trimethoprim-sulfamethoxazole (TMP-SMX), oral metronidazole (Flagyl), or dapsone may be considered.

Special Considerations

- Use erythromycin with pregnant and lactating women.
- Menopausal women experiencing flushing associated with hormonal fluctuations may benefit from hormone replacement therapy (HRT) or clonidine (Catapres) if HRT is contraindicated.

When to Consult, Refer, Hospitalize

- Refer to dermatology If the treatment response is suboptimal.

Follow-Up

- 2 to 4 weeks initially
- Annual follow-up is indicated once the condition has stabilized

Expected Course

- The initial response is usually within 3 weeks; the maximum response is within 9 weeks.

Complications

- Rhinophyma, as described above, may require surgical debulking or more intense therapy by laser or light-based treatments

HIDRADENITIS SUPPURATIVA

Description

- A chronic suppurative disease of the apocrine gland region of the axillae, anogenital region, breasts, and scalp with development of sinus tracts and scarring

- The classic presentation of hidradenitis suppurativa (HS) is a double-comedone blackhead.
- May also be referred to as acne inversa

Etiology

- Unknown
- Believed to be multifactorial with genetic, hormonal, lifestyle, and environmental components

Incidence and Demographics

- Race: all, more extensive involvement in African Americans
- Age: most common in those 18 to 30 years of age
- Sex: more common in females than males

Risk Factors

- Family history
- Nodulocystic acne
- Obesity
- Smoking/tobacco use
- Apocrine duct obstruction (antiperspirant use)

Prevention and Screening

- Management of obesity
- Avoid antiperspirants in those who have had previous problems with them

Assessment

History

- Recurrent painful lesions with suppuration in the intertriginous areas (e.g., groin, axilla, perineum)

Physical Exam

- Fluctuant, tender, and erythematous nodules
- Seropurulent/purulent drainage from single or multiple openings on the skin
- Hypertrophic scarring, keloid, and sinus tract formation
- Dilated open comedones, often characteristic double comedones

Diagnostic Studies

- Cultures are not usually indicated because multiple pathogens colonize.

Differential Diagnosis

- Furuncle or carbuncle
- Cat-scratch disease
- Lymphadenitis
- Acne vulgaris
- Epidermal inclusion cyst

In Anogenital Involvement

- Sinus tracts and fistulas associated with ulcerative colitis and enteritis
- Lymphogranuloma venereum

Management

Nonpharmacologic Treatment

- Local heat
- Keep the area clean and dry
- Weight loss
- Avoid antiperspirants
- Smoking cessation

Surgical Treatment

- Initially incision and drainage of acute abscesses
- Excision of nodules or marsupialization of sinuses in chronic cases
- Complete excision of axillae or involved anogenital area to the fascia with split-skin grafting for extensive, chronic disease

Pharmacologic Treatment

- Oral antibiotics until resolution (may take weeks). Examples include:
  - Erythromycin 250–500 mg four times a day
  - Minocycline (Minocin) 100 mg twice a day
  - Tetracycline 250–500 mg twice a day
  - Doxycycline 50–100 mg twice a day
- Intralesional triamcinolone (5 mg/mL) diluted with lidocaine injected into the wall of the lesion, followed by incision and drainage
  - Oral prednisone taper (60 mg once a day initially, tapered over 14 days)
  - Oral isotretinoin 0.5–1 mg/kg/day in two divided doses
  - Tretinoin cream (0.05%) may be used if tolerated as it is irritating to the skin.
  - Adalimumab (Humira)–TNF biologic

How Long to Treat

- Chronic and recurrent disease: treat episodic flares with oral antibiotics and corticosteroids as identified under pharmacologic treatment above.
- For frequent flares or extensive involvement, continuous antibiotics are indicated pending surgical intervention.

Special Considerations

- Erythromycin is recommended for pregnant and lactating women.
- Lesions with continuous discharge should be cultured.

When to Consult, Refer, Hospitalize

- Referral to a surgeon is indicated for extensive and/or chronic involvement.
- Referral to a rheumatologist or dermatologist when unresponsive to treatment or in severe cases

Follow-Up

- Weekly during flares

Expected Course

- Usually recurrent flares; patients often achieve resolution after surgery
- Often spontaneous remission toward the end of the third decade of life

Complications

- Fistulas to urethra, bladder, and/or rectum
- Anemia of chronic disease

Papulosquamous Eruptions

PITYRIASIS ROSEA

Description

- **Benign self-limited maculopapular, red scaly, sometimes pruritic rash that presents with a sentinel herald patch, salmon in color, and sometimes mistaken for tinea, with multiple eruptions a few days to several weeks later. Self-limiting with spontaneous remission.**

Etiology

- Unknown, presumed to be viral

Incidence and Demographics

- Most common in the spring and fall months and in temperate climates
- Most common in individuals 10 to 25 years of age and in women.

Risk Factors

- Sharing a household with an affected person
- Female sex
- Age 10 to 25 years

Prevention and Screening

- None

Assessment

History

- Single, large herald patch appearing most commonly on the trunk, followed in 1 to 2 weeks by generalized exanthem; mild to moderate pruritus
- No systemic symptoms but may be preceded by a viral-like illness

Physical Exam

- The initial lesion is a "herald patch": 2 to 6 cm, round, scaly plaque, usually on the trunk
- Generalized fine, oval, 3 to 7 mm papules and plaques with a fine "collarette" scale
- Distribution on the trunk, often in a Christmas tree pattern, following skin lines
- Individual lesions will be concentrated on the lower trunk. Individuals with darker skin may describe the lesions as hyperpigmented.

Diagnostic Studies

- Clinical diagnosis
- Potassium hydroxide (KOH) scraping may assist in excluding tinea
- If a herald patch is absent and secondary syphilis cannot be excluded, serological testing should be performed.

Differential Diagnosis

- Drug eruptions
- Secondary syphilis
- Guttate psoriasis
- Tinea corporis
- Tinea versicolor
- Seborrheic dermatitis
- Erythema migrans
- Viral exanthems
- Nummular eczema

Management

Nonpharmacologic Treatment

- UV or natural sunlight exposure, although there is insufficient evidence that UV exposure reduces the duration of symptoms

Pharmacologic Treatment

- None usually necessary, but may use oral antihistamines or topical corticosteroids to relieve pruritus

How Long to Treat

- Spontaneous remission in 6 to 8 weeks

Special Considerations

- Premature delivery is a concern for pregnant women diagnosed during the first trimester

When to Consult, Refer, Hospitalize

- Refer to an obstetrician-gynecologist for complications identified during pregnancy

Follow-Up

- For patient reassurance or when the diagnosis is in question

Fungal and Yeast Infections

FUNGAL (DERMATOPHYTE) INFECTIONS

Description

- Superficial fungal infection of the keratinized layer of the skin, including the stratum corneum (epidermomycosis), nails (onychomycosis), and hair (trichomycosis)
- Infections are named by body part involved or, in the case of tinea versicolor, for the multicolored appearance

Etiology

- Caused by several dermatophytes with a regional predominance
- Three common dermatophytes in the United States: *Microsporum, Trichophyton,* and Epidermophyton

Epidermophyton

- Spread is by direct contact with an active lesion on an animal or another human; with fomites such as clothing, linens, or gym mats; or, rarely, from the soil.

Incidence and Demographics

- Affects all ages, races, and genders.
- More common in tropical climates and in warmer months in temperate climates
- More common in immunocompromised patients, including when secondary to prolonged use of topical steroids, with a greater risk of intractable infection.

Risk Factors

- Heat and humidity
- Obesity
- Immunocompromised state (e.g., HIV)
- Diabetes
- Chronic topical or oral corticosteroid use
- Hyperhidrosis

Prevention and Screening

- Climate control as appropriate: air conditioning; loose, cotton clothing
- Obesity management
- Air drying or using an electric hair dryer to dry intertriginous areas
- Dry athletic shoes between wearing
- Avoid walking barefoot in public bathing areas
- Wear cotton socks
- Avoid sharing combs, brushes, or hair ornaments
- Avoid occlusive ornaments: acrylic nails; synthetic jewelry, belts, shoes

Assessment

History

- Known exposure to others with tinea or high-risk population
- Mild to moderately pruritic localized "rash" or isolated lesion

Physical Exam

- Presentation differs based on the location of the lesion: tinea capitis, scalp; tinea manuum, hand; tinea faciei, face; tinea corporis, body; tinea barbae, beard; tinea cruris, groin; tinea unguium, nails; and tinea pedis, feet.
- Scaling erythematous plaque ranging from less than 1 cm up to 20 cm
- Varying shapes: annular (round), arciform, or polycyclic
- With or without pustules/vesicles
- Usually has an elevated, sharp border with central clearing
- Color is erythematous or hyperpigmented.
- Tinea manuum may be bilateral (50%); may occur with tinea pedis or tinea cruris
- May be confused with granuloma annulare, which is similar in appearance but is a self-limiting condition of the hands, feet, elbows, and knees
- Tinea cruris (groin), commonly known as jock itch
  - Usually, arciform or polycyclic and duller red in coloring
  - Often coexists with tinea pedis; infection transferred from feet to the groin
  - Maceration common in intertriginous areas
- Tinea pedis (foot), commonly known as athlete's foot
  - Erythema, maceration between toes
  - Diffuse desquamation with superficial white scales and possible bulla formation
  - Hyperkeratosis of soles
  - Painful fissuring/cracking along lateral borders of the soles and toe webs
  - Usually, bilateral foot involvement
- Tinea versicolor (trunk and neck)—also known as pityriasis versicolor
  - Superficial *Pityrosporum orbiculare* yeast that colonizes on human skin
    - Clinically significant in only some persons
    - Hypopigmented or hyperpigmented nummular macules
    - Discrete, scattered, or confluent patches
    - Usually asymptomatic but may be mildly pruritic
- Trichomycosis (hair): tinea capitis (head), and tinea barbae (beard)
  - Involves dermatophyte invasion of the hair follicle by *Trichophyton* dermatophytes
  - Inflammation of the hair follicle, alopecia
  - Painful, boggy, suppurative nodules with crusting/kerion (scab)

- Onychomycosis (nail): tinea unguium
  - Nails become white, brown, yellow, or black; the surface becomes roughened; eventually the nail separates from the nail bed (onycholysis)

Diagnostic Studies

- KOH microscopy should be ordered first. Tinea will present as hyphae; tinea versicolor appears as long hyphae and buds commonly referred to as "spaghetti and meatballs"
- Wood's lamp
  - Tinea capitis fluoresces green.
  - Tinea versicolor fluoresces faint yellow-green scales.
  - Tinea cruris does not fluoresce, although Wood's lamp exam can differentiate erythrasma, a bacterial infection that fluoresces coral-red.
- Fungal cultures can identify a fungus but it usually take weeks to grow.
  - Indicated only when an infection is resistant to treatment
- Polymerase chain reaction (PCR) can be used to identify fungi in nail specimens.
- Periodic acid–Schiff test is used to detect fungal organisms. The sensitivity is higher than KOH microscopy.

Differential Diagnosis

Based on the location of lesions and can include many scaling skin disorders:

- Psoriasis
- Erythrasma
- Candidiasis
- Contact dermatitis
- Seborrhea
- Dyshidrotic eczema
- Atopic dermatitis
- Lichen simplex chronicus
- Lichen planus
- Pityriasis rubra pilaris

- Pityriasis rosea
- Erythema migrans
- Polymorphic light eruption
- Phototoxic drug eruption
- SLE
- Beard folliculitis
- Scabies
- Impetigo
- Ecthyma

Management

Nonpharmacologic Treatment

- Treat chronic, immunocompromising conditions.
- Follow the preventive measures described above.

Pharmacologic Treatment

- Tinea capitis–griseofulvin (children, 10–20 mg/kg/day for 6 weeks; adults, 500–1000 mg) daily for 4 to 6 weeks. Selenium sulfide shampoo 1% to 2.5% can be used as adjuvant therapy and applied twice a week for 2 weeks.
- Tinea barbae and tinea manuum—griseofulvin (children, 10–20 mg/kg/day for 6 weeks, adults, 500–1000 mg) daily for 4 to 8 weeks. Other options include itraconazole 200 mg daily for 2 to 4 weeks or terbinafine 250 mg daily for 6 weeks.
- Tinea faciei, tinea corporis, tinea cruris, tinea pedis—clotrimazole 1% (Lotrimin), ketoconazole 2% (Nizoral), terbinafine 1% (Lamisil); apply to the affected area, including a 2-cm peripheral border, and rub in twice a day
- Tinea unguium (onychomycosis)—terbinafine (Lamisil) 250 mg orally once daily for 12 weeks (toenails) or 6 weeks (fingernails). This treatment is indicated for adults and not for children
- Tinea versicolor—topical selenium sulfide 2.5% shampoo applied to the skin for 30 minutes, then washed off; repeat 2 weeks later
- Systemic antifungal agents should be used for widespread, recurrent, or resistant infections, as well as onychomycosis.

How Long to Treat

- Resolution is slow, and treatment length depends on the location of the dermatophytosis; all treatments take weeks to months.
  - Tinea capitis and tinea barbae: 4 to 6 weeks
  - Tinea corporis, tinea manuum, tinea faciei: 4 to 6 weeks
  - Tinea cruris: 2 to 4 weeks
  - Tinea versicolor: 4 to 6 weeks
  - Tinea pedis: 4 to 12 weeks
  - Tinea unguium: 8 to 12 months

Special Considerations

- Side effects from systemic antifungal agents include hepatotoxicity and lowering of serum testosterone. Hepatic function should be evaluated before initiating oral antifungal agents and every 4 weeks thereafter.
- Most antifungals are contraindicated in pregnancy and in breastfeeding women.
- Closely review the patient's medication history. Complications may occur due to drug interactions because the -azole medications are metabolized by the cytochrome P450 3A4 (CYP3A4) enzyme system.
- Additional considerations include interactions between terbinafine and CYP1A2 substrates, CYP3A4 substrates, CYP2C9 substrates, and CYP2D6 inhibitors.

When to Consult, Refer, Hospitalize

- Refer to a dermatologist for extensive involvement or unresponsive infection.
- Consider hospitalization for immunosuppressed patients with extensive disease.

Follow-Up

- Every 4 weeks for re-evaluation and to monitor hepatic function

Expected Course

- Relapse is common.

Complications

- Loss of hair and nails

CANDIDIASIS (MONILIASIS)

Description

- A pruritic rash on moist cutaneous and mucosal sites (caused by a yeast-like, superficial fungus) in vulnerable persons when local immunity is interrupted

Etiology

- *Candida* species (*Candida albicans* [most common], *Candida glabrata, Candida tropicalis*) are normal inhabitants of mucosal surfaces and intestinal tracts of healthy persons
- Infection occurs when local or systemic immunity of the host is disrupted

Incidence

- All ages, both sexes equally, and all races can be affected.
- In babies, it is most common in the perineal (diaper) region.

Prevention and Screening

- None

Risk Factors

- Predisposing factors that alter immunity
- Immunocompromised states (e.g., HIV and chronic debilitation)
- Chemotherapy or broad-spectrum antibiotic therapy
- Diabetes or poly endocrinopathies
- Maceration from repeated immersion in water, skin folds

- Occlusive clothing that traps moisture, such as diapers or rubber boots, diapers' plastic outer covering
- Hyperhidrosis (excessive sweating)
- Obesity with redundant skin folds
- Corticosteroid use
- Pregnancy and oral contraceptives

Assessment

History

- Pruritic and/or burning sensation and rash in characteristic locations such as intertriginous areas, anogenital region, and redundant skin folds
- Painful or sensitive white, "stuck on" lesions of the oral mucosa with decreased taste and odynophagia ("thrush")
- White curd-like vaginal discharge is usually associated with pruritus, external dysuria, and dyspareunia (vulvovaginitis)
- Painful fissuring of the foreskin of uncircumcised males with dysuria
- Painful, inflamed nail folds, discolored nails, and a creamy discharge (paronychial candidiasis)
- Painful, congested ear canal with moist exudate (otitis externa)

Physical Exam

- Bright red, smooth macules
- Maceration is typical of intertriginous infections
- Scaling elevated border
- "Satellite" lesions: similar macules outside of the main lesion
- Oral and vaginal candidiasis: white, stuck on but removable plaques on inflamed mucosa
- Balanoposthitis: flattened pustules, edema, erosions, fissuring on the erythematous surface of the penis
- Candida otitis externa: edematous ear canal with macerated appearance and moist, white, scaly exudate

Diagnostic Studies

- KOH preparation under the microscope will reflect buds and pseudo-hyphae in clusters.
- Fungal cultures can identify specific species but *usually* are not done because it can take 1 to 2 weeks for results.

Differential Diagnosis

Oral Candidiasis

- Hairy leukoplakia
- Pernicious anemia
- Geographic tongue
- Bite irritation

Genital Candidiasis

- Bacterial vaginosis
- Lichen planus
- Condyloma acuminatum
- Scabies
- Inverse pattern psoriasis
- Erythrasma

Intertriginous Areas

- Eczema
- Atopic dermatitis
- Contact dermatitis
- Dermatophytosis

Paronychial Candidiasis

- Herpetic whitlow
- S. *aureus* paronychia

Management

Nonpharmacologic Treatment

- Management of underlying predisposing factors such as obesity and diabetes
- Air exposure of affected areas, such as the diaper region in infants
- Careful drying of intertriginous areas and redundant skin folds
- Wear cotton undergarments.
- Avoid tight, synthetic clothing.

Pharmacologic Treatment

- Oral (thrush)
  - Nystatin (Mycostatin) oral suspension 4–6 mL (adults), 2 mL (children), swish and swallow four times a day
  - Clotrimazole 10 mg troches 3–5x/day (3 years and older), dissolve in the mouth
  - Systemic ketoconazole (Nizoral) 200 mg orally once to twice a day (adults; usually not recommended in children), fluconazole (Diflucan) 100 mg orally once. to twice a day (adults; check manufacturer literature for children), itraconazole (Sporanox) 100 mg orally once a day (adults; not recommended for children)
- Intertriginous and anogenital infections
  - Castellani paint × 1 (phenol topical)
- Topical antifungal: clotrimazole 1% cream, miconazole (Monistat) 2% cream, ketoconazole (Nizoral) 2% cream, econazole (Spectozole) 1% cream, terconazole (Terazol) 0.4 or 0.8% cream, terbinafine (Lamisil) 1% cream or solution twice a day, tolnaftate (Tinactin) 1% cream, solution, powder applied twice a day
  - Nystatin cream or ointment applied two to three times a day to diaper area in infants
  - Oral antifungal treatment, as described above, may be necessary for extensive or recurrent infections or when host immunity is suppressed.
  - Oral fluconazole (Diflucan 150 mg) × 1 has been successful in the treatment of vaginal candidiasis

How Long to Treat

- Oral candidiasis: 10 to 14 days
- Intertriginous and anogenital candidiasis: 1 to several weeks, depending on the extent of the infection and the immune status of the host
- Paronychial candidiasis: 2 to 4 weeks

Special Considerations

- Immunosuppressed and immunocompromised patients are subject to extensive and recurrent infections and may require a daily maintenance dose to limit recurrences.

When to Consult, Refer, Hospitalize

- Immunosuppressed patients with extensive or severe candidiasis, particularly oral/esophageal candidiasis, may require hospitalization or home IV infusion therapy of amphotericin B and nutrition supplementation.

Follow-Up

- Patients should be seen in 2 to 4 weeks and as needed to evaluate progress.

Expected Course

- Resolution can be expected in patients without immunosuppression, although predisposing factors such as obesity and poorly controlled diabetes may make recurrences common.

Complications

- Secondary infection of excoriated lesions
- Weight loss secondary to odynophagia with esophagitis

Bacterial Infections of the Skin

CELLULITIS

Description

- Acute bacterial infection of the dermis and subcutaneous tissues; can spread in a rapid, diffuse manner. Characterized by erythema, edema, warmth, and tenderness.
- Erysipelas is a type of superficial cellulitis caused by beta-hemolytic streptococci and accompanied by lymphatic involvement.

Etiology

- Usually caused by beta-hemolytic streptococci and *S. aureus*, although may also be caused by *Haemophilus influenzae* in children, *Pseudomonas aeruginosa* from hot tubs, and *Pasteurella* from animal bite wounds (e.g., cats)
- Occurs when a break in the skin allows bacteria to enter
- Non-purulent cellulitis is caused due to beta-hemolytic streptococci.

Incidence and Demographics

- Common in all age groups, genders, and ethnicities

Risk Factors

- Breaks in the skin from lacerations, abrasions, or excoriations, underlying dermatosis
- Prior diagnosis of cellulitis
- Diabetes mellitus
- Hematologic malignancies
- IV drug use
- Immunocompromised
- Lymphedema
- Venous insufficiency

Prevention and Screening

- Discourage scratching; maintain short, clean nails
- Meticulous diabetic foot care

Assessment

History

- May be unaware of the original break in the skin
- Possible history of fungal infection or dermatitis of the affected area
- Possible fever, malaise, anorexia, and pain increased with weight-bearing
- Possible airway occlusive symptoms if cellulitis involves the face (erysipelas), although airway involvement is rare

Physical Exam

- Puncture wound, fissure, or laceration may be visible.
- Erythematous plaque that is edematous, hot, and tender with sharply defined, irregular border
- Vesicles, bullae, and abscesses may be seen within the plaque.
- Possible erythematous streaking (lymphangitis)
- Regional lymphadenopathy
- Toxic signs may be present, especially if the involved area is large or the patient is immunocompromised or a child.
- *Necrotizing fasciitis: a* deep infection of subcutaneous tissue, appears as a large erythematous plaque with a central area of necrosis; beta-hemolytic streptococcus is usually the invading organism; staphylococcus may or may not be involved. Refer immediately to diminish tissue loss or death.

Diagnostic Studies

- Culture lesion
- Blood cultures may be indicated in toxic patients

- In facial cellulitis, consider a culture of cerebrospinal fluid
- A bone scan is indicated if the lesion is on the heel or hand to rule out osteomyelitis
- CBC lactate, CRP, and sedimentation rate indicated if the patient appears toxic

Differential Diagnosis

- Deep vein thrombosis or thrombophlebitis
- Contact dermatitis
- Giant urticaria
- Fixed drug eruption
- Necrotizing fasciitis
- Erythema migrans
- Early herpes zoster
- Insect bites and stings

Management

Nonpharmacologic Treatment

- Rest, immobilization, and elevation of the involved extremity
- Application of warm, moist compresses for 20 to 30 minutes four times a day

Pharmacologic Treatment

- Oral antibiotics that cover Gram-positive organisms:
  - Dicloxacillin (Dycill) 250–500 mg four times a day (children: 12.5–25 mg/kg/day,)
  - Erythromycin 250–500 mg (children: 30–50 mg/kg/day, four times a day)
  - Cephalexin (Keflex) 250–500 mg four times a day (children: 25–50 mg/kg/day, four times a day)
- For human bites, amoxicillin/clavulanate (Augmentin) 875/125 mg twice a day (adults; see manufacturer recommendations for children)
- Ceftriaxone (Rocephin) 250 mg to 1 g IM once a day (same in children)

- Ceftriaxone (Rocephin) 1 g IV once a day, Clindamycin (Cleocin) 600 to 900 mg IVthree times a day, or cefazolin 1 g IV once a day for moderate infections
- Nonsteroidal anti-inflammatory drugs (NSAIDs) and acetaminophen as needed for analgesia, fever, and to decrease inflammation (NSAIDS)

How Long to Treat

- 10 to 14 days, depending on the extent of involvement

Special Considerations

- Young children, immunocompromised patients, and patients with synthetic heart valves are at greater risk of toxicity and may warrant hospitalization.
- Medical management of predisposing conditions such as diabetes, IV drug use, malignancies, or chronic lymphedema will augment the treatment of cellulitis.

When to Consult, Refer, Hospitalize

- Hospitalize for toxicity, facial cellulitis, or if debridement is necessary.
- Refer to a surgeon or infectious disease specialist if the patient is not responding to therapy.

Follow-Up

- The erythematous plaque should be outlined with an indelible pen on the initial assessment, and the patient should return daily for the first few days to monitor the progression or regression of the involved area.

Expected Course

- Resolution is expected in 5 to 14 days

Complications

- Toxicity or septicemia
- Lymphedema may result from recurrent erysipelas.

IMPETIGO

Description

- Primary or secondary superficial bacterial infection of the skin leading to non-bullous or bullous lesions; may lead to ecthyma, a deeper infection involving the dermis
- The characteristic skin lesion is a honey-colored crust.
- Characterized by its auto-inoculable nature

Etiology

- *S. aureus*, group A beta-hemolytic streptococci, or mixed bacteria
- Organism gains access through breaks in the integrity of skin caused by trauma, scratching, scaling, or inflammation.
- Secondarily infected preexisting dermatitis is "impetiginization."

Incidence and Demographics

- Accounts for 10% of all skin problems in general outpatient pediatrics
- More prevalent in urban areas with poverty and overcrowding
- More common in young children ages 2 to 7 years of age

Risk Factors

- Young age; often endemic in day care centers or schools
- Contact sports
- Poor hygiene, crowded living conditions

Prevention and Screening

- Good hygiene (e.g., soap and water to reduce bacterial colonization)
- Avoid contact with infected patients

Assessment

History

- Rash that may or may not be pruritic that has been present for days to weeks
- Possible history of underlying dermatitis (atopic, contact)
- Possible exposure to household members or school or day care, sports exposure

Physical Exam

- Lesions can appear on the skin in which integrity has been disturbed.
- Commonly found on the face, torso, and extremities
- Non-bullous: small vesicles, pustules that rupture causing erosion and superficial honey-colored crusting, often caused by *Streptococcus pyogenes.*
- Bullous: large, transparent flaccid vesicle or bullae containing clear yellow fluid on an erythematous base; rupture easily and often caused by *S. aureus*; rupture leaves a rim surrounding a moist shallow ulcer; often found in clothing-covered areas

Diagnostic Studies

- Diagnosis is primarily clinical
- Cultures may be warranted if the diagnosis is in doubt or if the lesions fail to respond to an appropriate course of antibiotics

Differential Diagnosis

- Excoriations
- Perioral dermatitis
- Seborrheic dermatitis

- Contact dermatitis
- Herpes simplex or zoster
- Dermatophytosis
- Scabies
- Stasis or atherosclerotic ulcers
- Varicella
- Staphylococcal scalded skin syndrome
- Erysipelas

Management

Nonpharmacologic Treatment

- Wash the affected area with soap to remove crusts prior to applying a topical antibiotic
- Wash all linens, washcloths, etc., separately from other clothing
- Meticulous handwashing

Pharmacologic Treatment

- Mupirocin (Bactroban) 2% three times a day ointment topically to lesions (if limited) for 7 to 10 days
- Beta-lactamase–resistant oral antibiotics such as Augmentin if widespread lesions (larger than 0.3 cm) or if topical treatment is contraindicated
- Penicillin VK 250–500 mg four times a day × 10 days (children: 30–60 mg/kg/day four times a day × 10 days)
  - Erythromycin 250–500 mg four times a day × 10 days (children: 30–50 mg/kg/day four times a day × 10 days)
  - Dicloxacillin 500 mg four times a day × 10 days (children: 12.5–25 mg/kg/day four times a day × 10 days)
- If Pen VK or erythromycin is selected, cultures are warranted to ensure sensitivity to *S. aureus*.
- If the culture demonstrates methicillin-resistant *S. aureus* (MRSA), vancomycin (Vancocin) or SMP/TMZ is an alternative depending upon resistance within the community. However, vancomycin (Vancocin) would need to be administered intravenously and is therefore not recommended.

- Retapamulin (Altabax) 1% applied twice a day for 5 days, although it is contraindicated for oral, ophthalmic, intranasal, and intravaginal areas.

How Long to Treat

- 10 days is usually adequate.
- If there is no resolution at 10 days, obtain a culture to guide antibiotic therapy.

Special Considerations

- Penicillin VK or erythromycin is recommended in pregnant and lactating women.
- For the best penetration of topical antibiotics, soak the crusts with wet compresses for easier removal.
- Daily washing with an antimicrobial cleanser such as chlorhexidine gluconate is beneficial.

When to Consult, Refer, Hospitalize

- Hospitalization is warranted in toxic-appearing patients, although this is rare.

Follow-Up

Expected Course

- Generally resolved with a 10-day course of antibiotics
- Patients should be instructed to return sooner if symptoms do not appear to be resolving or if the condition appears to worsen/spread.

Complications

- With nontreatment or noncompliance with the medication regimen, the infection may progress to lymphangitis, cellulitis, erysipelas, bacteremia, or septicemia.
- GAS complications include guttate psoriasis, scarlet fever, and glomerulonephritis.
- Scarring often occurs after the healing of ecthyma.

FOLLICULITIS, FURUNCLE, AND CARBUNCLE

Description

- Folliculitis: local inflammation of hair follicles caused by infection or irritation; usually self-limiting
- Furuncle (boil or abscess): infection deep within a hair follicle
- Furunculosis: several discrete furuncles
- Carbuncle: deeper abscess involving subcutaneous tissue, arising in several contiguous hair follicles, interconnected by sinus tracts; may have several pustular openings onto skin; may be associated with systemic symptoms of fever and malaise

Etiology

- Usually due to *S. aureus*; hot tub folliculitis is caused by *P. aeruginosa*
- Most common in hairy areas exposed to friction, pressure, and moisture
- Folliculitis can present as a Gram-negative type. These include *Klebsiella*, *Enterobacter*, and *Proteus* and will appear as tiny pustules located on the chin or perinasal area as well as the cheeks.
- Fungal presentations are common and include candidiasis and tinea. Women who shave the upper thigh may experience Majocchi granuloma, which involves the entire hair follicle and is caused by *Trichophyton rubrum*.

Incidence and Demographics

- The exact incidence is unknown due to underreporting.
- Folliculitis is more common in adults than children due to more terminal hair growth.
- Herpes folliculitis is more common in men with beards.
- Malassezia folliculitis is more common in females.
- Pseudofolliculitis barbae is more common in African American men.
- Eosinophilic pustular folliculitis is more common in men around the age of 30.

Risk Factors

- Chronic staphylococcus carrier state (nares, axillae, anogenital, intestine)
- Obesity, poor hygiene, injection of drugs
- Immunocompromised state (e.g., HIV)
- Metabolic abnormalities (e.g., chronic granulomatosis, high serum IgE, diabetes)

Prevention and Screening

- Good hygiene
- Loose-fitting clothing
- Treatment of underlying immune and metabolic disorders

Assessment

History

- Folliculitis appears as single or multiple small pustules with possible mild erythema.
- Furuncle and carbuncles present as painful, warm, erythematous lesions with central pustulation developing over days.
- Carbuncles are sometimes accompanied by systemic symptoms of fever and malaise.
- History of predisposing factors or prior boils

Physical Exam

- Furuncle: firm, tender nodule with a central necrotic plug; nodule becomes fluctuant below the necrotic plug, usually with a pustule over the plug
- Carbuncle: several adjacent, coalescing furuncles with multiple, loculated abscesses, draining pustules, and necrotic plugs
- Vital signs may indicate fever and tachycardia.
- Local lymphadenopathy

Diagnostic Studies

- Laboratory studies are usually not indicated.
- Gram staining will often demonstrate Gram-positive cocci with multiple neutrophils.
- Culture and sensitivity may be done to confirm *S. aureus* or identify MRSA or other bacteria that may be resistant to treatment.
- Blood cultures are indicated if the patient remains febrile, appears toxic, or does not respond to treatment.

Differential Diagnosis

- Ruptured epidermal or pilar cyst
- Hidradenitis suppurativa
- MRSA
- Necrotizing herpes simplex virus
- Acne vulgaris
- Acne rosacea
- Pseudofolliculitis barbae
- Miliaris
- Superficial or dermatophyte fungal infections
- Cutaneous candidiasis

Management

Nonpharmacologic Treatment

- Warm, moist compresses or sitz baths for 10 minutes every 2 to 3 hours
- Incision and drainage is required for furuncle and carbuncle if large or pointing (pustule looks "ripe"); sterile packing is often necessary to allow the incision to continue to drain
- Wash daily with antibacterial soap; clean razors and personal items; change towels daily
- Superficial folliculitis, if left untreated, usually resolves on its own. Continue with warm moist compresses.

Pharmacologic Treatment

- Topical antibiotics are usually ineffective.
- Mupirocin ointment (Bactroban) three times a day to nares is helpful in eliminating chronic *S. aureus* carrier state or applied after a shower to prevent a recurrence.
- Systemic antibiotics are usually indicated for multiple furuncles and carbuncles, marked inflammation, or immunocompromised.
  - Dicloxacillin 250–500 mg four times a day; children: 12.5–50 mg/kg/day in divided doses
  - Cephalexin (Keflex) 250–500 mg four times a day; children: 25–50 mg/kg/day in divided doses
  - Amoxicillin and clavulanic acid (Augmentin) 250–500 mg; children: 20–40 mg/kg/ day in divided doses
  - Erythromycin ethylsuccinate (EES) 400 mg three times a day; children: 30–50 mg/kg/day in divided doses
  - Clarithromycin (Biaxin) 250–500 mg twice a day
  - Azithromycin (Zithromax) 250 mg once a day
  - Clindamycin (Cleocin) 150–300 mg four times a day
- Methicillin-resistant *S. aureus* (MRSA)
  - Minocycline (Minocin) 100 mg twice a day (adults); 4 mg/kg initially, then 2 mg/kg twice a day (children older than 8 years)
  - Trimethoprim-sulfamethoxazole DS twice a day; 8 mg/kg/day based on trimethoprim divided twice a day (children older than 2 months)
  - Ciprofloxacin (Cipro) 500 mg twice a day (18 and older only)
  - Linezolid (Zyvox) 600 mg twice a day
  - Vancomycin IV for severe infections
- For uncomplicated superficial folliculitis, topical benzoyl peroxide is the first-line treatment and should be applied twice daily until cleared.
- For fungal folliculitis, the primary treatment is itraconazole 100 mg twice a day for 4 days or terbinafine 250 mg once a day for 14 days or up to 3 weeks.
  - If *Candida* species, treatment is fluconazole 100–200 mg orally once a day for 14 to 21 days

How Long to Treat

- 7 to 10 days

Special Considerations

- Erythromycin should be used in pregnant or lactating women.

When to Consult, Refer, Hospitalize

- Consult with a physician if a large furuncle or carbuncle requires incision and drainage.
- Referral to a general surgeon is indicated for extensive abscess involvement or recurrence.

Follow-Up

- Daily follow-up initially to monitor response and to remove the packing from the surgical site

Complications

- Bacteremia and possible seeding of heart valves, joints, spine, long bones, and viscera
- Cavernous venous thromboses and meningitis

Viral Skin Infections

HERPES SIMPLEX VIRUS (HSV)

Description

- Recurrent viral mucocutaneous infection spread by skin-to-skin, skin-to-mucosa, or mucosa-to-skin contact; only known to affect humans
- Sites of involvement include the vermillion border of the lips, buccal mucosa, gingiva, cheeks, distal tips of fingers (herpetic whitlow), anogenital region.
- Genital HSV infection is a sexually transmitted disease.
- Requires break in normal skin integrity for initial cutaneous infection; asymptomatic until provoked

Etiology

- Herpes simplex virus type 1 and type 2—HSV replicates within epithelial cells, lyses them, and produces a thin-walled vesicle.
- HSV type 2 is usually associated with genital lesions.
- HSV type 1 is usually associated with vermillion border lesions.
- The virus migrates within several hours along sensory neurons to nerve root ganglia, where it then resides in a latent state.
- Viral reactivation occurs during periods of physical or emotional stress, although the exact mechanism of stimulating reactivation is unclear. When reactivated, the virus migrates back to the skin along sensory nerves, producing typical lesions.

Incidence and Demographics

- More common in women
- More common in younger adults, but can affect any age
- Affects all ethnicities

Risk Factors

- Intimate skin-to-skin or skin-to–mucous membrane contact with an infected person during stages of viral shedding; virus not stable at room temperature and therefore unlikely to spread through fomites or aerosol
- Contagious during the prodromal and vesicular stages
- Sun exposure to face; viral upper respiratory infection
- Altered hormonal status (menstruation)
- Immune status alteration (HIV, malignancy, chemotherapy, systemic corticosteroids, irradiation)

Prevention and Screening

- Safe sex practices (e.g., avoiding sexual contact when lesions are present)
- Avoidance of close contacts while symptomatic

Assessment

History

- May not be aware of contact with an infected person (incubation period 2 to 20 days; average 6 days)
- The initial or primary outbreak may range from very minor to severe, with grouped vesicles at the site of exposure.
- Commonly associated with regional lymphadenopathy, malaise, muscle pain, headaches, and possibly fever
- In childhood, it most often presents as acute gingivostomatitis with multiple shallow, painful ulcers, fever, hypersalivation, and lymphadenopathy.
- Recurrences preceded by prodromal tingling or aching at the site of previous lesions; may be less severe, no systemic symptoms

Physical Exam

- Thin roof, grouped vesicles on erythematous bases, often at border of lips, penis, labia, buttocks
- Vesicles burst, shallow ulcer exposed with crusting and ulcerations, then crust and dry over 1 week
- Regional lymphadenopathy, malaise, muscle pain, headaches, and possible fever

Diagnostic Studies

- HSV PCR or viral cultures may be useful when lesions are present to confirm the diagnosis.
- Tzanck smear microscopic exam (Wright's or Giemsa's stain) would demonstrate giant, multinucleated epidermal cells.
- Little clinical value from HSV serology

Differential Diagnosis

- Aphthous stomatitis
- Herpangina
- Chancroid

- Syphilis
- Pyoderma
- Trauma
- Hand, foot, and mouth disease
- Impetigo
- Herpes zoster
- Erythema multiform
- Monkeypox
- Behcet's disease

Management

Nonpharmacologic Treatment

- Sitz baths, cool compresses, Burow's solution for comfort
- Safe sex practices are of limited value; condoms do not reduce the risk of transmission as viral shedding occurs along a wide area of the groin/perineal region
- Sunscreen may prevent outbreaks

Pharmacologic Treatment

- Oral antivirals are usually not indicated for adults unless the infection is genital. (See Chapter 13 for genital herpes treatment.)
- Acyclovir (Zovirax) 15 mg/kg per day divided in five doses × 7 days in children with gingivostomatitis: for adults, 200 mg 5 times daily or 800 mg three times a day or valacyclovir 1,000 mg twice a day or famciclovir 250 mg three times a day
- Topical 5% acyclovir q.2.h. (only approved indication is for treatment of initial outbreak in immunocompromised patients) × 5 days
- Penciclovir (Denavir) cream q.2.h. × 4 days (indicated for the treatment of recurrent orolabial herpes; only been shown to reduce average attack from 5 to 4.5 days)
- Prophylactic acyclovir 400 mg twice a day; valacyclovir 500 mg once a day or famciclovir 125–250 mg twice a day when risk of triggers is high (UV light exposure, dental or oral surgery)
- Docosanol (Abreva) is the only FDA-approved over-the-counter topical treatment.

Special Considerations

- Treatment of an initial outbreak of herpes genitalis during pregnancy is recommended because the risk to the fetus of complications from a severe and prolonged outbreak outweighs the risk of complications from medications.
- Patients with frequent outbreaks should be evaluated for other sexually transmitted infections (STIs), including HIV.
- HIV+ patients with CD4 less than 50 should be prescribed prophylactic oral therapy; topical therapies are not effective.
- HSV is lifelong. Suppression of the virus is key in the management of outbreaks, especially if outbreaks surpass five per year. Valacyclovir suppression dosing is 500 mg daily.

When to Consult, Refer, Hospitalize

- Consult with a physician if hospitalization is required for IV therapy if the patient is immunocompromised with widespread disease.

Follow-Up

- Routine follow-up is not necessary unless severe

Expected Course

- Usual resolution of symptoms within 2 weeks for the first occurrence, 5 to 7 days for recurrences
- Recurrences become less frequent over time

Complications

- Secondary infection of lesions
- Post-inflammatory hyperpigmentation
- Erythema multiforme

HERPES ZOSTER

Description

- "Shingles"; acute, painful, unilateral, localized vesicular cutaneous infection in a dermatomal pattern

Etiology

- Varicella zoster virus (VZV), usually contracted in childhood as chickenpox
- Lies dormant in a nerve ganglion; reactivation of the virus causes eruption along the course of the nerve; cause of reactivation unclear

Incidence and Demographics

- Incidence increases with age.
- Affects women more than men
- No seasonal variation
- Less common in African Americans than in other ethnicities

Risk Factors

- Advanced age (e.g., ≥50 years and older)
- Female sex
- Chronic corticosteroid use
- Immunosuppression
- Prior varicella infection
- Trauma to the sensory ganglia

Prevention and Screening

- Varicella vaccine now included in routine childhood immunization schedule; may prevent the development of herpes zoster in later life

- Varicella vaccine (Shingrix) is now recommended by the Centers for Disease Control and Prevention (CDC) Advisory Committee on Immunization Practices (ACIP) for the prevention of herpes zoster in adults ≥50 years. Requires two doses, 2 to 6 months apart.
- Patients who previously received Zostavax should receive Shingrix at least 2 months after their initial vaccination
- Adults: No screening for previous varicella disease is indicated.

Assessment

History

- Pain (piercing, stabbing, boring), paresthesia (tingling, burning, itching), and allodynia (heightened sensitivity to mild stimuli) along neuronal pathway preceding eruption by 3 to 5 days; may mimic internal pathology
- Generalized malaise, fever, and headache in approximately 5% of patients

Physical Exam

- Initially, grouped vesicles along a unilateral dermatomal pathway, followed by bullae within 2 days (more than one contiguous dermatome may be involved but noncontiguous dermatome involvement is rare)
- By day 4, vesicles become pustules, followed by crusting in 7 to 10 days.
- Lesions occur on an erythematous, edematous cutaneous base.

Diagnostic Studies

- Diagnosis is primarily based on history and physical examination.
- Tzanck smear, serum VZV antibodies, or viral culture may be considered if the diagnosis cannot be determined clinically

Differential Diagnosis

- Herpes simplex
- Contact dermatitis
- Erysipelas

- Bullous impetigo
- Poison ivy or oak
- Necrotizing fasciitis
- Ulcerative keratitis

Management

Nonpharmacologic Treatment

- Moist dressings (water, normal saline, or Burow's solution) may decrease pain.

Pharmacologic Treatment

- Acyclovir (Zovirax) 800 mg 5 times daily
- Valacyclovir (Valtrex) 1,000 mg three times a day
- Famciclovir (Famvir) 500 mg three times a day
- IV acyclovir 10 mg/kg three times a day
- IV foscarnet (Foscavir) for acyclovir-resistant strains
- Topical clobetasol can be used to decrease the vesiculation of herpetic lesions.
- Pain management with narcotic pain medications or NSAIDs
- Postherpetic neuralgia (PHN) treatment could include topical capsaicin or lidocaine, which have been used successfully. Gabapentin and pregabalin (anticonvulsants) are effective for the treatment of postherpetic neuralgia.

How Long to Treat

- 7 to 10 days

Special Considerations

- The most common risk factor is decreasing immunity, which puts those with advancing age and immunocompromised conditions most at risk
- Long-term effects associated with PHN can be devastating to the patient; early treatment may help in decreasing long-term effects.

When to Consult, Refer, Hospitalize

- Disseminated infection may require hospitalization or in-home IV therapy.
- Herpes ophthalmicus and patients with corneal involvement will need an immediate referral to an ophthalmologist.
- Uncontrolled PHN will need to be referred to pain management, infectious disease, or neurology.

Follow-Up

- Follow-up in 2 weeks to ensure the infection is resolving

Expected course

- The initial course is generally resolved in 2 to 3 weeks

Complications

- PHN
- Local hemorrhage, gangrene, or secondary infection
- Systemic meningoencephalitis, cerebral vascular syndrome, cranial nerve syndromes (ophthalmic, trigeminal, facial, and auditory), peripheral motor weakness

HUMAN PAPILLOMAVIRUS/VERRUCA/WARTS

Description

- Discrete, benign, epithelial hyperplasia on the skin and mucous membranes
    - ◇ Vulgaris: common wart; can affect all locations
    - ◇ Plantaris: plantar wart, plantar surface of the foot; plana: flat wart
- Discrete benign, epithelial neoplasms caused by various types of the human papillomavirus (HPV), a group of double-stranded DNA viruses belonging to *Papillomaviridae* family.

Etiology

- Infection caused by human papillomaviruses, DNA viruses of which at least 70 types have been described; incubation period of 1 to 6 months; 65% spontaneous resolution in 12 to 24 months, but some persist for years
- Several varieties have been identified; specific morphology and predilection can vary by anatomic site.
- Most are benign; subtypes that infect the cervix are known to have oncogenic potential and are sexually transmitted.
- Approximately 40 of 150 subtypes of HPV affect mucosal surfaces. These include areas of the oral cavity, vulva, vagina, anus, and penis. Sixteen of these are considered oncogenic viruses, which can develop into cancer.
- Warts that affect the hands and feet typically do not affect the genitalia.

Incidence and Demographics

- Affects all ages and ethnicities
- Eighty five percent (85%) of people will have an HPV infection in their lifetime.
- More common in children and young adults
- More common in those with an immunocompromised state (e.g., HIV or receiving chemotherapy)

Risk Factors

- Skin-to-skin contact
- Household contact
- Occupations involving the handling of meat or fish
- Immunocompromised state (e.g., HIV)

Prevention and Screening

- Education about the contagious nature of the virus and avoidance of contact
- For the prevention of HPV, two doses of Gardasil 9 are recommended beginning at age 11.

ASSESSMENT

History

- Painless skin lesions that present from days to months, possibly with known exposure (incubation period 2 to 9 months)
- Plantar warts generally painful with weight-bearing
- May bleed if disrupted by shaving or scratching
- May be mildly pruritic, especially if secondarily infected

Physical Exam

- Verruca vulgaris or "common warts": firm, hyperkeratotic 1 to 10 mm papules with surface cleft
  - Usually flesh-colored and discrete
  - May be vegetative
  - Characteristic black puncta, or "dish-brown dots," are thrombosed capillary loops, best seen with a hand lens; may only be apparent after paring callused surface
  - Common on hands, fingers, and knees (sites of trauma), pressure points on feet
- Verruca plantaris or "plantar warts": flesh-colored, rough, hyperkeratotic papules or plaques (possible mosaic configuration) with black puncta on the plantar surface of feet
- Verruca plana or "flat warts": small, skin-colored, flat-topped ("mesa-like") 1 to 5 mm papules
  - Usually round or oval
  - Always discrete and closely set multiple lesions that sometimes appear in a linear configuration (autoinoculation from scratching)
  - Found on face, hands, or shins
- Common warts include filiform, which are recognized by fine, finger-like projections.
- Anogenital warts (condyloma acuminata) appear as unobtrusive, small, skin-colored papules to large, cauliflower-like growths.

Diagnostic Studies

- Diagnosis is often clinical; black puncta are pathognomonic.
- Suspicious lesions should be sent for pathology evaluation.

Differential Diagnosis

- Molluscum contagiosum
- Seborrheic keratosis
- Actinic keratosis
- Clavus or callus of feet
- Condyloma lata
- Squamous cell carcinoma
- Embedded foreign body

Management

Nonpharmacologic Treatment

- Warts of the hand: laser surgery, electrodesiccation, cryotherapy (liquid nitrogen)
- Apply opaque ("duct") tape to verruca plantaris or planus, change weekly (shown to be as effective as other treatments)

Pharmacologic Treatment

- Verruca vulgaris: keratolytic agents (salicylic, trichloroacetic acid [TCA] 90%, or lactic acids); over-the-counter (OTC) salicylic acid (Compound W, Duoplant, Mediplast pads) preparations applied nightly; soak in warm water for 10 minutes, dry and "sand" lesion with an emery board before applying the product; cover with Band-Aid or tape to increase effectiveness; silver nitrate 10% has been effective and cost-effective
- Verruca plantaris: same as with verruca vulgaris, except use higher potency product
- Verruca planus: retinoic acid A or salicylic acid applied daily
- Anogenital warts: podophyllin topical application every 1 to 2 weeks; bio trichloroacetic acid (TCA) topical application every 1 to 2 weeks; imiquimod 5%
- Systemic H-2 blockers such as cimetidine (Tagamet) or ranitidine (Zantac) twice a day for persistent warts in children along the vermillion border of lip or eyelid, if outbreak is very extensive, or if treatment is painful.

How Long to Treat

- 4 to 12 weeks, depending on the location and severity

Special Considerations

- Immunocompromised patients should be treated aggressively because some HPV strains have a high risk of transformation into squamous cell carcinomas.
- Podophyllin is contraindicated in pregnant and lactating women.
- *Molluscum contagiosum* is another cutaneous viral infection (poxvirus) with characteristic 1 to 2 mm, pearly white papules with an umbilicated center.
    - Spontaneous regression occurs in 6 months unless the patient is immunocompromised.
    - Widespread involvement in the immunocompromised requires treatment as noted in pharmacologic treatment section above.
    - If molluscum is found in the anogenital region of a child, there should be suspicion for sexual abuse.

When to Consult, Refer, Hospitalize

- Consult with a dermatologist for inadequate resolution with the above regimens.

Follow-Up

- As needed

Expected Course

- 50% to 60% of cases regress spontaneously within 2 years.
- 65% of patients have recurrences regardless of treatment.

Complications

- Scarring, post-inflammatory hyperpigmentation

Prevention

- Two doses of Gardasil 9 are recommended beginning at age 11 for boys and girls.

Parasitic Infestations and Bites

SCABIES

Description

- Infestation by scabies mite, spread by direct contact; leads to generalized pruritus, a hypersensitivity reaction to the scabies excretions

Etiology

- *Sarcoptes scabiei* that thrive and multiply only on human skin; spread by human-to-human contact; may live up to 2 days on clothing and bed linens
- Sensitization to *S. scabiei* must occur before developing the generalized pruritus associated with an infestation. For people with an initial infestation, sensitization takes about 10 days; subsequent infestations progress to the pruritic stage much more quickly.

Incidence and Demographics

- Occurs in children younger than age 5 primarily through direct contact, and in adults through sexual contact
- Higher incidence in colder seasons and in overcrowded living conditions
- Epidemics occur in cycles; incubation is 4 to 6 weeks
- Affects all genders and ethnicities equally

Risk Factors

- Institutional living
- Sexual contact with new or multiple partners
- Living in close quarters

- Low socioeconomic status
- Immunocompromised state

Prevention and Screening

- Education is important to prevent reinfestation.

Assessment

History

- Close contacts with similar symptoms
- Severe generalized pruritus sparing head and neck, with initial infestation about 1 month after exposure
- Pruritus and scratching often interfere with sleep

Physical Exam

- Characteristic scattered vesicles, burrows, or nodules: gray or skin-colored ridge, serpiginous or straight, 2 mm to a few centimeters in length; with excoriations
- Common distribution: axillae, anogenital region, wrists, hands (webs of fingers), waist, and flexor surfaces of elbows
- May develop generalized erythroderma or lichen simplex chronicus
- Eczematous dermatitis is common in atopic persons
- Post-inflammatory hyperpigmentation may be present
- Secondary infections to denuded sites common
- Crusted vesicles or burrows may present after an infestation of several months

Diagnostic Studies

- Diagnosis is clinical
- Ectoparasite prep
- Skin biopsy can identify mite, eosinophilic infiltrates. Eggs and mite fecal material are rarely identified via biopsy.

- A dermatoscope can be used to identify a "delta sign" reflecting a dark triangular shape identifying the head of the scabies mite. The "delta wing jet with contrail sign" is associated with the head of the mite and the burrowing trail.

Differential Diagnosis

- Drug eruption dermatitis
- Atopic or contact dermatitis
- Pityriasis rosea
- Herpetiform dermatitis
- Pediculosis dermatitis
- Xerotic dermatitis
- Insect bites
- Impetigo
- Delusions of parasitosis
- Metabolic pruritus

Management

Nonpharmacologic Treatment

- Wash all bedding and clothing in a washing machine with hot soapy water and hot dry cycle at the time of treatment; seal non-washable clothing and articles in a plastic bag for 1 week.
- Lubricants may help to reduce itching.

Pharmacologic Treatment

- Pharmacologic treatment is required for the eradication of mites and their eggs.
- First-line treatment is ivermectin/permethrin topical (1%). Apply to the hair and scalp as directed; leave for 10 minutes before rinsing.
- Secondary treatments include:
  - ◇ Precipitated sulfur 5%–10%. Apply for 8 hours on days 1–3. Considered safe in neonates and during pregnancy; limited efficacy data; inexpensive.

    - ◊ Ivermectin 200 µg/kg taken orally on days 1 and 8 has shown to be very effective and has a good safety profile. It should not be given to children weighing less than 15 kg or to pregnant or lactating women.
- Topical steroids should be used for severely pruritic areas.
- Systemic antihistamines such as diphenhydramine (Benadryl) 25–50 mg every 4 to 6 hours for pruritus

How Long to Treat

- One-time treatment with lindane or permethrin may be effective, but a repeat treatment in 10 to 14 days is often necessary to eliminate infestation.
- Systemic steroids are generally tapered over 10 to 14 days.
- Systemic antihistamines are used on an as-needed basis.

Special Considerations

- For children under 2 months of age, mechanical removal, treatment of contacts, and supportive measures are the mainstays of treatment. Pharmacologic therapy is not recommended.
- Lindane 1% lotion has a black box warning from the FDA due to its neurotoxic effects and is not recommended.

When to Consult, Refer, Hospitalize

- Refer to a dermatologist when resolution is not achieved with the above regimens.

Follow-Up

- Re-evaluation in 1 to 2 weeks, and then at weekly intervals if there is extensive dermatitis.

Expected Course

- Mites may be eradicated with 1 or 2 treatments, although generalized pruritus may persist for several weeks because it is a hypersensitivity reaction to the mite.

Complications

- Secondary infection due to scratching

INSECT BITES AND STINGS

Description

- Common injury caused by flying or crawling insects, including ticks, bees or wasps, fleas, and chiggers, or from arachnids

Etiology

- Bites occur from the mouth of insects and arachnids.
- Stings occur from ovipositors (stingers) and physical structures or injection of noxious chemicals from insects.
- Many bites cause allergic reactions with local or systemic symptoms, immediate or delayed.
- Anaphylaxis is possible.

Incidence and Demographics

- Incidence is unknown due to underreporting.
- Affect all ages, genders, and ethnicities
- More common in the late spring and summer months.
- Flea bites occur year-round.

Risk Factors

- Camping, landscaping, gardening, or playing in grassy or wooded areas.
- Geographic exposure (e.g., some organisms are found in distinct locations)

Prevention and Screening

- Avoid infested areas.
- Apply insect repellents (containing less than 10% diethyltoluamide [DEET] or permethrin) before going outside
- Wear neutral-colored clothing.
- Avoid scented products.
- Apply permethrin to clothing.
- Wear protective clothing such as long pants and shirts.
- Carefully check for ticks after a hike in potentially tick-infested areas.
- Eliminate fleas from living areas with powders or spray.

Assessment

History

- Recent exposure to insect-infested areas; report of feeling a bite or sting
- Swelling, pain, or pruritus of the affected area
- May report nausea, vomiting, diarrhea, headache, fever, lightheadedness, flushing, hives, dyspnea, wheezing

Physical Exam

- Presentation varies due to different insects and individual reactions.
- Mosquitoes: scattered erythematous pruritic wheals with central puncta
- Fleas: irregularly grouped or linear urticarial wheals or papules with central puncta
- Bees and wasps: redness, edema, pain, pruritus, induration
- Chiggers: discrete bright red papules on legs and belt line
- Distribution usually on exposed areas of skin, except fleas—areas where clothing is snug
- Spiders: swelling and erythema at the site, and may develop more severe reactions in areas of fatty subcutaneous tissue; necrosis can develop within 4 hours
- Wheezing, hypotension, and change in mental status may present in anaphylaxis

Diagnostic Studies

- None

Differential Diagnosis

- Varicella
- Impetigo
- Scabies
- Cellulitis
- Abscess
- Necrotizing fasciitis
- Folliculitis
- Drug reaction
- Atopy

Management

Nonpharmacologic Treatment

- Cool compresses or ice; colloidal oatmeal baths to assist with pruritis
- Remove stinger or tick if visible

Pharmacologic Treatment

- Symptomatic treatment of pruritus: pramoxine (topical anesthetic), topical steroids, oral antihistamines
- Oral corticosteroids can be used for more severe pruritus and swelling.
- Update tetanus prophylaxis as needed.
- Epinephrine and other emergency measures for anaphylactic reactions
  - Dose of epinephrine 1:1,000 (aqueous) 0.01 mL/kg per dose administered subcutaneously.

- ◇ In infants/children: 0.01 mg/kg, max 0. 3 mg/dose; adults: 0.1–0.5 mg, max dose 1 mg.
- ◇ If life-threatening systemic anaphylaxis occurs, call 911 and emergency transport; give epinephrine as above; start IV, oxygen, and inhaled albuterol (Proventil) nebulizer if bronchospasm is severe.

How Long to Treat

- Until symptoms are relieved; usually 48 hours

Special Considerations

- Papular urticaria, a hypersensitivity reaction, may develop secondary to bites from mosquitoes, fleas, or other insects—grouped urticarial papules with central puncta, vesicles, pustules, or bullae. This reaction usually occurs in the first decade of life and may last for 1 to 2 years.

When to Consult, Refer, Hospitalize

- Transfer to an acute care facility for anaphylactic reactions and for bites by brown recluse or black widow spiders.

Follow-Up

- Monitor for secondary infections.

Complications

- Spider bites by brown recluses or black widows can cause tissue necrosis.

PEDICULOSIS CAPITIS AND PUBIS

Description

- Infestation with one of the three species of parasitic lice (wingless and blood-sucking) that affect humans: *Pediculus humanus capitis, Pediculus humanus corporis*, or *Pthirus pubis*
- Infestation of the scalp, body, or pubic hair causing mild pruritus and excoriation

Etiology

- Pediculosis pubis is spread through close physical or sexual contact, sharing bed linens.
- Pediculosis capitis is spread through head-to-head contact.
- The incubation period from egg to hatching is 7 to 14 days.
- Hatched nymphs grow for 9 to 12 days, mate, and then females lay eggs. Females live for 3 to 4 weeks and can lay 10 eggs per day.
- Lice need to ingest blood every few hours and rarely survive for more than 24 hours off the host.

Incidence and Demographics

- All ages and genders are affected.
- Pediculosis pubis more common in young adults
- Pediculosis capitis more common in children and uncommon in African Americans

Risk Factors

- Shared hats, combs, and head-to-head contact for pediculosis capitis; can be an epidemic in schools and daycares
- Sex with multiple partners and poor personal hygiene for pediculosis pubis

Prevention and Screening

- Education of parents, children, and school personnel about modes of transmission and to avoid sharing hats, combs, etc.
- Educating young adults about the modes of transmission and avoiding sex with multiple partners

Assessment

History

- Mild pruritus of the scalp and nape of the neck, pubis, or axilla for days to weeks
- The only symptom in children may be restlessness.
- Sexual contact with an affected person
- Poor personal hygiene

Physical Exam

- Pediculosis capitis
  - 2 to 5 mm mobile lice often difficult to find; usually fewer than 10 per infestation
  - More commonly found are small (1.0 mm), creamy, yellowish-white nits adherent to the shaft of hair as it emerges from the scalp; a few to thousands of nits may be found on one scalp.
  - White nits farther from the scalp indicate longer-standing infection. (Hair grows approximately 0.5 mm/day.)
  - Excoriations, crusting, purulent exudate (plica polonica), eczematous dermatitis, or papular urticaria and lichen simplex chronicus along the nape of the neck
  - Regional lymphadenopathy may be found with a longstanding infestation or extensive excoriations and crusting.
- Pediculosis pubis
  - Lice: appear as 1 to 2 mm brownish-gray adherent dots on hair in the pubic region, perineum, axillae, and torso
  - Nits: whitish-gray dots on the hair shaft
  - Papular urticaria: slate-gray or bluish-gray 0.5 to 1 cm non-blanching macules
  - Excoriations, crusting, purulent exudate, regional adenopathy

Diagnostic Studies

- Mainly a clinical diagnosis, but may be confirmed by microscopic exam of lice, which demonstrates a 1 to 4 mm six-legged insect with a gray-white body that may be engorged with blood, or nits that are yellowish-white eggs less than 0.5 mm, or in the case of an older nit, an empty, translucent white egg
- Wood's lamp will demonstrate pearly fluorescence of live nits
- Bacterial cultures can confirm secondary infection and guide antibiotic therapy

Differential Diagnosis

- Hair spray/lacquer
- Eczema
- Tinea cruris
- Dandruff
- Neurotic excoriation
- Impetigo
- Contact or seborrheic dermatitis
- Scabies

Management

Nonpharmacologic Treatment

- Vacuuming carpets and furniture; washing clothing and linens in hot water and using a hot dryer; and soaking combs, brushes, and hair ornaments in rubbing alcohol are all effective means of controlling the environment to prevent the spread or reinfection with lice.
- Hair should be combed with a fine-toothed comb after treatment to remove adherent nits.
- Wetting the hair with white vinegar before combing loosens nits and facilitates removal.
- In resistant cases, applying oily substances such as mayonnaise, leaving it on overnight, and shampooing out in the morning may be effective.
- Children may return to daycare or school on the day after treatment.
- Seal items that are not washable in a plastic bag for 10 days.

Pharmacologic Treatment

- First-line treatment is ivermectin/permethrin topical (1%). Apply to the hair as directed and leave for 10 minutes before rinsing. Re-treat in 1 week.
    - Ivermectin topical 0.5% lotion (Sklice) is approved by the FDA for 6 months or older.
- Secondary treatments include:
    - Precipitated sulfur 5%–10%. Apply for 8 hours on days 1 to 3. Considered safe in neonates and during pregnancy; limited efficacy data; inexpensive.

- ◊ Ivermectin 200 µg/kg taken orally on days 1 and 8 has shown to be very effective and has a good safety profile. It should not be given to children weighing less than 15 kg or to pregnant or lactating women.
- ◊ Spinosad (Natroba) topical suspension 0.9% is FDA approved for the treatment of head lice for people 6 months or older and does not require nit combing. Re-application is required if lice are seen after 7 days from the first application.
- ◊ Secondarily infected lesions should be treated with appropriate antibiotics.
- ◊ Treat nits on eyebrows and eyelashes with petroleum jelly. Apply three times a day for 8 to 10 days and comb out nits.

How Long to Treat

- Once, with retreatment in 1 week

Special Considerations

- For children younger than 2 months of age, mechanical removal, treatment of contacts, and supportive measures are the mainstays of treatment. Pharmacologic therapy is not recommended.
- Lindane 1% lotion has a black box warning from the FDA due to its neurotoxic effects and is not recommended.

When to Consult, Refer, Hospitalize

- Consider referral for sexually transmitted infection (STI) testing for children with pediculosis pubis.

Follow-Up

- Patients should be re-evaluated in 1 week and re-treated if any nits or lice remain.

Expected Course

- Reinfection is likely if schools are not notified, other children are not evaluated and treated, or if sexual contacts or bed partners are not treated.

Complications

- Secondary infection from excoriated lesions

Tumors

BASAL CELL CARCINOMA

Description

- Slow-growing carcinoma commonly presents as a papule or nodule with central umbilication and progresses to significant ulceration.
- There is no risk of metastasis
- Most common skin cancer, on sun-exposed areas

Etiology

- Due to proliferating atypical basal cells with various amounts of stroma
- Excess sun exposure, particularly in fair-skinned persons
- Slow growing with rare metastasis, but may become invasive if located on the face, in the ear canal, or in the posterior auricular sulcus

Incidence and Demographics

- Men are affected more than women
- Affects all ethnicities, although less common in African Americans and Asians
- More common in adults over the age of 45

Risk Factors

- Fair skin
- Adults over the age of 45
- Male sex
- Sun/UV radiation exposure

- Prior x-ray surface therapy for acne
- Prior radiation therapy treatment

Prevention and Screening

- Sun-exposure precautions (e.g., sunscreen, wide-brimmed hats, sunglasses, protective clothing, and avoiding tanning beds and sunbathing)
- Monthly skin self-exams and yearly clinical exams

Assessment

History

- Patient may or may not be aware of suspicious lesions

Physical Exam

- Pearly, translucent papule on sun-exposed skin (80% on the face and neck); visible telangiectasia
- "Ulcer" or "sore" with a rolled border ("rodent bite ulcer"); central umbilication possible; central depression of the lesion possible
- Crusting may be present; pink or red; pigmented lesions may be brown, blue, or black
- Use of dermoscopy may identify blue globules, arborizing/branched vessels

Diagnostic Studies

- Biopsy is effective demonstrating atypical basal cells

Differential Diagnosis

- Molluscum contagiosum
- Warts
- Cysts
- Other benign lesions

- Squamous cell carcinoma
- Microcystic adnexal carcinoma
- Trichoepithelioma
- Merkel cell carcinoma

Management

- Excision, cryosurgery, or electrosurgery
- Mohs surgery: microscopically controlled surgery for lesions in the danger zones of nasolabial folds, around eyes, as well as in the ear canal and posterior auricular sulcus
- Radiation therapy is an alternative in areas of possible cosmetic disfigurement

How Long to Treat

- Radiation treatment, if required, will be determined by a radiation oncologist.

Special Considerations

- Reoccurrence or development of a new lesion may occur within 5 years.

When to Consult, Refer, Hospitalize

- Refer all suspected skin cancer to a dermatologist for biopsy

Follow-Up

- Monthly skin self-exams
- All patients should be monitored every 6 to 12 months for newly appearing and changing lesions; any lesion that is itchy or tender for more than 2 weeks should be evaluated.

Expected Course

- Resolution is expected with the therapies noted above

Complications

- Scarring following excision

SQUAMOUS CELL CARCINOMA

Description

- Skin malignancy that occurs on sun-exposed areas and results from atypical, transformed keratinocytes.
- Four types:
  - Actinic keratosis
  - Squamous cell carcinoma in situ (Bowen disease)—confined to the outer layer of skin
  - Invasive squamous cell carcinoma—invasion into deep skin layers
  - Metastatic squamous cell carcinoma—distant metastasis

Etiology

- Skin exposure to an exogenous carcinogen such as sunlight, ionizing radiation
- Arsenic ingestion, tobacco, human papillomavirus
- Malignant growth of epithelial keratinocytes developing on the skin and mucous membranes
- May begin as an actinic keratosis lesion resulting in malignant changes.

Incidence and Demographics

- Second most common nonmelanoma skin cancer
- Men affected more than women
- More common in those with sun exposure and those living in sunbelt states, adults over the age of 45, and those with fair skin

Risk Factors

- Fair skin
- Adults over the age of 45
- Male sex
- Sun/UV radiation exposure
- Arsenic ingestion, tobacco use, radiation exposure
- Preexisting solar keratosis
- Organ transplant recipients
- Immunosuppression

Prevention and Screening

- Sun-exposure precautions (e.g., sunscreen, wide-brimmed hats, sunglasses, protective clothing, and avoiding tanning beds and sunbathing)
- Monthly skin self-exams and yearly clinical exams

Assessment

History

- Suspicious lesion developing over 3 to 6 months
- Most often on sun-exposed skin (face, lips, hands, and forearms)

Physical Exam

- Originate with small red nodule, papule, or plaque; progresses to induration
- Thick, adherent, keratotic scale
- Honey-colored exudate extruded from the periphery
- May be eroded, crusted, ulcerated, hard, erythematous; isolated, or multiple

Diagnostic Studies

- Biopsy is effective in identifying atypical squamous cells

Differential Diagnosis

- Basal cell carcinoma
- Malignant melanoma
- Actinic keratosis
- Paget's disease
- Seborrheic keratosis
- Prurigo nodularis
- Other benign lesions
- Psoriasis
- Eczema
- Fungal infection
- Tinea corporis

Management

- Immediate surgery or radiation depending on the size, shape, and location of the tumor
- Strict sun precautions for rest of life; lesions 2 cm or greater are prone to recur

How Long to Treat

- Radiation treatment, if required, will be determined by a radiation oncologist.

Special Considerations

- Any slowly evolving isolated keratotic lesion in a high-risk patient that persists for more than 1 month is to be considered carcinoma until proven otherwise with a biopsy.

When to Consult, Refer, Hospitalize

- Refer all suspected skin cancer to a dermatologist for biopsy.

Follow-Up

Expected Course

- Remission is achieved in 90% of cases
- Monitor for reoccurrence annually, and if the patient reports change in any existing lesion; photographs of lesions can be kept for comparison of appearance.

Complications

- Scarring following excision

MALIGNANT MELANOMA

Description

- Malignant tumor arising from melanocytes with a high risk of metastasis
- Classifications: superficial spreading melanoma (most common with a long phase of superficial extension before deep penetration); nodular melanoma (poor prognosis); lentigo maligna melanoma (slow growing and affecting sun-damaged skin); acral lentiginous melanoma (rare, presents on the palms, soles, or nails); desmoplastic melanoma, amelanotic melanoma, and mucosal melanoma

Etiology

- Malignant growth of melanocytes
- Genetic and environmental factors:
    - Genetic—inheritance of sun-sensitive skin, red hair, blue eyes
    - Environmental—excessive exposure to solar and IV radiation, proximity to the equator, history of frequent sunburns

Incidence and Demographics

- Fifth most common form of skin cancer
- Accounts for two-thirds of skin cancer deaths
- Affects men and women equally
- Affects all ethnicities equally
- Cases with lymph node involvement at the time of diagnosis have a 5-year survival rate of 30%; with distant metastasis, less than 10%
- More common in areas close to the equator

Risk Factors

- Family or personal history of melanoma or other skin cancer
- History of atypical nevi
- Red or blond hair
- Dysplastic nevi syndrome
- Excessive sun exposure
- Recurrent sunburns
- Fair skin

Prevention and Screening

- Sun-exposure precautions (e.g., sunscreen, wide-brimmed hats, sunglasses, protective clothing, and avoiding tanning beds and sunbathing)
- Monthly skin self-exams and yearly clinical exams

Assessment

History

- New pigmented lesion or recent change in longstanding skin lesion, demonstrating signs of evolution

- Lesion that burns, itches, is painful, or bleeds
- Constitutional symptoms may be present with a late presentation and is concerning for metastatic disease

Physical Exam

- Macule, papule, or nodule
- Colors ranging from pink to brown, blue, or black
- Borders are most often irregular.
- Size can vary from a few millimeters to centimeters.
- The five cardinal signs of malignant melanoma are:
  - A: Asymmetry
  - B: Border is irregular and often scalloped.
  - C: Color is mottled with a variegated display of brown, black, gray, and/or pink.
  - D: Diameter is large (greater than 6.0 mm).
  - E: Elevation is almost always present with subtle or obvious surface distortion; best assessed by side-lighting of the lesion.
- Five histopathologic types:
  1. Superficial spreading malignant melanoma (most common)
  2. Nodular malignant melanoma
  3. Acral-lentiginous melanoma (palms of hands, soles of feet, nail beds)
  4. Malignant melanomas of mucous membranes
  5. Melanomas arising from blue or congenital nevi

Diagnostic Studies

- Dermoscopy
- Biopsy, including margins and depth of invasion assessment
- Sentinel lymph node biopsy to rule out metastatic disease may be indicated.

Differential Diagnosis

- Benign nevi
- Seborrheic keratosis
- Vascular skin lesions
- Squamous cell carcinoma
- Basal cell carcinoma
- Dermatofibroma

Management

- Aggressive surgical management by excision with margins intact and sentinel lymph node biopsy
- Chemotherapy for patients with high-risk metastatic melanomas, to be managed by an oncology specialist

How Long to Treat

- To be determined by an oncologist

Special Considerations

- Patients with skin phototype 1 or 2 should *never* sunbathe and always use sunscreen with a sun protection factor (SPF) of more than 30. (See Table 5–4 for skin phototype classifications.)

When to Consult, Refer, Hospitalize

- Refer all suspected malignant melanomas to a dermatologist for a biopsy.

Follow-Up

- Monthly skin self-exams
- All patients should be monitored every 6 to 12 months for newly appearing and changing lesions; any lesion that is itchy or tender for more than 2 weeks should be evaluated.

TABLE 5–4.
SKIN PHOTOTYPE CLASSIFICATIONS

SKIN PHOTOTYPES		
1	Pale white	Does not tan; burns easily
2	White	Tans poorly; burns easily
3	White	Tans after initial burn
4	Light brown	Tans easily
5	Brown	Tans easily
6	Dark brown	Blackens

Complications

- Lung, liver, brain, bowel metastasis

Expected Course

- Prognosis based on staging of the initial lesion

Other Integumentary Conditions

ALOPECIA AREATA

Description

- Autoimmune disease resulting in inflammation of hair follicles and resultant non-scarring hair loss, often in discrete oval patches
- Severity varies; may affect eyelashes, eyebrows, body hair, and nails
- Alopecia areata totalis involves whole scalp; alopecia areata universalis involves all body hair
- In 10%–20% of those affected there may be pitting, brittleness, and/or striations on the surface of the nails.

Etiology

- Not fully known, but thought to be due to an autoimmune process
- Genetic link identified through the genome-wide association studies (GWAS)

Incidence and Demographics

- Rarely occurs before age 4
- More common in children and young adults
- Lifetime incidence is 2%
- Affects men and women equally
- Affects all ethnicities equally

Risk Factors

- Family history of autoimmune disease
- Associated with trisomy 21, atopy, and other autoimmune disorders (thyroid is most common)

Prevention and Screening

- None

Assessment

History

- Usually asymptomatic except for sudden (overnight or over a few days) loss of hair
- Occasionally burning or itching of the scalp just before hair loss

Physical Exam

- Sudden appearance of one or more well-circumscribed patches of hair loss
- Underlying skin will have a normal appearance.

- "Exclamation point hairs"—short hairs at periphery with an attenuated bulb is pathognomonic
- Fine nail pitting in present in approximately 20% of cases

Diagnostic Studies

- Usually none except to exclude other diagnoses; consider fungal cultures, KOH, and/or scalp biopsy

Differential Diagnosis

- Tinea capitis
- Systemic disease, drugs, and toxins
- Trichotillomania
- Telogen effluvium
- Syphilitic alopecia
- Traumatic alopecia from cosmetic treatments
- Traction alopecia—tight braids, rollers
- Androgenic (male pattern hair loss)

Management

Nonpharmacologic Treatment

- Education of child and parents about disease and course
- Support groups
- Hair pieces, hats, or head coverings
- Psychological counseling

Pharmacologic Treatment

- Controversial, as spontaneous resolution often occurs, but may include topical, systemic, or intralesional steroids, or topical minoxidil or anthralin

- Baricitinib (Olumiant), a JAK inhibitor, is FDA approved for severe alopecia areata. Be sure to review the black box warning with patients related to development of serious infections

Special Considerations

- More diffuse, non-scarring hair loss may occur due to androgen hormonal changes, systemic disease, weight loss, certain medications and toxins, thyroid disease, lupus, and congenital syndromes.
- Scarring hair loss can occur with connective tissue diseases, skin diseases, burns, radiation, congenital disorders, and tumors.
- Trichotillomania is a type of traction alopecia due to self-pulling of hair.

When to Consult, Refer, Hospitalize

- Refer to a dermatologist to guide diagnosis and treatment.

Follow-Up

- Routine health maintenance exams
- Monitor and reassess for regrowth in 6 to 12 months

Expected Course

- Course and prognosis are extremely variable
- Hair that regrows is often hypopigmented and fine

Complications

- Usually none

PSORIASIS

Description

- Chronic inflammatory skin disease characterized by scaling papules and plaques

Etiology

- Etiology is unknown, although there are suspected genetic, immunologic, and infective causative factors.
- Infection associated with recurrent upper respiratory infections (e.g., streptococcal pharyngitis) and HIV
- Immunology—triggered by external insults in genetically susceptible individuals resulting in an alteration in cell kinetics of keratinocytes with shortening of cell turnover rate. Increased production of epidermal cells and normal maturation of the skin cells cannot take place leading to the development of keratinization.

Incidence and Demographics

- Affects 3% of the U.S. population
- Prevalence is similar in men and women
- Uncommon in children
- Peak incidence is until age 40 with a second peak after age 50
- More common in White individuals and African Americans
- Race: 1% to 2% of White population affected

Risk Factors

- Trauma (Köbner's phenomenon—lesions develop in areas of trauma)
- Recurrent upper respiratory infections (e.g., streptococcal pharyngitis) and HIV can lead to Guttate psoriasis.
- Medications: corticosteroids, lithium, interferon, and beta-adrenergic blockers can cause psoriasis drug eruptions.
- Stress
- Genetic predisposition

Prevention and Screening

- Stress management

Assessment

History

- Skin lesions usually with insidious onset, but may be acute
- Pruritus may or may not be present.
- May be associated with acute systemic illness with fever and malaise
- May be associated with arthralgias/arthritis

Physical Exam

- Morphology: silvery-white scaling papules and plaques
- Distribution: usually symmetrical; involves scalp, extensor surfaces, and areas subject to trauma (Köbner's phenomenon)
- Associated symptoms: may involve pitting of nails, yellowing of the nail at distal end, separation of nail plate from the bed
- Characteristic scale attaches to skin at only one point; drop of blood where scale peels off (Auspitz sign).
- Variations: Guttate psoriasis (drop-like lesions), pustular psoriasis, psoriatic arthritis

Diagnostic Studies

- Diagnosis is clinical.
- Rheumatoid factor will be negative in psoriatic arthritis.

Differential Diagnosis

- Seborrheic dermatitis
- Tinea infections
- Candidal infections

- Drug eruptions
- Eczema
- Lichen simplex chronicus
- Lichen planus
- Pityriasis rosea

Management

Nonpharmacologic Treatment

- Phototherapy can be used for moderate to severe psoriasis.
- Avoid rubbing or scratching lesions.
- Oatmeal baths for pruritus
- Avoid excessive sun exposure.

Pharmacologic Treatment

- Topical treatments are the mainstay of therapy, and the formulation depends on the area treated.
- Systemic steroids should be avoided as they can cause rebound flares.
- Topical corticosteroids should be covered with an occlusive dressing (Cordran tape) for localized areas
- Systemic therapy options include methotrexate, anthralin, oral retinoids, cyclosporine, and sulfasalazine but should be reserved for severe cases with treatment managed by a dermatologist
- Apremilast (Otezla) is an oral phosdiesterase-4 (PDE-4) inhibitor approved for the treatment of psoriasis and psoriatic arthritis. It does not require any routine lab monitoring and can be used in patients 18 years and older.
- Biologic therapy should be considered for moderate to severe cases. Biologics work at the cellular level and target the immunologic processes resulting in psoriatic activity.
- Tumor necrosis factor-alpha (TNF-α) inhibitors include adalimumab, certolizumab, infliximab, and etanercept
  - Interleukin (IL) inhibitors including tildrakizumab, risankizumab, and guselkumab inhibit IL-23, whereas ustekinumab inhibits IL-12 and IL-23. Ixekizumab, secukinumab, and brodalumab inhibit IL-17.

How Long to Treat

- Treatment duration depends on the type of psoriasis diagnosed.
- Treatment should continue until the flare-up subsides.

Special Considerations

- Von Zumbusch acute pustular psoriasis is a life-threatening problem with acute onset requiring hospitalization. There is no known precipitating factor, and the patient may or may not have had stable plaque-like psoriasis in the past.
- Tuberculosis, HIV, hepatitis B, and hepatitis C screening is recommended prior to initiating biologic therapy. Ustekinumab and IL-17 inhibitors are recommended for patients with hepatitis B infection or latent tuberculosis. TNF inhibitors should be used cautiously.
- Certolizumab may be used during pregnancy if clinically indicated.
- TNF inhibitors are not recommended in patients with multiple sclerosis.

When to Consult, Refer, Hospitalize

- Patients should be referred to a dermatologist for moderate to severe cases requiring systemic therapy or biologics.
- Collaboration with a rheumatologist is recommended for suspected or concomitant psoriatic arthritis

Follow-Up

- Routine, with laboratory monitoring if systemic medications are utilized

Expected Course

- Chronic condition requiring initial treatment and maintenance therapy

Complications

- Secondary infection

BURNS

Description

- Thermal, electrical, or chemical injury causing damage to the epidermis, dermis, and/or subcutaneous tissue

Etiology

- Exposure to intense heat of fire or steam, damaging chemicals, electrical voltage; the longer the contact with the skin, the greater the burn injury

Incidence and Demographics

- Common injuries, although the prevalence is unknown as many do not seek care
- Flame burns most common in adults; scald burns more common in children
- Scald, tar, chemical, and electrical burns more common in the workplace

Risk Factors

- Firefighters
- Unsupervised children
- Workplace exposure to scalding liquids (tar, steam) and chemicals or electricity
- Male sex

Prevention and Screening

- Education on fire safety and safe handling of hot liquids, chemicals, and electricity in the community and workplace

Assessment

History

- Exposure to fire, chemicals, scalding liquids, or electricity
- Intense pain at site of exposure; third-degree burns are usually painless

Physical Exam

- Burns are classified by the extent and depth of tissue involvement, patient age, and associated illness or injury.
- Depth of injury described as first, superficial second, deep second, third, or fourth-degree burns:
  - First-degree: superficial burns involving the epidermis only; redness and blanching erythema (demonstrating capillary refill) of affected area with no initial blistering
  - Second-degree, further classified as superficial or deep: partial-thickness burns involve entire epidermis and variable portions of the dermis. Superficial second-degree burns expose superficial parts of the dermis. With deep second-degree burns, both the epidermis and the superficial dermis are destroyed. Red, moist, and edematous skin with small or large bullae.
  - Third-degree: full-thickness burn involving entire dermis and subcutaneous tissue; pale, white, tan, or charred wound that may appear dry and depressed below surrounding skin; skin may feel tight and leathery.
  - Fourth-degree: the entire skin is destroyed with damage to subcutaneous and deeper tissues.
- Extent of involvement can be measured by using the "rule of nines:"
  - Anterior head and neck = 4.5%
  - Posterior head and neck = 4.5%
  - Torso and abdomen = 18%
  - Back = 18%
  - Anterior arms = 4.5% each
  - Posterior arms = 4.5% each
  - Genitalia = 1%
  - Anterior legs = 9% each
  - Posterior legs = 9% each
- Equate the patient's palm size as 1% of total body size

Diagnostic Studies

- Dependent on the severity of the burn.

Differential Diagnosis

- Contact dermatitis
- Herpes zoster
- Atopic dermatitis
- Child abuse
- Scalded skin syndrome
- Stevens-Johnson syndrome

Management

Nonpharmacologic Treatment

- Burns involving the eye should be irrigated with saline or lactated Ringer's solution.
- Wounds should be cleaned and debrided using plain soap and water, Betadine diluted with water, or saline solution.
- Elevate involved extremities, avoiding constricting dressings.

Pharmacologic Treatment

- Topical silver sulfadiazine (Silvadene) 1/16-inch layer over the entire surface, covered with non-absorbent gauze (Kerlix or Telfa), and wrapped in at least a 3-inch–thick non-adhesive wrap
- Analgesia with narcotics or NSAIDs as needed
- Tetanus prophylaxis
- Antibiotic coverage for secondary infection

How Long to Treat

- Dressing changes twice a day with frequent re-evaluation until resolution to assess for secondary infection

Special Considerations

- Very young, older, and debilitated patients are at a higher risk for hemodynamic compromise.

When to Consult, Refer, Hospitalize

- *Refer patients with the following characteristics to a burn center:*
    - Deep second-degree or third-degree burns
    - Burns of greater than 10% total body surface area (TBSA) in patients younger than 10 years and older than 50 years
    - Burns of greater than 20% TBSA in all other patients
    - Burns of the face, hands, and feet; over a joint or of the perineum; or that are circumferential
    - Burns resulting from child or adult abuse
    - Inhalation injury, electrical burns, chemical burns
    - Suspected toxic epidermal necrolysis syndrome

Follow-Up

- Daily follow-up is recommended initially to ensure proper wound management and evaluation for infection, and then weekly until the burn has healed.

Expected Course

- Depends on extent and location of burn

Complications

- Hemodynamic compromise, multi-organ failure, sepsis
- Scarring
- Posttraumatic stress
- Increased photosensitivity of healed skin

CASE STUDIES

CASE 1

A 15-year-old boy presents to your clinic after a camping trip with his parents. Two days after the trip, he noticed a rash on his legs. During your examination, you identify an erythematous linear rash on both lower extremities.

Past Medical History: asthma

Medications: Montelukast 10 mg orally daily and Albuterol inhaler 1 puff every 4 hours as needed

1. What pertinent history should be obtained?
2. What is the most likely diagnosis based on the information provided?
3. What additional assessment findings would you expect to find on physical examination?
4. Is the patient contagious?
5. What treatment plan would you recommend?

CASE 2

A 26-year-old White man presents to your clinic with a complaint of a "funny rash" on his back and across his shoulders. The rash has been present for 6 months, further described as "brown and white patches," worse when he is hot or outside in the heat. His girlfriend adds that the rash is slowly spreading.

Social history: employed in an automobile factory; recently joined a church volleyball league

Past Medical History: healthy, non-smoker, drinks beer 2 to 3 nights per week with friends

1. What pertinent history should be obtained?
2. During your physical examination, you note discrete, scattered, or confluent patches. Wood's lamp exam reveals faint yellow-green scales. What is the most likely diagnosis?
3. What laboratory tests would you order to confirm your suspected diagnosis?
4. What treatment plan would you recommend?

CASE 3

A 5-year-old girl presents to your clinic with skin lesions. Her mother reports that the lesions were initially vesicular but are now honey-crusted in various stages of healing on the patient's face, arms, and legs. The patient attends daycare and has remained afebrile.

Past Medical History: no hospitalizations; two to three episodes of otitis media each year

1. What pertinent history should be obtained?
2. What is the most likely diagnosis based on the information provided?
3. What additional assessment findings would you expect to find on physical examination?
4. Is the patient contagious?
5. What laboratory tests would be indicated?
6. What treatment plan would you recommend?

CASE STUDIES DISCUSSION

CASE 1

1. What pertinent history should be obtained?

   Has the patient had a fever, systemic symptoms, bites, or other exposure? Does the patient have a history of irritant dermatitis or other rashes? Does the patient have environmental, food, seasonal, and/or drug allergies?

2. What is the most likely diagnosis based on the information provided? Contact dermatitis, likely due to a plant (e.g., poison ivy).

3. What additional assessment findings would you expect to find on physical examination?

   Eruptions along areas of skin exposure on the arms and legs, possibly linear. Papules, dry scaling, and erythema. Possibly scratch marks. Later in the course of contact dermatitis, may see weeping and excoriation.

4. Is the patient contagious?

   No, contact dermatitis is not contagious unless the clothing or other items are contaminated with oil from the plant. All clothing or shoes with oil from the plant should be washed to remove the irritant.

5. What treatment plan would you recommend?

   Identify and remove the offending agent. Symptomatic care with colloidal oatmeal, astringent, topical corticosteroids (do not use over large areas or if infected), oral steroids if a large area is involved, antihistamines, and antibiotics (for cellulitis or impetigo only).

CASE 2

1. What pertinent history should be obtained?

   Has the patient used any new products? Does he have any allergies or take any medications daily? Has he had any prior episodes of similar symptoms? Is there any itching, scaling, or flaking?

2. During your physical examination, you note discrete, scattered, or confluent patches. Wood's lamp exam reveals faint yellow-green scales. What is the most likely diagnosis?

   Tinea versicolor

3. What laboratory tests would you order to confirm your suspected diagnosis? Microscopic examination with KOH preparation. A skin biopsy may be considered.

4. What treatment plan would you recommend?

   Topical selenium sulfide 2.5% shampoo to skin for 10 minutes daily for 7 days.

CASE 3

1. What pertinent history should be obtained?

   How long have the lesions been present? Has she had a fever? Have any home remedies been tried? Does the patient live in crowded conditions or attend daycare? Has the patient been exposed to anyone with similar symptoms? Are her vaccines up to date? Fever?

2. What is the most likely diagnosis given this presentation? Impetigo.

3. What additional assessment findings would you expect to find on physical examination?

   Possible poor hygiene evident in child's grooming; breakdown and secondary infection (impetiginizing) of neglected skin lesions; honey-colored fluid oozing from open lesions and others with a crusted covering; bullous (large vesicle or bullae containing clear yellow fluid on erythematous base); ecthyma (ulceration with thick adherent crust); possible tenderness; possible regional lymphadenopathy.

4. Is the patient contagious?

   Yes.

5. What laboratory tests would be indicated?

   Diagnosis is primarily clinical. Wound cultures may be warranted if the diagnosis is in doubt or if the lesions fail to respond to an appropriate course of antibiotics. Cultures may demonstrate *S. aureus,* group A streptococci, or methicillin-resistant *S. aureus.* If the infection is recurrent, serology for anti-DNase B may be indicated to assess for prior strep infection.

6. What treatment plan would you recommend?

   Wash the affected area with soap to remove crusts prior to applying topical antibiotics. Topical Mupirocin should be used for small lesions. Penicillin should be used for streptococci and dicloxacillin for staphylococcus. Erythromycin may be used if the patient is allergic to penicillin.

REFERENCES

Arcangelo, V. P., Peterson, A. M., Wilbur, V., & Kang, T. P. (2021). *Pharmacotherapeutics for advanced practice.* (5th ed.). Philadelphia, PA: Wolters Kluwer.

Borda, L. J., Perper, M., & Keri, J. E. (2019). Treatment of seborrheic dermatitis: A comprehensive review. *Journal of Dermatological Treatment, 2,* 158–169. https://doi.org/10.1080/09546634.2018.1473554

Bunik, M., Hay, W. W., Levin, M. J., & Abzug, M. J. (2022). *Current diagnosis & treatment: Pediatrics* (26th ed.). New York, NY: McGraw-Hill.

Dinulos, J. G. (2021). *Clinical dermatology: A color guide to diagnosis and therapy* (7th ed.). Edinburgh, Scotland: Elsevier.

Domino, F. J., Baldor, R. A., Barry, K. A., Golding, J., & Stephens, M. B. (2022). *The 5-minute clinical consult.* Philadelphia, PA: Wolters Kluwer.

Facts and Comparisons. (2017). *Drug facts and comparisons 2017.* St. Louis, MO: Wolters Kluwer Health.

Frazier, W., & Bhardwaj, N. (2020). Atopic dermatitis: Diagnosis and treatment. *American Family Physician, 101*(10), 590–598.

Gilbert, D. N., Chambers, H. F., Saag, M. S., Pavia, A. T., Boucher, H. W., Black, D., Freedman, D. O., Kim, K., & Schwartz, B. S. (2022). *The Sanford guide to antimicrobial therapy.* Hyde Park, VT: Antimicrobial Therapy, INC.

Goroll, A. H., & Mulley, A. G. (2021). *Primary care medicine* (8th ed.). Philadelphia, PA: Wolters Kluwer

Habif, T. P., Dinulos, J. G., Chapman, M. S., & Zug, K. A. (2018). *Skin disease: Diagnosis and treatment* (7th ed.). Philadelphia, PA: Elsevier.

Kang, S., Amagai, M., Brucker, A. L., Enk, A. H., Margolis, D. J., McMichael, A. J., & Orringer, J. S. (2019). *Fitzpatrick's dermatology in general medicine* (9th ed.). New York, NY: McGraw-Hill.

Lee, S., & Shin, M. (2017). Prevalence and causes of childhood urticaria. *Allergy, Asthma and Immunology Research, 9*(3): 189–90. doi: 10.4168/aair.2017.9.3.189

Leung, A. K., Barankin, B., Lam, J. M., Leong, K. F., & Hon, K. L. (2019). Dermatology: How to manage acne vulgaris. *Drugs in Context, 10,* 1–18. https://doi.org/10.7573/dic.2021-8-6

Oge, L. K., Broussard, A., & Marshall, M. D. (2019). Acne vulgaris: Diagnosis and treatment. *American Family Physician, 100*(8), 475–484.

Papadakis, M. A., McPhee, S. J., Rabow, M. W., eds. (2022). *Current medical diagnosis & treatment 2022* (61st ed.). New York, NY: McGraw-Hill.

Rajabi, F., Drake, L. A., Senna, M. M., & Rezaei, N. (2018). Alopecia areata: A review of disease pathogenesis. *British Journal of Dermatology, 179*(5), 1033–1048. https://doi.org/10.1111/bjd.16808

Shinkai, K. & Fox, L. P. (2022). Dermatologic disorders. In M. A. Papadakis, S. J. McPhee, & M. W. Rabow (Eds.), *Current medical diagnosis and treatment* (61st ed.). New York, NY: Lange Medical Books/ McGraw Hill.

Wolff, K., Johnson, R. A., & Saavedra, A. P., & Roh, E. K. (2017). *Fitzpatrick's color atlas and synopsis of clinical dermatology* (8th ed.). New York, NY: McGraw-Hill.

Woo, T. M., & Robinson, M. V. (2019). *Pharmacotherapeutics for nurse practitioner prescribers* (5th ed.). Philadelphia, PA: F. A. Davis Co.

Zuberbier, T. et al. (2021). The international EAACI/GA²LEN/EuroGuiDerm/APAAACI guideline for the definition, classification, diagnosis, and management of urticaria. *Allergy, 77*(3), 734–766. https://doi.org/10.1111/all.15090

CHAPTER 6

EYE, EAR, NOSE, AND THROAT DISORDERS

Aaron M. Sebach, PhD, DNP, MBA, AGACNP-BC, FNP-BC, NP-C, CP-C, CEN, CPEN, CLNC, CGNC, CNE, CNEcl, SFHM

General Approach

- Assessing visual acuity is the single most important test in evaluating eye complaints in primary care.
- Obtain a good history of the presenting illness to make a correct diagnosis.
- The emergence of increasingly resistant microorganisms makes it imperative to be judicious in prescribing antibiotics for ear, nose, and throat (ENT) complaints.
- Proper equipment, including an otoscope with a pneumatic attachment and an ophthalmoscope, is critical for performing a proper physical exam.

RED FLAGS

Eyes

- Sudden acute onset of vision loss—immediate referral to emergency care is needed.
- Herpetic keratitis—use topical steroid eye preparations cautiously as they may increase intraocular pressure. Use caution because herpetic keratitis may present similarly to viral conjunctivitis.
- Chemical burns—irrigate immediately and copiously before evaluation.
- History suggestive of ocular foreign body with no visible findings—refer to ophthalmologist. Many eye problems require evaluation and management by a specialist. (See Table 6–1 for signs and symptoms that should be referred immediately to an ophthalmologist.)

TABLE 6–1.
RED FLAG SIGNS AND SYMPTOMS OF VISION-THREATENING DISORDERS

SYMPTOMS	SIGNS
Blurred vision that does *not* clear with blinking	Ciliary flush
Acute loss or decreased vision	Corneal damage (opacities, trauma)
Halos around sources of lights	Abnormal pupils
Flashing lights	Increased intraocular pressure
Sudden floating spots or sensation of "cob-webs" across field of vision	Shallow anterior chamber
Photophobia	Severe green-yellow discharge from eye
Periocular headache	Erythema, chemosis, and lid edema
Ocular pain	Absent red reflex
Nystagmus	Proptosis (forward displacement of the eye globe within the orbit

- *Acute angle-closure glaucoma* results in permanent vision loss if not treated *immediately*.
- *Retinoblastoma* (malignant tumor of retina) may present as white pupils (leukocoria), esotropia, exotropia, or anisocoria; refer to ophthalmologist for prompt evaluation.
- Contact lens wearers are at higher risk for corneal damage.

Ears

- Complications of ear infections: Otitis media or externa with spreading infection, mastoid tenderness, lymphadenopathy, and neurologic abnormalities are urgent for referral.
- Suspected perforated tympanic membrane is a contraindication for removal of cerumen impaction; refer to a specialist.
- Coronavirus disease 2019 (COVID-19) symptoms can include vertigo, tinnitus, peripheral facial palsy, and hearing loss. Consider COVID-19 testing based on exposure history, review of systems, and physical examination.

Nose and Sinuses

- Important, serious findings pointing to complications of sinusitis include external facial swelling, erythema, or cellulitis over an involved sinus (periorbital or forehead); vision changes such as diplopia; difficulty moving eyes (extraocular movements [EOMs]); proptosis; and any abnormal neurologic signs. *Urgent for referral.*

- COVID-19 symptoms can include nasal congestion, anosmia, cacosmia, hyposmia, and rhinorrhea. Consider COVID-19 testing based on exposure history, review of systems, and physical examination.

Throat/Mouth

- *Epiglottal spasm:* in cases of suspected epiglottitis, attempting to examine the oral cavity or insert a tongue blade for visualization of the pharynx can result in acute airway obstruction and potential asphyxiation.
- Consider *peritonsillar abscess* when the patient with severe tonsillitis (usually more pronounced unilaterally) appears toxic with fever, trismus, "hot potato" voice, palatal bulge, and uvula deviation.
- Avulsed teeth should be rinsed in water and immediately reinserted before sending for emergency dental referral. Tooth can be transported in milk or saline, or inside the cheek if no risk of accidentally swallowing exists, as with children.
- COVID-19 symptoms can include hypogeusia and sore throat. Consider COVID-19 testing based on exposure history, review of systems, and physical examination.

TABLE 6–2.
ACUTE AND CHRONIC EYE DISORDERS

ACUTE	CHRONIC
Acute angle-closure glaucoma	Cataracts
Blepharitis	Ketoconjunctivitis sicca (dry eye syndrome)
Conjunctivitis	Open-angle glaucoma
Corneal ulcer	Strabismus
Hordeolum	
Iritis	
Keratitis	
Nasolacrimal duct obstruction	
Ocular trauma (Ocular foreign body, corneal abrasion, hyphema, subconjunctival hemorrhage)	
Retinoblastoma	
Uveitis	

Disorders of the Eyes

BLEPHARITIS

Description

- Inflammatory disease process of the eyelid(s)—chronic or acute
  - Anterior blepharitis involves the eyelashes and follicles; usually subdivided into staphylococcal, *Demodex* mite infestation, and seborrheic types
  - Posterior blepharitis involves meibomian gland orifices; is more common than anterior blepharitis

Etiology

- Seborrheic: sebaceous gland dysfunction with accelerated shedding of skin cells
- Staphylococcal: super infection of Zeis glands of lid margin and meibomian glands posterior to lashes with *Staphylococcus aureus*; usually part of mixed blepharitis
- Meibomian gland dysfunction: obstruction and inflammation of the gland; associated with acne rosacea, acne vulgaris, and oral retinoid therapy
- Blepharitis may develop as a late manifestation of COVID-19.

Incidence and Demographics

- One of the most common (20% 45 years and older, 68% 60 years and older) eye disorders in adults; not common in children
  - Males and females affected equally
  - Mixed (seborrheic and infectious) blepharitis most common type

Risk Factors

- History of skin problems: seborrheic dermatitis, contact dermatitis, acne rosacea, dry eye syndrome
- Poor hygiene, including improper cleaning of the face using old or contaminated eye makeup; contact lens use
- Immunocompromise due to chemotherapy, diabetes, or HIV

Prevention and Screening

- Maintenance of long-term regimen of lid hygiene can decrease risk of recurrence.

Assessment

History

- Unilateral or bilateral eye irritation; itching, erythema, flaking, or crusting of the lids; changes in the eyelashes
  - Common complaints: burning, watering, gritty sensation, crusting and matting of the lashes and medial canthus, red lids, red eyes, photophobia, and impaired vision
  - Symptoms worse upon awakening (typically in the morning)
  - Additional complaints of purulent drainage if infection has developed (conjunctivitis, stye)
  - History of recurrent stye, acne, rosacea, or eczema
  - History of COVID-19 diagnosis.

Physical Exam

- All types: eyelid erythema, collarettes of inflammation around lashes, change in eye-lash pattern (broken, missing, misdirected)
- Seborrheic type: dandruff-like flaking, scaling, waxy surface of lid margin
- Infectious: purulent discharge, concurrent papules or pustules, punctate ulcerations
- Mixed: all signs listed above
- Chronic: thickening of lid with or without above concurrent symptoms
- Conjunctiva may be infected.
- Visual acuity unaffected; exam of cornea and pupil normal

Diagnostic Studies

- Rarely, a culture of secretions may be indicated if treatment failure with usual antibiotics

Differential Diagnosis

- Chalazion, hordeolum, conjunctivitis, and keratitis may result from blepharitis.
- Styes and chalazion: consider blepharitis if no response to treatment after 1 month.
- Sebaceous cell carcinoma of eyelid: initial presentation similar to blepharitis (usually unilateral), styes, and chalazion; consider if no response to treatments after 1 month.
- COVID-19

Management

Nonpharmacologic Treatment

- Warm, moist compresses four times a day x 15 minutes to soften encrustations
- Gentle lid massage with circular motion following warm compress application
- Daily lid hygiene using dilute tear-free shampoo with warm, damp cotton tip (cotton swab or ball)
- Discontinue use of contact lens or eye makeup while symptomatic or being treated
- Maintenance: long-term regimen of lid hygiene helps prevent outbreaks of more symptomatic disease.

Pharmacologic Treatment

- Topical ophthalmic antibiotics: choice of bacitracin, sodium sulfacetamide, erythromycin, and ofloxacin depending on sensitivities, allergies; frequency and duration of treatment guided by severity
- Severe cases: consider oral antibiotic use—choice of doxycycline 100 mg/day or tetracycline 1,000 mg/day in divided doses, tapered after clinical improvement (2–4 weeks) to doxycycline 50 mg/day or tetracycline 250–500 mg/day. For pregnant women or children consider erythromycin or azithromycin (500 mg on day 1, followed by 250 mg on days 2–5)
- Short-term topical corticosteroids for acute eyelid or ocular surface inflammation may be useful. Should be evaluated by ophthalmologist prior to use and 2 weeks after use.

Special Considerations

- A herpes simplex virus (HSV) infection of the eyelid may appear very similar to *Staphylococcus* blepharitis but has acute onset.

When to Consult, Refer, Hospitalize

- Refer to ophthalmologist if treatment fails or if concurrent or additional symptoms develop that require surgical treatment (meibomian gland drainage or extraction)

Follow-Up

Expected Course

- Alleviate chronic inflammatory symptoms with lid hygiene.
- Infectious component should resolve with treatment as above

Complications

- Spread of infection to conjunctiva, cornea, or both
- Scarring of eyelid margin

NASOLACRIMAL DUCT OBSTRUCTION

Description

- Dacryostenosis: "blocked tear ducts" with tear drainage cut off between lacrimal sac and nose
- Most common cause of persistent tearing and ocular discharge in infants

Etiology

- Blockage caused by residual epithelial membranes; canalization of the nasolacrimal duct is incomplete
- Generally, not completely occluded

Incidence and Demographics

- Occurs in up to 6% of newborns; however, 5% to 20% of healthy infants may have symptoms at sometime during the first year of life.

Risk Factors

- Prematurity, parent may report excessive tearing

Prevention and Screening

- No known prevention

Assessment

History

- Parent reports chronic or intermittent tearing and debris on eyelashes (matting) from one or both eyes
- Redness of the conjunctiva is not typical; mild redness of lower lid may be present from chronic rubbing of eyes.

Physical Exam

- Note presence of watery or mucous discharge; may be purulent if infected; eyes look wet, tearing over lid; increase in size of tear meniscus; palpation of lacrimal sac may cause reflux of tears or mucoid discharge
- Maceration of eyelids from excessive tearing; crusting on lashes

Diagnostic Studies

- None indicated; diagnosis based on history and physical exam; if area is infected, may perform culture and sensitivity
- May perform fluorescein study (dye disappearance test)

Differential Diagnosis

- Congenital glaucoma
- Entropion
- Conjunctivitis
- Corneal abrasion or foreign body
- Blepharitis
- Uveitis
- Dacryocystocele

Management

Nonpharmacologic Treatment

- Observe for up to 6–7 months if asymptomatic other than watery eyes.
- Lacrimal sac (Crigler) massage: Apply moderate pressure downward on lacrimal sac to expel buildup 2–3 times per day until symptoms resolve.
- Lacrimal duct probing and irrigation: should be performed by an ophthalmologist, usually if unresolved by 12 months of age; may be done sooner if recurrent infection or lid irritation
- Nasolacrimal duct (NLD) intubation (stent) or balloon dacryocystoplasty have been used in treatment failure and in children older than 12 months of age

Pharmacologic Treatment

- Treat secondary infections with topical antibiotics (tobramycin, moxifloxacin, gentamycin, erythromycin, sulfacetamide, or fluoroquinolones); short course, 3–5 days.
- Moxifloxacin is not recommended for treatment of secondary infections.

How Long to Treat

- Depends on response to treatment

Special Considerations

- None

When to Consult, Refer, Hospitalize

- Re-evaluate at 6–7 months; refer to ophthalmologist if patient remains symptomatic; signs and symptoms of dacryocystitis or dacryocystocele; or signs of amblyopia or anisometropia.

Follow-Up

Expected course

- 90% of cases will resolve spontaneously by 6 months of age.

Complications

- Acute or chronic dacryocystitis
- Secondary infection of conjunctivae or eyelids due to excessive drainage

KETOCONJUNCTIVITIS SICCA

Description

- Known as dry eye disease (DED)
- Aqueous deficient dry eye (ADDE) due to limited tear production
- Evaporative dry eye disease (EDE) due to tear evaporation
- One of the most common reasons for eye complaints

Etiology

- ADDE—reduced tear production from the lacrimal glands
- EDE—meibomian gland dysfunction results in excessive evaporation of the tear film.
- May be related to Sjögren syndrome.

Incidence and Demographics

- More common in women than men, 2:1 ratio
- More common in adults 50 years and older
- 10% to 30% of the population affected
- Prevalence increasing in young adults due to contact lens and technology use

Risk Factors

- Vitamin A deficiency can cause lacrimal acinar damage and goblet cell disruption
- Aging
- Certain medications can impair aqueous production—isotretinoin, diuretics, anticholinergics, antihistamines, beta blockers, oral contraceptives, and phenothiazines.
- Sjögren syndrome
- Eyelid palsy, malposition, or margin abnormality
- Contact lens use
- Ocular surface disease
- Recent laser vision correction (e.g., LASIK).

Prevention and Screening

- Annual screening for patients wearing contact lens

Assessment

History

- Redness
- Dryness
- Itching
- Photophobia
- Burning or gritty sensation

- Mucoid discharge
- History of Sjögren syndrome

Physical Exam

- Conjunctival injection
- Breakdown of the ocular surface
- Excessive reflex tearing from irritation due to dryness
- Reduced blink rate
- Malposition of the eye lids

Diagnostic Studies

- Symptom questionnaires (e.g., Ocular Surface Disease Index, Dry Eye Questionnaire, Symptom Assessment of Dry Eye, Contact Lens Dry Eye Questionnaire, Contact Lens Impact on Quality of Life)
- Schirmer test—assesses aqueous tear production
- Tear breakup time—most used to assess tear film instability
- Impression cytology
- Thermography—measures cooling of the ocular surface due to evaporation
- Epithelial staining—assesses ocular surface damage

Differential Diagnosis

- Blepharitis
- Ocular rosacea
- Toxic keratopathy
- Conjunctivitis
- Bell's palsy
- Contact lens complication
- Floppy eyelid syndrome

Management

Nonpharmacologic Treatment

- Reduce technology use.
- Ophthalmology to treat lid disease
- Essential fatty acid supplementation
- Proper lid hygiene and warm compresses
- Ophthalmology procedures (e.g., pulsed light therapy, heating, and expression of meibomian glands)

Pharmacologic Treatment

- Artificial tears (gel formulations are preferred)
- Topical or systemic omega-3 fatty acids
- Cyclosporine 0.05% ophthalmic emulsion 1 drop OU two times a day
- Lifitegrast 5% ophthalmic solution 1 drop OU two times a day
- Doxycycline 100 mg QD or BID for meibomian gland dysfunction

When to Consult, Refer, Hospitalize

- Refer to ophthalmology for cases unresponsive to pharmacologic treatment and those requiring surgical procedures

Follow-Up

Expected Course

- Most patients experience improvement with lubricants
- Severe cases require surgical management

Complications

- Prolonged dry eye can result in corneal ulceration or corneal perforation
- Corneal ulceration and corneal perforation can cause blindness

HORDEOLUM (STYE) AND CHALAZION

Description

- Inflammatory disorders of the lubricating glands of the eyelids and eyelashes
- Hordeolum (stye): acute inflammation or infection of the eyelid margin involving the sebaceous gland of an eyelash or meibomian gland
- Chalazion: chronic inflammation that develops when a Zeis or meibomian gland becomes obstructed

Etiology

- Obstructed glands (Zeis, Moll, or meibomian) cause inflammatory papule, pustule, or granulomatous papule.
- Hordeolum: 90%–95% caused by infection with *S. aureus*
- Chalazion: chronic inflammation that develops when a Zeis or meibomian gland becomes obstructed; more often internal eyelid

Incidence and Demographics

- Predominant age: none, seen in all ages
- Predominant sex: male and female equally affected

Risk Factors

- Poor eyelid hygiene
- Previous hordeolum
- Wearing contact lenses
- Applying makeup
- Blepharitis and rosacea

Prevention and Screening

- Eyelid hygiene

Assessment

History

- Patient complains of a sudden onset of localized tenderness, swelling, or redness of the eyelid.
- Foreign body sensation
- History of prior episodes

Physical Exam

- Localized or generalized inflammation or erythema of the eyelid
- Erythematous papule or pustule may be visible on outer or conjunctival aspect of eyelid.
- Possible ulceration at base of lash follicle where infectious head has ruptured
- Conjunctiva may be infected.
- Visual acuity unaffected; exam of cornea and pupil normal

Diagnostic Studies

- Usually none indicated, culture of eyelid margins usually not necessary

Differential Diagnosis

- Sebaceous cell carcinoma (rare)
- Trauma
- Blepharitis
- Dacryocystitis
- Periorbital cellulitis

Management

Nonpharmacologic Treatment

- Warm compresses for 15 minutes 4 times per day
- Daily lid hygiene until resolved (see section on blepharitis)
- Educate patient not to squeeze or express hordeolum.

Pharmacologic Treatment

- Ophthalmic antibiotics on eyelid margin: erythromycin ointment (Ilotycin) up to 6 times daily for 7–10 days
- Artificial tears for underlying dry eyes
- Oral dicloxacillin or cephalexin for 2 weeks if refractory to topical antibiotics

How Long to Treat

- Lid hygiene and warm compresses continued until resolution
- Antibiotic ointment for 7–10 days

Special Considerations

- None

When to Consult, Refer, Hospitalize

- Refer nonresponding conditions to an ophthalmologist for excision and drainage or curettage.
- Although rare, the initial presentation of cancer is similar to that of blepharitis, styes, and chalazion; consider if no response to treatment after 1 month and refer to ophthalmology.

Follow-Up

Expected Course

- Usually resolves with good hygiene and warm compresses
- May be recurrent or develop in clusters that do not heal well; consider diabetes mellitus
- If no improvement, assess need for surgical treatment

Complications

- Cellulitis of the eyelid

STRABISMUS

Description

- Abnormal ocular alignment; commonly referred to as "crossed eyes"
- Can occur in one or both eyes, and in any direction
- Described as "esotropia" when eyes are crossed inward (nasal deviation); "exotropia" when eyes are crossed outward (temporal deviation); "hypertropia" or "hypotro pia" when the eyes deviate upward or downward, regardless of which eye is fixated.
- If uncorrected, it may result in amblyopia (loss or lack of development of central vision in one eye). When eyes are misaligned, the brain will receive two images instead of one; the brain manages this by "shutting down" or not processing one of the images. Left untreated, this eventually becomes permanent, leading to loss of depth perception. Children do not outgrow strabismus.

Etiology

- Unknown cause in most children
- May be congenital or acquired (disease-induced); may be caused by diseases including cranial nerve palsies, orbital mass, orbital fractures, Graves' ophthalmopathy, retinoblastoma, neurologic disorders such as cerebral palsy, and certain genetic conditions
- May be paralytic (paralysis of one or more ocular muscles) or nonparalytic (unequal muscle tone)

- Viral infections can affect cranial nerves, causing development of strabismus; in case of viral illness, strabismus may resolve spontaneously.
- Results from an inability of the visual cortex to use the eyes together, or a disorder of the cranial nerves (III, IV, or VI) or the extraocular muscles
- An intermittent phoria—esophoria or exophoria—is common in the first 6 months of life. It may be noted by parents particularly when infant is tired; parents may report that child's eyes are "crossed" for a few seconds to minutes. Phorias resolve spontaneously by 6 months of life and do not require referral before that time.

Incidence and Demographics

- Genetic: Parents with strabismus have a 12%–17% chance of having a child with strabismus.
- Occurs in approximately 4% of children

Risk Factors

- Family history of strabismus
- Prematurity
- Low birth weight with a history of retinopathy of prematurity or neurologic complications
- Any other disease that causes vision loss may also cause strabismus.

Prevention and Screening

- Alignment of eyes should be assessed at birth and on all well-child checkups; visual acuity should be assessed in routine exams as soon as children are capable of using pediatric eye charts, at age 3 years and 5 years (sooner if indicated).

Assessment

History

- Parent reports that the child's eyes "don't move together," "are crossed"
- Developmental/birth history
- Family history of strabismus or other eye disorders

- History of trauma, other medical problems, or exposure to toxins or medications
- Onset of deviation (early infancy); duration and severity of deviation; whether deviation is constant or intermittent and what exacerbates the deviation (fatigue, positions of gaze)

Physical Exam

- Assess general health, developmental level, neurologic status, and the presence of a head tilt.
- Assess visual acuity and function, pupillary reactivity, and eyelid position.
- Extraocular movements (EOMs): Six cardinal positions of gaze (CN III, IV, and VI) would detect primarily a paralytic strabismus, but in each position the corneal light reflex can be used to assess for nonparalytic strabismus.
- Corneal light reflex (Hirschberg): demonstrates a nonparalytic tropia.
- Cover test: No movement is detected if the patient has normal ocular alignment. Strabismus is present if the eye that is not occluded shifts to re-fixate.
- Cover/uncover test: The patient stares at a fixed point. A cover is placed over one eye for a few seconds and then is rapidly removed. The eye that was under the cover is carefully observed for movement or deviation; if detected, latent strabismus is present.
- Brückner test: The provider stands about 20 inches from the child in a darkened room, looks at both eyes through the ophthalmoscope, and notes symmetry of red reflexes bilaterally.
    - Note presence of nystagmus or other involuntary eye movements.
- Perform a funduscopic exam; note fullness of red reflex.

Diagnostic Studies

- Neuroimaging studies (visual evoked response, electroretinogram, and electrooculography) may be ordered by an ophthalmologist
    - Consider in children with craniofacial malformations, neurologic abnormalities, trauma, or acute onset of paralytic or restrictive strabismus
- Computerized tomography (CT) scan and magnetic resonance imaging (MRI) studies of the orbits and head may be helpful to exclude an intra- cranial mass (bleed or tumor) if onset is acute or if associated with trauma, craniofacial abnormalities, or neurologic disease.

Differential Diagnosis

- Pseudostrabismus
- Amblyopia
- Ocular instability of infancy
- Cranial nerve palsies
- CNS or orbital tumor
- Orbital fractures
- Graves' ophthalmopathy

Management

Nonpharmacologic Treatment

- Treatment should be started as soon as a diagnosis is made.
- Management depends on the cause.
- Goal of treatments is to improve ocular alignment and binocularity.
- Any child in whom strabismus is suspected must be evaluated and treated by a pediatric ophthalmologist.
- Use of optical devices (prisms and glasses). Eyeglasses may be sufficient to induce binocular function and correct refractive errors.
- Surgery on the eye muscles is successful up to 80% of the time; some patients (20%–25%) may require a second surgery.
- The unaffected eye may be patched, alone or before glasses or surgery, to prevent amblyopia.
- Visual training exercises may be useful.

Pharmacologic Treatment

- Topical miotic drops to manipulate accommodation (atropine 1% daily or on weekends) may be helpful in some forms of esotropia. This is only prescribed by the ophthalmologist.
- Botulinum toxin A (Botox) injection: produces a dose-dependent duration of paralysis to the extraocular muscle. Two or more injections are usually necessary for lasting effects.

Special Considerations

- None

When to Consult, Refer, Hospitalize

- Constant strabismus at any age
- Corneal light reflex test or cover test abnormality
- Persistent esodeviations after 4 months of age
- Asymmetry of pupil with Brückner test
- Any change in deviation
- Parental concern of ocular alignment
- Refer to an ophthalmologist *as soon as strabismus is observed,* especially in infancy; in an infant younger than 1 year, amblyopia can occur with as little as 1 week of abnormal visual input.

Follow-Up

Expected Course

- Depends on type and treatment modality employed; once alignment is achieved, patients are followed by ophthalmologist every 3–6 months (depending on age and type of strabismus).
- Decompensation and reappearance may occur in up to 40% of patients in adulthood.

Complications

- Amblyopia, diplopia (in acquired strabismus in patients 3 years of age or older)
- Secondary contracture of the extraocular muscles, limiting extraocular mobility and binocular visual fields
- Secondary contracture develops over a course of weeks to months if strabismus is not treated
- Adverse psychosocial and vocational consequences

RETINOBLASTOMA

Description

- Rare malignant tumor originating from the retina; most common intraocular tumor of childhood; can be unilateral (75%) or bilateral (25%)

Etiology

- Genetic mutations of nerve cells in the retina originate in retinoblasts following loss, mutation, deletion, or rearrangement of retinoblastoma gene on chromosome 13.
- Hereditary retinoblastoma is autosomal dominant and tends to affect both eyes.
- Unaffected parents who have one child with retinoblastoma have a 4%–7% risk of having a subsequent child with the disease.

Incidence and Demographics

- Occurs in 1:15,000 to 1:16,600 live births in the United States and Northern Europe
- Ninety percent of all retinoblastoma cases are diagnosed by 3 years of age.
- Forty percent inherited; 60% noninheritable type
- Accounts for 3% of all malignancies in children younger than 15

Risk Factors

- Family history of retinoblastoma or retinomas (nonmalignant)

Prevention and Screening

- None known; genetic testing can identify individuals with the retinoblastoma mutation only about 5% of the time (not helpful).
- Red reflex checks at all well baby and well child visits
- Assess all children with strabismus to rule out retinoblastoma.
- Siblings and children of parents with retinoblastoma should have thorough ophthalmic examinations (which can be done under anesthesia) shortly after birth, every 3 months until age 3–4, and every 6 months until age 5–6.

Assessment

History

- Parents may note crossed eyes or outward deviation of eyes.
- Leukocoria may be noticed in a photograph.
- Pain and redness are rare; usually no complaints of visual problems because the unaffected eye maintains the vision.
- Note family history of malignancies, particularly of the eyes.

Physical Exam

- "Cat's eye reflex" (leukocoria): white pupil seen when observing the red reflex; may be unilateral or bilateral; not necessary for diagnosis
- Presence of strabismus, anisocoria, decreased vision, ocular inflammation, or proptosis (late finding)

Diagnostic Studies

- All studies should be done by an ophthalmologist and an oncologist.
- Dilated indirect ophthalmoscopic examination performed under anesthesia.
- Aqueous cytology (rarely used as it can increase risk of extraocular spread of retino blastoma); CT scan of the head and orbits.
- MRI to confirm the presence of an intraocular mass
- Ocular ultrasonography

Differential Diagnosis

- Retinopathy of prematurity
- Coats' disease
- Hypopyon
- Iritis
- Uveitis

- Toxoplasmosis, other ocular infections
- Strabismus

Management

- By ophthalmology and oncology; treatment will depend on extent of disease and may include intraocular or intravenous chemotherapy, radiation, radioactive plaques (I-125 brachytherapy), cryotherapy, laser photoablation, and surgery (enucleation).
- Fractionated external beam radiation therapy (EBRT): reserved for eyes with residual or recurrent retinoblastoma following a complete course of intravenous chemotherapy. EBRT is associated with fatal bony and soft tissue secondary malignant neoplasms.

When to Consult, Refer, Hospitalize

- All children with retinoblastoma should be referred immediately to ophthalmology.

Follow-Up

- Frequently by ophthalmology; every 3 months for the first year after treatment; if stable, follow-up visits can be tapered to every 4 to 6 months until age 6 or 7, and then annually
- Long-term by multidisciplinary team

Future evaluations for:

- Contralateral eye developing retinoblastoma (in about 15%)
- Metastasis: occurs before 5 years
- Second malignancies; may include osteosarcoma (most common), bladder, breast, lung cancer, and melanoma; occurs in about 10% of children

Expected course

- Ninety-four percent overall 5-year survival rate in the United States
- Development of metastatic disease usually seen within 1 year of diagnosis
- Poor prognosis for children with metastatic disease
- Vision salvageable in a large percentage of children diagnosed at early stages

Complications

- Increase risk of cancer returning in eye and other areas
- Death
- Blindness

CONJUNCTIVITIS

Description

- Acute inflammation of the palpebral and/or bulbar conjunctival layer of the eyes
- Commonly referred to as "pink eye" or "red eye"; may be bilateral or unilateral
- Conjunctivitis in first month of life is most commonly caused by infections passed through vaginal delivery; known as ophthalmia neonatorum.

Etiology

- Many causative organisms; *Chlamydia trachomatis* and *Neisseria gonorrhoeae* most common in newborns
- Viral:
  - adenoviruses (most common)
  - herpes zoster
  - herpes simplex virus (HSV) type 1 and type 2
  - enterovirus
  - Zika
- Bacterial:
  - Adults:
    - *S. aureus*
    - *C. trachomatis*
    - *N. gonorrheae*
    - *Neisseria meningitidis* as STDs

- ◇ Children:
  - *Haemophilus influenzae*
  - *Streptococcus pneumoniae*
  - *Moraxella catarrhalis*
- ◇ Allergic: allergic rhinitis ("hay fever"), seasonal allergies, atopy, contact blepharitis, nonspecific
- ◇ Irritative: topical medications, wind, dry eye, contact lens solutions, UV light exposure, smoke
- ◇ Autoimmune: Sjögren's syndrome, Wegener's granulomatosis, pemphigoid
- ◇ Rare: fungal, parasitic, rickettsia, tuberculosis, syphilis, Kawasaki disease, gout, Graves' disease, sarcoidosis, psoriasis, Stevens-Johnson syndrome, Reiter syndrome
- ◇ Conjunctivitis is the most common ophthalmic manifestation of COVID-19.

Incidence and Demographics

- ♦ Common eye disorder in all ages
- ♦ Pediatric: viral, bacterial
- ♦ Adult: viral, bacterial, allergic
- ♦ Increased incidence in the fall because of higher incidence of viral infections and exposure to seasonal allergens

Risk Factors

- ♦ History of contact with infected people
- ♦ Contact lenses: especially wearing lenses overnight
- ♦ STD contact: gonococcal (rate in adults), *Chlamydia*, syphilis, or herpes
- ♦ Exposure to infectious agents, chemical agents, wind, extreme temperatures, allergens

Prevention and Screening

- ♦ Avoid known allergens, irritants, and others with conjunctivitis.
- ♦ Frequent handwashing and good hygiene to reduce risk of transmission
- ♦ Provide gonorrhea prophylaxis for newborns: 1% silver nitrate, 0.5% erythromycin, or 1% tetracycline ointment.

Assessment

History (see Table 6–2)

- Irritated eyes with redness, mild pain, or itching in one or both eyes, or spread from one to the other (bilateral more common with bacterial infections)
- Gritty, scratching, or burning sensation; sensation of fullness around the eyes; itching; and photophobia
- Watery or purulent drainage, crusting on eyelashes upon awakening. Watery (more common with viral, less copious with allergic) or purulent drainage (bacterial)
- Visual complaints limited to complaints of blurry vision that clears with blinking
- Assess for associated symptoms that may indicate systemic disease, such as rash, lesions, joint pain, fever, genitourinary complaints, constitutional symptoms.
- Ascertain recent international travel to Zika zones.

Physical Exam

- Must document visual acuity
- Pupillary reaction and EOMs intact
- Edema of eyelids and matted eyelashes
- Red eye, conjunctival injection
- Foreign body sensation
- *Note:* ciliary flush, corneal changes, pupil abnormalities, and photophobia are not associated with simple conjunctivitis; must rule out keratitis, iritis, or other serious conditions through urgent referral (see Box 6–1)

Diagnostic Studies

- Eighty-eight percent of children have bacterial conjunctivitis if four criteria present: younger than 6 years old, no watery discharge, morning "glue eyes," winter months.
- Consider conjunctival scrapings for microscopic examination and culture; confer with a specialist in ophthalmology for purulent, membranous, or pseudomembranous.
- Enzyme immunoassays for *Chlamydia* organisms if suspected as etiology

TABLE 6–2. DIFFERENTIATING CHARACTERISTICS OF CONJUNCTIVITIS

CAUSE	SYMPTOMS
Bacterial	Children under 6 years old Often starts in one eye, spreads to both In young children, one-third have concurrent acute otitis media Occasionally associated with sore throat or fever +/- mild pruritus Moderate tearing Generalized hyperemia Copious nonwatery exudate; eyelids adherent ("glue eye") Preauricular adenopathy uncommon Stained scrapings/exudates: bacteria or polymorphonuclear cells (PMNCs) Conjunctival chemosis/edema If patient wears contact lenses, rule out microbial keratitis; *Pseudomonas* common organism
N. gonorrhea	Rare in adults, vertical transmission with newborns Copious amounts of purulent discharge Chemosis/conjunctival/lid edema
Chlamydia	Mild pruritus Moderate tearing Hyperemia generalized Profuse exudates: copious and eyelids "stuck together" Preauricular lymphadenopathy common with inclusion conjunctivitis Stained scrapings/exudates: PMNCs, plasma cells, inclusion bodies Never associated with sore throat or fever Genitourinary symptoms may be evident Photophobia (indicator of advanced infection)
Viral	Minimal pruritus Profuse tearing Generalized hyperemia Minimal exudate Preauricular lymphadenopathy common

Continued

TABLE 6–2.
(CONTINUED)

CAUSE	SYMPTOMS
	Stained scrapings/exudates: monocytes Occasionally associated with sore throat and fever Herpetic type may be associated with cold sores, burning sensation; rarely—itching
Allergic	Severe itchy eyes Moderate tearing (stringy discharge; usually bilateral) Generalized hyperemia Minimal exudates Preauricular lymphadenopathy: not present Stained scraping/exudates: eosinophils Never associated with sore throat or fever +/- associated allergy type symptoms (rhinitis, sneezing, scratchy throat) Seasonal or dander allergies Chemosis/conjunctival/eyelid edema "Cobblestone" appearance of conjunctival edema

- May consider fluorescein staining to assess for epithelial integrity (corneal abrasion, keratitis, ulcer).
- COVID-19 testing as appropriate based on history and review of systems.

Differential Diagnosis

- Acute uveitis
- Foreign body/corneal ulcers
- Acute glaucoma
- Scleritis, episcleritis
- Blepharitis
- Pingueculitis
- Keratitis
- Rubeola, rubella
- Herpes simplex virus (HSV 1)

- Zika virus syndrome
- COVID-19

Management

Nonpharmacologic Treatment

- Apply warm or cool moist compresses
- Replace eye makeup, especially mascara
- Patient should avoid wearing contact lenses until conjunctivitis resolves and consider replacement with new lenses.
- Educate patient on proper use of eye drops.
- Patient should avoid irritants (smoke, wind, sun).

Pharmacologic Treatment

- Allergic and atopic:
  - Ketotifen (Zaditor, Alaway) 0.25%, 1 drop two times a day
  - Cromolyn (Opticrom) 4%, 1 drop four times a day
  - Epinastine (Elestat) 0.05%, 1 drop two times a day
  - Ketorolac (Acular) 0.1%, 1 drop four times a day
  - Emedastine 0.05%, 1 drop four times a day
  - Azelastine (Optivar) 0.05%, 1 drop two times a day
  - Olopatadine (Patanol) 0.1%, 1 drop two times a day, or 0.2%, 1 drop daily
  - Oral nonsedating antihistamines: cetirizine (Zyrtec), fexofenadine (Allegra), for nasal and urticarial symptoms
  - Oral antihistamine (diphenhydramine) in severe cases
- Bacterial:
  - Young children: *H. influenzae* most common, *S. pneumoniae* less common if child received pneumococcal conjugate vaccine 13 (PCV13); check vaccine status.
    - Trimethoprim/polymyxin (Polytrim) ophthalmic 1–2 drops four times a day x 7 days
    - Moxifloxacin ophthalmic solution more than 4 monthS old: 1 drop three times a day x 7 days (quicker response, but more expensive)

- Oral: If concurrent acute otitis media (AOM) Augmentin 80 mg/kg/day x 10 days (not amoxicillin) or Cefdinir 14 mg/kg/day x 10 days to cover both infections

◊ Adults:

- Trimethoprim/polymyxin (Polytrim) ophthalmic 1–2 drops four times a day x 7 days
- Erythromycin (Ilotycin) ophthalmic ointment ½ inch two to four times a day x 5 days (not as effective for young children with haemophilus influenzae (H. Flu) or staphylococcus aureus (Staph)
- Sulfacetamide sodium (Bleph-10) 2 drops every 4 hours while awake x 5 days
- Tobramycin 3% (Tobrex) ophthalmic drops every 4 hours; ointment every 8 hours
- Moxifloxacin ophthalmic solution 1 drop three times a day x 7 days (quicker response, but more expensive)

◊ Gonococcal

- Hospitalize and treat with systemic ceftriaxone (Rocephin) 25–50 mg/kg/day IV or IM, or cefotaxime (Claforan) 25–50 mg/kg/day IV or IM every 12h x 7 days; if no corneal lesions, ceftriaxone 1 g IM x1 and topical bacitracin ophthalmic ointment ½ inch four times a day x 7 days

◊ Chlamydial:

- Adults—doxycycline (Vibramycin) 100 mg orally two times a day x 3 weeks; children—erythromycin 50 mg/kg/day orally ÷ 4 doses x 14 days
- Neonates: erythromycin ethylsuccinate 30 mg/kg/day every 6 hours orally x 14 days

◊ If other bacteria suspected, base treatment on culture and sensitivity results

♦ Viral (non-herpetic):

◊ Artificial tears for symptomatic relief

◊ Vasoconstrictor/antihistamine (naphazoline/pheniramine) four times a day for severe itching

◊ May consider topical antibiotics (see above)

♦ Viral (herpetic): Refer to ophthalmologist for treatment.

How Long to Treat

♦ Length of treatment determined by etiology and responsiveness to treatment

◊ Bactericidal agents resolve symptoms more quickly but are more expensive

◊ Bacteriostatic agents (trimethoprim/polymyxin) take longer but are less expensive

- If not resolved in 5–7 days, consider alternate diagnosis/ophthalmologic consultation
- Refer to ophthalmologist if condition is worse in 24 hours.

Special Considerations

- Geriatric: suspect autoimmune, systemic, or irritative conditions
- Pregnancy or lactation: Do not use doxycycline.
- Day care regulations may require a child to be treated with a topical antibiotic despite lack of evidence.

When to Consult, Refer, Hospitalize

- Hospitalization for hyperacute bacterial conjunctivitis requiring IV antibiotics or for penetrating ocular trauma
- Immediate referral to ophthalmologist if moderate to severe pain, ciliary flush, change in visual acuity, abnormal eye exam, evidence of keratitis or uveitis, contact lens–related bacterial conjunctivitis, or signs of herpetic etiology
- Referral to ophthalmologist if symptoms worsen within 24 hours

Follow-Up

Expected Course

- Bacterial conjunctivitis: 2–5 days with treatment, 5–7 days without treatment
- Viral conjunctivitis: 5–14 days
- Herpes simplex virus: 2–3 weeks
- Allergic: seasonal

Complications

- Potential for spread of infection to surrounding areas (blepharitis, keratitis, iritis)
- Corneal ulcers or perforation (gonococcal infection)
- Scars on cornea, lids, with eyelids or lashes misdirected
- Hypopyon

IRITIS/UVEITIS/KERATITIS

Description

- Iritis: inflammation of the iris
- Keratitis: corneal inflammation or infection that is potentially vision-threatening; result of infection or direct irritation
- Uveitis: acute intraocular inflammation of one or more of the components of uveal tract (iris, ciliary body, choroids, and retina)
  - Anterior uveitis: inflammation of the iris (iritis) or iris and ciliary body (iridocyclitis); approximately 90% of patients with uveitis
  - Intermediate uveitis: inflammation of structures posterior to the lens (pars planitis or peripheral uveitis)
  - Posterior uveitis: inflammation of the choroid (choroiditis), retina (chorioretinitis), or vitreous near the optic nerve and macula
- Panuveitis: all components affected
  - May be acute or chronic

Etiology

- Uveitis (caused by trauma, infections, inflammation, or, rarely, neoplasms); isolated eye disease (lens-induced uveitis, trauma, pars planitis, acute retinal necrosis); masquerade syndromes (ocular lymphoma, leukemia, retinoblastoma); idiopathic (approximately 25%)
- Cause differs by location
- Anterior uveitis (iritis): trauma is common; 50% of non-traumatic causes are idiopath ic; 20% are caused by seronegative spondyloarthropathies (ankylosing spondylitis, reactive arthritis, psoriatic arthritis, inflammatory bowel disease); 10% are caused by juvenile idiopathic arthritis. Less common infections include herpes, syphilis, and tuberculosis.
- Intermediate: most are idiopathic.
- Posterior: toxoplasmosis is the most common, followed by idiopathic.
- Panuveitis: idiopathic (22% to 45%) and sarcoidosis (14% to 28%). Unilateral panuveitis is often endophthalmitis (endogenous or related to trauma or surgery). Bilateral panuveitis can be caused by sarcoidosis or syphilis.
- Keratitis: frequently associated with trauma, history of HSV, bacterial infections, or contact lens wear

Incidence and Demographics

- Noninfectious uveitis accounts for 10% of legal blindness in the United States.
- Eighty percent of uveitis cases seen in children are caused by juvenile rheumatoid arthritis.
- Affects all ages
- Affects males more than females (2.5:1) in HLA-B27 anterior uveitis; otherwise males and females equally affected
- Iritis is 4 times more prevalent than posterior uveitis.

Risk Factors

- Immunocompromised status
    - Autoimmune and inflammatory systemic conditions (Behçet's disease and ankylosing spondylitis, associated with the gene for human leukocyte antigen [HLA] B51/B5 and B27, respectively)
    - Contact lenses
    - HSV history or close contact with an HSV-infected person

Prevention and Screening

- High-risk groups: screened routinely by ophthalmology
- Contact precautions with active HSV lesions; varicella vaccination

Assessment

History

- Determine history of autoimmune diseases, STDs, tubercu losis, AIDS.
- Note decreased visual acuity.
- Usually unilateral eye pain, redness, tearing, photophobia, and decreased vision; 360-degree perilimbal injection
- History of eye trauma, an associated systemic disease, or risk factors for infection
- Anterior uveitis: acute onset of deep eye pain, redness, photophobia, visual loss

TABLE 6–3.
CHARACTERISTICS OF KERATITIS/IRITIS/UVEITIS

	DEFINITION	CAUSES	EXAM FINDINGS	PLAN
Keratitis	Corneal inflammation or infection that is potentially vision-threatening; due to infection or direct irritation	Trauma, contact lens use, and refractive corneal surgery are common causes of bacterial keratitis; herpes simplex virus types 1 and 2 or varicella zoster virus	Ciliary injection often with constricted pupils, watery or purulent discharge, photophobia, possible corneal clouding or lesions, vision loss depending on the location, extraocular herpetic rash	Refer to ophthalmology
Iritis/ Uveitis	Inflammation of the uveal tract, including the iris and the ciliary body (anterior) and/or choroid (posterior)	Often associated with immunologic disorders; infection with tuberculosis (TB), syphilis, cytomegalovirus (CMV), toxoplasmosis, herpes, Lyme disease; may be idiopathic	Deep eye pain, ciliary flush, photophobia, redness, tearing, decreased vision, 360-degree perilimbal injection	Refer to ophthalmology; consider human leukocyte antigen B27 (HLA-B27), antinuclear antibody (ANA), purified protein derivative (PPD), Lyme serology, rapid plasma regain (RPR) if severe or recurrent

- Intermediate uveitis and posterior uveitis: insidious onset; presents with altered vision or floaters; typically no pain, redness, tearing, or photophobia
- Keratitis: history of varicella or herpes simplex infection; prodromal period of fever, malaise, headache, and eye pain before eruptions or lesions may be common; acute onset of eye pain, headache, photophobia, tearing, ocular redness, decreased or blurred vision

Physical Exam

- Slit-lamp exam and indirect ophthalmoscopy are necessary for precise diagnosis.
- Assess visual acuity and extraocular movement; perform funduscopic exam.

- Anterior (iritis): tenderness to palpation, diffuse redness with perilimbal erythema; constricted pupil; frequently unilateral
- Iritis: opacities or haziness on the cornea and within the aqueous (may hinder funduscopic exam). If visualized, funduscopic findings may include keratic precipitates ("mutton fat"), nodules on the iris, hypopyon, macular changes (lesions, edema), and optic neuropathy (rare).
- Posterior uveitis: Funduscopic findings will vary with the offending organism; com monly bilateral.
- Keratitis: diffuse redness with ciliary injection, often with constricted pupil; eye discharge; and pain, photophobia, and vision loss depending on the location of ulcer ation; typically unilateral

Diagnostic Studies

- Usually unnecessary, but may need studies to determine whether an undiagnosed underlying cause exists
- Slit-lamp exam, dilated fundus exam, and intraocular pressure measurements by ophthalmologist

Differential Diagnosis

See Table 6–3

- Conjunctivitis
- Acute angle-closure glaucoma
- Retinal detachment
- Intraocular tumors
- Scleritis/episcleritis
- CNS lymphoma

Management

Nonpharmacologic Treatment

- Educate patient on proper method for instilling eye drops.
- Instruct patient to wear dark glasses if photophobia is a problem.

TABLE 6–3.
SELECTED DIFFERENTIAL DIAGNOSES OF THE RED EYE

CONDITION	PAIN	DISCHARGE	PHOTOPHOBIA	PUPILS	VISION LOSS	FLUORESCEIN STAIN	ANTERIOR CHAMBER
Acute Angle-Closure Glaucoma	Moderate to severe	No	Yes	Mid-sized, dilated, nonreactive	Yes	Normal	Shallow
Anterior Scleritis	Severe boring and piercing—worse at night and with eye movements	None	Possible	Equal	Occasional	Peripheral keratitis	Clear
Anterior Uveitis	Moderate to severe	None	Consensual	Constricted	Occasional	Dendrites	Cells or flares
Conjunctivitis	Minimal to none	Yes	None	Equal	No	Normal	Clear
Episcleritis	Mild	None	None	Equal	Occasional	Normal	Clear
Subconjunctival Hemorrhage	None	None	None	Equal	No	Normal	Clear

Adapted from: Alattas, O. A., Hamdi, A. A., Mudarba, F. M., Alsheheri, A. M., Al-Yahya, M. S., Almotairi, S. A., Saeed, R. A., Buamer. M. M., Alsuwailem, M. S., & Alamri, I. A. (2019). Red eye diagnosis and management in primary health care. *Archives of Pharmacy Practice, 10*(3), 1–5.

- Avoid all contact with nonimmune people
- Avoid contact lenses during treatment period
- Cool compresses

Pharmacologic Treatment (Under Management of an Ophthalmologist)

- Identify and treat any infections
- Artificial tears; oral pain medications
- Corticosteroids with or without cycloplegics
- Antimicrobials, systemic immunosuppression, chemotherapy,
- Anti-inflammatory therapy, treatment of underlying cause

When to Consult, Refer, Hospitalize

- Refer all patients immediately with red eye and vision loss to an ophthalmologist.
- Iritis and viral keratitis: urgent referral
- Bacterial keratitis: emergent referral

Follow-Up

Expected Course

- Uveitis/iritis: variable depending on underlying disease and tolerance to medications; need to evaluate other associated systemic disease
- Viral keratitis: patients monitored with slit-lamp exam every 1–2 days until improve ment, then every 3–4 days until epithelial defect improves, and then weekly until antiviral drops have been completed

Complications

- Loss of vision
- Cycloplegia: paralysis of ciliary muscle
- Cataract formation

- Glaucoma
- Recurrence of viral infection

GLAUCOMA

Description

- An optic neuropathy that leads to progressive, irreversible vision loss; frequently associated with increased intraocular pressure (IOP)
- Second leading cause of blindness
- Many different types—two main types are open-angle and angle-closure glaucoma
  - Open-angle: most common form in the United States (90% of all cases); optic neuropathy with progressive peripheral visual field loss followed by central field loss usually (not always) in the presence of elevated IOP; can be primary or chronic
  - Angle-closure glaucoma: narrowing or closure of the anterior chamber angle resulting in aqueous humor drainage leading to elevated IOP and damage to the optic nerve; also known as acute or narrow-angle glaucoma

Etiology

See Table 6–4

Incidence and Demographics

See Table 6–4

Risk Factors

See Table 6–4

Prevention and Screening

- Screening eye exam starting at age 40 biannually; sooner if high risk
- IOP screening age 40–65; intervals controversial
- Prophylactic laser treatment to second eye for prevention of damage

TABLE 6–4. CHARACTERISTICS OF OPEN-ANGLE GLAUCOMA AND ANGLE-CLOSURE GLAUCOMA

	OPEN-ANGLE GLAUCOMA	ANGLE-CLOSURE GLAUCOMA
Etiology	Slow clogging of the drainage canals, resulting in increase in IOP Develops slowly and is a lifelong condition Wide-open angle between the iris and cornea	Blocked drainage canals (anatomically predisposed, mass, or hemorrhage), resulting in sudden increase in IOP Develops suddenly Demands immediate medical attention Closed or narrow angle between the iris and cornea
Incidence/ Demographics	Usually older than 40 years Increases with age Male = female European and African descent more than Asian descent 44 million people affected worldwide	Age older than 40–50 years Female more than male Inuit and Asian more than African and European Most common form worldwide, but only 10% in the United States 20 million people affected worldwide (75% Asian)
Risk Factors Symptoms	Increased IOP Myopia Diabetes mellitus African American Older age Hypothyroidism Hypertension Diabetes Cardiovascular disease Family history Prolonged use of corticosteroids Painless, slowly progressive visual loss; central visual acuity remains unaffected until late in disease	Hyperopia (farsightedness) Age older than 40–50 years old shallow anterior chamber Female Family history Asian or Inuit descent Medications: antihistamines, adrenergic agents, antipsychotics, antidepressants, anticholinergic agents Emotional stress or sudden papillary dilation Severe unilateral ocular pain, blurred vision, lacrimation, photophobia, halos around lights/objects, frontal ipsilateral headaches, nausea, and vomiting

Continued

TABLE 6–4. (CONTINUED)

	OPEN-ANGLE GLAUCOMA	ANGLE-CLOSURE GLAUCOMA
Physical Exam	Detected incidentally during comprehensive ophthalmic examination Normal (8–20 mmHg) or increased IOP Fixed, mid-dilated pupil (higher than 20 mmHg) Increased cup-to-disc ratio Normal pupil	Elevated IOP (40–80 mmHg) Corneal and lid edema, conjunctival hyperemia, ciliary flush Pain with eye movement Shallow anterior chamber
Differential Diagnosis	Normal tension glaucoma Optic nerve pits Anterior ischemic optic neuropathy Compressive lesions of optic nerve or chiasm Posthemorrhagic (shock optic neuropathy)	Acute orbital compartment syndrome Traumatic hyphema Conjunctivitis, episcleritis Corneal abrasion Herpes zoster ophthalmicus Iritis and uveitis Glaucoma, malignant/neovascular Orbital/periorbital infection Lens-induced angle closure

Adapted from Domino, F. J. (2022). *The 5-minute clinical consult premium 2022.* (30th ed.). Philadelphia, PA: Wolters Kluwer.

Assessment

History

- Variable presentation depending on type; see Table 6–4
- Thorough history to identify precipitating events, other medical problems, medications

Physical Exam

- Findings are presented in Table 6–4 below as they correlate to the classifications of glaucoma.

- Screening exams include visual acuity, peripheral vision by confrontation, inspection of outer eye and sclera, pupillary response, and funduscopic exam to assess optic cup-to-disc ratio.
- Further examination by a specialist is required to assess with slit lamp.

Diagnostic Studies (Performed by Ophthalmologist)

- Tonometry: intraocular pressure measurement; IOP normal range is 10–20 mmHg; greater than 20 indicates need for further specialist evaluation
- Ophthalmoscopy: shape and color of optic nerve
- Perimetry: complete examination of field of vision
- Gonioscopy: angle in the eyes where iris meets cornea
- Pachymetry: thickness of the cornea

Differential Diagnosis

See Table 6–4, pages 378–379.

Management

Nonpharmacologic Treatment

- Open-angle glaucoma: argon laser trabeculoplasty; trabeculectomy (filtering surgery); shunt surgery, canaloplasty
- Angle-closure glaucoma: laser peripheral iridotomy after medical stabilization; surgical peripheral iridectomy if laser is not possible, cataract surgery with anterior lens implant
- Patient education: avoidance of certain medications (over-the-counter decongestants, motion sickness medications, adrenergic agents, antipsychotics, antidepressants, and anticholinergic agents) to prevent angle-closure attack; medication counseling and administration; instruction to seek emergency medical attention if there are changes in visual acuity, blurred vision, eye pain, or headache

Pharmacologic Treatment

- Open-angle glaucoma: ophthalmic and oral maintenance medications to reduce IOP
  - Decrease aqueous formation (timolol [Timoptic] 0.5%, acetazolamide [Diamox] 250 mg, or brimonidine tartrate 0.1%).
  - Increase aqueous outflow (pilocarpine [Isopto Carpine] 1–4%).
  - Enhance uveoscleral outflow (latanoprost [Xalatan] 0.005%).
- Angle-closure glaucoma: goal is to prevent or reverse angle closure, control IOP, and prevent damage to optic nerve
  - Beta-adrenergic blockers: 0.5% timolol maleate
  - Alpha-adrenergic agonists: 1% apraclonidine (Iopidine)
  - Prostaglandin analogs: latanoprost
  - Miotics: 2% pilocarpine
  - Carbonic anhydrase inhibitors: acetazolamide
  - Systemic hyperosmotic agents: mannitol (Osmitrol)

How Long to Treat

- Medical management is ongoing.

Special Considerations

- Medications must be used with caution in patients who are on diuretics or who have renal failure, asthma, chronic obstructive pulmonary disease (COPD), heart failure, cirrhosis, diabetes, or acidosis.
- Monitor for glaucoma/increased ocular pressure following laser vision correction. SMILE (Small Incision Lenicule Extraction) uses a smaller incision and lower incidence of increased ocular pressure. Post-operative steroids following photorefractive keratectomy (PRK) can increase the incidence of glaucoma. LASIK has the highest incidence of glaucoma risk among laser vision correction surgery.

When to Consult, Refer, Hospitalize

- Angle-closure glaucoma: requires immediate initiation of medication and referral to an ophthalmologist for surgical treatment

- Open-angle glaucoma: requires consult/referral to an ophthalmologist for examination and monitoring of the condition

Follow-Up

- Angle-closure glaucoma: postsurgical, chronic monitoring post-acute attack per ophthalmologist
- Open-angle glaucoma: every 3–6 months as directed by ophthalmologist

Expected Course

- Varies greatly depending on severity, duration, early/late diagnosis
- If treated surgically and in a timely manner, recurrence of acute attack is rare
- Medical management of open-angle glaucoma may prevent visual loss if initiated early and treated adequately.

Complications

- Loss of visual fields and visual acuity, leading to blindness if untreated
- Corneal damage: chronic edema, fibrosis, vascularization, or cataracts
- Atrophy of the iris, malignant glaucoma, central retinal vein occlusion

CATARACT

Description

- Progressive, painless clouding (opacity or discoloration) of the lens of the eye, resulting in localized or generalized partial or total blindness
- Leading cause of blindness worldwide

Etiology

- Age-related or senile (90% of the cause)
- Congenital (intrauterine infections, inborn errors of metabolism)
- Ocular trauma, infectious or inflammatory conditions (uveitis/scleritis)
- Secondary to systemic disease (diabetes, thyroid, parathyroid, sarcoid, myotonic dystrophy, atopic dermatitis)
- Systemic or inhaled corticosteroids
- Physical (radiation or infrared heat) exposure
- Protein (crystalline) changes in the normally transparent lens, causing opacity and scattering of light

Incidence and Demographics

- Leading cause of treatable blindness in the world
- Approximately 30 million blind people worldwide, 50% because of cataracts
- Cataracts present in 90% of those ages 65–74, and in 50% of those age 75 years and older have vision loss.
- Predominant sex: variable, some believe females more than males (CDC, 2023)

Risk Factors

- Aging
- Cigarette smoking
- Ultraviolet B sunlight exposure
- Diabetes, metabolic syndrome
- Prolonged high-dose steroids
- Positive family history
- Poor lifestyle habits (malnutrition and physical inactivity)
- Alcohol consumption

Prevention and Screening

- No definite measures to prevent cataract formation
- Theoretical measures to slow the process include using glasses with ultraviolet protection in sunny conditions; antioxidants such as vitamins C or E; avoiding tobacco products; controlling diabetes; care with high-dose, long-term steroid use.
- Screening for cataracts is part of every routine annual eye exam after age 40–50.
- Screening for cataracts is routine at birth for infants and at each well-child visit.

Assessment

History

- Painless, progressive decline in vision that is highly variable among individuals
- Typically bilateral, although often asymmetrical
- Complaints of problems with night driving, reading road signs, or fine print; nearsightedness occurs before opacity
- Symptoms associated with worsening vision related to falls, injuries, or accidents
- Non–aging-related cataracts have several etiologies; history must be thorough.

Physical Exam

- Comprehensive eye exam: visual acuity testing will establish baseline; follow-up visits to track changes
- Funduscopic exam reveals altered red reflex (dark spots or generally diminished) and clouding of the lens; at highly advanced stage, pupil will appear white or leukocoria will be evident in congenital cataracts
- All other aspects of the outer eye exam are unremarkable.
- Dilated funduscopic exam may detect other age-related changes that also affect vision (macular degeneration, diabetic or hypertensive retinopathies).

Diagnostic Studies

- Visual quality assessment by ophthalmologist: glare test, contrast sensitivity, and retinal or macular function assessment

Differential Diagnosis

- Corneal scarring/edema
- Lens opacities
- Tumor
- Retinal scar
- Retinal detachment
- Macular degeneration

Management

Nonpharmacologic Treatment

- Laser vision correction in early stages or after surgery for some patients
- Surgery necessary when cataract markedly decreases visual acuity (i.e., cataract extraction and artificial lens implant)
- Wear eye protection from UV light

Pharmacologic Treatment

- No drugs will halt the progression of the aging process in the eye.
- Postoperatively, topical antibiotic and ophthalmic steroids under direction of ophthalmologist

Special Considerations

- The presence of other diseases (e.g., macular degeneration, diabetic or hypertensive retinopathy) influences the decision to perform corrective surgery.
- Make surgeon aware if patient is taking an alpha-1 antagonist (tamsulosin, doxazosin, terazosin, or alfuzosin) before surgery because of the increased risk of intraoperative floppy iris syndrome.
- If possible, patients on anticoagulants may need to be temporarily discontinued for 1–2 weeks before surgery.

When to Consult, Refer, Hospitalize

- All patients with cataracts should be referred to an ophthalmologist for eye assess ment, management, and treatment.

Follow-Up

Expected Course

- Surgical extraction with lens implant improves vision in the absence of other diseases in 95% of the cases
- Ophthalmologists' follow-up postoperatively: day 1, 1 week, and 1 month later.
- Change in prescriptive glasses is determined 1–3 months after surgery

Complications

- Vary widely: delay in visual recovery, protracted visual discomfort, blindness, to loss of eye
- Retinal detachment, glaucoma, hemorrhage, infection postoperatively, lens malposition/dislocation, cystoid macular edema, endophthalmitis

Ocular Trauma

SUBCONJUNCTIVAL HEMORRHAGE (SCH)

Description

- Bleeding beneath the conjunctiva from small vessels

Etiology

- May occur spontaneously or by trauma
- Improper contact lens placement/cleaning
- Valsalva maneuvers (sneezing, coughing, vomiting, straining)

- Hypertension: most common cause in patients older than 60 years of age
- Atherosclerotic disease, diabetes, bleeding factors (thrombocytopenia, elevated prothrombin time)
- Rupture of conjunctival blood vessel causes bright red, sharply delineated area sur rounded by normal-appearing conjunctiva.

Risk Factors

- Age
- Contact lens wearer
- Systemic diseases
- Bleeding disorders
- Recent cataract surgery

Prevention and Screening

- Correct cleaning and maintenance of contact lenses
- Protective eyewear in sports/hobbies
- Control of systemic diseases (atherosclerosis, hypertension, diabetes)
- Control of prothrombin time in patients on warfarin therapy

Assessment

History

- Generally asymptomatic
- Report of sudden appearance of blood in the eye
- Obtain history of trauma, contact lens usage, cataract surgery, and comprehensive past medical history.
- Sometimes noticed upon awakening
- No reports of pain, blurred vision, or other related symptoms

Physical Exam

- Normal-appearing external eye; PERRLA (pupils equal, round, reactive to light and accommodation) and normal funduscopic exam and visual acuity; no discharge or exudates present with SCH
- Blood noted under part or the entire conjunctiva; usually unilateral but may be bilateral
- Evaluate blood pressure

Diagnostic Studies

- Usually none if suspected
- Fluorescein stain if foreign body is expected
- Workup for bleeding disorder if repeated episodes

Differential Diagnosis

- Foreign body
- Hyphema
- Penetrating trauma
- Acute-angle glaucoma
- Conjunctivitis
- Iritis

Management

Nonpharmacologic Treatment

- Self-limiting—no treatment required. Warm compresses and eye lubricants may be useful.
- Control blood pressure, blood glucose, international normalized ratio; use of protective eyewear as indicated

Pharmacologic Treatment

- None indicated unless there are associated infectious findings (conjunctivitis)

Special Considerations

- May be seen in hypertension and in neonates or their mothers as a result of labor and delivery

When to Consult, Refer, Hospitalize

- Refer to ophthalmologist if suspicious or associated with history of blunt trauma, patient complains of decreased visual acuity or disturbances, or no resolution of SCH within 2 weeks.
- Refer to hematologist if recurrent to evaluate for bleeding disorders.

Follow-Up

Expected course

- Hemorrhages resorb in 1–2 weeks.

HYPHEMA

Description

- Hemorrhage (gross visible blood) into the anterior chamber of the eye
- Frequently accompanies penetrating eye injuries
- Can result in permanent vision loss

Etiology

- Blunt or penetrating injury to eye such as from a rock, paintballs, BB gun pellet, dart, stick, fists, belt, elastic bungee cords, air bag deployment, or baseball; or from a fall
- Child abuse
- Traumatic eye injury during sports
- Intraocular surgery
- Spontaneous (uncommon): secondary to neovascularization (e.g., diabetes mellitus, ischemia, cicatrix formation), ocular neoplasms (e.g., retinoblastoma), coagulation disorders, uveitis, and vascular anomalies

Incidence

- Approximately 17–20 injuries/100,000 population
- Males 3–5 times more than females
- Approximately 70% occur in children, with peak incidence between 10 and 20 years of age

Risk Factors

- Blunt trauma to the eye, especially penetrating type
- Anticoagulant therapy
- Hemophilia
- Sickle cell anemia

Prevention and Screening

- Use of protective eyewear in high-risk situations
- Maintenance and control of hematologic disorders

Assessment

History

- Obtain details regarding precipitating event (recent eye trauma).
- Eye pain usually is present from trauma or increased intraocular pressure.
- Decreased or blurred vision; diplopia common with orbital fracture
- Ache around the affected eye
- Photophobia
- Nausea and vomiting may accompany injury.
- Patient or family history of hemophilia, blood disorders (including sickle-cell disease); medications (especially those that would affect clotting such as aspirin, nonsteroidal anti-inflammatory drugs (NSAIDs), and herbal preparations such as ginkgo biloba)

- History of sickle-cell disease or trait increases risk of rebleeding and the development of complications; usually needs more aggressive management.
- Children, especially young children, often are somnolent; needs to be differentiated from decreased level of consciousness associated with a head injury.

Physical Exam

- Open globe must be ruled out prior to any examination procedure that causes pressure to the eyeball (eyelid retraction, IOP measurement).
- Comprehensive eye exam (inspection of eyelids, lashes, lacrimal ducts, and cornea; extraocular movement, and visual fields by confrontation)
- Decrease visual acuity, photophobia
- Eye pain with papillary constriction to bright light (direct and consensual)
- Blood in the anterior chamber is visible to varying degrees, from partial filling seen as a visible fluid level line to a completely filled chamber. (Bleeds are graded according to the amount of blood in the anterior chamber, with grade 4 being the worst—entire chamber filled. Incidence of complications increases with higher grades.)
- Damage to adjacent structures or abnormal IOP
- May have increased ocular pressure (32%), may occur several days after injury
- Obtain a neurological exam if patient is somnolent.
- Assess for other signs of bleeding (e.g., bruising).
- Direct ophthalmoscopy is useful for closer visualization of anterior structures and lens.
- Funduscopic examination may be difficult because of miosis (pupillary constriction) and photophobia, or with a large hyphema
- Fluorescein examination should be deferred if the ruptured globe is highly suspected or evident.

Diagnostic Studies

- Clotting times (prothrombin time [PT], partial thromboplastin time [PTT], international normalized ratio [INR]), complete blood count (CBC) with differential if indicated
- Possible sickle cell prep (African, Hispanic, or Mediterranean descent)
- Orbital CT scan without contrast as indicated (globe rupture, intraocular foreign body)
- Cranial CT scan may be needed in other facial/head trauma.

Differential Diagnosis

- Globe trauma
- Eye contusion
- Systemic disease
- Melanoma
- Retinoblastoma
- Medication-induced anticoagulation

Management

Nonpharmacologic Treatment

- Apply bilateral eye patches to limit additional injury or blinking during transport to an emergency facility or ophthalmologist (put no pressure on the globe); eye shield to affected eye should always be worn until the hyphema resolves or for at least 1 week to avoid further injury to the affected eye.
- Grade 2: Inpatient rest and monitoring
- Grade 1 and after discharge: Limit activity—no screen time, TV viewing, or reading; elevate head. Some experts recommend that patients remain ambulatory versus bed rest for 5–7 days.
- If severe or developing complications, surgery may be done to evacuate blood.
- The goal is to prevent secondary hemorrhage and intraocular hypertension.
- Monitor intraocular pressure daily.

Pharmacologic Treatment

- Acetaminophen with or without codeine may be used as needed for pain.
- Avoid NSAIDs and aspirin.
- Other topical or oral agents may be used to suppress aqueous flow and decrease intraocular pressure or inflammation.

Special Considerations

- Aspirin products, miotics, and mydriatics should not be used.
- Sedation may be needed to ensure complete rest, especially in children.

When to Consult, Refer, Hospitalize

- Immediate referral to emergency facility, hospital, or ophthalmologist
- Greater than 50% affected require intervention by an ophthalmologist
- Outpatient management is acceptable if low grade and the patient is compliant with treatment plan
- If at home, must follow-up daily to check intraocular pressure and for rebleeds

Follow-Up

Expected course

- Variable, dependent on severity; ophthalmologist may manage patient at home or as inpatient
- Followed by ophthalmologist daily for 5 or more days
- Blood usually reabsorbs in 5–10 days (if no rebleeding)

Complications

- Decreased visual acuity
- Recurrent bleeding (approximately 25%): most common time is ≥5 days post injury; increases risk of complications
- Retinal detachment or ocular rupture
- Permanent corneal staining (from the hemorrhage) and subsequent haziness
- Glaucoma (immediately or later in life)
- Optic atrophy

CORNEAL ABRASION

Description

- Defect in the epithelial layer of the cornea caused by mechanical trauma to the surface of eye

Etiology

- Traumatic: fingernails, paws, paper or cardboard, branches, etc. (64% of cases)
- Foreign body: rust, wood, glass, plastic, fiberglass, etc.
- Contact lens related: removal of an over-worn, improperly fitting, or improperly cleaned contact lens (12% of cases)
- Spontaneous (recurrent erosions): occurs with no immediate injury or foreign body; seen in previous traumatic eye abrasions or eyes that have an underlying defect in the corneal epithelium

Incidence and Demographics

- Common in all ages; more males treated for corneal abrasion than females

Risk Factors

- Contact lens wear
- Foreign body in eye
- Any abrasive injury
- Lack of protective eyewear
- Contact sports
- Blepharitis
- Dry eye syndrome
- Entropion
- Autoimmune disorders
- Chronic corneal exposure (Bell's palsy, exophthalmos)

- Chronic topical steroid use or abuse of topical anesthetics
- Recent eye surgery
- Flash burn (welding burn)

Prevention and Screening

- Use of eye protection during high-risk activities
- Proper contact lens handling
- Use of artificial tears
- Lenses to block UV rays (welding helmets)

Assessment

History

- Complaints of excruciating eye pain, inability to open eye, photophobia, tearing, foreign body sensation, blurred vision, or conjunctival injection
- Usually unilateral
- History of contact lens use, dry eyes, trauma from foreign body or chemical burn
- History of connective tissue disorder
- Excessive tearing

Physical Exam

- Conjunctival injection, photophobia, increased lacrimation on affected side, blepharospasm
- Altered integrity of normally smooth cornea seen as irregular light reflex; actual abrasion may be visible with the naked eye or only upon fluorescein staining.
- Visual acuity may be decreased if abrasion is centrally located, pupils are reactive, and funduscopic exam is normal.
- Invert upper eyelid to assess for foreign body.

Diagnostic Studies

- Fluorescein staining will reveal epithelial disruption on the cornea.
- Slit-lamp exam by ophthalmologist may be required to determine corneal penetration.

Differential Diagnosis

- Foreign body
- Unilateral iritis
- Keratitis
- Acute or chronic glaucoma
- Herpes simplex or zoster
- Corneal ulcer
- Scleritis

Management

Nonpharmacologic Treatment

- Irrigation with normal saline to flush any nonpenetrating particles or foreign body after applying topical anesthetic (proparacaine or tetracaine)
- Patching of eye no longer recommended
- Avoid wearing contact lenses until abrasion healed and person is pain free.

Pharmacologic Treatment

- Topical antibiotic ointment or solution to prevent infection: ofloxacin, ciprofloxacin, sulfacetamide 10%, erythromycin, gentamicin, or polymyxin B/trimethoprim; continue until eye pain resolves
- Topical NSAIDs: help relieve pain; use with caution, may cause corneal melting and perforation
- Analgesics for pain (systemic)
- Never treat with topical steroids; may delay healing
- Tetanus booster if indicated

How Long to Treat

- Topical antibiotics for 3–5 days or until eye pain is resolved

Special Considerations

- Topical analgesics are used for evaluation of the eye in a clinic setting only and should not be prescribed for pain management at home.
- Advise patients of the risk of severe complications and need for follow-up next day.

When to Consult, Refer, Hospitalize

- Referral to an ophthalmologist if injury is extensive, signs of infection, severe ocular pain not explained by apparent pathology, or no improvement in 24 hours

Follow-Up

- Contact lens wearers: reevaluate daily with slit-lamp exam
- Minor abrasions: reevaluated only if they become more painful
- Large abrasions (larger than 4 mm): reevaluate in 24 hours

Expected Course

- Variable depending on severity; simple corneal abrasion resolves in 24–48 hours

Complications

- Recurrence
- Scarring of the cornea
- Corneal perforation
- Infection, ulceration
- Loss of vision

CORNEAL ULCER

Description

- Defect in the epithelial layer of the cornea involving the underlying stroma.

Etiology

- Bacterial—most common etiology of corneal ulcers. Common pathogens include *S. aureus*, coagulase-negative *Staphylococcus*, and *Pseudomonas aeruginosa*.
- Viral—herpes simplex virus most common. Less common viruses include varicella zoster and cytomegalovirus.
- Fungal—represent less than 10% of corneal infections. Common fungi include *Aspergillus*, *Fusarium*, *Scedosporium apiospermum*, *Candida albicans*, and *Phaeohyphpmycetes*
- Protozoan—acanthamoeba.
- Autoimmune disease—Wegener granulomatosis, relapsing polychondritis, polyarteritis nodosa, microscopic polyangiitis, Churg-Strauss syndrome.

Incidence and Demographics

- Common in all age groups
- More common in contact lens wearers, particularly with prolonged contact lens use
- 30,000 to 75,000 cases annually

Risk Factors

- Contact lens use
- Corneal abrasion
- Ocular trauma
- Chronic ocular disease
- Contaminated ocular medication
- Diabetes

- Autoimmune disorders
- Abrasive ocular injury
- Chronic topical steroid use or abuse of topical anesthetics
- Recent ocular surgery
- Flash burn (welding burn)

Prevention and Screening

- Use of eye protection during high-risk activities
- Proper contact lens handling and use
- Use of artificial tears
- Lenses to block UV rays (welding helmets)

Assessment

History

- Bacterial: rapid onset of unilateral pain, photophobia, conjunctival infection, and decreased visual acuity.
- Viral: foreign body sensation, conjunctival injection, blurred vision, and photophobia.
- Fungal: mild to no conjunctival injection
- Protozoan: pain out of proportion, severe photophobia
- History of contact lens use, dry eyes, trauma from foreign body or chemical burn
- Recent ocular trauma
- Personal history of or exposure to herpes
- Immunosuppressant therapy

Physical Exam

- Pupillary response.
- Invert eyelids to assess for foreign body.

- Assess conjunctiva for injection and ciliary flush.
- Increased lacrimation on affected side.
- Photophobia.

Diagnostic Studies

- Visual acuity.
- IOP: Only assess if there is no concern for perforated ulcer or globe rupture.
- Slit-lamp exam to determine characteristics of the lesion(s).
- Ulcers will present as clearly defined infiltrates as well as stroma edema and inflammation.
- Seidel's test to identify the site of an ocular leak due to rupture.
- Culture and sensitivity will guide pharmacologic therapy.

Differential Diagnosis

- Corneal abrasion
- Nonulcerative keratitis
- Foreign body
- Iritis
- Chemical burn
- Scleritis
- Anterior uveitis
- Episcleritis

Management

Nonpharmacologic Treatment

- Patching of eye not recommended
- Avoid wearing contact lenses until ulcer is healed

Pharmacologic Treatment

- Bacterial: topical options include ciprofloxacin and ofloxacin. Systemic: ceftriaxone for gonococcal ulcers. Corticosteroids should only be ordered by ophthalmology.
- Viral, topical: trifluridine, ganciclovir. Oral: acyclovir, valacyclovir. Valganciclovir is recommended for CMV.
- Fungal, topical: natamycin, amphotericin B.
- Protozoan, topical: chlorhexidine, poligexametilen biguanide
- Systemic analgesics for pain
- Tetanus booster if indicated

Special Considerations

- Valganciclovir requires monitoring for aplastic anemia.
- Concurrent autoimmune disorders require systemic immunosuppressants and cytotoxic agents with management by ophthalmology and rheumatology

When to Consult, Refer, Hospitalize

- Emergent ophthalmology referral
- Consider hospitalization for patients who are unable or unwilling to comply with treatment

Follow-Up

- Follow-up care should be provided and directed by ophthalmology

Expected Course

- Variable depending on severity

Complications

- Corneal scarring or perforation
- Glaucoma

- Irregular astigmatism
- Cataracts
- Vision loss
- Endophthalmitis

OCULAR FOREIGN BODY

Description

- Abnormal substance (foreign body) on the epithelium of the eye surface such as dust, dirt, metal, glass, lost contact lens, or organic material

Etiology

- Accidental trauma
- Foreign body becomes lodged in the corneal epithelium or stroma
- Disruption in the epithelial integrity of the cornea causes symptoms
- If foreign body penetrates further than the epithelial surface, ophthalmologist referral is indicated.

Incidence and Demographics

- Commonly occurring condition
- Males more than females

Risk Factors

- Lack of or improper use of protective eyewear during at-risk activities
- Living or playing in dusty or sandy environment (e.g., desert, beach)

Prevention and Screening

- Use of protective eyewear in appropriate or at-risk situations

Assessment

History

- Patients may complain of pain, foreign body sensation, photophobia, tearing, red eye.
- Determine event, timing, and place of injury; some projectiles puncture the eye and become lodged in the deeper layers, leaving only a relatively minor injury apparent. If history suggests this, immediate referral is advised.

Physical Exam

- Comprehensive eye exam. Include visual acuity, inspection of the outer eye, and both the outer and inner aspect of the upper and lower eyelids; check pupillary response and EOMs; and do funduscopic examination.
- Evert the eyelids for visualization of inner aspect of the eyelids.
- Findings may include a quiet eye (no tearing, discharge, injection, or edema), dark specks on the iris, "rust ring" at site of entry of steel or iron projectile, diffuse injection, or abrasion or tear of the epithelial layer.

Diagnostic Studies

- Fluorescein staining detects defects on the epithelial lining of the conjunctiva and cornea.
- Slit-lamp exam to assess inner eye thoroughly if no foreign body found

Differential Diagnosis

- Corneal abrasion
- Infection
- Herpetic ulcer
- Keratitis, bacterial
- Foreign body, intraocular
- Keratitis, fungal

Management

Nonpharmacologic Treatment

- Goal is to relieve pain, avoid infection, and prevent permanent loss of function.
- Irrigate eye with normal saline solution for 10 minutes or more.
- After application of eye anesthetic drops (proparacaine HCl [e.g., Ophthaine]), foreign bodies that are superficial may be dislodged with irrigation alone, or gentle touch with a moistened cotton-tipped applicator. Evert the eyelid to remove foreign bodies under eyelids.
- *Note:* Use moistened cotton-tipped applicator *only* if object is not embedded.
- Application of patch to injured eye is no longer recommended.

Pharmacologic Treatment

- Topical ophthalmic anesthetic is reserved for examination *only*, not treatment.
- Topical antibiotics are applied for prophylaxis until the epithelial defect heals; see corneal abrasion for list of pharmacologic treatments.
- Provide a tetanus booster if indicated.

Diagnostic Studies

- Fluorescein staining will detect a concurrent corneal abrasion.
- A slit-lamp exam may be necessary to assess for intraocular penetration of foreign body.

How Long to Treat

- Depends on extent of injury; patient seen by ophthalmologist for follow-up if necessary

Special Considerations

- Do not prescribe ophthalmic anesthetics for home pain control; use systemic analgesics (acetaminophen with codeine as needed).

When to Consult, Refer, Hospitalize

- Urgent referral to an ophthalmologist if a corneal foreign body cannot be removed, or if there is suspicion of corneal infection or penetrating injury
- Presence of a rust ring requires referral to ophthalmologist for treatment.
- Patients with a suspected intraocular foreign body must be referred emergently to an ophthalmologist.

Follow-Up

Expected Course

- Depends on type of foreign body and severity of the injury

Complications

- Penetration of foreign body
- Infection, corneal abrasion, tissue necrosis
- Glaucoma secondary to intraocular inflammation, cataract formation

Problems of the Ears

HEARING LOSS

Description

- Diminished or absent sense of hearing with inability to detect or comprehend sound or speech
- Can be partial, complete, unilateral, or bilateral
- Categorized as either conductive or sensorineural or both

Etiology

- *Conductive hearing loss (CHL):* dysfunction of the external or middle ear; decreased hearing by air conduction
  - ◇ Common causes in adults include: cerumen impaction, otosclerosis, cholesteatoma, and tympanic membrane perforation secondary to chronic otitis media
  - ◇ Common causes in children: otitis media and related conditions such as middle ear effusion and eustachian tube dysfunction
  - ◇ Often correctable with medical therapy, surgical therapy, or both
- *Sensorineural hearing loss (SNHL):* deterioration of the cochlea (inner ear) or eighth cranial nerve or both; decreased hearing through bone conduction; can be congenital or acquired and hereditary or nonhereditary; affects older adults (approximately 90%) more than children (less than 10%)
  - ◇ There are many different causes of SNHL, Presbycusis the most common, followed by noise-induced hearing loss. Other causes include pharmacologic toxicity (aminoglycosides, loop diuretics, antimalarials, salicylates), trauma (head injury, noise, barotraumas, irradiation), infections (otitis media, CMV, syphilis, labyrinthitis), and other disorders (multiple sclerosis, migraine, sickle-cell disease, blood dyscrasia, polyarteritis nodosa, HIV, meningioma).
  - ◇ Presbycusis: the most common cause of SNHL is due to the aging process; nonpathological, high-frequency hearing loss, etiology unknown. SNHL usually is not correctable with medical or surgical therapy; however, it may be preventable or stable.
- *Mixed:* both air and bone conduction impaired

Incidence and Demographics

- Is the third most common chronic condition in older Americans after hypertension and arthritis
- Twenty-eight million Americans have some degree of hearing loss
- Affects between 25% and 40% of patients 65 years and older
- All ages are affected; males and females affected equally
- Affects approximately 1.4 million children (under18 years)
- 1 of every 1,000 newborns in the United States is completely deaf; over 3 million children have hearing loss
- Congenital hearing loss affects newborns at rate of approximately 1–6 cases per 1,000; more than 60% are genetic causes and occur before speech development.
- 15% of children 6–19 years of age

- Otosclerosis is the most common cause of conductive, slowly progressive hearing loss in people aged 30–40 years; caused by bone dyscrasias; can be unilateral or bilateral.
- 7.6% of patients diagnosed with COVID-19 experience hearing loss.

Risk Factors

- Conductive:
  - Chronic sinusitis; allergy
  - Cigarette smoking
  - Sleep apnea with CPAP use
  - Eustachian tube dysfunction
  - Neuromuscular disease
  - Family history/heredity
  - Prematurity and low birth weight
  - Adenoid hypertrophy; nasopharyngeal mass
- SNHL:
  - Aging/older age
  - Loud noise/acoustic trauma
  - Dizziness/vertigo
  - Medications (aminoglycosides, loop diuretics, quinine, aspirin, chemotherapeutic agents)
  - Bacterial meningitis
  - Head trauma
  - Infectious diseases (chickenpox, measles, encephalitis, influenza, mumps)
  - Neoplasm, bone disorders, immune disorders, neurologic disorders, and vascular and hematologic disorders

Prevention and Screening

- Mandatory newborn screening: 25% of premature infants weighing less than 2,500 g have hearing loss.
- Audiologic testing after major intracranial infection (meningitis)
- Hearing screening repeated at age 3 or older often if high risk

- Routine screening for patients 65 years and older
- Limiting noise exposure—using hearing protection
- Avoiding ear canal instrumentation (e.g., cotton swabs, hairpins)
- Limiting ototoxic medications
- Vaccination for *H. influenzae* type b meningitis and for measles, mumps, and rubella (MMR)

Assessment

See Table 6–5

Diagnostic Studies

- Tympanometry: assessing tympanic membrane (TM) mobility and middle ear's ability to receive sound waves
    - Antinuclear antibody and sedimentation rate to screen for autoimmune disease if indicated

TABLE 6–5.
CHARACTERISTICS OF HEARING LOSS

	CONDUCTIVE	SENSORINEURAL
Etiology	Cerumen impaction Acute otitis externa Acute otitis media Otitis media with effusion TM perforation Otosclerosis Cholesteoma Traumatic ossicular chain disruption	Presbycusis Noise-induced hearing loss Meniere's disease Acoustic neuroma Sudden sensorineural hearing loss
Pattern of Loss	Decreased low tones	Decreased high-frequency pitch
History	Unilateral loss, although cerumen impaction, otosclerosis, and traumatic ossicular chain disruption can be bilateral	Unilateral loss, although noise-induced hearing loss and presbycusis can be bilateral

- ◊ Audiometry evaluation for all chronic hearing loss and for acute hearing loss of un-known etiology
- ◊ Vestibular testing if tinnitus or vertigo is involved
- ◊ CT scan if tumors/bony lesions are suspected
- ◊ MRI of the brain and internal auditory canal (IAC) with contrast if acoustic neuroma is suspected

Differential Diagnosis

- Presbycusis
- Infectious, vascular, metabolic problems
- Meniere's disease
- Acoustic neuromas
- Ototoxicity (aspirin, quinine, aminoglycosides)
- Viral labyrinthitis
- Conductive problems: obstruction of canal, TM impairment, otosclerosis, cholestea toma, cochlear damage
- COVID-19

Management

Nonpharmacologic Treatment

- Depends on etiology; remove obstructing wax or foreign body (ceruminolytics, such as Debrox, and irrigation), treat underlying infections, discontinue ototoxic medications, surgical treatment (e.g., cochlear implants, tympanostomy and tube placement, tympa-noplasty, mastoidectomy, stapedectomy/stapedotomy, canaloplasty), hearing aids, adaptive measures (lip-reading, sign language)

Pharmacologic Treatment

- Antibiotics if indicated
- Steroid therapy may be indicated for sudden sensorineural loss of unknown etiology

How Long to Treat

- Variable depending on underlying cause

Special Considerations

- Sign language interpreters should be considered in the primary care office for communication with patients with hearing impairments.
- Otosclerosis can worsen during pregnancy.
- Loss of communication produces emotional stress and is a physical risk for older adults.
- Some medications used to treat COVID-19 can cause hearing loss
- Hearing loss is rarely a symptom at the onset of a COVID-19 infection.

When to Consult, Refer, Hospitalize

- Emergent referral for SNHL with sudden acute hearing loss. Appointment should be made within 1–2 days.
- Otolaryngologist for hearing loss of unknown etiology
- Audiology if hearing loss is suspected; also provides hearing aid options and maintenance
- Genetics if congenital syndrome or familial hearing loss is suspected
- Speech therapist if speech delay or speech impediment is present
- Endocrinology if associated endocrine disorders are suspected
- Neurotology and neurosurgery if intracranial lesions are suspected or intracranial complication of middle ear disease

Follow-Up

Expected Course

- ◊ Presbycusis and SNHL are usually permanent and may be progressive.
- ◊ Temporary hearing alterations are reversible when related to minor problems such as congestion, otitis, cerumen, or foreign body obstruction that is responsive to treatment.

Complications

- ◇ Potential for serious sequelae with cholesteatoma, including balance problems, facial nerve paralysis, meningitis, brain abscess
- ◇ Neurologic abnormalities, perforations, cholesteatoma, tinnitus, vertigo, deafness

IMPACTED CERUMEN

Description

- Obstruction of the external auditory canal due to accumulation of cerumen (ear wax), a naturally occurring lubricant that serves as a protective lining of the canal

Etiology

- Excessive production of ear wax beyond what can be cleared by natural mechanisms
- Manipulation of canal (e.g., introduction of cotton-tipped applicator) that pushes cerumen deeper into canal, resulting in a buildup that is beyond the ability of the natural process of clearing

Incidence and Demographics

- Farmers and industrial workers around grains, powders, and textiles; greater incidence among older adults

Risk Factors

- Ear hygiene practices that compact cerumen in ear canal (i.e., cotton swabs)
- Age, occupation (wearing headphones, ear plugs), use of hearing aids

Prevention and Screening

- Gentle cleaning of external opening with washcloth without entering canal itself may be helpful.
- Avoid pushing cerumen further into external canal.

Assessment

History

- Decreased or partial hearing loss
- Feeling of fullness or pressure, itching
- Dizziness/tinnitus
- Pain if pushed against tympanic membrane

Physical Exam

- Dark brown wax, may be moist or dry
- Partial or complete obstruction of ear canal
- Visualization of canal and TM may be partially or completely blocked by the wax

Differential Diagnosis

- Foreign body in canal
- Otitis media
- Otitis externa

Management

Nonpharmacologic Treatment

- Removal of the cerumen can be achieved by use of a curette. Irrigation is no longer recommended due to the risk of tympanic membrane perforation. If irrigation is used, it should be done with caution.
- Contraindications for irrigation: tympanostomy tube, perforated tympanic membrane, previous or current history of otitis media, severe otitis externa, organic foreign body (e.g., legumes swell in contact with water)

Pharmacologic Treatment

- Soften hardened cerumen by instilling 3 drops of hydrogen peroxide and water (1:1), 1–2 drops of baby oil or ceruminolytic solvents (Debrox) for 10–30 minutes before irrigation.
- Optional: Have patient use Debrox at home the day before irrigation.

How Long to Treat

- May require ongoing maintenance indefinitely

Special Considerations

- Provide education about proper ear hygiene.

When to Consult, Refer, Hospitalize

- Referral to a specialist is required if the affected ear is the only ear with intact hearing, there is suspected perforation of the TM, or coexisting problems of the ear are present, such as severe infection, unexplained hearing loss, or hearing loss that did not clear with treatment of the impaction.

Follow-Up

Expected Course

- Acute impaction is generally resolved completely following treatment.
- Ongoing potential for repeated impaction is minimized by maintenance.

Complications

- Pain, bleeding, TM perforation

OTITIS EXTERNA (OE)

Description

- Inflammation or infection of the external auditory canal
- Commonly called "swimmer's ear"

Etiology

- Excessive water exposure
- Ruptured TM
- Traumatized external auditory canal (as with a cotton-tipped swab)
- Bacterial infection (90%): *P. aeruginosa* (67%), *S. aureus, Streptococcus pyogenes*
- Fungal infection (10%): *Aspergillus* (90%) or *Candida* infection
- Eczematous conditions: seborrheic dermatitis, atopic dermatitis, psoriasis, neurodermatitis

Incidence and Demographics

- Unknown; higher in summer months and in warm, wet climates
- All ages
- Males and females equally affected

Risk Factors

- Trauma to external ear canal
- Swimming
- Hot, humid weather
- Hearing aid use
- Eczema
- Advanced age, diabetes, AIDS, debilitating disease, leukopenia, malnutrition for necrotizing OE

Prevention and Screening

- Avoiding prolonged exposure to moisture
- Using preventive antiseptics (2% acetic acid solution [over-the-counter, OTC] 1–2 drops) or alcohol to dry out canal after swimming or bathing, and/or use blow-dryer on cool setting held several inches away from ear
- Cleaning earplugs with alcohol after use
- Treating predisposing skin conditions
- Eliminating self-inflicted trauma to canal with cotton swabs
- Diagnosing and treat underlying system conditions
- Using earplugs when swimming

Assessment

History

- Reports of itching, plugging of ear, ear pain, and discharge from ear

Physical Exam

- Ear canal is red, containing purulent discharge and debris; is edematous.
- Look for the presence of alive or dead insects.
- Pain on manipulation of pinnae
- Possible periauricular adenitis
- Possible eczema of pinna
- May have cranial nerve VII, IX–XII involvement (extremely rare)
- TM normal or dull
- Indicators of advanced infection or necrotizing malignant otitis externa: ulcerations, facial nerve palsy, mastoid tenderness, cellulitis, fever, chills, malaise; requires *immediate referral.*

Diagnostic Studies

- For general uncomplicated otitis externa, no diagnostic studies are indicated.
- Resistant infections may warrant Gram stain and culture of canal discharge.
- An erythrocyte sedimentation rate (ESR) will be significantly increased in malignant otitis externa.

Differential Diagnosis

- Idiopathic ear pain
- Acute otitis media with perforation
- Hearing loss
- Insect foreign body
- Wisdom tooth eruption
- Basal cell or squamous cell carcinoma
- Mastoiditis
- Temporomandibular joint (TMJ) problems
- Cranial nerve (VII, IX–XII) palsy with necrotizing OE

Management

Nonpharmacologic Treatment

- Removal of debris for enhancing examination by cleansing using a curette or cotton- tipped swab with saline or 1:1 hydrogen peroxide/water solution (may sting). (*Note*: Do not irrigate.)
- Placement of a wick or gauze strip in canals with greatly narrowed lumen to draw in otic drops
- Application of local heat (water bottle, warm pack) to outer ear for pain relief
- Avoidance of swimming with active infection

Pharmacologic Treatment

- OTC pain management (acetaminophen, NSAIDs); may need opioids
- First-line topical otic antibiotic: ofloxacin (Floxin), polymyxin B sulfate/neomycin sulfate/hydrocortisone (Cortisporin); acetic acid (VosoL HC) to fight infection in combination with a corticosteroid to decrease inflammation
- Second-line topical otic antibiotics: betamethasone 0.05% solution; azole antifungals for fungal otitis externa
- Topical acidifying agent such as acetic acid to inhibit growth of bacteria and fungi (Vosol)
- Oral antibiotics in combination with topical otic antibiotics indicated only if associated otitis media or if cellulitis of outer ear is present

How Long to Treat

- Usually 5–7 days
- Complicated case or malignant otitis externa requires prolonged therapy (6–8 weeks).

Special Considerations

- Necrotizing malignant otitis externa is typically found in patients 65 years and older, diagnosed with diabetes or immunocompromised, and requires *immediate specialist referral.*

When to Consult, Refer, Hospitalize

- Referral to a specialist is indicated for patients who do not respond to treatment or patients with severe infections, systemic involvement, cellulitis, or malignant external otitis.
- Hospitalization is required for necrotizing otitis media requiring parenteral anti-pseudomonal antibiotics.

Follow-Up

Expected Course

- Forty-eight hours after therapy to assess improvement
- Simple cases will resolve with treatment; however, reoccurrence or chronic problems will require ongoing monitoring and prophylactic measures (earplugs, acetic acid 2% after bathing or swimming).

Complications

- Mastoiditis, malignant external otitis, cellulitis, chondritis

OTITIS MEDIA

Description

- Acute otitis media (AOM): moderate to severe bulging of the TM or new onset of otorrhea not due to acute otitis externa with acute signs of illness or signs and symptoms of middle ear inflammation, often associated with recent viral upper respiratory infection.
- Otitis media with effusion (OME) also called "serous otitis media": presence of middle ear effusion in the absence of acute signs of infection; in children, may follow AOM; in adults, associated with Eustachian tube (ET) dysfunction

Etiology

- Acute otitis media:
  - Typically follows viral upper respiratory infection, causing ET dysfunction
  - Involved bacterial organisms include *Streptococcus pneumoniae* (20%–35%), *H. influenzae* (20%–30%), *M. catarrhalis* (15%), group A beta-hemolytic *Streptococcus* (3%), *S. aureus* (12%)
- Viral: involves respiratory syncytial virus (RSV), parainfluenza, influenza, enterovirus es, adenovirus, human metapneumovirus; 15%–44% of AOM

- Otitis media with effusion:
  - ◊ Residual fluid in middle ear following AOM
  - ◊ Eustachian tube dysfunction: The typically short, narrow, flexible, and horizontal ET found in children predisposes them to accumulation of nasopharyngeal secretions in the ET and middle ear. Supine bottle feeding and sucking may also contribute to reflux of fluid from the nasopharynx.

Incidence and Demographics

- AOM: predominant age: 6–24 months; declines in children over 7 years; rare in adults; male more than female; increased incidence in the fall and winter months
- OME: Nearly 90% of children ages 6 months to 4 years have had at least one episode.

Risk Factors

- Premature birth
- Bottle feeding while supine
- Routine day care attendance
- Frequent pacifier use after 6 months of age
- Smoking in household
- Male gender
- Native American, Inuit, or Alaskan native ethnicity
- Low socioeconomic status
- Family history of recurrent otitis
- Underlying ear, nose, or throat disease (adenoid hypertrophy, cleft palate, allergic rhinitis, Down syndrome)

Prevention and Screening

- Breastfeeding for more than 6 months is protective.
- Avoiding supine bottle feeding, passive smoke, and pacifiers after 6 months may be helpful.
- Pneumococcal vaccination: reduces AOM cases by 6%–28%

- Influenza vaccination: reduces AOM by approximately 30% in children older than 2 years of age
- Hib vaccination series starting at age 2 months

Assessment

History

- Acute otitis media
  - Rapid onset
  - Symptoms: otalgia, ear pulling, fever, irritability, otorrhea, sleeplessness, hearing loss, balance problems, anorexia, vomiting, diarrhea
  - Fever common but not universal
  - Patient may report extreme pain that is suddenly relieved with popping sensation, indicative of ruptured TM.
  - Precedes or accompanies symptoms of upper respiratory infection
- Otitis media with effusion
  - Symptoms variable, from none to severe with pain, vertigo, and ataxia
  - Patient typically complains of a sense of fullness in the ear and decreased hearing; popping or crackling sounds in the ear with yawning, chewing, swallowing, or blowing nose
  - Is transient in most children and may not be diagnosed
  - May report recent history of upper respiratory infection, allergy symptoms, or airplane travel

Physical Exam

- Acute otitis media
  - Fever
  - Decreased TM mobility; TM bulging, opaque, often yellowish or inflamed; TM may be red or injected
  - OM with effusion—presence of air/fluid behind TM
  - Redness alone does not indicate AOM.
  - Otorrhea if perforated TM
  - Bullae on the TM are indicative of *Mycobacterium pneumoniae.*

- ◇ May be preauricular or have cervical lymph node tenderness and enlargement
- ◇ An entirely normal exam warrants further examination of related structures for conditions that may present with referred ear pain (e.g.,TMJ dysfunction, sinusitis, cranial nerve abnormalities, dentition problems, nasopharyngeal carcinoma).

- ♦ Otitis media with effusion
  - ◇ TM often dull but not bulging; blunting of landmarks and diffuse light reflex
  - ◇ Presence of air/fluid level
  - ◇ TM may be retracted
  - ◇ Presence of bubbles
  - ◇ Speech unclear or unintelligible
  - ◇ Pneumatic otoscopy: decreased mobility ofTM
  - ◇ Weber test is positive to affected ear

Diagnostic Studies

- ♦ Pneumatic otoscopy
- ♦ Tympanometry to confirm tympanic membrane mobility
- ♦ Audiometry when hearing loss persists more than 3 months or at any time that language delay, significant hearing loss, or learning problems are suspected
- ♦ No routine testing is indicated, although CBC may be done if complicated or systemic infection is suspected

Differential Diagnosis

- ♦ Otitis externa
- ♦ Tympanosclerosis
- ♦ Otitis-conjunctivitis syndrome
- ♦ Redness because of crying
- ♦ Referred pain from jaw, teeth, or throat
- ♦ Bullous myringitis
- ♦ Trauma
- ♦ Nasopharyngeal carcinoma

Management

Nonpharmacologic Treatment

- Observation
- Valsalva maneuver (have child hold nose and blow with lips closed) or chewing gum to facilitate opening of Eustachian tubes for draining middle ear
- Warm pack to ear
- Oral analgesics for pain

Pharmacologic Treatment

- Acute otitis media
  - Disagreement exists regarding the usefulness of antibiotic treatment because most cases are self-resolving.
  - American Academy of Pediatrics/American Academy of Family Physicians (AAP/AAFP) Guidelines:
    - Infants 6 months of age and younger: antibacterial therapy is recommended regardless of degree of diagnostic certainty.
    - Children older than 6 months: antibacterial therapy is recommended when the diagnosis of AOM is certain and illness is severe.
    - Observation for 48–72 hours is an option when the diagnosis is certain, but illness is mild, and in patients with uncertain diagnosis
- If antibiotic therapy is used: penicillins, cephalosporins, macrolides, sulfonamides (see Table 6–6)
- CDC guidelines for antibiotic therapy:
  - First-line therapy: amoxicillin 80–90 mg/kg/day, in divided doses; 5–7 day treatment for children 2 years old or older with no complications and 10-day course for children younger than 2 years old; adult dose: 500 mg orally three times a day
  - Consider use of a cephalosporin (cefdinir, cefpodoxime, cefuroxime), azithromycin, clarithromycin, or sulfamethoxazole-trimethoprim in the event of penicillin allergy.
  - When choosing an antibiotic, consider risk of infection with resistant strains of bacteria.
  - For clinically defined treatment failures after 3 days of therapy, an alternative agent should be selected after considering risk of infection with resistant strains. Choose a drug effective against drug-resistant *S. pneumoniae* (DRSP) and beta-lactamase-producing pathogens, such as oral amoxicillin-clavulanate (Augmentin XR), cefuroxime axetil (Ceftin), or intramuscular ceftriaxone (Rocephin) x 3 days.

TABLE 6–6.
ANTIBIOTICS FOR ACUTE OTITIS MEDIA

DRUG/BRAND NAME	ADULT DOSAGE	PEDIATRIC DOSAGE
Amoxicillin (Amoxil, Trimox, Wymox)	500 mg three times a day, 3.5 g/day	80–90 mg/kg in 2–3 divided doses two times a day x 5–7 days in children 2 years or older and 10 days for children younger than 2 years
Amoxicillin-clavulanate (Augmentin) Augmentin XR Augmentin is also available in chewable tablets and suspension in a variety of dose ranges.	875 mg every12 h (based on amoxicillin component) 2 tabs every12 h	90 mg/kg in 6.4 mg/kg/day divided doses two times a day
Azithromycin (Zithromax)	250 mg (2) to start, then 1 once a day x 4 days	10 mg/kg/day on day 1, then 5 mg/kg/day on days 2–5
Cefaclor (Ceclor)	250–500 mg every8 h	40 mg/kg/day in 3 divided doses
Cefdinir (Omnicef)	300 mg every12 h (for 5 days in adults)	14 mg/kg/day in 1 dose or 2 divided doses (for 5 days in children >2 years old)
Cefixime (Suprax)	400 mg once a day	8 mg/kg/day once a day
Cefpodoxime (Vantin)	200 mg every12 h for 5 days	10 mg/kg/day in 2 divided doses for 5 days
Cefprozil (Cefzil)	250–500 mg every12 h	30 mg/kg/day in 2 divided doses
Ceftibuten (Cedax)	400 mg once a day	9 mg/kg/day once a day
Ceftriaxone (Rocephin)	1 g q12h IM or IV	50 mg/kg IM x 1–3 days
Cefuroxime axetil (Ceftin)	250–500 mg b.i.d.	30 mg/kg/day in 2 divided doses
Clarithromycin (Biaxin)	500 mg every12 h	15 mg/kg/day in 2 divided doses
Erythromycin-sulfisoxazole (Pediazole)	Not indicated	50 mg/kg in 3 or 4 divided doses (based on erythromycin component)
Loracarbef (Lorabid)	200 mg every12 h	30 mg/kg in 2 divided doses

Continued

TABLE 6–6.
(CONTINUED)

DRUG/BRAND NAME	ADULT DOSAGE	PEDIATRIC DOSAGE
Trimethoprim-sulfamethoxazole (Septra, Bactrim)	1 double-strength tablet q 12 h (160 mg trim. + 800 mg sulfa)	8 mg/kg trim + 40 mg/kg sulfa in 2 divided doses x 10 days. Do not use if group A streptococcus is suspected.
Trimethoprim (Trimpex, Proloprim)	Not indicated	10 mg/kg in 2 divided doses

- ◇ Pain management with OTC preparations such as acetaminophen or NSAIDs; codeine additionally if needed; warm compresses over affected ear
- ◇ Decongestants for the associated congestion of the nose or sinuses. (*Note*: Does not affect otitis media but provides symptom relief for congestion.)
- ◇ Antihistamines *only* if patient has allergies with increased watery secretions

- ♦ Otitis media with effusion
  - ◇ Antibiotic therapy is not routinely indicated for serous otitis media.
  - ◇ AAP/AFPP recommend watchful waiting for 3 months

How Long to Treat

- ♦ Antibiotic therapy is generally for 7–10 days except for azithromycin (Zithromax), cefpodoxime (Vantin), and cefdinir (Omnicef), which are given for 5 days.

Special Considerations

- ♦ Accurate diagnosis is essential to avoid overuse of antibiotics.
- ♦ Airplane travel in patients with ET dysfunction may cause painful barotraumas, bleeding intoTM, orTM perforation. Chewing gum or food (or sucking of pacifier or bottle in infants) may help equalize pressure.

When to Consult, Refer, Hospitalize

- ♦ Refer to ENT specialist for surgery in recurrent AOM if more than 3 episodes in 6 months, more than4 episodes in 12 months with at least one occurring in the past 6 months, or AOM episodes occur while patient is on chemoprophylaxis.

- Complications of severe infection such as mastoiditis or cholesteatoma
- Refer to ENT specialist for chronic middle ear effusion.
- Referral to ENT specialist for OME is individualized: if bilateral OME more than 3 months, unilateral OME more than 6 months, hearing loss more than 25 dB, or for high-risk individuals any time.
  - If a child is at risk for speech, language, or learning problems
  - Refer to ENT specialist for perforation of the TM that is nonresponsive to treatment within 48–72 hours, or a hearing loss of 20 dB or more post-treatment.

Follow-Up

Expected Course

- Simple cases are resolved in 7–10 days for AOM and should be reevaluated after treatment is completed to monitor resolution of middle ear effusion.
- Middle ear effusion commonly persists after course of treatment for AOM.
- Recheck can be made in 2–8 weeks depending on reliability of patient/parent.
- Follow-up in 48–72 hours in children who fail to improve on antibiotic therapy.

Complications

- Permanent conductive hearing loss, pain, balance disturbance, and tinnitus
- Speech and language disabilities can occur with OME.
- Perforation of TM, facial nerve paralysis, otitis hydrocephalus
- Cholesteatoma, tympanosclerosis
- Advanced infection (acute mastoiditis, meningitis, epidural abscess)
- Atrophy and scarring of eardrum, chronic perforation and otorrhea, cholesteatoma, and permanent hearing loss are possible in recurrent AOM and OME.

TINNITUS

Description

- Perception of sound without external auditory stimulus.
- Can be intermittent or constant, described as ringing, buzzing, clicking, or pulsing.

Etiology

- Subjective: due to otologic conditions including presbycusis, cerumen impaction, otitis media, sensorineural hearing loss,TM perforation, otosclerosis, vestibular schwannoma, ototoxic medications, and Ménière's disease
- Objective: arteriovenous malformations (AVMs), anemia, thyrotoxicosis, vascular neoplasm, intracranial hypertension, otitis media, partial stenosis of cervical vessels, and palatal myoclonus.

Incidence and Demographics

- Affects 300 to 600 million people worldwide; 50 million in the United States
- Most cases reported in adults ages 40 to 70.
- 10 million American report their symptoms as severe and debilitating.
- Equal incidence among genders and ethnicities.
- 14.8% of patients diagnosed with COVID-19 experience tinnitus.

Risk Factors

- History of noise exposure
- Old age
- Vestibular schwannoma
- Hearing loss
- Ototoxic medications (e.g., aspirin, NSAIDS, furosemide, quinine, cisplatin)

Prevention and Screening

- Use hearing protection when working around loud sounds
- Avoid noisy environments.
- Avoid ototoxic medications wherever possible; assess the risk/benefit ratio.

Assessment

History

- Common: noise exposure, hearing loss, vertigo, ototoxic medication use, perception of sound without external auditory stimulus.
- Perception of sound can be described as ringing, hissing, clicking, pulsing, humming, buzzing, or throbbing.
- Symptoms may be intermittent or constant.
- Patient questionnaires can be used to assess severity of symptoms (e.g., tinnitus severity index, tinnitus handicap inventory, and tinnitus handicap questionnaire).

Physical Exam

- Examination may be normal.
- Hearing loss, unilateral or bilateral
- Rinne and Weber tests to assess for conductive or sensorineural hearing loss

Diagnostic Studies

- Audiometry is the gold standard, used to assess for hearing loss, the most common cause of tinnitus.
- Other diagnostic studies are used to rule in or out differential diagnoses.

Differential Diagnosis

- Ménière's disease
- Acoustic neuroma
- Globus tumor
- Dehiscent jugular bulb
- Otitis media
- Otosclerosis
- Myoclonus

- Cerebrovascular disease
- Patulous Eustachian tube
- Multiple sclerosis
- AVM
- Dural arteriovenous fistula
- Salicylate overdose
- Benign intracranial hypertension
- COVID-19

Management

Nonpharmacologic Treatment

- Mainstay of therapy is supportive care and reassurance.
- Avoid ototoxic medications.
- Limit or avoid exposure to loud noises.
- Cognitive behavioral therapy
- Limit or avoid caffeine, alcohol, simple sugars, aspartame, food colorings and dyes, tobacco, NutraSweet, and monosodium glutamate.
- Tinnitus retraining therapy
- Integrative therapy (e.g., hypnosis, acupuncture)

Pharmacologic Treatment

- Antidepressants and/or anxiolytics may be indicated for concomitant depression and anxiety.

Special Considerations

- Tinnitus is non-specific. Rule out life-threatening conditions.

When to Consult, Refer, Hospitalize

- Refer to ENT for audiometry if not available in office.
- Refer to ENT if tinnitus is unilateral as it could indicate acoustic neuroma.
- Refer to mental health specialist for cognitive behavioral therapy as clinically indicated.

Follow-Up

- Annual audiometry is recommended to assess for asymmetry or progression.

Expected Course

- Variable depending on severity and underlying etiology.

Problems of Nose/Sinuses

RHINITIS

Description

- Inflammation of the nasal mucous membranes, accompanied by itchy eyes, nose, and palate, postnasal drip, cough, irritability, fatigue, and edema of mucosa; may be allergic, nonallergic (vasomotor rhinitis), or infectious

Etiology

- *Allergic rhinitis* is an IgE-mediated hypersensitivity reaction, related to inhaled seasonal pollen allergens (tree, grass, weeds) and perennial allergens of dust mites, pet dander, cockroaches, molds, indoor pollutants, and cigarette smoke.
- *Infectious rhinitis (common cold)* is most commonly due to the rhinovirus, as well as coronavirus, influenza, parainfluenza, and adenoviruses, or, less commonly, bacteria.
- *Nonallergic or vasomotor rhinitis* etiologies are not well understood but are thought to be autonomic responses that result in dilation of the nasal submucosal vessels. Influencing or triggering factors include temperature/humidity change, odors, selected drugs, emotional response, and body positions such as lying down.

- *Other causes*: The perennial form of nonallergic rhinitis is associated with atrophy of the nasal bones and nasal lining in the geriatric population; nasal polyps, benign over growths of the nasal mucous membrane, and connective tissue disorders; abuse of nasal decongestants oxymetazoline (Afrin) with rebound edema of the nose after continuous use; and transient rhinitis associated with pregnancy due to hormonal influences in women or foreign body in children.

Incidence and Demographics

- Increased incidence since the industrial revolution
- Affects 1 in 5 Americans
- Forty-four percent to 87% of patients have mixed rhinitis (allergic and nonallergic).
- Infectious: common in all ages, especially children

Risk Factors

- Family history of atopy
- Higher socioeconomic status
- Tobacco smoke
- Other allergies (asthma)
- Pets in house; cockroaches in home
- Genetics (80% have family history of allergic conditions)
- COVID-19 exposure

Prevention and Screening

- Avoid environmental allergens.
- Frequent handwashing to reduce risk of infection
- Environmental control measures indoors: frequent vacuuming with particulate filters, air cleaners (HEPA filters), mattress and pillow encasements, removal of carpeting, air conditioner, dehumidifier to reduce indoor humidity (less than50%), closing doors and windows during allergy season

Assessment

See Table 6–7

TABLE 6–7.
COMPARISON OF RHINITIS PRESENTATIONS

	ALLERGIC RHINITIS	INFECTIOUS RHINITIS (COLD)	VASOMOTOR RHINITIS	ATROPHIC RHINITIS
Onset	Age 8–11	Anytime	Adulthood	Older adulthood
Common Primary Symptoms	Nasal congestion, sneezing, itchy nose, clear rhinorrhea	Congestion or obstruction, sneezing, scratchy sore throat, nasal crusting, cloudy or colored drainage	Abrupt onset congestion and pronounced rhinorrhea and postnasal drip, sneezing	Nasal congestion, thick postnasal drip, frequent clearing of throat, bad smell in nose
Associated Symptoms	Cough, sore throat, itching and puffy eyes, headache	Cough, hoarseness, malaise, headache, fever higher than 100°F, may complain of facial or sinus tenderness	Watery eyes	May have nasal discomfort
Physical Exam Findings	Nasal mucosa pale and boggy, blue-gray nasal mucosa Enlarged turbinates Clear, watery discharge Postnasal discharge "Allergic shiners" Transverse nasal crease Nasal salute mouth-breathing Pharyngeal cobbling Mold may have white discharge	Edema and hyperemia of mucous membranes, throat erythema without edema, rhinorrhea (clear, yellow or green), postnasal drainage, dull TMs, lungs clear, cervical lymph nodes tender and enlarged	Turbinates pale and edematous, rhinorrhea No other findings	Nasal mucosa dry, smooth, and shiny Studded with crust Foul odor may be present Non-edematous Airway patent No other findings

Diagnostic Studies

- Based on history and physical
- Skin testing for allergies
- Nasal smear for eosinophils, mold
- Serum IgE levels (test has limited value)
- CBC if infectious process
- Rapid flu test if influenza is suspected

Differential Diagnosis

- Upper respiratory infection (URI)
- Foreign body
- Hormonal: oral contraceptives or pregnancy
- Sinusitis
- COVID-19
- Nasal polyps or overgrowths
- Adenoid hypertrophy
- Otitis media
- Endocrine disease (hypothyroidism)

Management

Nonpharmacologic Treatment

- General measures for all types: hydration, humidification (except for allergic), intranasal saline spray or irrigation
- Avoidance of known triggers

Pharmacologic Treatment

- **Allergic:**
  - **Glucocorticoid nasal sprays** are most effective for maintenance therapy. Examples include: first generation—beclomethasone (Beconase AQ), flunisolide (Nasarel), budesonide (Rhinocort Aqua), trimacinolone (Nasacort). Second generation—fluticasone propionate (Flonase), mometasone furoate (Nasonex), fluticasone furoate (Veramyst), ciclesonide (Ominaris or Zetonna). Refer to packaging for age-appropriate use and dosage.
  - **Oral antihistamines** can be used to treat sneezing, rhinorrhea, and itching. Second-generation antihistamines are preferred as they are non-sedating. Examples include cetirizine (Zyrtec), levocetirizine (Zyzal), loratadine (Claritin), fexofenadine (Allegra), desloratadine (Clarinex). First-generation sedating antihistamines include diphenhydramine (Benadryl), hydroxyzine (Vistaril), and brompheniramine (Bromfed).
  - **Oral antihistamine/decongestant combinations** can be used to provide enhanced symptom relief. Examples include loratadine/pseudoephedrine, cetirizine/pseudoephedrine, and fexofenadrine/pseudoephedrine.
  - **Antihistamine nasal sprays** can improve nasal congestion due to their anti-inflammatory properties. Examples include azelastine (Astelin) and olopatadine (Pataday).
  - **Otc nasal spray decongestant** is not recommended as monotherapy in chronic rhinitis due to the risk of rebound congestion. Use for the shortest period of time.
  - **Oral decongestants** can be used to decrease mucosal edema and decrease blood supply to the nasal mucosa. Example includes pseudoephedrine (Sudafed). Use with caution as they can cause insomnia, irritability, headache, and hypertension.
  - **Cromolyn sodium** is a mast cell stabilizer and can be used 2–3 sprays 3–4 times per day.
  - **Ipratropium bromide** can be used to decrease rhinorrhea but should not be used as first-line therapy.
  - **Montelukast (Singulair)** is a leukotriene receptor antagonist. Reserve for patients who cannot tolerate nasal sprays.
  - **Systemic glucocorticoids** not recommended as routine therapy. Reserve for severe cases for the shortest amount of time.
  - **Allergen immunotherapy** can be considered as an adjuvant therapy. Refer to an allergist for injections.
- **Infectious:**
  - NSAIDS or acetaminophen for pain or fever. Consider oral or nasal decongestants, antihistamines.
- **Atrophic:**
  - Guaifenesin (Naldecon Senior EX syrup) for stimulation of mucus, or intranasal saline solution spray

How Long to Treat

- Infectious rhinitis: for symptom relief only
- Allergic rhinitis: usually daily throughout allergy season
- Nonallergic rhinitis: daily may be needed to prevent symptoms

Special Considerations

- Use medications (especially decongestants and antihistamines) with caution in the older adult population; medications commonly produce adverse reactions or may interact with other medications that older adults take routinely.
- Use OTC decongestants with caution in patients with diabetes, hypertension, or glaucoma.

When to Consult, Refer, Hospitalize

- Referral to an allergist for allergen immunotherapy for allergic rhinitis that is not easily managed by medications or avoidance of known allergens
- Referral to ENT for those with complications, nasal polyps, or growths, or symptoms unmanageable with above-described treatments.

Follow-Up

- Routine generally 2–4 weeks after initiation of treatment for allergic and nonallergic rhinitis
- If infectious rhinitis has not resolved in 10 days

Expected Course

- Viral rhinitis usually resolves within 7–10 days.
- Allergic, vasomotor, and atrophic rhinitis are ongoing problems that are managed, not cured.

Complications

- Rhinitis medicamentosa (rebound)
- Worsening of related pulmonary conditions (e.g., COPD, asthma)
- Spread of infection: otitis media, acute sinusitis, pneumonia, bronchitis
- Nasopharyngeal lymphoid hyperplasia
- Epistaxis
- Sleep disturbance

EPISTAXIS

Description

- Hemorrhage from the nostrils, nasopharynx, or nasal cavity (anterior or posterior); "nosebleed"
- May be a symptom of an underlying problem

Etiology

- Primarily idiopathic, but may have many other causes; less than 10% related to neoplasm or coagulopathy
- Trauma: nose picking, foreign body, septal perforation, sinus fracture, abuse of inhaled recreational drugs (cocaine)
- Localized inflammation or irritation: infection, irritant inhalation, topical steroid use, septal deviation, low humidity
- Vascular abnormalities such as aging sclerotic vessels, AVMs
- Hypertension (bleeding worsened by but not caused by hypertension)
- Coagulation problems from diseases such as von Willebrand disease, leukemias, blood dyscrasias, platelet dysfunction; medications such as warfarin (Coumadin), clopidogrel (Plavix), NSAIDs; or aspirin, alcoholism
- Neoplasm: rare, but consider in persistent unilateral cases
- Low humidity heated indoor air in winter climates

Incidence and Demographics

- Common in the United States
- Estimated lifetime incidence approximately 60%
- Bimodal: peaks in children up to age 15 and in adults over 50
- Rare in children under age 2

Risk Factors

- All of the concomitant or precipitating problems listed under Etiology

Prevention and Screening

- Adequate moisturizing of the mucous membranes (humidifier, saline nasal spray); keeping nails clipped short and away from nose
- Petroleum jelly or antibiotic ointment applied to the anterior nasal septum
- Control of underlying nasal and systemic problems
- Protective athletic equipment, safety precautions to prevent trauma
- Avoid trauma and irritants

Assessment

History

- Patients may present with actively bleeding nose or may consult for episodes that were resolved with self-care.
- Ascertain precipitating events; from which nostril blood first appeared; associated symptoms, including nausea and vomiting, URI indications.
- Inquire about trauma (including nose picking), previous episodes, comorbid conditions, current medications (including OTC and supplements).

Physical Exam

- Inspect for site of bleed; note localized or diffuse mucosal irritation, bleeding from 1 or 2 nostrils, venous or arterial source (Table 6–8); obtain vital signs, do complete ENT exam.

TABLE 6–8.
CHARACTERISTICS OF NASAL BLEEDING SITES

	ANTERIOR EPISTAXIS	POSTERIOR EPISTAXIS
Presentation	Typically unilateral	Unilateral or bilateral
Timing	Lasts between a few to 30 minutes, in isolation or recurrently	Intermittent
Source of Bleed	Typically venous from Kiesselbach's plexus 90% are located here	Typically arterial from posterior nasopharynx More common location in older adults
Other	Usually less severe, easier to treat More common in young patients	Can result in significant hemorrhage May have nausea or coffee-ground emesis

Diagnostic Studies

- Only recurrent or severe cases warrant extensive evaluation with head radiograph or CT scan.
- CBC, platelet count, PT for recurrent or intractable cases
- PT/PTT if patient is taking warfarin or other medications affecting coagulation
- Cross-match when appropriate
- Toxicology screen when illicit drug use is suspected

Differential Diagnosis

- Drug-related as an anticoagulant side effect or from abuse (nasal cocaine inhalation)
- Symptom of one of the etiologic agents identified above
- Localized, isolated, benign event

Management

Nonpharmacologic Treatment

- For simple (anterior) nosebleeds, application of direct pinching-type pressure just below the bridge of the nose for 5–20 minutes will stop the bleeding; can be taught to the patient for self-care in the event of recurrence of a simple nosebleed. Keep the patient in an upright position and apply ice packs over the bridge of the nose.

- If not responsive to above measures, most anterior venous bleeds can be controlled by placing a cotton ball moistened with 1:1,000 epinephrine *or* vasoconstrictor nose drops (e.g., phenylephrine) just inside the nares and then applying pressure for 5–10 minutes. Some practitioners may also initiate cauterization with silver nitrate sticks or chemical cautery with chromic acid beads to the site of the bleeding.
- For maintenance of nasal hygiene and to avoid recurrence, apply petroleum jelly (Vaseline) to nares routinely for lubrication. Use humidifiers, cut fingernails, and avoid picking.
- For arterial (posterior) bleeds or epistaxis not responding to above acute treatment, immediate referral to an emergency department (ER) or ENT specialist for further treatment procedures, which may include cauterization via silver nitrate stick, bead of chromic acid, or 25% trichloroacetic acid, or electrocautery or thermal cautery followed by packing with ribbons of gauze impregnated with petroleum jelly, nasal tampons, or balloon inflation compression.

Pharmacologic Treatment

- Vasoconstrictors and topical anesthetics for bleeding cessation and analgesia
- Cocaine 4%, phenylephrine 0.25%, epinephrine 1:1,000, lidocaine laryngeal spray, lidocaine jelly 2%, lidocaine solution 4%, viscous lidocaine 2%
- Treatment of underlying disorders

How Long to Treat

- Episodic for the actual bleeding incident
- Ongoing monitoring and treatment as indicated for the associated underlying disorders

Special Considerations

- Pediatrics: more likely anterior, idiopathic, and recurrent
- Older adults: more likely to be posterior bleed

When to Consult, Refer, Hospitalize

- Posterior bleeding: frequently requires otolaryngology consultation
- Intractable bleeding: may require endoscopic laser or electrocauterization or angiography with arteriolar embolization; therefore, immediate referral to an emergency facility or ENT
- Recurrent epistaxis: refer to an ENT specialist

Follow-Up

Expected Course

- Excellent prognosis for isolated, idiopathic epistaxis
- Variable outcome depending on underlying cause

Complications

- Septal perforation from cauterization therapy
- Toxic shock syndrome with packing
- Arrhythmias triggered by packing
- Pressure-induced tissue necrosis of nasal mucosa

SINUSITIS

Description

- Symptomatic inflammation of the nasal cavity and paranasal sinuses, categorized as acute, recurrent, subacute, or chronic
- *Acute*: an infection of one or more paranasal sinuses of less than 4 weeks' duration; considered recurrent if more than 3 acute episodes per year
- Subacute: ongoing symptoms of purulent nasal discharge and inflammation of the sinuses for 4–12 weeks
- Chronic: prolonged inflammation of the sinuses with or without associated infection more than 12 weeks; irreversible damage to the mucosa is possible

Etiology

- Viral: vast majority of cases (rhinovirus, influenza A and B, parainfluenza virus, respiratory syncytial, adenovirus, coronavirus, enterovirus)
- Bacterial: more likely if symptoms worsen after 5–7 days or do not improve after 10 days (*S. pneumoniae, H. influenzae, M. catarrhalis*); often over-diagnosed, leading to overuse of antibiotics and an increase in antibiotic resistance
- Fungal: seen in immunocompromised hosts (uncontrolled diabetes, neutropenia, use of corticosteroids) or nosocomial infection. Increased incidence in humid climates

Incidence and Demographics

- Highest in early fall through early spring
- Affects 31 million Americans each year
- About 2% of viral rhinosinusitis episodes have bacterial superinfections.

Risk Factors

- Viral URI
- Allergic rhinitis
- Asthma
- Cigarette smoking
- Dental infections and procedures
- Anatomic variations: tonsillar and adenoid hypertrophy, turbinate hypertrophy, nasal polyps, deviated septum, cleft palate
- Immunodeficiency (HIV)
- Cystic fibrosis
- COVID-19 exposure

Prevention and Screening

- Handwashing to prevent transmission of viral infection

Assessment

History

- Major challenge is to distinguish between viral and bacterial disease
- Predictive symptoms of bacterial infection: worsening symptoms more than 5–7 days after initial improvement; persistent symptoms for more than 10 days; persistent purulent nasal discharge; unilateral upper tooth or facial pain; unilateral maxillary sinus tenderness; fever
- Other associated symptoms: headache, nasal congestion, retro-orbital pain, otalgia, hyposomia, halitosis, chronic cough worse at night

Physical Exam

- Complete HEENT (head, eyes, ears, nose, throat) and pulmonary exam, with typical findings in the case of acute sinusitis:
  - Fever
  - Edema and erythema of nasal mucosa and turbinates causing nasal obstruction
  - Purulent discharge
  - Tenderness to palpation over sinus(es)
  - Presence of white fungal balls
- Chronic sinusitis merits a more detailed examination for underlying risk factors
- *Note*: Important serious findings include external facial swelling, erythema, or cellulitis over an involved sinus (periorbital or forehead); vision changes such as diplopia; difficulty moving eyes (EOMs); proptosis; and any abnormal neurologic signs. *These are all indicative of serious complications requiring urgent referral and treatment.*

Diagnostic Studies

- Diagnostic tests are not routinely recommended; no diagnostic test can differentiate between viral and bacterial rhinosinusitis.
- Lab: none indicated in routine evaluations; transillumination of sinuses may confirm fluid in sinuses (helpful if asymmetric; not helpful if symmetric)
- Imaging: value of imaging studies is limited; they do not distinguish between viral and bacterial etiology

- Limited coronal CT scan can be useful in recurrent infection or failure to respond to medical therapy
- Rhinoscopy by ENT specialist

Differential Diagnosis

- Dental disease
- Nasopharyngeal tumor
- Wegener's syndrome
- HIV infection
- Immotile cilia syndrome
- Kartagener syndrome
- Headache, tension or migraine
- Trauma, foreign body
- Cystic fibrosis
- Granuloma
- COVID-19

Management

Nonpharmacologic Treatment

- Hydration
- Steam inhalation 20–30 minutes, three times a day
- Saline irrigation (Neti pot, Navage) or nose drops/spray
- Sleeping with head of bed elevated
- Avoiding exposure to cigarette smoke or fumes
- Avoiding caffeine and alcohol
- Warm facial packs

Pharmacologic Treatment

- Analgesics: acetaminophen, aspirin, NSAIDs, acetaminophen with codeine (severe cases)
- Decongestants: pseudoephedrine HCl, phenylephrine nasal spray (limit use), oxymetazoline nasal spray (Afrin; limited to 3-day use)
- Antibiotics: indicated only when findings suggest bacterial infection (symptoms that persist more than 10 days or worsen in 5–7 days)
- First-line antibiotics:
  - Amoxicillin: 1 g three times a day (adults) and 80–90 mg/kg/day divided every8 h (children)
  - Trimethoprim-sulfamethoxazole (TMP/SMX): 160/800 mg every12 h (adults) and 8–12 mg/kg/day of trimethoprim component divided every12 h (children)
  - Doxycycline: 100 mg orally two times a day (adults only)
- Second-line antibiotics: use if no response to first-line therapy after 72 hours or if patient has had antibiotics within the past 4–6 weeks
  - Amoxicillin-clavulanate: 875/125 mg every 12 h (adults) and 30 mg/kg/day of amoxicillin component divided two times a day (children)
  - Augmentin XR two times a day in adults and Augmentin ES-600 in children (for beta-lactam and penicillin-binding protein resistance)
  - Other second-line antibiotics: cefpodoxime, cefuroxime axetil, azithromycin, clarithro mycin, levofloxacin (Levaquin). Use levofloxacin (Levaquin) with caution due to black box warning. See specific dosages in Table 6–6 as for otitis media.
- If lack of response after 3 weeks of antibiotics, consider CT scan, ENT referral
- Oral antihistamines: loratadine, fexofenadine, cetirizine, desloratadine (Clarinex) or levocetirizine (Xyzal), diphenhydramine
- Leukotriene inhibitors: montelukast, zafirlukast (Accolate), especially in patients with asthma
- Nasal steroids: fluticasone. Refer to Rhinitis section for a list of intranasal glucocorticoids.

How Long to Treat

- Recommendations are not consistent; however, a 10–14-day course is typical for acute sinusitis.
- Chronic sinusitis should be treated until the patient is well for 7 days.

Special Considerations

- Avoid prolonged use of topical decongestants to prevent rebound congestion and dependence.
- Resist the urge and patient demand to treat viral URIs with antibiotics.
- Pregnancy: avoid clarithromycin and levofloxacin as they may cause fetotoxicity; other safer alternatives are available.

When to Consult, Refer, Hospitalize

- Complications or failure of treatment

Follow-Up

Expected Course

- Improvement of symptoms within 72 hours and resolution of sinusitis within 10–14 days
- Follow-up if no improvement after 72 hours or no resolution after 10 days of antibiotic use

Complications

- Serious complications are rare: brain abscess, meningitis, osteomyelitis, orbital cellulitis, cavernous sinus thrombosis, subdural empyema

Problems of the Pharynx

PHARYNGITIS/TONSILLITIS

Description

- Inflammation of the pharynx commonly caused by acute viral infection; infection by group A beta-hemolytic streptococci is of greatest concern, because of the potential preventable rheumatic sequelae (scarlet fever, rheumatic fever, glomerulonephritis)

Etiology

- Spread by person-to-person contact via droplets of oral, respiratory, and nasal secretions
- Viral infection accounts for 90% of pharyngitis.
- Viral agents include: rhinovirus, adenovirus, parainfluenza, coxsackie, echovirus, herpes simplex virus, Epstein-Barr, cytomegalovirus.
- Most common bacterial agents: Group A beta-hemolytic streptococci, *N. gonorrhoeae*, *Corynebacterium diphtheriae*, *H. influenzae*, *M. catarrhalis*, groups C and G *Streptococcus* (rarely)
- Infectious mononucleosis: Epstein-Barr virus; affects adolescents most frequently
- Chronic causes: more likely noninfectious; irritation from postnasal discharge of chronic allergic rhinitis or reflux; referred pain, chemical irritation, or smoking; neoplasms and vasculitis

Incidence and Demographics

- Commonly occurring illness; approximately 30 million cases per year estimated
- Group A *Streptococcus* is the most common bacterial cause, approximately 15%–30% of cases in children and 5%–10% of cases in adults
- Rheumatic fever is rare in the United States; greatest incidence is in children ages 5–18 years

Risk Factors

- Epidemics of group A beta-hemolytic streptococcal disease
- Age (the young are most susceptible)
- Family history
- Communal living (dormitories, barracks)
- Immunosuppression; diabetes mellitus
- Recent illness; fatigue
- Excess alcohol consumption, smoking, receptive oral sex
- Inadequate immunization status against diphtheria-tetanus and pertussis, (DTaP, Td, or Tdap)
- COVID-19 exposure

Prevention and Screening

- Frequent handwashing, especially in situations of contact with infected people
- Avoiding contact with infected people

Assessment

History

- Complaint of sore throat, cough, hoarseness, lower respiratory symptoms, fever, anorexia, chills, malaise, headache; contacts with similar symptoms or diagnosed infection are common

Physical Exam

- Enlarged tonsils, pharyngeal erythema, tonsillar exudates, soft palate petechiae, cervical adenopathy, fever (temperature greater than102.5°F)
- Scarlet fever rash: streptococcal pharyngitis
- Gray pseudomembrane found in diphtheria and, occasionally, mononucleosis
- Erythematous-based clear vesicles are found in herpes stomatitis.
- Conjunctivitis is found with adenovirus infections.
- Immunization status

Diagnostic Studies

- Diagnostic testing for Streptococcus is done only in patients with history of fever, tonsillar exu dates, and tender anterior cervical adenopathy, without presence of cough
- Rapid strep antigen screen: 50%–80% sensitivity; more than 95% specificity; do not culture if positive
- Throat culture remains the "gold standard" for diagnosis of group A beta-hemolytic streptococcus.
- If a negative rapid strep screen is found in a patient with a high probability of streptococcus, culture to confirm.
- Monospot is indicated for suspicion of mononucleosis: in addition to sore throat, fatigue, malaise, fever chills, rash, lymphadenopathy (particularly posterior cervical).

- Table 6–9 characterizes pharyngitis types, symptoms and exam findings
- Culture of the pathogen may help identify causative organism; however, may not be cost-effective or influence outcome.
- Monospot is indicated for suspicion of mononucleosis.
- CBC with differential reveals increased white blood cell (WBC) count if bacterial, decreased if viral (not rou tinely done)
- If indicated, culture for gonorrhea and/or *Chlamydia* infection.
- Potassium hydroxide (KOH) wet mount reveals pseudohyphae and budding spores in candidiasis.

Differential Diagnosis

- Strep "carrier state"
- Etiologic agents identified above
- Epiglottitis
- Thyroiditis
- Peritonsillar abscess (rare)
- Postnasal drip related to rhinitis or sinusitis
- Diphtheria
- COVID-19

Management

- Goal: identify and treat group A beta-hemolytic streptococcal pharyngitis to decrease risk of acute rheumatic fever

Nonpharmacologic Treatment

- Symptomatic treatment includes: force fluids, salt water gargles, OTC analgesics (ac etaminophen, NSAIDs if no contraindications), throat lozenges, cool-mist humidifier
- Rest and contact sports avoidance advisable with pharyngitis associated with mononucleosis.

TABLE 6–9. CHARACTERISTICS OF PHARYNGITIS BY ETIOLOGY

	SYMPTOMS	EXAM FINDINGS
VIRAL		
Coxsackievirus and others	Sore throat, malaise, fever, headache	Small oral vesicles, ulcers on posterior pharynx, tonsils, buccal mucus
Epstein-Barr	Above + fatigue	Exudative tonsillitis, palatial petechiae, posterior cervical adenopathy; possible maculopapular rash
Primary HIV	Above + myalgia, photophobia lasting a few days to 2 weeks	Posterior cervical lymphadenopathy Similar to Epstein-Barr with rash
BACTERIAL		
Group A streptococcus	Sore throat, fever, odynophagia (primarily) Abdominal pain, vomiting, headache	Fever (temperature higher than 101°F) Erythema and white or yellow exudate of tonsils and/or pharynx Anterior cervical lymphadenopathy Absence of other URI symptoms/ signs generally but not always
Scarlet fever	Abrupt-onset fever, pharyngitis, headache	Sandpaper-like fine, erythematous rash on trunk and extremities (absent on face) that blanches on pressure Appears within 24–48 hours, lasts 4–10 days
Rheumatic fever	Symptoms develop1–6 months after strep infection	Various manifestations: heart murmur, polyarthritis, rash (see Chapter 4, Infectious Diseases)
STD		
Chlamydia or Gonorrhea	Chronic sore throat History of oral sex or sexual abuse in children	Exudative, erythematous pharynx Anterior cervical lymphadenopathy
Mycoplasma	Same as strep	Same as strep

Continued

TABLE 6–9. (CONTINUED)

	SYMPTOMS	EXAM FINDINGS
FUNGAL		
Candida albicans	History of antibiotic use, immunosuppression, use of inhaled corticosteroids	Thin, diffuse, or patchy white plaques on red base on mucous membranes, pharynx, tongue
Peritonsillar abscess Dysphagia, dysphonia, drooling, trismus (difficulty opening mouth because of pain and inflammation)	Unilateral throat and ear pain	Erythema and swelling of soft palate Uvula and soft palate edema such that it may appear that the uvula "points" toward side of Abscess Exquisitely tender, palpable, fluctuant abscess on tonsil Similarly tender, enlarged anterior cervical lymph nodes

- *Note*: Peritonsillar abscess requires urgent referral to otolaryngologist for possible IV antibiotics, incision, and drainage; tonsillectomy may be recommended as definitive treatment after the acute episode resolves. With children criteria include snoring, sleep apnea.

Pharmacologic Treatment

- First-line therapy:
  - Penicillin V (Pen-Vee K) 250 mg three times a day (less than 27 kg) or 500 mg two or three times a day (more than 27 kg) is the drug of choice for *Streptococcus*; children: 25–50 mg/kg/day, divided b.i.d–q.i.d all for 10 days *or*
  - Amoxicillin 50 mg/kg/day once daily x 10 days (use with caution, because EBV infection may induce rash)
- If allergic to penicillin:
  - Cephalexin (Keflex) 250 mg orally three times a day for adults and 30 mg/kg/day two times a day x 10 days for children
  - Cefadroxil 30 mg/kg/day (max 1 g)
  - Clindamycin 7 mg/kg/dose three times a day (max 300 mg/dose)

- Second-line therapy: first-generation cephalosporins, azithromycin, clarithromycin
- Intramuscular penicillin G benzathine (single dose) for patients who are unable to complete the full 10-day dose or for those who are at increased risk for rheumatic fever
- Eradication of carrier state: Clindamycin 20 mg/kg/day in 3 divided doses x 10 days (most effective)
  - Cephalexin 25–50 mg/kg/day two times a day x 10 days
  - Penicillin + rifampin: use above penicillin doses + rifampin 20 mg/kg/day two times a day for final 4 days
  - Consider repeat throat culture after treatment to document eradication of group A strep
  - Asymptomatic carriers: generally, no treatment indicated
- For *Chlamydial* or mycoplasmal infections, which, when present, are usually accompanied by lower respiratory tract symptoms: children—erythromycin 30–50 mg/kg two times a day x 10 days; adults—doxycycline 100 mg two times a day x 10 days or azithromycin 500 mg for 1 day followed by 250 mg for 4 days
- For gonococcal pharyngitis: ceftriaxone 125–250 mg IM (consider treatment for *Chlamydia* as well)
- For candidiasis pharyngitis: nystatin (Mycostatin) 100,000 U/mL oral suspension 4–6 mL four times a day

Frequent resistance in some communities to azithromycin

- *Not recommended*: Erythromycin, first-generation cephalosporins, azithromycin, clarithromycin

Eradication of carrier state:

- Penicillin V dosage: 50mg/kg/day in 4 doses x 10 days

How Long to Treat

- Patients being treated with penicillin should complete the full 10 days of oral antibiotic. Five-day therapy is acceptable with cefpodoxime, cefdinir, or azithromycin.

Special Considerations

- Patient must complete full course of antibiotics for group A streptococcus regardless of symptom response
- Household and close personal contacts of the patient with strep are treated only if symptomatic.
- Children may return to school once afebrile and taking antibiotics for at least 24 hours.
- Advise those diagnosed with mononucleosis to avoid contact sports for 4 weeks to avoid possible splenic rupture.
- Dispose of toothbrush once on antibiotics.

When to Consult, Refer, Hospitalize

- Any patient with peritonsillar or retropharyngeal abscess requires urgent referral.
- Patients with symptoms or edema affecting the ability to breathe or swallow (e.g., inability to swallow their own saliva) require immediate transfer to hospital.

Follow-Up

- No follow-up necessary unless not resolving

Expected Course

- Strep pharyngitis typically lasts for 5–7 days, with fever peaking at second to third day; will spontaneously resolve, but early treatment of strep pharyngitis decreases symptomatic period by ½–2 days and decreases risk of rheumatic complications.
- Viral pharyngitis will resolve spontaneously.
- Symptoms of rheumatic complications develop in weeks to months following resolution of pharyngitis.

Complications

- Otitis media, mastoiditis, septicemia, rhinitis, sinusitis, pneumonia
- Rheumatic fever
- Poststreptococcal glomerulonephritis, peritonsillar abscess, systemic infection

EPIGLOTTIS

Description

- Rapid development of inflammation and edema of the supraglottic structures, epiglottis, vallecula, aryepiglottic folds, and arytenoids leading to narrowed airway and respiratory compromise
- *Note:* **An acute and sudden onset of a potentially life-threatening illness**

Etiology

- Infectious etiology:
  - Bacterial: *H. influenzae* type b (Hib), *S. pyogenes, S. pneumoniae, S. aureus, Haemophilus parainfluenzae, Escherichia coli,* and many more
  - Fungal (*Candida* spp.)
  - Viral: HSV-1, varicella zoster, parainfluenza type 3, influenza B, Epstein-Barr
- Traumatic (caustic ingestion, thermal injury, foreign body ingestion)
- Allergic reactions

Incidence and Demographics

- Has decreased dramatically since the introduction of Hib vaccine
- Predominant age shifting to older children (median age, 7 years) and adults
- Predominant sex: male more than female (1.8:1)

Risk Factors

- Patient has not had Hib vaccine
- Immunocompromise
- Associated with comorbid conditions (hypertension, diabetes mellitus, substance abuse)

Prevention and Screening

- Immunization with *H. influenzae* type B vaccine, although not 100% effective; available only for children up to age 5
- Rifampin 20 mg/kg/day x 4 days (max daily dose 600 mg) for close contacts (may be carriers) of invasive Hib

Assessment

History

- Sudden onset of severe pain with swallowing *or* already unable to swallow own saliva by time of examination
- Fever, toxic appearing, respiratory distress (stridor, tachypnea, anxiety, refusal to lie down, and labored breathing)
- Dysphagia, refusal to eat, drooling, sore throat, anterior neck pain
- Muffled "hot potato" voice/cry (vs. hoarseness in croup)
- Minimal cough (vs. barking cough in croup); usually no precipitating URI (vs. positive history in croup)
- In adults, presentation more indolent (sore throat and odynophagia are predominant symptoms)
- Past medical history including immunization history and current medications
- Drooling

Physical Exam

- Toxic appearance/shock
- Marked restlessness, irritability, and anxiety
- Airway obstruction resulting in respiratory distress
- Marked substernal and subcostal retractions and labored breathing indicate impending respiratory failure
- Stridor softer and less prominent than in croup
- Anterior neck exam may reveal tender adenopathy.

- Classic posturing of sitting up and leaning forward, tongue hanging out, often holding something (a cup) to spit their saliva out as they cannot swallow it without severe pain
- Cyanosis indicates poor prognosis.
- *Note*: Examination of the pharynx should be carried out *only* with equipment and personnel in place for emergency intubation or tracheotomy for airway maintenance. Insertion of a tongue blade into the oral cavity may precipitate laryngeal spasm and acute airway obstruction.

Diagnostic Studies

- Blood and epiglottis cultures (obtained under the same conditions as examination described above)
- Blood cultures are positive in 75%–90% of children.
- CBC positive for leukocytosis with left shift
- Hib antigen test in serum/urine is useful in children with previous antibiotic treatment.
  - Lateral neck X-ray is consistent with enlarged edematous epiglottitis (the thumbprint sign) but contraindicated because of the risk of sudden complete airway obstruction. If obtained, ensure adequate staff in case complete airway obstruction occurs.
  - Chest X-ray for screening of pneumonia (25% occurrence rate) and placement of endotracheal tube

Differential Diagnosis

- Viral croup
- Acute angioneurotic edema
- Foreign body aspiration
- Peritonsillar abscess
- Retropharyngeal abscess
- Diphtheria in unimmunized patients
- Lingual tonsillitis
- Sepsis
- Uvulitis
- Angioedema
- Viral croup (laryngotracheobronchitis)

Management

- Immediately arrange for monitoring, IV, and maintenance of secure airway with appropriate personnel and equipment and transport to an emergency setting or hospital with intensive care unit (ICU).
- Monitor vital signs, oxygen saturation, and be alert for potential abrupt deterioration.
- Begin IV antibiotics.
- Monitor patient in the ICU.
- Two goals: maintain airway and administer antimicrobial agents

Special Considerations

- Incidence decreasing in children since use of Hib vaccine

When to Consult, Refer, Hospitalize

- All patients with epiglottitis require immediate transport to the hospital.

Follow-Up

Expected Course

- With prompt and appropriate treatment, morbidity and mortality rates are low.
- Airway management measures are usually discontinued within 24–48 hours of treatment.
- Immunization recommended

Complications

- Pneumonia, meningitis, cervical adenitis, septic arthritis, cellulitis
- Progression of infection to deep neck tissue
- Epiglottic abscess
- Septic shock
- Pneumothorax
- Death from airway obstruction (asphyxia)

Problems of the Mouth

ORAL CANDIDIASIS (THRUSH)

Description

- Fungal infection of the oral mucous membranes

Etiology

- *C. albicans* is part of the normal flora of the oral cavity that causes overt infection when there is a reduction in the competitive oral microflora.

Incidence and Demographics

- Essentially a disease of infants; in adults it may be a sign of immunosuppression.
- Common with immunodeficiency, persons with obesity, diabetes, hyperhidrosis

Risk Factors

- Most common cause in infants and children is long-term use of broad-spectrum antibiotics.
- May also arise in immunosuppressed patients (HIV).
- Conditions that cause decrease in the host resistance—stress, diabetes, malnutrition, prematurity, use of inhaled corticosteroids (ICS)
- Denture wear
- Use of inhaled steroids, e.g., metered dose inhaler (MDIs)

Prevention and Screening

- Judicious use of antibiotics
- Patient should rinse mouth after inhaled steroid use.
- Dentures should be cleaned appropriately and fit well.
- Control of diabetes, weight loss, decrease in stress, proper nutrition

Assessment

History

- White coating in the mouth
- Decreased sucking or appetite because of discomfort, sore throat
- Ask about recent antibiotic use

Physical Exam

- White, raised, distinct patches in the mouth—particularly the tongue, buccal mucosa, and hard palate—which rub off easily, leaving an underlying red, raw surface
- Membrane consists of an almost pure colony of fungus
- Immunocompromised hosts: oral lesions are white, raised, nontender, distinct patches; red, slightly raised patches; thick, dark-brownish coating; deep fissures
- Angular chelitis: infection in corners of the mouth

Diagnostic Studies

- KOH preparation for microscopy of plaque can be made but is not necessary
- Culture for rare types of fungal/yeast infections or alternative infection if first-line treatment fails

Differential Diagnosis

- Exudative pharyngitis
- Hairy leukoplakia (adults), does not rub off
- Lichen planus
- Geographic tongue
- Herpes simplex erythema multiforme
- Pemphigus
- Baby formula or breast milk

Management

Nonpharmacologic Treatment

- Determine and treat underlying cause (e.g., antibiotic use, immune problem).
- Boil pacifiers and bottle nipples; assess mother's breasts/nipples for *Candida* infections.
- Disinfect dentures.

Pharmacologic Treatment

- First-line therapy:
  - Clotrimazole (Mycelex) troches 10 mg (suck on for 20 minutes), 5x day for 7–14 days
  - Nystatin pastilles: 200,000 U each, four times a day for 7–14 days
  - Denture wearers: nystatin ointment 100,000 U/g on fitting surfaces of denture and corners of mouth for 3 weeks; remove dentures at night; clean 2x/week with diluted (1:20) bleach or soaking solution containing benzoic acid, 0.12% chlorhexidine gluconate, or alkalize proteases
  - Moderate to severe disease: fluconazole (Diflucan) 100–200 mg (3 mg/kg) daily x 7–14 days or itraconazole (Sporanox) solution or capsules
- Second-line therapy:
  - Nystatin oral suspension (100,000 U/mL: Infants: 0.5 mL in each cheek q.i.d x 10 days; children: 5–10 mL q.i.d x 10 days; adults: swish and swallow 5–10 mL four times a day x 14 days; prophylaxis—same dosages x 2–5 days
  - Fluconazole 100 mg daily for 7–14 days (load immunocompromised patient with 200 mg)
  - Itraconazole (Sporanox) suspension: 200 mg (20 mL) daily; swish and swallow for 7–14 days; capsules 200 mg daily with food for 2–4 weeks
  - Miconazole (Daktarin) oral gel (20 mg/mL) four times a day, swish and swallow
  - Amphotericin B (Fungizone) oral suspension (100 mg/mL), 1 mL four times a day daily, swish and swallow; use between meals
  - Ketoconazole (Nizoral): 200–400 mg orally daily for 14–21 days
- Probiotics: *Lactobacillus* and *Bifidobacterium* may be beneficial

How Long to Treat

- Usually 7–14 days or continue until 2 days after disappearance of infection

Special Considerations

- Miconazole is usually the drug of choice in pregnancy.
- Use caution when prescribing oral agents because possible severe allergic reactions (renal failure or hepatoxicity) may occur.

When to Consult, Refer, Hospitalize

- Consult with physician or infectious disease specialist for immunocompromised patient, esophageal infection, or failure to resolve as expected.

Follow-Up

Expected Course

- Resolves in 1–2 weeks depending on severity and host immune status

Complications

- Feeding problems, weight loss
- Immunocompromised hosts: complications depend on severity of immunosuppression

GINGIVOSTOMATITIS

Description

- Inflammation of the mucosal lining of the oral cavity—that may involve the gingiva, mouth, cheeks, lip, tongue, and floor or roof of mouth—that leads to painful sores.

Etiology

- Many oral lesions are caused by viruses.
- Children:
  - Primary herpetic lesions
  - Hand-foot-mouth disease (HFMD)

- ◇ Herpangina
- ◇ Angular stomatitis
- ◇ Aphthous stomatitis (peak onset age 10–19 years)

- ♦ Teenagers and adults:
  - ◇ Vincent stomatitis (trench mouth),
- ♦ Acute necrotizing ulcerative gingivitis
  - ◇ Behçet's disease
  - ◇ Nicotinic stomatitis
  - ◇ Chronic ulcerative stomatitis
- ♦ Smoking
- ♦ Food hypersensitivity (citrus, nuts, coffee, chocolate, potatoes, cheeses, figs, gluten)
- ♦ Nutritional deficiencies: vitamin B6, vitamin B12, folic acid, vitamin C, iron
- ♦ Malnutrition
- ♦ Hormonal, bacterial, traumatic, uremic; ill-fitting dentures; chemotherapy or radiation
- ♦ Allergic or toxic drug reactions

Incidence and Demographics

See Table 6–10

Risk Factors

- ♦ Poor oral hygiene or oral trauma
- ♦ Dietary deficiencies and malnutrition
- ♦ Chronic systemic disease (celiac disease, Crohn's disease, Behçet's syndrome, HIV, reactive arthritis)
- ♦ Medications (NSAIDs, beta-blockers, angiotensin-converting enzyme inhibitors [ACEIs])
- ♦ Vitamin deficiencies (zinc, iron, B_{12}, folate)
- ♦ Food and chemical sensitivities
- ♦ Immune deficiencies
- ♦ Poor denture fit/quality
- ♦ Smoking

- Cancer therapies
- Crowded living conditions, day care
- Sunlight exposure
- Stress

Prevention and Screening

- Avoiding causative factors
- Good oral hygiene
- Good nutrition
- Avoiding/discontinuing smoking
- Properly fitting dentures
- Avoiding contact with infected individuals
- UV protection
- Decrease stress
- Proper nutrition
- Frequent handwashing, avoidance of scratching

Assessment

History and Physical Exam

- Patient will complain of burning sensation, intolerance to temperature, and irritating foods. Diagnosis depends on etiology:
  - Varies from minimal to severe pain
  - Fever, malaise, headaches
- Physical exam should include comprehensive oral examination along with cervical, submandibular, and submental lymph node evaluation. (See Table 6–10.)

Diagnostic Studies

- Viral cultures and polymerase chain reaction (PCR) testing can be done but are not usually necessary

TABLE 6–10.
DIFFERENTIATING CHARACTERISTICS OF COMMON GINGIVOSTOMATITIS

COMMON GINGIVOSTOMATITIS	DESCRIPTION
Herpes simplex virus ("cold sores")	♦ Viral: HSV-1 (90%) and HSV-2 (10%) ♦ Affects: all ages; acquired in childhood (6 months–5 years of age) ♦ Contagious—transmitted through infectious saliva ♦ Can occur anytime and is recurrent ♦ Lesion location: buccal mucosa, anterior tonsillar pillars, inner lips, tongue, and gingiva; spares posterior pharynx ♦ History and physical exam findings: ◊ Poor oral intake, drooling ◊ Fever + irritability precede development of lesions ◊ Swollen, erythematous friable lesions, then vesicles that break down and become gray ulcers that bleed ◊ Tender cervical adenopathy ◊ Associated symptoms (common in primary disease): fever, headache, malaise, abdominal pain, and myalgia
Hand, foot, and mouth disease (HFMD)	♦ Viral: Coxsackievirus A16 and enterovirus A7 are the most common ♦ Affects children less than 5 years of age; more common in infants and ♦ toddlers ♦ Highly contagious through aerosolized droplets and/or oral secretions through fecal–oral route, or contact with skin lesions ♦ Seasonal: spring and summer ♦ Lesion location: any area of mucosa, most common on tongue and buccal mucosa; spares posterior pharynx; includes rash on hands and feet ♦ History and physical exam findings: ◊ Low-grade fever (2–3 days), decreased appetite, malaise, vague abdominal pain, mouth or throat pain, and mild URI, evolving to lesions ◊ Painful oral lesions rupture to form ulcers ◊ Usually not pruritic ◊ Cervical or submandibular adenopathy may be present. ◊ Associated symptoms: cutaneous lesions on palms of hands, soles of feet, and buttocks; may cause CNS symptoms

Continued

TABLE 6–10. (CONTINUED)

COMMON GINGIVOSTOMATITIS	DESCRIPTION
Herpangina	♦ Viral: Coxsackievirus group A 16 most common ♦ Affects: all ages; common in children 3–10 years of age ♦ Highly contagious through aerosolized droplets and/or oral secretions through fecal–oral route, or contact with skin lesions ♦ Seasonal: summer and early fall ♦ Lesion location: tonsils and soft palate; spares anterior pharynx ♦ H & P: ◊ Painful vesicles, fever, sore throat, difficulty swallowing, and dysphagia; gray, pinhead-sized vesicles rupture and form large, fibrin-covered ulcers ◊ Associated symptoms: headache, vomiting, and abdominal pain may occur
Aphthous ulcers ("canker sores")	♦ Etiology unknown; stress, systemic disease, medications, oral trauma, etc. ♦ Affects any age; common in ages 10–19 years ♦ Not contagious ♦ Not seasonal: can occur any time ♦ Lesion location: labial and buccal mucosa, ventral tongue; spares gingiva and hard palate ♦ H & P: ◊ Burning sensation, hurts to eat and swallow, especially foods and drinks with a high acid content ◊ Obtain history of GI symptoms, genital ulcers, HIV risk fac tors, and joint pain ◊ Recurring, one or more ulcers covered by painful oral lesions appear as localized, round-to-oval ulcers with a grayish base

- Consider:
  - ◊ Tzanck test (HSV), does not differentiate HSV-1 from HSV-2
  - ◊ Serologic test for syphilis
  - ◊ CBC, cultures to determine secondary infection
  - ◊ Ferritin, B12, folate
  - ◊ ESR
  - ◊ KOH

- ◇ Skin biopsy
- ◇ HIV testing

Differential Diagnosis

- Etiologies mentioned above
- Pharyngitis/tonsillitis
- Oral trauma
- Syphilis
- Squamous cell carcinoma
- Stevens-Johnson syndrome
- Scarlet fever
- Burning mouth syndrome

Management

- Treatment depends on causative factors.

Nonpharmacologic Treatment

- Palliative and supportive because many cases are self-limiting
- Fluids, popsicles may be beneficial; gargle/swish with mild mouthwash or 1:1 hydrogen peroxide and water; maintain good oral hygiene; stop smoking; refit dentures; avoid specific allergens; replace vitamin deficiencies.
- Avoid salty, acidic, or sharp foods.

Pharmacologic Treatment

- Acetaminophen or ibuprofen for analgesia; narcotics may be necessary
- "Miracle mouth rinses": swish, gargle, and spit out. (Viscous lidocaine 2%, Maalox, and diphenhydramine is one formulation used).
- 2% viscous lidocaine (Xylocaine); swish and spit for local discomfort (generally not recommended because of risk of swallowing and associated seizures).

- Liquid diphenhydramine by mouth or swish and spit, for allergic reactions.
- Oral anesthetics, but can be harmful and result in self-injury when children chew on anesthetized lips
- Antibiotics for gangrenous stomatitis (penicillin and metronidazole IV recommended)
  - Topical valacyclovir (Valtrex) or penciclovir (Deavir); docosanol (Abreva; sold OTC) is often used in treatment of recurrent oral herpes to decrease the duration of HSV shedding but has minimal effect on symptoms.
  - Consider oral acyclovir: primary herpetic stomatitis in children—5 mg/kg divided 5x/day x 7 days; adults—400 mg three times a day x 7–10 days.
  - Recurrence: acyclovir 400 mg orally three times a day x 5 days or 800 mg two times a day x 5 days or 800 mg three times a day x 2 days or famciclovir (Famvir) 250 mg three times a day x 5 days
  - Suppression: use 400 mg two times a day daily.
  - Sucralfate (Carafate) suspension 1 tsp; swishing in mouth or placing on ulcers four times a day may be helpful.
- Possible corticosteroids in severe cases
- Severe cases may require parenteral fluids and antiviral therapy, particularly in children and immunocompromised patients.

How Long to Treat

- Continue symptomatic treatment until resolution; depends on etiology
- Lesions to be followed until resolved; if they fail to resolve, continuously recur, or appear suspicious, biopsy may be needed.

Special Considerations

- Herpetic (primary), HFMD, herpangina, and traumatic ulcers are common causes in pediatric population
- Ill-fitting dentures, nutritional deficiencies seen in older adult population
- HSV is always present in dormant state and can reactivate.

When to Consult, Refer, Hospitalize

- If dehydration is caused by decreased fluid intake or immunocompromised state, patient may require hospitalization for IV fluids or IV acyclovir therapy.

Follow-Up

- Follow-up visit in 3–7 days if case is severe
- Extensive/primary cases should be rechecked in 1 week
- Monitor for secondary bacterial infections

Expected Course

- Most cases are self-limiting and resolve in 7–14 days.
- Consider long-term suppression therapy (HSV).

Complications

- Usually none
- Recurrent scarifying stomatitis may result in intraoral scarring with restriction of oral mobility.
- Behçet's disease may result in vision loss, pneumonia, colitis, vasculitis, or encephalitis.
- Herpetic stomatitis may be complicated by ocular or CNS involvement; herpes pneumonia.

Problems of the Neck

CERVICAL ADENITIS

Description

- Inflammation of one or more cervical lymph nodes; most common cause is infection
- Most common site is submandibular and anterior cervical
- Also called "cervical lymphadenitis"

Etiology

- Infection: local (dental caries or periodontal disease, URI, otitis media, pharyngitis, stomatitis) or systemic infection
  - ◊ Viral (most common cause in children): Epstein-Barr virus (EBV), cytomegalovirus (CMV), varicella zoster, HIV, HSV, adenovirus, rhinovirus, enterovirus,

- ◇ Bacterial: beta-hemolytic streptococcal (70%), staphylococci (20%); methicillin-resistant *S. aureus* (MRSA) must also be considered
- ◇ Other infections: Cat-scratch disease (*Bartonella henselae*), atypical mycobacteria, toxoplasmosis

- Malignant neoplasms (80% of isolated solitary neck masses in adults 40 years of age) or older
- Manifestation of systemic autoimmune diseases such as lupus, rheumatoid arthritis, or sarcoidosis
- Rarely due to trauma
- Easily mistaken for goiter or thyroid nodule or parotitis

Incidence and Demographics

- More commonly found in children
- About 55% of healthy children in all age groups have palpable cervical nodes that are not associated with acute infection or systemic illness
- Can occur at any age

Risk Factors

- Infection
- Systemic disease
- Cat scratch
- Tobacco and alcohol use (associated with squamous cell carcinoma and 80% of cervical lymphatic tumors)

Prevention and Screening

- Avoid use of tobacco and abuse of alcohol.
- Maintain general health with strategies such as adequate nutrition, exercise, and rest
- Avoid contact with those known to have contagious viral infections.
- Good handwashing hygiene
- Immunization with MMR vaccine

Assessment

History

- History of recent or current upper respiratory infection
- History of MMR immunization
- Duration and mode of onset of node enlargement, any tenderness, warmth, or change in size
- Pain with eating suggests parotid gland involvement.
- Patient with malignancy—describes lymphadenitis as being present for an undetermined time (gradual enlargement) and becoming larger, nontender, and firm
- Fever, sore throat, ear pain, toothache, rash, unexplained weight loss, night sweats, irritability, cough, and wheezing
- Exposure to cats (cat-scratch disease)

Physical Exam

- A thorough examination of the teeth, gingiva, oropharynx, and ears is required, assessing for indicators of infection.
- All lymph nodes should be assessed to differentiate between an isolated and localized adenitis versus the generalized, diffuse lymphadenopathy associated with systemic disease.
- Assess whether the node(s) are soft, firm, hard; assess for matting, adherence to skin or to deeper tissues; fluctuant
- Physical findings vary depending upon the etiology.
- Infection-related lymphadenitis is typically found in the anterior cervical chain and the submandibular nodes. These are soft, tender, and warm, and may reveal erythema of the overlying skin. The size of enlargement is variable (2–6 cm) and is usually bilateral.
- Malignancy-related lymphadenitis is often found in the supraclavicular area with a firm texture that is fixed to the skin and underlying tissue. Exam may reveal one or several enlarged nodes along the anterior cervical chain. Lesions may be found in the oral cavity, nose (e.g., unilateral obstruction), or pharynx.
- Examination should carefully differentiate among other structures (thyroid, parotid, or salivary glands).

Diagnostic Studies

- Suspected infectious lymphadenitis may be diagnosed clinically.
- Tests to consider in the workup include:
  - Rapid group A streptococcal test and culture
  - CBC with differential
  - TB skin testing
  - Rapid mononucleosis test
  - Serologic testing for EBV, CBV, toxoplasmosis, *Bartonella henselae*, HIV, and fungi
  - Chest X-ray
  - Large fluctuant nodes are aspirated for culture and sensitivity if unresponsive to therapy or worsening.
  - Node biopsy if there is no improvement or malignancy is suspected
  - CT scan, ultrasound, or MRI can be done to differentiate among solid, fluctuant, or cystic mass.
- Refer to a specialist if the patient is *over* 40 years of age.

Differential Diagnosis

- Malignancy
- Localized infection
- Lymphatic malformation
- Thyroid enlargement
- Cat-scratch disease
- Parotid or salivary gland inflammation
- Mumps
- Rubella
- Rubeola

Management

Nonpharmacologic Treatment

- For localized infection, warm compresses for 15 minutes four times a day
- Good handwashing and washing cat scratches/bites with warm soapy water

Pharmacologic Treatment

- OTC analgesics such as NSAIDs or acetaminophen for fever or pain
- Most cases of cervical lymphadenopathy or lymphadenitis do not require specific therapy because they often represent reactive enlargement or viral infection.
- Suppurative cases can be treated for suspected bacterial infections and should cover *S. aureus* and *S. pyogenes*. Immunocompromised patients should always be treated with antibiotics.
  - First-line therapy: amoxicillin plus clavulanic acid, 30–40 mg/kg/day divided two times a day (500 mg three times a day for adults) or clindamycin (30–40 mg/kg/day divided three to four times a day for 10 to 14 days)
  - Failure to improve in 36 to 48 hours should prompt reassessment of diagnosis and therapy.
  - Second-line therapy: erythromycin 10 mg/kg/dose four times a day, cephalexin 10–20 mg/ kg/dose four times a day or (500 mg two times a day for adult), dicloxacillin (Dynapen) 25 mg/kg/day
- For atypical mycobacteria and atypical tuberculosis:
  - Surgical excision is the treatment of choice for nontuberculous mycobacterial lymphadenitis.
- For cat-scratch disease:
  - Usually a self-limiting disorder requiring no specific treatment
  - Controlled studies have not shown antibiotics to affect course, but they can be used.
- Azithromycin x 5 days
- Rifampin 5–10 mg/kg/dose every12–24 hours or
- TMP-SMX (Bactrim) 5 mg ofTMP/kg/dose two times a day
- Ciprofloxacin (Cipro) 500 mg two times a day (not recommended for patients younger than 18)
- Erythromycin, clarithromycin, doxycycline, and gentamicin are other agents used.

How Long to Treat

- Antibiotic therapy should be continued for 1–2 weeks.

Special Considerations

- Have a high index of suspicion for malignancy in patients who abuse alcohol or tobacco, or who present with weight loss and night sweats.
- In patients with risk factors, screen for HIV infection.

When to Consult, Refer, Hospitalize

- Follow-up in clinic if symptoms do not resolve 48–72 hours after treatment is initiated.
- Refer immediately to an emergency facility if the patient has difficulty swallowing or breathing.
- Refer to surgeon or ENT specialist for excision biopsy if malignancy is suspected (nodes that are matted, hard, or painless without source of regional infection).

Follow-Up

Expected Course

- Benign lymphadenitis will resolve over time, sometimes within days of treatment, other times over the course of 2–3 weeks with or without treatment; if not resolved after 4 weeks, refer to ENT as biopsy may be indicated.

Complications

- Localized infection that spreads hematologically with sepsis
- Obstruction of airway from extending edema and inflammation
- Malignancy and death

CASE STUDIES

CASE 1

A 16-year-old girl presents with a "severe cold" for 4–5 days.

History of Present Illness: Was previously well. Until last week, she had a cold, which is persisting without much improvement. Patient's mother is very concerned that she needs antibiotics; claims that previous providers had always used them to treat her daughter's head colds.

Patient feels feverish, has dry cough, runny nose, mostly clear drainage with some yel low mucus in the mornings, scratchy sore throat, and ears "popping." Tried ibuprofen cold and sinus product with benefit.

Past Medical History: Is in general good health, single, and sexually active with boyfriend x 2 months.

Denies food, drug, or environmental allergies; smokes 5 cigarettes per day.

Medications: Oral contraceptives; took amoxicillin 500 mg two times a day yesterday—left over from a prescription she was given 2 months ago for "sinusitis."

1. What additional history do you need?
2. What are the risk factors for possible diagnoses?

   Exam: Temp is 99.0°F. Thin-appearing White female in no acute distress; looks mildly ill. Voice quality is "nasal." Posterior oropharynx has mild erythema, no lesions or exudate, tonsils not enlarged, neck supple with no lymphadenopathy, ear canals and TMs are clear bilaterally. Nasal turbinates are mildly erythematous and edematous with watery discharge. Heart: regular rate and rhythm (RRR) at 88 BPM; lungs are clear.

3. What diagnostic tests would you order?
4. What is your differential diagnosis?
5. What treatment plan will you carry out?

CASE 2

A 22-year-old female college student presents with sore throat and earache.

V: Sore throat began 3 days ago. She was seen at student health center 2 days ago and treated with penicillin V potassium 250 mg four times a day Sore throat was worse last night and patient especially complained of severe right ear pain. Notes fever and chills but did not take temperature; overall feels very tired and achy. Hurts to swallow, only drinking liquids. Lives in the dormitory. Denies problems with shortness of breath, chest pain, rash, joint pains, nausea, vomiting, or diarrhea.

Past Medical History: Healthy, denies any preexisting medical problems.

Medications: Pen V K, ibuprofen p.r.n. for fever and pain x 3 days; last dose 4 hours ago

Exam: Young Asian female; looks ill. Temp 102.3°F, sinuses nontender, nasal mucosa clear. Ear canals and TMs negative. Throat 4+ erythema on posterior wall, white-yellow pu rulent exudate on right tonsillar area. Positive trismus, palatal bulge on the right. Neck positive for anterior cervical lymphadenopathy; tender, soft, and mobile. Chest clear. Heart: RRR at 110 BPM.

1. What are the most likely possibilities for a differential diagnosis?
2. What information in the history is the most significant?
3. What physical examination components are especially useful for this presentation?
4. Are the findings from the history and physical adequate to make the diagnosis?
5. What diagnostic studies will rule in or out any of the possibilities?
6. What treatment plan will you carry out?

CASE 3

A 6-year-old boy presents with severe right ear pain.

V: Child was well until this morning, when he awoke at 6 a.m. crying with right ear pain. Mother noted that he felt very hot; she did not take temp. Gave children's acetaminophen and he slept a little. Mother later noted drainage from the ear on his pillow.

PAST MEDICAL HISTORY: Frequent otitis media as an infant/toddler, which he seemed to "grow out of"; never required long-term antibiotics or ventilation tubes; last otitis media was about 2 years ago.

Exam: Young Black male child, looks moderately ill. Temp 101.2°F orally. Right ear canal has whitish crust and is moist, no erythema or edema, tragus nontender with manipulation.

TM red and bulging, small perforation present. Oropharynx clear, nose clear, neck supple, no lymphadenopathy. Heart: RRR 110, respirations 32, lungs clear.

1. What additional history is important?
2. What is the differential diagnosis?
3. What historical and physical exam features support the differential?
4. What are the risk factors for otitis media?
5. How will you treat this child?

CASE STUDIES DISCUSSION

CASE 1

1. What additional history do you need?

   Details on history of frequent head colds (review the symptoms and signs, number of episodes in past few years, how treated, whether the episodes resolved). Any change in environment (dusty or damp, pets)? Has she ever had allergy tests or radiographic sinus imaging or endoscopy? Does she have asthma or allergic symptoms? Any symptoms/ signs of systemic disease (diabetes)? Any intranasal (or other) drug use? Alcohol use? OTC nasal decongestants? Does she use condoms? Assess her STD risk.

2. What are the risk factors for possible diagnoses?

   Cigarettes predispose to allergic rhinitis and sinusitis. Allergic rhinitis predisposes to sinusitis. Oral contraceptives may cause vasomotor rhinitis. Oral sex and new partner may cause gonococcal pharyngitis, risk for HIV, and immunosuppression.

3. What diagnostic tests would you order?

   Probably none currently unless the history and physical exam suggests HIV risk or other systemic disease (diabetes, anemia)

4. What is your differential diagnosis?

   Infectious rhinitis, probably viral; allergic rhinitis; acute bacterial sinusitis; vasomotor rhinitis.

5. What treatment plan will you carry out?

   Patient/family education on various types of rhinitis/sinusitis and what treatment is appropriate in this case versus indiscriminate use of antibiotics; also prevention measures and maintenance care. Suggest saline lavage four times a day, intranasal corticosteroid spray, non-sedating antihistamine, OTC oral decongestants, infection prevention, and allergy control in her environment.

CASE 2

1. What are the most likely possibilities for a differential diagnosis?

   Peritonsillar abscess, streptococcal tonsillitis, infectious mononucleosis, antibiotic non-compliance, acute otitis media, antibiotic-resistant infection.

2. What information in the history is the most significant?

   Failure to improve on antibiotics; symptoms worse with ear pain, which may be referred from pharynx.

3. What physical examination components are especially useful for this presentation?

   Fever, erythematous posterior pharynx with exudative tonsil, trismus, palatal bulge, ten-der lymphadenopathy, negative ear findings.

4. Are the findings from the history and physical adequate to make the diagnosis, and what diagnostic studies will rule in or out any of the possibilities?

   The history and physical are very revealing for peritonsillar abscess; however, CBC with differential, mono screen test, quick streptococcal screen, throat culture, and possibly blood cultures will help define her diagnosis.

5. What treatment plan will you carry out?

   Start parenteral antibiotics (ceftriaxone is a good choice) and consult with ENT specialist for urgent evaluation and possible admission. If urgent referral to ENT is not possible, make arrangements for her to be seen at the nearest emergency department for evaluation and treatment.

CASE 3

1. What additional history is important?

   Any recent URI? Cigarette smoke exposure? Is the child in day care? Any siblings? Recent swimming? Has he ever had otitis externa or TM rupture? Has he ever put anything in his ear?

2. What is the differential diagnosis?

   Acute otitis media with perforation, acute otitis externa, foreign body.

3. What historical and physical exam features support the differential diagnosis?

   The external auditory canal is without erythema or edema, no tragal tenderness, so otitis externa is ruled out; the red, bulging TM with a perforation and acute illness supports acute otitis media; the whitish crust in the ear canal is from the perforation of the TM with extrusion of exudate.

4. What are the risk factors for otitis media?

   Male, day care, Eustachian tube dysfunction, second hand cigarette smoke exposure.

5. How will you treat this child?

   Amoxicillin 80–90 mg/kg/day in divided doses; or ofloxacin (Floxin) otic 5 gtts two times a day; acetaminophen or ibuprofen for pain and fever; follow-up in 2 weeks but instructed to return if not improving in 48–72 hours

REFERENCES

Alattas, O. A., Hamdi, A. A., Mudarba, F. M., Alsheheri, A. M., Al-Yahya, M. S., Almotairi, S. A., Saeed, R. A., Buamer. M. M., Alsuwailem, M. S., & Alamri, I. A. (2019). Red eye diagnosis and management in primary health care. *Archives of Pharmacy Practice, 10*(3), 1–5.

American Academy of Pediatrics. (2021). *2021 recommendations for preventative pediatric health care.* https://publications.aap.org/pediatrics/article/147/3/e2020049776/33378/2021-Recommendations-for-Preventive-Pediatric

American Cancer Society. (2020). *Retinoblastoma.* https://www.cancer.org/cancer/retinoblastoma/about/key-statistics.html

Arcangelo, V. P., Peterson, A. M., Wilbur, V., & Kang, T. M. (2021). *Pharmacotherapeutics for advanced practice.* (5th Ed.). Philadelphia, PA: Wolters Kluwer.

Boyd, K. (2021). *Corneal abrasion and erosion.* https://www.aao.org/eye-health/diseases/what-is-corneal-abrasion

Cabana. M. D. (ed). (2018). *The 5-minute pediatric consult premium.* (8th Ed.). Philadelphia, PA: Wolters Kluwer.

Centers for Disease Control and Prevention. (2023). Common eye disorders and diseases. https://www.cdc.gov/visionhealth/basics/ced/index.html#.

Centers for Disease Control and Prevention. (2019). Zika virus: Clinical evaluation & disease. https://www.cdc.gov/zika/hc-providers/preparing-for-zika/clinicalevaluationdisease.html

Domino, F. J. (2022). *The 5-minute clinical consult* premium 2022. (30th ed.). Philadelphia, PA: Wolters Kluwer.

Ferri, F. F. (ed.). (2022). *2022 Ferri's clinical advisor.* Philadelphia, PA: Elsevier.

Gervasio, K., & Peck, T. (2021). *The Willis eye manual: Office and emergency room diagnosis and treatment of eye disease.* (8th ed.). Philadelphia, PA: Wolters Kluwer.

Gilbert, D. N., Chambers, H. F., Saag, M. S., Pavia, A. T., Boucher, H. W., Black, D., Freedman, D. O., Kim, K., & Schwartz, B. S. (2021). *The Stanford guide to antimicrobial therapy 2021.* (51st ed.). Hyde Park, VT: Antimicrobial Therapy, Inc.

Goroll, A. H., & Mulley, A. G. (2020). *Primary care medicine: Office evaluation and management of the adult patient.* (8th ed.). Philadelphia, PA: Wolters Kluwer.

Hay, W., Levin, M., Abzug, M., & Bunik, M. (2020). *Current diagnosis and treatment pediatrics 2020–21.* (25th ed.). New York, NY: McGraw Hill.

Kimberlin, D. W., Barnett, E. D., Lynfield, R., & Sawyer, M. H. (eds.). (2021). *Red book (2021): Report of the committee on infectious diseases.* (32nd ed.). American Academy of Pediatrics.

Kliegman, R. M., & St. Geme, J. W. (2019). *Nelson textbook of pediatrics* (21st ed.). St. Louis, MO: Elsevier.

Maaks, D. L. G., Starr, N. B., Braby, M. A., Gaylord, N. M., Driessnack, M., & Duderstadt, K. G. (2019). *Burns pediatric primary care.* (7th ed.). St. Louis, MO: Elsevier.

Papadakis, M., McPhee, S., Rabow, M., & McQuaid, K. (2022). *Current medical diagnosis and treatment 2022.* (61st ed.). New York, NY: McGraw Hill.

Rhoads, J., & Penick, J. (2022). *Formulating a differential diagnosis for the advanced practice provider.* (3rd ed.). New York, NY: Springer.

Tintinalli, J. E., Stapczynski, J. S., Ma, O. J., Cline, D. M., Meckler, G. D., & Yealy, D. M. (2019). *Tintinalli's emergency medicine: A comprehensive study guide.* (9th ed.). New York, NY: McGraw-Hill.

Usatine, R., Smith, M. A., Mayeaux, E. J., & Chumley, H. (2019). *The color atlas and synopsis of family medicine.* (3rd ed.). New York, NY: McGraw-Hill.

Visovsky, C. G., Zambroski, C. H., & Lutz, R. M. (2022). *Edmunds' pharmacology for the primary care provider.* (5th ed.). Philadelphia, PA: Elsevier.

Yan, H. (ed.). (2022). *Management on complicated ocular trauma.* New York, NY: Springer.

Zheng, X. Y., Choy, B.N.K., Zhou, M. M., Shi, C. P., & Zhao, Z. Y. (2020). Lacrimal sac bacteriology and susceptibility pattern in infants with congenital nasolacrimal duct obstruction in the 1st year of life: A cross-sectional study. *BMC Pediatrics, 20,* 1–9. https://doi.org/10.1186/s12887-020-02358-5

CHAPTER 7

RESPIRATORY DISORDERS

Nikiya Lewis, DNP, APRN, FNP-C

General Approach

Note: Some respiratory infections can be found in Chapter 4, "Infectious Diseases."

- Through careful history and physical examination, determine the etiology of the problem: infectious (bacterial, viral, or other), allergic, occupational, environmental, or congenital defect.
- Most respiratory infections are viral. Treat empirically with antibiotics only if the patient has a secondary bacterial infection, underlying respiratory condition, or prolonged symptoms.
- Determine whether symptoms are acute or chronic to guide management.
- For dyspnea, determine patient's position at onset of symptoms, relationship to activity, and any factors that improve or exacerbate symptoms.
- Assess rate, depth, rhythm, work of breathing, and symmetry of chest movement. Rate is a critical indicator of respiratory status, especially in children (see Table 7–1).
- Obtain smoking history and smoking exposure.
- Is cough productive or nonproductive? Note color, amount, and consistency of sputum.
- Note nature of cough: paroxysmal, continuous, or staccato.
- Assess exercise tolerance and activity level.
- In infants, assess ability to take bottle or nurse.
- Antitussives should not be given in conditions in which retention of respiratory secretions may be harmful.
- Encourage patients to stay well hydrated.
- Assess lung status with pulmonary function testing and spirometry. (This can usually be obtained beginning at age 5.)

TABLE 7–1.
NORMAL RESPIRATORY RATES (COUNTED FOR 1 MINUTE AT REST)

	PRETERM	BIRTH–1 YEAR	OLDER THAN 1–3 YEARS	OLDER THAN 3–6 YEARS	OLDER THAN 6–12 YEARS	OLDER THAN 12–18 YEARS	ADULTS	ADULTS 65 YEARS OR OLDER
Normal rate (breaths/ minute)	40–70	30–60	20–30	20–25	18–30	12–18	16–20	12–30

- Patients with cardiovascular disease, peripheral vascular disease, hyperthyroidism, diabetes mellitus, urinary retention, prostatic hypertrophy, hypertension, and increased intraocular pressure should avoid decongestants.
- In pediatric patients, assess appetite; fluid intake (hydration status); change in sleep pattern; activity in home, school, and day care environment; and immunization history.

RED FLAGS

Post-tussive emesis and signs and symptoms of respiratory distress should be quickly evaluated, treated with oxygen and bronchodilators, if appropriate referred to an emergency department.

- *Community-acquired pneumonia*—consider hospitalization in:
  - Adult patients age 50 and older with history of comorbid conditions, altered mental status, leukopenia (less than 4,000 per microliter), leukocytosis (greater than 30,000 per microliter), tachycardia, tachypnea, systolic blood pressure less than 90 mmHg, and temperature 35°C (95°F) or lower or 40°C (104°F) or higher
  - Pediatric patients appearing toxic, who have immunodeficiencies or cardiac or pulmonary disease, or are in respiratory distress or dehydrated
- *Hemoptysis*: Older patients, smokers, and patients who do not respond to treatment for infection have a high index of suspicion for lung cancer. Obtain chest X-ray and refer for bronchoscopy and further workup.
- *Asthma*: Acute exacerbation may present as diminished breath sounds without audible wheezing, but a patient may be in severe respiratory distress. Begin treatment, monitor closely, and be on the alert to transfer to an emergency facility.

Acute Conditions

ACUTE BRONCHITIS

Description

- Self-limited inflammation of the bronchi due to upper airway infection associated with cough lasting more than 5 days with or without production of mucus. Causes injury to epithelial, surfaces causing increased production of mucus and thickening of bronchiole wall. Most common cause of antibiotic abuse.

Etiology

- Viruses most common (95% of cases): rhinovirus, coronavirus types 1 to 3, adenovirus, influenza A and B, parainfluenza virus, respiratory syncytial virus (RSV), human metapneumovirus
- Bacterial infections are uncommon causes: *Bordetella pertussis, Chlamydia pneumoniae*, and *Mycoplasma*
- Possible fungal infections
- Chemical irritants

Incidence and Demographics

- Affects all ages: Severity and frequency increases with cigarette smoking and preexisting pulmonary disease.
- The incidence is highest in the late fall and winter seasons.

Risk Factors

- Infants
- Older adults
- Air pollutants/environmental changes
- Smoking/secondhand smoke
- Chronic bronchopulmonary diseases, chronic sinusitis, bronchopulmonary allergy
- Tracheostomy

- Immunosuppression: immunoglobulin deficiency, HIV infection, alcoholism
- Gastrointestinal reflux disease (GERD)
- Environmental changes; hypertrophied tonsils and adenoids in children

Prevention and Screening

- Avoid smoking and secondhand smoke.
- Control underlying risk factors (asthma, sinusitis, GERD).
- Avoid exposure, especially in day care.
- Get pneumovax and influenza immunizations.

Assessment

History

- Acute and persistent cough lasting more than 5 days (typically 1 to 3 weeks). The cough may be associated with purulent or non-purulent sputum production or with purulent-appearing sputum production.
- Mild dyspnea, bronchospasm, wheeze, fever, and fatigue may be present; smoking status of patient or household members; infectious illness of household members; past medical history of respiratory diseases
- Acute bronchitis due to pertussis causes a paroxysmal "whooping" cough.

Physical Exam

- Afebrile or low-grade temperature less than 101°F (38°C)
- Tachypnea
- Pharynx injected
- Respiratory wheezes or rhonchi; rales should not be present.
- No physical findings of lower airway congestion or consolidation. In children, upper airway congestion may be heard in the lungs; to differentiate, listen to breathing and then compare to auscultation sounds.

Diagnostic Studies

- Diagnosis generally based on clinical presentation
- Chest X-ray to exclude pneumonia for patients with severe respiratory symptoms and temperature over 38°C (100.4°F), pulse over 100/min, respiratory rate over 24, and abnormal lung exam
- Complete blood count (CBC) and sputum culture: not generally performed unless uncertain of diagnosis or suspicious for coronavirus disease 2019 (COVID-19), influenza, or pertussis
- Influenza titers during seasonal peaks
- Nasopharyngeal culture and polymerase chain reaction (PCR), if necessary, to exclude pertussis
- Purified protein derivative (PPD) if at risk for tuberculosis
- Pulmonary function tests (PFTs) if asthma or obstructive disease suspected (seldom needed during acute phases)
- Pulse oximetry if available
- Arterial blood gases: hypoxemia (rarely)

Differential Diagnosis

- Pneumonia
- Asthma
- COVID-19
- Angiotensin-converting enzyme (ACE) inhibitor use
- Pulmonary embolism
- Lung cancer
- Heart failure
- Upper respiratory infection
- Influenza
- Post-nasal drip
- GERD
- Tuberculosis

Management

Non-pharmacologic Treatment

- Rest, adequate hydration, steam inhalations, vaporizers, smoking cessation or avoid smoke, treat associated illnesses

Pharmacologic Treatment

- Acute bronchitis is a common diagnosis resulting in antibiotic overprescribing. It is most commonly caused by viral infection. Antibiotics should be used only when indicated. Empiric antibiotic therapy is not recommended. See Table 7–2.
- The American College of Chest Physicians (CHEST) does not recommend the use of codeine to decrease cough symptoms in patients with upper respiratory tract infections.
- Avoid antihistamines; they dry out secretions.
- Decongestants if accompanied by sinus condition
- Antipyretic analgesics: aspirin (avoid in children), acetaminophen, ibuprofen
- Cough suppressants for troublesome cough (not with chronic obstructive pulmonary disease [COPD]); guaifenesin or dextromethorphan
- Mucolytic agents not recommended
- Inhaled beta-agonist (albuterol) or in combination with steroids for cough with bronchospasm
- Consider steroids for bronchospasm
- Cough and cold preparations should not be used in children younger than age 6.

TABLE 7–2
ACUTE BRONCHITIS: STRATEGIES TO REDUCE ANTIBIOTIC USE

- Address patients' concerns in therapeutic manner
- Reassure patients that condition is self-limiting, and symptoms usually resolve in 1 to 3 weeks
- Use shared decision-making
- Offer other non-antibiotic medications for symptom control
- Use delayed prescription strategies
- Explain to patients that antibiotic use will not shorten the duration of symptoms or prevent complications and has the potential to lead to severe adverse reactions
- Refer to acute bronchitis as "chest cold"

Adapted from *Acute Bronchitis* by Kinkade & Long, 2016.

How Long to Treat

- If uncomplicated, generally self-limiting, recovery 7 to 21 days
- Cough may linger for several weeks.
- In children, if recurrent, need to consider other diagnoses (asthma)

Special Considerations

- Geriatrics: Monitor closely for complications such as pneumonia.
- Other: Symptoms and duration may be worse in smokers.
- Adults with pertussis may transmit it to unimmunized children.

When to Consult, Refer, Hospitalize

- Outpatient treatment unless an older adult or complicated by severe underlying disease
- Refer if hypoxia, severe bronchospasm present, or exacerbation of underlying disease.
- Refer to pulmonologist or asthma specialist for further evaluation if no improvement in 4 to 6 weeks or if more severe symptoms.

Follow-Up

- If no improvement or symptoms worsen after 72 hours

Expected Course

- Generally, symptoms resolve in 7 to 21 days, but cough may persist for 3 to 4 weeks.

Complications

- Secondary bacterial infection, pneumonia, bronchiectasis, hemoptysis, acute respiratory failure, chronic cough

BRONCHIOLITIS

Description

- Acute inflammation and obstruction of small airways and reactive airways, generally affecting infants and young children
- Leading cause of illness and hospitalization in infants and children

Etiology

- RSV is the most common cause, followed by rhinovirus
- Other causes: parainfluenza virus, adenovirus, influenza virus, *Mycoplasma pneumoniae*, coronavirus, and *C.* (or *Chlamydophila) pneumoniae*

Incidence and Demographics

- Common cause of illness and hospitalization in children younger than 2 years of age
- Predominant age: newborn to 2 years (peak age less than 6 months)
- Predominant sex: male more than female
- Seasonal occurrence, more common during the fall and winter

Risk Factors

- Prematurity (gestational age less than 37 weeks)
- Age less than 12 weeks
- Smoking exposure
- Low birth weight
- Immunodeficiency
- Formula feeding (not breastfed)
- Contact with infected person (primary mode of transmission)
- Children in day care environment
- Heart–lung transplant patient (immune compromise)

- History of bronchopulmonary dysplasia, congenital heart disease, neurologic disease
- Adults: exposure to toxic fumes, connective tissue disease (respiratory epithelial damage)

Prevention and Screening

- Handwashing
- Minimize passive exposure to cigarette smoke
- Contact isolation of infected babies
- Contact with infants to a minimum for people with colds
- Palivizumab (Synagis) administered monthly (October through May), 15 mg/kg IM in high-risk patients
  - 32 to 35 weeks of gestation and younger than 3 months old at start of RSV season with at least one risk factor: either attending day care or with a sibling younger than 5 years old at home
  - 28 to 32 weeks of gestation and younger than 6 months old
  - Less than 28 weeks of gestation and younger than 12 months old
  - Moderately severe bronchopulmonary dysplasia and up to 2 years of age
  - Hemodynamically significant congenital heart disease (until age 6 months)
  - Once begun, continue through end of season, regardless of age attained
- RSV immunoglobulin can also be used in at-risk patients; monthly infusions of 750 mg/kg, October through May
- Influenza vaccine for children 6 to 59 months of age and their household contacts

Assessment

History

- Exposure to upper respiratory infection
- 1- to 3-day history of upper respiratory symptoms (nasal discharge, congestion, and mild cough)
- Diminished appetite, irritability, noisy breathing, cough, grunting, vomiting
- Afebrile or low-grade temperature present
- Apnea or cyanosis (apnea may be only symptom in very young infants), respiratory distress

Physical Exam

- Afebrile or low-grade fever
- Nasal congestion with thick, purulent secretions; nasal flaring; rhinorrhea; pharyngitis; conjunctivitis; otitis may be present
- Cough; tachypnea; retractions
- Hyper-resonance
- Wheezing; prolonged expiratory phase; fine crackles (wheezing may not be audible if airways are profoundly narrowed)
- Tachycardia and/or mild hypoxemia
- Signs of dehydration: depressed fontanels, tacky mucous membranes, crying without tears
- Cyanosis of oral mucosa and nail beds
- Hepatosplenomegaly (due to hyperinflated lungs)

Diagnostic Studies

- Usually diagnosed by clinical presentation
- Pulse oximetry to monitor respiratory status (less than 94% significant)
- Laboratory studies and radiographic images are usually not necessary for diagnosis; however, they may be useful to evaluate complications and other comorbid infections.
- Chest X-ray: increased anteroposterior (AP) diameter, flattened diaphragm, air trapping, patchy infiltrates, focal atelectasis (right upper lobe common), peribronchial cuffing
- CBC with differential
- Urine specific gravity to monitor hydration
- Nasopharyngeal washings for RSV enzyme immunoassay (rapid results) and culture (usually not necessary during RSV season, but may be useful)
- Consider sweat test for chronic reoccurrence to exclude cystic fibrosis.

Differential Diagnosis

- Pneumonia
- COVID-19

- Aspiration
- Foreign body
- Vascular rings asthma
- Croup
- GERD
- Cystic fibrosis
- Pertussis
- Heart failure

Management

Goal: supportive to prevent hypoxia and dehydration

Nonpharmacologic Treatment

- In uncomplicated cases, supportive care and anticipatory guidance are recommended: frequent offerings of clear fluids or diluted milk; frequent suctioning of secretions with saline and a bulb syringe, and monitoring of disease progression
- Cool, humidified oxygen if hypoxemic

Pharmacologic Treatment

- Humidified oxygen if needed for pulse oximetry less than 94% on room air
- Nebulized albuterol (0.15 mg/kg) in 2 ml of saline every 20 minutes for 1 hour with continual reevaluation; refer if no response or respiratory distress apparent after treatments; not routinely prescribed for the first episode in children
- Racemic epinephrine may reduce wheezing and reduce tachypnea.
- Oral dexamethasone (1 mg/kg loading dose, then 0.6 mg/kg twice a dayx 5 days); not routinely prescribed for the first episode in children.
- Nebulized dexamethasone (2–4 mg in 3 mL normal saline) may be beneficial; not routinely prescribed for the first episode in children.
- Antibiotics only if secondary bacterial infection present

How Long to Treat

- Depends on age, severity of illness, associated high-risk conditions, and causative agent
- Inhaled bronchodilators should be continued only if there is a documented clinical response and then given every 4 to 6 hours; discontinue once signs and symptoms of respiratory distress improve.
- Most infants show marked improvement in 3 to 5 days in respiratory status; however, wheezing may persist for weeks.
- If patient is receiving home care, follow daily by telephone for 2 to 4 days; patient may need frequent office visits.

Special Considerations

- Glucocorticoids are not recommended routinely in the treatment of previously healthy infants hospitalized with the first episode of bronchiolitis but may be beneficial to those with chronic lung diseases and those with recurrent episodes of wheezing suggestive of asthma.
- Bronchiolitis can be associated with apnea in children younger than 6 weeks of age.

When to Consult, Refer, Hospitalize

- Respiratory rate over 45/minute with respiratory distress or apnea
- Hypoxia (pulse oximetry less than 94%)
- Ill or toxic appearance, dehydration
- Underlying heart, respiratory condition, or immune suppression

Follow-Up

Expected Course

- Most children who do not require hospitalization recover by 28 days.

Complications

- Bacterial superinfection
- Bronchiolitis obliterans

- Apnea
- Respiratory failure
- Death
- Increased incidence of development of reactive airway disease (asthma)

CROUP (LARYNGOTRACHEOBRONCHITIS)

Description

- Acute inflammatory disease of larynx and subglottic airway, with characteristic "barking" cough, inspiratory stridor, and hoarseness. Is the most common cause of upper-airway obstruction or stridor in children.

Etiology

- Parainfluenza the most common organism in all age groups (75% to 80% of cases)
- RSV (infants)
- *M. pneumoniae* and influenza virus (children over 5 years)
- Paramyxovirus, adenovirus, rhinovirus, enterovirus reovirus, measles virus (where vaccination not common)
- Viral infection causes inflammation, edema of subglottic space

Incidence and Demographics

- Most prevalent in late fall and early winter, but can occur any time of the year
- Most common in children 6 months to 3 years of age, with peak at 2 years; rare among children older than 6 years
- More common in boys: male-to-female ratio ranges from 1.4:1 to 2:1.

Risk Factors

- History of croup
- Recurrent upper respiratory infections

Prevention and Screening

- No specific prevention measures except proper handwashing and other measures aimed at decreasing transmission of respiratory viruses

Assessment

History

- Acute onset of "seal-like" barky cough, inspiratory stridor, and chest-wall indrawing
- History of 2 to 3 days of nonspecific prodromal syndrome (low-grade fever, coryza, and rhinorrhea)
- Cough is worse at night; symptoms often resolve en route to the hospital as the child is exposed to cool night air.
- Symptoms progress rapidly (upper airway obstruction after fewer than 12 hours of onset)
- Changes in activity level, alertness, fluid intake, or voiding patterns
- Underlying abnormalities of the upper airway
- History of neuromuscular disorders
- Inquire about *Haemophilus influenzae* immunization status.

Physical Exam

- Signs and symptoms are variable, depending upon age, degree of airway obstruction, hydration status, and level of fatigue.
- Level of consciousness, irritability, lethargy, struggling to breath
- Work of breathing: labored, tachypnea, nasal flaring, retractions, prolonged expiratory phase
- Inspiratory stridor or stridor at rest; wheezing; short sentences; hoarseness
- Breath sounds may be diminished from airway narrowing, crackles, or rhonchi.
- "Barking" cough is characteristic.
- Tympanic membranes, throat, and sinus may be involved.
- Low-grade or moderate fever
- Tachycardia caused by fever, respiratory distress, and hypovolemia.

Diagnostic Studies

- Diagnosis is usually made on clinical presentation without testing.
- Minimize laboratory testing, imaging, procedures as they may agitate child and worsen tachypnea.
- Pulse oximetry (often normal)
- White blood cell (WBC) counts may be low, normal, or elevated.
- Anteroposterior and lateral X-ray of neck shows funnel-shaped subglottic region with normal epiglottis: "steeple," "hourglass," or "pencil point" sign (present in 40% to 60% of children).
- Computerized tomography (CT) scan may be more sensitive for defining cause for obstruction in difficult cases.

Differential Diagnosis

- COVID-19
- Epiglottitis
- Foreign body aspiration
- Subglottic stenosis
- Bacterial tracheitis
- Trauma
- Simple upper respiratory infection (URI)
- Asthma
- Airway anomalies
- Anaphylaxis
- Peritonsillar abscess
- Spasmodic croup

Management

Nonpharmacologic Treatment

- Mild cases can be managed at home.
- Deliver humidified air by cool mist vaporizer or steam-filled bathroom.

- Take patient outside into cool night air.
- Keep patient quiet; crying may exacerbate symptoms.

Pharmacologic Treatment

- Cornerstone: immediate nebulized epinephrine and dexamethasone
- Racemic epinephrine: 0.05 mL/kg/dose (max 0.5 mL) of 2.25% solution nebulized in normal saline; total volume 3 mL
- L-epinephrine: 0.5 mL/kg/dose (max 5 mL) of a 1:1,000 dilution; onset in 1 to 5 minutes, duration 2 hours; repeat as necessary if side effects tolerated; observe child for 3 to 4 hours
- Corticosteroids:
  - Dexamethasone (Decadron) 0.15–0.6 mg/kg; single dose IM/IV/PO have equal efficacy
  - Other steroids: prednisolone can be used, but not as good as dexamethasone
  - Nebulized budesonide can also be effective.
- Antibiotics not indicated, subsequent bacterial infection possible, but uncommon.
- Oxygen as needed
- Amantadine for influenza A: 100 mg by mouth twice a day for 3 to 5 days
- Probiotics may decrease incidence of upper respiratory tract infections.

How Long to Treat

- Length of treatment is based on clinical response.
- Concern about a rebound phenomenon from racemic epinephrine exists; patients who are clinically stable can be discharged safely if 4 hours have elapsed since the last dose of racemic epinephrine and systemic corticosteroids have been given, as long as patient has reliable caretakers and good access to medical services.

Special Considerations

- Close monitoring of disease progression, stridor, respiratory rate, pulse oximetry, hydration status, and mental status is critical.
- Must exclude epiglottitis; watch for preferred sitting position (tripod position with hands extended), drooling, and muffled voice.

- When examining, do not place supine or use tongue blade to examine throat until epiglottis excluded.

When to Consult, Refer, Hospitalize

- Admit patients who do not respond to therapy or have recurrent stridor at rest after epinephrine wears off.
- Admission also indicated for patients with hypoxia, pneumonia, congestive heart disease.

Follow-Up

Expected Course

- Symptoms may worsen over the first 3 days, so parents/guardian should be advised to return to the clinic for increasing stridor or respiratory distress.
- For children with moderately severe croup who are discharged, phone contact or clinic follow-up is warranted in 8 to 24 hours.
- Up to one-third of patients will have a recurrence.
- Usually full recovery without lasting effects

Complications

- Rare
- Subglottic stenosis in intubated patients
- Bacterial tracheitis
- Cardiopulmonary arrest
- Pneumonia

PERSISTENT COUGH

Description

- Productive or nonproductive cough—subacute cough lasting 3 to 8 weeks; chronic cough persists longer than 8 weeks; in children, chronic cough is defined as cough longer than 4 weeks
- Chronic cough affects respiration, sleep, and social function.

Etiology

- Multiple etiologies; most related to bronchial irritation
- Coughing helps defend against pathogens and clear the tracheobronchial tree of foreign particles, noxious aerosols, and mucus.
- Etiology of persistent cough may not be readily apparent, due to the wide variety of infectious, mechanical, and physiologic causes (see Table 7–3).

Incidence and Demographics

- Common and frequent presenting complaint in all age groups
- Occurs in males and females equally

Risk Factors

- Cigarette smoking or exposure
- Occupational exposure
- Allergens
- Pulmonary diseases

Prevention and Screening

- Smoking cessation
- Removing respiratory irritants
- Therapeutic lifestyle changes

Assessment

History

- Characteristics and timing of cough: onset and duration
  - ◊ Cough at night suggests sinusitis with postnasal drainage, asthma, congestive heart failure (CHF)

TABLE 7–3.
MOST COMMON ETIOLOGY OF CHRONIC COUGH BY AGE

INFANTS	TODDLER/ PRESCHOOL	SCHOOL-AGE/ ADOLESCENT	ADULTS
Infection ♦ Viral (RSV, adenovirus, influenza, parainfluenza) ♦ ***Bordetella pertussis*** ♦ ***Chlamydia trachomatis*** ♦ ***Mycobacterium tuberculosis*** Congenital Anomalies ♦ Cleft palate ♦ Tracheo-esophageal fistula ♦ Tracheobronchomalacia ♦ Vascular ring Other ♦ Cystic fibrosis ♦ Irritants, passive smoke ♦ Asthma ♦ Foreign body ♦ Neurologic impairment ♦ GERD ♦ Immunodeficiency	Infection ♦ Viral (RSV, adenovirus, influenza, parainfluenza) ♦ *B. pertussis* ♦ *Mycoplasma pneumoniae* ♦ *M. tuberculosis* Other ♦ Foreign body ♦ Asthma ♦ Cystic fibrosis ♦ Irritants, passive smoke ♦ Immunodeficiency, ciliary dyskinesia, GERD ♦ Sinusitis, postnasal drip ♦ Immunodeficiency	Infection ♦ Viral ♦ *M. pneumoniae* ♦ *M. tuberculosis* Other ♦ Asthma ♦ Sinusitis, postnasal drip ♦ Irritants, smoking ♦ Allergic rhinitis ♦ Cystic fibrosis ♦ Ciliary dyskinesia ♦ Psychogenic (habit)	♦ Smoking, passive smoke ♦ Postnasal drip from sinusitis, allergic rhinitis ♦ GERD ♦ Asthma ♦ Chronic bronchitis Bronchiectasis pneumonia ♦ Drug-induced (ACE inhibitors) ♦ Irritant foreign body Tuberculosis ♦ Lung malignancy Psychogenic factors ♦ Congestive heart failure (CHF) ♦ Sleep apnea ♦ Interstitial lung disease ♦ *B. pertussis* ♦ Nonasthmatic eosinophilic bronchitis

- ◇ Paroxysmal coughing longer than 14 days: pertussis, cystic fibrosis
- ◇ Cough at school, not while at home or on weekends: psychogenic, consider allergy (e.g., mold in building)

- Productive or nonproductive cough (presence or absence of sputum production not used as sole basis for treatment)
- Productive: bronchitis, cystic fibrosis, tuberculosis, infection (mucopurulent), pneumococcal pneumonia (rust colored), asthma (thick, tenacious, clear)
- Frequent respiratory infections: cystic fibrosis
- In children, poor weight gain, delayed milestones: cystic fibrosis, immunodeficiency
- Foul-smelling, steatorrhea bowel movements: cystic fibrosis
- Family history of cystic fibrosis (genetic disorder, primarily in White children)
- Exercise-induced cough associated with asthma, bronchiectasis, or cardiac disease
- Associated symptoms: fatigue, weight loss, night sweats, fever, indigestion, rhinitis, epistaxis, hemoptysis (consider cancer, tuberculosis, foreign body obstruction, cystic fibrosis, HIV, sinusitis, or GERD)
- Precipitating factors: exercise, cold temperatures, laughing; seasonal irritants may indicate asthma
- Past medical history may be significant for bronchitis, pneumonia, asthma, allergy, choking episodes, or heartburn: GERD
- Family members ill: infection; family history of atopy/asthma
- Smokers: lung tumor, emphysema, chronic bronchitis
- Medication history: ACE inhibitors or beta blockers

Physical Exam

- Appearance/nutritional status
- Nasal discharge, throat clearing, and mucus or mucopurulent drainage in posterior pharynx: postnasal drip rhinitis, sinusitis
- Respiratory rate, evidence of distress, wheezing, adventitious sounds: asthma, cystic fibrosis, foreign body, bronchitis, pneumonia, tuberculosis
- Tracheal shift suggests mediastinal mass or foreign body
- Observe for clubbing: lung malignancy, cardiac source, COPD
- In children, evaluate height and weight and plot on growth curve.

Diagnostic Studies

- Tuberculosis skin testing: PPD
- Chest X-ray for cough in smokers, cough longer than 8 weeks in nonsmokers, patients with hemoptysis, and in children and patients 40 years of age and older
- Sinus imaging for suspected acute or chronic sinusitis (paranasal sinuses only in children 18 months to 6 years) is not necessary.
- Pulmonary function testing for asthma
- Methacholine bronchoprovocation testing may be positive in absence of clinical findings of asthma.
- Barium swallow/esophageal pH monitoring for suspected GERD
- CBC with differential if infection is suspected
- Wright and Gram stains, culture of sputum for productive cough
- Bronchoscopy/endoscopy (particularly useful in children from birth to 18 months)
- Sweat test for suspected cystic fibrosis
- Allergen testing if needed
- Echocardiogram for suspected cardiac etiology
- Sleep study for suspected sleep apnea

Differential Diagnosis

See Table 7–3 above.

Management

It is important to determine the underlying disorder causing the cough and treat accordingly. While determining cause, consider the following to manage.

Nonpharmacologic Treatment

- Eliminate irritant exposure (smoke, occupational agents); discontinue ACE inhibitors or beta blockers; increase humidification.

- Therapeutic lifestyle changes for GERD (e.g., stop smoking, avoid reflux-inducing foods, small frequent meals, avoid eating 2 to 3 hours before lying down, elevate head of bed)
- Warm fluids, hard candy (for adults), or nasal drops; bulb syringe suction in infants and children

Pharmacologic Treatment

- Nasal steroids, antihistamines, antacids, bronchodilators, inhaled corticosteroids, proton-pump inhibitors (PPIs), and antibiotics are some treatments used for cases of chronic cough. The cause guides the therapeutic management.
- Initial empiric treatment: oral antihistamine/decongestant therapy with first-generation antihistamine or nasal steroid spray
- Ipratropium bromide therapy for chronic bronchitis
- Central-acting anti-tussive drugs (dextromethorphan or narcotics) are recommended for short-term symptomatic relief of nonproductive cough. Use with caution; these should not be given in conditions in which retention of respiratory secretions may be harmful; may reserve for nighttime use only. American Academy of Pediatrics (AAP) does not recommend for pediatric use.
    - Dextromethorphan: patients older than 12 years: 10–20 mg by mouth every 4 hours; patients 6 to 12 years: 5–10 mg by mouth every 4 hours (use with caution as pediatric recommendations are not available)
    - Narcotics: codeine 3–600 mg by mouth every 4–6 hours; hydrocodone 5 mg by mouth every 6 hours; hydrocodone (Tussionex Pennkinetic) 10 mg (5 mL) by mouth every 12 hours in patients older than 12 years; narcotic cough suppressants recommended for cough associated with lung cancer.
- Peripherally acting anti-tussive: benzonatate (Tessalon Perles) 100–200 mg by mouth three times a day for patients older than 10 years
- Amiloride 0.625 mg/kg/day may improve cough clearance of sputum in patients with cystic fibrosis.

How Long to Treat

- May take weeks to months for cough to resolve; resolution depends on treatment of underlying cause of cough

Special Considerations

- Geriatrics: Use decreased dose of antihistamines in allergy; observe and use caution with first-generation antihistamine because of increased sedation.
- Pediatrics: Avoid over-the-counter (OTC) cough and cold medicines (antitussives, expectorants, nasal decongestants, antihistamines, or combinations) in children younger than 2 years of age.

When to Consult, Refer, Hospitalize

- Refer undiagnosed patients with risk factors to specialist.
- Consult with pulmonologist for signs of respiratory distress or if unresponsive to treatment.

Follow-Up

Expected Course

- Depends on patient status; patients with negative workup; follow every 1 to 3 months if cough continues.

Complications

- Cardiovascular: arrhythmias, syncope
- Stress urinary incontinence
- Abdominal and intercostal muscle strain
- Gastrointestinal: emesis, hemorrhage, herniation
- Neurologic: dizziness, headache, seizures
- Respiratory: pneumothorax, laryngeal, or tracheobronchial trauma
- Skin: petechiae, purpura, disruption of surgical wounds
- Medication side effects
- Other: negative impact on quality of life

HEMOPTYSIS

Description

- Expectoration of gross blood or blood-stained sputum originating from lungs or bronchial tubes is a symptom of underlying disease or pulmonary injury.
- Classifications: non-massive (blood loss less than 200 mL/day) or massive (more than 200 mL/day)
- Pseudo-hemoptysis: blood expectorated from the upper respiratory tract or upper gastrointestinal tract

Etiology

- Most common cause: acute and chronic bronchitis, pneumonia, tuberculosis (TB), and lung cancer
- Inflammation of tracheobronchial mucosa due to minor erosion from bronchiectasis, sarcoidosis, Wegner's granulomatosis, lupus pneumonitis
- Broncho-vascular fistula
- Injury to pulmonary vasculature due to lung abscess, aspergillomas, or pulmonary emboli causing pulmonary infarction; trauma; foreign body
- Increased pulmonary capillary pressure due to pulmonary edema, mitral stenosis, arteriovenous malformations, or granuloma formation
- Bleeding disorders or anticoagulant therapy
- Nonpulmonary sources: nose or gastrointestinal tract
- Cryptogenic hemoptysis: negative workup; etiology unknown in 30% to 40% of patients, 90% resolve in 6 months
- Major cause in children: lower respiratory tract infection, followed by foreign body aspiration (younger than 4 years of age), bronchiectasis (secondary to cystic fibrosis). Primary pulmonary tuberculosis or blunt-force trauma, although rare, should also be considered.

Risk Factors

- COPD
- Cigarette smoking

- Crack cocaine inhalation
- Trauma
- Bleeding disorders

Prevention and Screening

- Avoid smoking tobacco and crack cocaine use.

Assessment

History

- Identify patients at risk for hemoptysis from bronchitis, pneumonia, TB, and lung cancer.
- Smoking and travel history
- Onset and duration of symptoms; amount, frequency, and characteristics of sputum; is there white or purulent phlegm mixed with blood?
- Determine if non-pulmonary source of bleeding: vomiting, expectoration from naso-pharynx, anticoagulant drug use, substance use, chest trauma
- Associated symptoms: weight loss, night sweats, dyspnea, fever, fatigue, bruising, hematuria, rash, joint pain or swelling
- Tuberculosis (TB) exposure, dates of last TB test and chest X-ray
- Past cardiac, pulmonary, hematological, or immunological history
- Environmental exposure, asbestos
- Family history of respiratory, cardiac, or hematologic disease

Physical Exam

- Fever and tachypnea, tachycardia, cyanosis, fatigue, diaphoresis
- Nail clubbing: indicates severe disorder such as lung abscess, tumor, bronchiectasis
- Skin: bruising, rash, palpable purpura
- Ears, nasal, pharyngeal exam to determine bleeding source
- Jugular venous distention and ankle edema: heart failure

- Chest exam for pulmonary and cardiac findings: wheezing, diffuse crackles, use of accessory muscles, heart murmur
- Lymphadenopathy: TB, carcinoma, sarcoidosis
- Extremities: peripheral edema, joint effusions, or periarticular warmth

Diagnostic Studies

- Directed by history and physical findings
- Chest X-ray
- CT for initial evaluation of patients with high risk of malignancy
- Tuberculin skin test (PPD), unless positive in the past
- CBC with differential and platelets
- Gram stain of sputum: infection; acid-fast stain: TB
- Sputum cytologic exam: malignancy
- Renal function, urinalysis, liver function tests, brain natriuretic peptide (BNP)
- Serologic testing: antinuclear antibodies, antineutrophil cytoplasmic antibodies, anti-glomerular basement membrane antibodies, anticardiolipin antibodies
- Coagulation studies: prothrombin time (PT), partial thromboplastin time (PTT), bleeding time if bleeding present in more than one site
- High-resolution chest CT: complementary to bronchoscopy (test of choice for suspected small peripheral malignancies)
- Ventilation–perfusion scan/angiography: pulmonary embolism

Differential Diagnosis

See Etiology.

- Must differentiate from epistaxis, hematemesis, and bleeding from nasopharyngeal sources

Management

Goal: bleeding cessation, aspiration, prevention, and treat underlying cause; initial step is to manage ABCs (airway, breathing, circulation).

Nonpharmacologic Treatment

- Surgical interventions: flexible bronchoscopy; angiography for embolization if indicated

Pharmacologic Treatment

- Treat underlying illness or infection; refer to specific conditions in text.

Special Considerations

- In older adult smokers, think lung cancer until proven otherwise.

When to Consult, Refer, Hospitalize

- Refer patients at high risk for malignancy to pulmonologist or if bronchoscopy is indicated.
- Refer if blood persists more than 2 to 3 days after treatment initiated for respiratory infection.
- Hospitalization for patient with massive hemoptysis or unstable condition

Follow-Up

Expected Course

- Mild streaking due to infection should resolve in 2 to 3 days; with true hemoptysis, patient should follow-up in 12 to 48 hours.

Complications

- Massive hemoptysis is life-threatening.

PNEUMONIA

Description

- An acute inflammation of the lungs caused by infection
- Etiology, presentation, risk factors, management, and prognosis differ depending on if the infection is acquired in the community, hospital, or other health care facility.
- Community-acquired pneumonia (CAP): Lower-respiratory tract infection not acquired in a hospital, long-term care facility, or during other recent contact with the health care system; is acquired in the community setting—described as "typical" pneumonia when caused by bacteria; "atypical" when caused by *Chlamydia, Mycoplasma,* or viruses
- Health care–associated pneumonia (HCAP): Lung infection that develops at least 48 hours after hospital admission, in a long-term care facility, or any recent contact with health care facility
- Other forms of pneumonia not discussed in this chapter include aspiration pneumonia, pneumonia in immune-compromised patient, *Pneumocystis jirovecii* pneumonia

Etiology

Community-Acquired Pneumonia

Infants and Children

- Birth to 20 days: *Escherichia coli,* group B streptococci, *Listeria monocytogenes*
- 3 weeks to 3 months: *Chlamydia trachomatis, Streptococcus pneumoniae*
- 4 months to 18 years:
  - Typical: *S. pneumoniae*
  - Atypical: *C. pneumoniae, M. pneumoniae*

Adults

- Typical: *S. pneumoniae, H. influenzae, Staphylococcus aureus,* group A
- *Streptococcus, Moraxella catarrhalis*
- Atypical: *Legionella* species, *M. pneumoniae, Chlamydophila pneumoniae*
- Although bacterial causes are the most common, viral, fungal, and chemical aspiration all contribute.

Health Care–Associated Pneumonia

- Enteric gram-negative bacilli (*Enterobacter, Klebsiella pneumoniae, E. coli, Serratia marcescens, Proteus,* and *Acinetobacter*), *Pseudomonas aeruginosa,* methicillin-sensitive *S. aureus,* and methicillin-resistant *S. aureus* (MRSA) most common

Incidence and Demographics

- Common and increasing in both groups
- CAP: Eighth leading cause of death in the United States, 16 to 23 cases per 1,000 people; increased incidence in winter months

Risk Factors

- CAP: 65 years and older; pulmonary, cardiac, liver, renal disease; preceding influenza; alcohol abuse; tobacco abuse; immunosuppression; HIV/AIDS; chronic corticosteroid use
- HCAP: mechanical ventilation; intensive care unit (ICU) admission; aspiration risks: swallowing dysfunction, supine positioning, tracheal intubation, tracheostomy; oropharyngeal microbial colonization; elevated gastric pH; immunosuppression; hyperglycemia/poor glycemic control

Prevention and Screening

- Good handwashing
- Routine pneumococcal conjugate vaccine 13 (PCV-13) to all children 2 to 59 months of age: given at 2, 4, 6, and 12 to 15 months of age
- PCV-13 is recommended for patients 65 years of age and older, followed by a dose of 23-valent pneumococcal polysaccharide (PPSV23) vaccine 6 to 12 months later.
- PPSV23 vaccination
  - First dose is given if the patient is 65 years or older; give second dose if patient received first dose 5 years prior and was younger than 65 years of age
  - Age 19 to 64 with history of chronic cardiovascular disease, chronic pulmonary disease including asthma, diabetes mellitus, chronic liver disease, alcoholism, cochlear implants, cerebrospinal fluid (CSF) leaks, tobacco use, or live-in long-term care facilities.

  - ◊ Revaccination not recommended if younger than 65 years of age.
  - ◊ Age 19 to 64 with history of immunosuppression: second dose recommended if more than 5 years elapsed since first dose
- Influenza and pertussis vaccines
- RSV prophylaxis in high-risk children younger than 2 years
- Avoid invasive mechanical ventilation
- Infection-control measures
- Elevate head of bed
- Subglottic suctioning
- Oral/pharyngeal decontamination
- Maintain gastric acidity
- Treat comorbidities
- Avoid smoking

Assessment

History

See Table 7–4.

- Onset either abrupt, insidious; or current, or recent stay at health care–related facility
- Recent or concurrent URI, fever, cough (productive or nonproductive), dyspnea, chills, sweats, rigors, fatigue, malaise, myalgias, chest discomfort, headache, anorexia, abdominal pain; pleuritic chest pain; patients generally feel unwell
- Pediatrics: atypical pneumonia: slowly progressive; malaise, low-grade fever, sore throat, and cough developing over 3 to 5 days
- Older adults: often present with weakness and mental status change
- History of chronic obstructive pulmonary disease or HIV infection
- Occupation, animal exposures, and sexual history helpful to identify specific infectious agent
- Recent travel history (within 2 weeks) may help identify *Legionella* pneumonia (seen on cruise ships and hotel stays).
- Influenza suggested with typical symptoms during peak influenza season
- ICU admission, mechanical ventilation, or aspiration history

TABLE 7–4.
CLINICAL EVALUATION PNEUMONIA BY ETIOLOGY

	BACTERIAL	VIRAL	MYCOPLASMA (ATYPICAL)
Onset	Acute	Insidious	Gradual
Common symptoms	Fever/chills Cough Sputum production Pleuritic chest pain Confusion in the older adult	Flu-like early symptoms followed by: Increasing shortness of breath Myalgia Weakness Worsening cough	Commonly asymptomatic Headache, malaise Low-grade fever Sore throat Cough (productive or nonproductive)
Common Physical Exam Findings	Higher temperature Tachypnea, tachycardia Flat to dull sounds on percussion Crackles, rales, and bronchial breath sounds	Lower temperature Tachycardia or tachypnea out of proportion to the temperature	Low temperature Sputum production Lung sounds unremarkable initially; rales and wheezes may develop Dullness on percussion Rales
Chest X-ray	Unilateral lung findings Dense lobar consolidations, alveolar infiltrates with air bronchograms	Bilateral lung findings Interstitial infiltrates Patchy distribution	Unilateral or bilateral findings Reticular nodular opacities and/or patchy consolidations
Laboratory Findings	Positive cultures	Positive viral test (such as + flu) Low procalcitonin (less than0.25 ng/mL) Negative cultures	Hemolysis

Physical Exam

- Fever with temperature higher than 100.4°F (38°C), tachypnea, tachycardia
- Lungs: rales, rhonchi, egophony, increased tactile fremitus, bronchial breath sounds, dullness to percussion, asymmetric breath sounds, use of accessory muscles, nasal flaring

- **Red flag**: respirations in 2 to 6 months old higher than 50; 7 to 35 months old higher than 40; over 35 months old higher than 35
- Abdominal tenderness
- Cardiac evaluation is normal unless underlying disease
- Signs of dehydration
- Assess mental status
- Increased respiratory secretions and leukocytosis also seen in HCAP

Diagnostic Studies

- Chest X-ray: infiltrates confirmed
- Routine laboratory testing usually unnecessary to establish an etiology in outpatients with CAP
- Suctioned or expectorated sputum gram stain
- Nasopharyngeal washings for RSV enzyme immunoassay (children)
- CBC, two sets of blood cultures (usually reserved for hospitalized patients), C-reactive protein (CRP), procalcitonin levels, comprehensive metabolic panel (CMP)
- WBC count elevated (may be low in older adults or immunocompromised patients)
- *Legionella* urine antigen test if *Legionella* suspected
- Bronchoalveolar lavage or protected specimen brush with quantitative cultures
- Serial chest X-rays or chest CT scans if health care–associated pneumonia

Differential Diagnosis

- Pulmonary edema
- COVID-19
- Asthma exacerbation
- Atelectasis
- Acute bronchitis
- Bronchiolitis
- Bronchiectasis
- COPD

- Foreign body aspiration
- Fungal pneumonia
- Lung abscess
- Respiratory failure
- Viral pneumonia
- *P. jirovecii* pneumonia
- Pulmonary tuberculosis
- Lung cancer

Management

Nonpharmacologic Treatment

- Hydration, high humidity
- Monitoring of respiratory status, rest
- Smoking cessation, avoidance of secondhand smoke
- Chest physiotherapy for bacterial pneumonia
- Oxygen, if needed
- Semi upright or upright positioning
- Noninvasive ventilation using continuous positive airway pressure (CPAP) or bilevel positive airway pressure (BiPAP) with endotracheal intubation
- Incentive spirometry to help prevent postoperative pneumonia

Pharmacologic Treatment

- Empiric treatment often necessary because often not able to identify pathogen
- Adult CAP outpatient:
  - ◊ American Thoracic Society (ATS) and Infectious Diseases Society of America (ATS/IDSA) Recommendations:
    - Healthy adults, younger than 65 years of age, no antibiotics in past 3 months
      - Beta-lactam: amoxicillin 1 g three times daily (preferred initial therapy)
      - Suggestive alternative: doxycycline 100 mg twice daily or a macrolide (azithromycin 500 mg on first day then 250 mg daily or clarithromycin 500 mg twice daily or clarithromycin ER 1000 mg daily)

- ◇ For adults ≥65 years, or with comorbidities, or with antibiotic use in the past 3 months:
  - Combination therapy with:
    - amoxicillin/clavulanate 500 mg/125 mg three times daily, or amoxicillin/clavulanate 875 mg/125 mg twice daily, or 2000 mg/125 mg twice daily, or a cephalosporin (cefpodoxime 200 mg twice daily or cefuroxime 500 mg twice daily); and
    - macrolide (azithromycin 500 mg on the first day and then 250 mg daily, clarithromycin [500 mg twice daily or extended release 1000 mg once daily]) (strong recommendation, moderate quality of evidence for combination therapy), or doxycycline 100 mg twice daily (conditional recommendation, low quality of evidence for combination therapy), or
  - Monotherapy with:
    - fluoroquinolone (levofloxacin 750 mg daily, moxifloxacin 400 mg daily, or gemifloxacin 320 mg daily)

- ♦ Pediatric outpatient (more than 3 months):
  - ◇ Antibiotic treatment in preschool-age children is not routinely recommended, as viral pathogens are more common.
  - ◇ For typical bacterial pneumonia: amoxicillin 90 mg/kg/day by mouth twice a day (max 4 g/day); amoxicillin-clavulanate 90 mg/kg/day by mouth twice a day (max 4 g/day); levofloxacin 16–20 mg/kg/day (ages 6 months to 5 years) and 8–10 mg/kg/day (over 5 years old) max 750 mg/day
  - ◇ For atypical bacterial pneumonia: azithromycin 10 mg/kg by mouth on day 1, then 5 mg/kg/day on days 2 through 5; clarithromycin 15 mg/kg/day by mouth twice a day (max 1 g/day); erythromycin 40 mg/kg/day by mouth daily
- ♦ CAP, inpatient (non-ICU): IV antibiotic initially, then switch to oral after clinical improvement
  - ◇ Cefotaxime, ceftriaxone, or ampicillin-sulbactam plus macrolide (clarithromycin or erythromycin) x 14 days
  - ◇ Gatifloxacin or levofloxacin x 14 days
- ♦ For pseudomonas CAP:
  - ◇ Piperacillin/tazobactam (Zosyn), cefepime, imipenem/cilastatin (Primaxin), meropenem (Merrem), or doripenem (Doribax) plus either ciprofloxacin (Cipro) or levofloxacin (Levaquin); or
  - ◇ Piperacillin/tazobactam (Zosyn), cefepime, imipenem/cilastatin (Primaxin), meropenem (Merrem), or doripenem (Doribax) plus an aminoglycoside and azithromycin; or
  - ◇ Piperacillin/tazobactam (Zosyn), cefepime, imipenem/cilastatin (Primaxin), meropenem (Merrem), or doripenem (Doribax) plus aminoglycoside and an anti-pneumococcal respiratory fluoroquinolone
- ♦ HCAP: anti-pseudomonal beta-lactams, antipseudomonal fluoroquinolones, aminoglycosides, vancomycin, or linezolid are used

- Viral pneumonia
  - ◊ Bronchodilator if wheezing is present
  - ◊ Consider amantadine (Symmetrel) or rimantadine (Flumadine) 100 mg by mouth twice a day for influenza A
- Antitussives
  - ◊ Generally, cough should not be suppressed, and antitussives should be avoided; however, in patients with severe chest discomfort and persistent cough, may consider use of nonnarcotic or low-dose narcotic antitussive for night use only; see the section on Persistent Cough.

How Long to Treat

- For mild to moderate CAP: a short course of antimicrobial agents is sufficient.
- Patients should be afebrile for 48 hours and clinically stable before therapy is discontinued.
- Some symptoms (cough, fatigue, and dyspnea) may be present for 2 to 4 weeks. Infiltrates on chest X-ray may last up to 30 days.
  - ◊ Most patients improve within 2 weeks. Older adults or very sick patients may need longer treatment.

Special Considerations

- Drug resistance: Suspect drug-resistant *S. pneumonia* in communities with increased prevalence. Risk factors include patients younger than 2 year of age or 65 years and older, beta-lactam or macrolide treatment within the past 3 to 6 months, alcoholism, medical comorbidities, immunosuppression, and exposure to day care.

When to Consult, Refer, Hospitalize

- Consider hospitalization for adult patients 65 years and over, with history of comorbid conditions, altered mental status, leukopenia (less than 4,000), leukocytosis (more than 30,000), tachycardia, tachypnea, systolic blood pressure less than 90 mmHg, and temperature lower than 35°C (95°F) or higher than 40°C (104°F).
- Consider hospitalization in pediatric patients who are less than 3 to 6 months; look toxic; immunocompromised, cardiac, or pulmonary disease; are in respiratory distress; or are dehydrated.

- Consider chest CT scan if patient fails to improve on current management.
- Consult specialist if there is little improvement or deterioration after 48 to 72 hours of therapy.

Follow-Up

- 24-hour follow-up contact for patients moderately to severely ill, and 72 hours after beginning antimicrobials for reevaluation
- For patients who are improving, routine follow-up in 2 to 3 weeks
- Patients 40 years and older, and all smokers, follow-up chest X-ray in 4 to 8 weeks to rule out underlying bronchogenic carcinoma, which may present as pneumonia
- In children with recurrent pneumonia, repeat chest X-ray in 4 to 6 weeks

Expected Course

- Dependent upon pathogen, patient response, comorbidities, and complications

Complications

- Necrotizing pneumonia, respiratory failure, empyema, abscesses, cavitation, broncho-pleural fistula, sepsis

PRIMARY LUNG MALIGNANCIES

Description

- Cancer that forms in tissues of the lung, usually in the cells lining air passages
- Non–small cell lung cancer (NSCLC): over 85% of all lung cancers; includes adenocarcinoma, squamous cell carcinoma, large cell
- There are three broad categories:
  - ◊ Adenocarcinoma: most common in United States and in nonsmokers; about 40% of NSCLC, metastasizes early, poor prognosis
    - Squamous cell carcinoma: less than 25% of NSCLC, dose-related effect with smoking, slower growing

- Large cell carcinoma: about 10% of NSCLC, poor prognosis
- Lung carcinoid tumor (also called *lung neuroendocrine* tumors): 5% of lung cancers; most of these tumors grow slowly and rarely spread.

♦ Small cell lung cancer (SCLC), also known as *oat cell carcinoma*: 15% of all lung cancers; centrally located; early metastases; aggressive

♦ Other: mesothelioma, sarcoma

♦ Most metastasize to lymph nodes (pulmonary, mediastinal), then liver, adrenal, bone, kidney, brain.

Etiology

♦ Cigarette smoking, most important cause in both men and women in the United States

♦ Other causes: secondhand smoke, ionizing radiation (radon gas, therapeutic radiation), asbestos exposure, heavy metals (nickel, chromium), industrial carcinogens

♦ Possible causes: lung scarring, air pollution, genetic factors

♦ Carcinogen causes chromosomal damage, abnormal cell growth, leads to malignancy

♦ Besides direct damage to the airways, lung cancers cause complications through direct extension, metastasis, and paraneoplastic syndromes such as syndrome of inappropriate antidiuretic hormone (SIADH).

Incidence and Demographics

♦ Lung cancer is the leading cause of cancer death for both men and women.

♦ Approximately 236,740 new cases of lung cancer in the United States (2022 estimate)

♦ 1.8 million deaths worldwide in 2020

♦ Predominant sex: men more than women

♦ Predominant age: over 45 years; peak at 70 years

Risk Factors

♦ Smoking (cigarette, pipe, cigars)

♦ Secondhand smoke

♦ Radon

- Environmental and occupational exposures: asbestos exposure, air pollution, ionizing radiation, mutagenic gases (halogen ethers, mustard gas, aromatic hydrocarbons), metals (inorganic arsenic, chromium, nickel)
- Lung scarring from tuberculosis
- Radiation therapy to the breast or chest

Prevention and Screening

- Aggressive smoking-cessation counseling and therapy (20% to 30% risk reduction occurs within 5 years of cessation)
- Avoid supplemental beta-carotene and vitamin E in smokers.
- Avoid hormone replacement therapy in postmenopausal smokers or former smokers.
- Avoid industrial exposures.
- Screening controversial: annual low-dose CT of chest annually compared to chest X-ray alone until age 74 decreased lung cancer mortality but did not increase life expectancy

Assessment

History

- May be asymptomatic for most of course
- Pulmonary: cough (new or change in chronic cough), wheezing and stridor, dyspnea, hemoptysis, pneumonitis (fever and productive cough)
- Constitutional: malaise, bone pain (metastatic disease), fatigue, weight loss, anorexia, fever, anemia, clubbing of digits
- Other: chest pain (dull, pleuritic), shoulder/arm pain (Pancoast tumors), dysphagia, plethora (redness of face or neck), hoarseness, Horner syndrome, neurologic abnormalities (headaches, syncope, weakness, seizures, recent change in mental status), pericardial tamponade (pericardial invasion)

Physical Exam

- General: pain, performance status, weight loss
- Head, eyes, ears, nose, and throat (HEENT): Horner syndrome, dysphonia, stridor, sclera icterus

- Neck: supraclavicular/cervical lymph nodes, mass
- Lungs: effusion, wheezing, airway obstruction, pleural effusion
- Abdomen/groin: hepatomegaly or lymphadenopathy
- Extremities: signs of hypertrophic pulmonary osteoarthropathy, deep vein thrombosis (DVT)
- Neurologic: exclude cognitive and focal motor defects

Diagnostic Studies

- Initial lab tests: CBC, blood urea nitrogen (BUN), serum creatinine, liver function tests, lactate dehydrogenase (LDH), electrolytes (hypercalcemia; paraneoplastic syndrome; hyponatremia: SIADH), sputum cytology
- Chest X-rays: most important initial diagnostic test in predicting whether lung cancer is potential cause of chronic cough (compare with old films); possible findings: nodule or mass, persistent infiltrate, atelectasis, mediastinal widening, hilar enlargement, pleural effusion
- CT scan of chest (with IV contrast): nodule or mass, lymphadenopathy, and for cancer staging
- Fine needle aspiration (FNA) biopsy
- Other test to evaluate for metastatic disease and staging:
    - Brain magnetic resonance imaging (MRI): necrotic or bleeding lesions
    - Abdomen: hepatic, adrenal, renal masses
    - Positron emission tomography (PET) scan: to determine metastasis
    - Bone scan: advanced disease or bone pain
- Fiberoptic bronchoscopy when the chest X-ray suggests that a tumor or an inflammatory pulmonary parenchymal process is present

Management

- Treatment options for patients are determined by histology, stage, general health, and comorbidities.
- Chemotherapy is the mainstay of treatment for SCLC and advanced NSCLC.
- Adjuvant chemotherapy following surgery is used in patients with fully resected stage II-III NSCLC.
- Radiation is used in some unresectable diseases in combination with chemotherapy.

Nonpharmacologic Treatment

- Palliative therapy includes general care of the patient, with particular attention to pain control, symptom control, maintenance of adequate nutrition/hydration, and psychological support.
- Acupuncture has been found effective in the management of chemotherapy-associated nausea and vomiting, and in controlling pain associated with surgery.
- Oxygen may be necessary in some patients experiencing dyspnea.

Pharmacologic Treatment

- Multiple therapies are used in lung cancer treatment including surgery, chemotherapy, radiation therapy, targeted therapy, laser therapy, photodynamic therapy, cryosurgery, electrocautery, watchful waiting. For more complete information, see http:// www.cancer.gov/cancertopics/types/lung

How Long to Treat

- Duration of treatment depends on type and stage of cancer.

Special Considerations

- Discuss end-of-life care with patients and family members.
- Consider bisphosphonates or denosumab in patients with bone metastases.

When to Consult, Refer, Hospitalize

- Any patient with suspected lung malignancy should be referred to a pulmonologist for evaluation, with subsequent referral to a thoracic surgeon and/or oncologist for treatment.

Follow-Up

Expected Course

- Depends on clinical history: postoperative visits every 3 to 6 months with physical exam and chest X-ray

- Follow-up CT scans as indicated
- Overall, 5-year survival rate for all types and stages is 17.4% (NSCLC: 17%; SCLC: 6%); patients with SCLC rarely live 5 years (4%)

Complications

- Development of metastatic disease (brain, bones, adrenals, and liver)
- Local recurrence of disease
- Postoperative complications
- Side effects of chemotherapy and radiation

TUBERCULOSIS (TB)

Description

- Contagious bacterial infection (*Mycobacterium tuberculosis*) that involves the lungs, but may spread to other organs (skin, kidneys, bones, genitourinary, meninges, peritoneum, and heart)
- Classified as tuberculosis disease (disease from initial infection; active tuberculosis is the older term) or tuberculosis infection (asymptomatic with positive PPD, negative chest X-ray, noninfectious; latent TB is the older term)

Etiology

- Caused by *M. tuberculosis* from inhaling aerosolized droplets from a cough or sneeze of an infected person
- Reactivation may occur years later, and symptoms of active disease appear.
- Structure of the bacterium *M. tuberculosis* makes it relatively resistant to destruction by macrophages and drugs; it multiplies slowly and may lay dormant for a long period.

Incidence and Demographics

- 22% of world's population are infected with TB.
- More likely to develop in people who are infected with HIV than people without HIV.

- Second leading infectious killer after COVID-19
- 9.9 million people diagnosed worldwide in 2020 and 1.5 million TB-related deaths
- TB incidence 2020: U.S. 2.2 case/100,000 persons
- In 2021, 71% of reported TB cases in the United States occurred among foreign-born persons.
- In the United States, the highest rates are in people of Asian, African American, and Hispanic/Latino descent.

Risk Factors

- HIV infection is the strongest known risk factor.
- For infection:
  - Homeless, minority, residents and employees in institutionalized settings, close contact with infected persons, people from high-risk countries (Asia, Africa, Latin America), health care workers, travel to high-risk areas, medically underserved areas, low income, substance abuse
- For development of disease once infected:
  - HIV, lymphoma, silicosis, diabetes mellitus, chronic renal failure, cancer of head/neck/lung, children younger than 5 years of age, malnutrition, systemic corticosteroids, immunosuppressive drugs, IV drug abuse, alcohol abuse, cigarette smokers, less than 2 years since infection with *M. tuberculosis*, history of gastrectomy or jejuna bypass, less than 90% ideal body weight, conversion from negative to positive tuberculin skin test (PPD) or interferon-gamma release assay (IGRA) within previous 2 years

Prevention and Screening

- Treat tuberculosis infection and report to health department; test and treat all close contacts.
- Tuberculin skin tests (TST): Mantoux (PPD) is standard test, establishes exposure to TB; see Table 7–5 for PPD interpretation.
- A whole-blood IGRA (e.g., QuantiFERON-TB Gold In-Tube test (QFT-GIT) or T-SPOT TB Test (T-Spot)
- The Centers for Disease Control and Prevention (CDC) recommend that IGRAs QFT-GIT test can be used in place of TST in all circumstances in which the TST is currently used. IGRAs are preferred for testing in people who have received Bacillus Calmette–Guérin (BCG) and in people from groups with low rates of return for TST reading.

- A positive TST or IGRA result only indicates if someone has been infected with *M. tuberculosis.* These tests cannot identify if a person has TB disease.
- Practice appropriate infection control procedures in the workplace. The Bacillus Calmette–Guérin (BCG) vaccine: Consider use in United States for children with negative PPD and HIV tests with unavoidable high risk and for health care workers at high risk for drug-resistant infection; used in countries with endemic TB; may cause persistent positive PPD.

Assessment

History

- Assess for history of TB, exposure to TB, or treatment for active or latent disease.
- Assess HIV status and other risk factors.
- Often a person with latent TB infection does not feel sick, is asymptomatic, cannot spread TB to others, and is at risk of developing TB disease.
- TB disease: Patient will feel sick, usually will have one or more symptoms, and may spread TB bacteria to others.
- General symptoms of TB disease: chills, night sweats, weight loss, appetite loss, fatigue, malaise
- Symptoms of pulmonary TB disease: cough lasting 3 or more weeks, chest pain, hemoptysis
- Symptoms of extrapulmonary TB disease depend on part of body affected:
  - ◇ Back pain: TB of spine
  - ◇ Hematuria: TB of kidneys
  - ◇ Lymphadenopathy: TB of lymph nodes
- Children are usually asymptomatic at initial infection; symptoms may occur 1 to 6 months later.
- Extrapulmonary TB symptoms depend on site affected.

Physical Exam

- Often entirely normal
- Specific findings vary based on system involved

- May find weight loss, adenopathy, apical rales/crackles on lung exam
- Evaluate for extrapulmonary TB
- HIV testing and counseling should be offered regularly to all patients during a physical examination.

Diagnostic Studies

- PPD to assess exposure (see Table 7–5); 5 U (0.1 mL) intradermal injection into volar forearm; measure induration at 48 to 72 hours; repeat second test in 1 to 3 weeks after initial test for persons with no recent PPD, age 55 years and older, nursing home resident, prison inmate, health care worker, or IGRAs.
- Chest X-ray: infiltrate in middle and lower lobes in primary TB; fibronodular upper lobe infiltrate in reactivation of disease; see small, homogenous infiltrates, cavitation, hilar, and paratracheal lymph node enlargement
- Three different morning sputum samples for acid-fast bacilli (AFB) stain and culture; if positive treat right away. TB is a reportable disease. Positive results must be reported within 24 hours to the state or local TB control program.
- Nucleic acid amplification (NAA) test identifies *M. tuberculosis* by amplifying tuberculous DNA and RNA segments found in the patient's specimen. If NAA test and AFB smears are both positive, patients are presumed to have TB disease and should begin treatment. If NAA test is negative and AFB smears are positive, patients may be infected with nontuberculous mycobacteria (NTM).
- Drug susceptibility testing is done when culture is found to be positive and is important because it determines which drugs can kill the tubercle bacilli, which can prevent further drug resistance.
- CBC with differential and platelets, creatinine, aspartate transaminase (AST), alanine transaminase (ALT), bilirubin, alkaline phosphatase
- HIV testing; if positive, need baseline CD4 count
- CT chest bronchoscopy

Differential Diagnosis

- COPD
- Asthma
- Pneumonia

TABLE 7–5.
GUIDELINES FOR DETERMINING A POSITIVE TUBERCULIN SKIN TEST AND NEED FOR PREVENTIVE TREATMENT

INDURATION ≥5 MM	INDURATION ≥10 MM	INDURATION ≥15 MM
HIV-positive people	Recent immigrants (within the last 5 years) from high-prevalence countries	All persons with no known risk factors for TB
Fibrotic changes on chest X-ray consistent with old TB	IV drug users	
Patients with organ transplants, other immunosuppressed patients (e.g., receiving the equivalent of more than 15 mg/day of prednisone for more than 1 month)	Residents and employees of high-risk congregate settings: prisons, jails, nursing homes, and other health care facilities; residential facilities for AIDS patients; and homeless shelters	
Recent contact of a person with TB disease	Mycobacteriology laboratory personnel Preexisting medical conditions: weight loss more than10% below ideal body weight, silicosis, diabetes mellitus, gastrectomy, jejunal bypass, silicosis, chronic renal failure, malignancy Any child younger than 5 years; infants, children, and adolescents exposed to adults in high-risk categories	

Adapted from *Tuberculin skin testing,* by the Centers for Disease Control and Prevention, 2020. Retrieved from https://www.cdc.gov/tb/publications/factsheets/testing/skintesting.htm

- Cancer
- Pleurisy
- Histoplasmosis
- Silicosis
- Interstitial lung disease

Management

Nonpharmacologic Treatment

- Education and counseling regarding the importance of adherence; consider use of community resources such as directly observed therapy (DOT) to ensure adherence
- Review transmission of disease and need for good hygiene, handwashing, secretion precautions, and no sharing of utensils, glasses, etc., for active disease.
- Education on the symptoms caused by adverse reactions of the TB treatment medications (no appetite, nausea, vomiting, jaundice, fever longer than 3 days, abdominal pain, neuropathy of fingers and toes, skin rash, easy bleeding, aching joints, dizziness, easy bruising, blurred or changed vision, ringing in ears, hearing loss, tingling/numbness around mouth). If symptom(s) are present, stop medication and contact health care provider immediately.

Pharmacologic Treatment

- In 2017, the CDC updated recommendations for the treatment of latent tuberculosis infection (LTBI). (See Table 7-6.) The CDC continues to recommend a once weekly dose of rifapentine plus isoniazid for 12 weeks (3HP) for treatment of LTBI in adults. Recommendations now include the use of 3HP:
  - In people with LTBI 2–17 years of age;
  - In people with LTBI who have HIV infection including AIDS and are taking antiretroviral medications with acceptable drug–drug interactions with rifapentine; and
  - By DOT or self-administered therapy (SAT) in people ≥2 years.
  - Patients should be given documentation of treatment upon completion.
- TB disease treatment regimen: See Table 7–7. DOT is required for children, institutionalized patients, risk for nonadherence, and nondaily regimens. Current recommendations can be obtained from http://www.thoracic.org and www.cdc.gov
  - TB disease must be treated for at least 6 to 9 months, 18 to 24 months or longer to treat multidrug-resistant TB (MDR-TB).
  - Regimens for treating TB have an initial phase of 2 months, followed by a continuation phase of either 4 or 7 months.
- Continuation phase: 4 months used in the large majority of patients
- Treatment completion is determined by the number of doses ingested over a given period of time, not by number of weeks or months on the regimen.

TABLE 7–6.
LATENT TB INFECTION TREATMENT REGIMENS

DRUG(S)	DURATION	FREQUENCY	TOTAL DOSES
Isoniazid (INH) and Rifapentine (RPT) Not recommended for: ♦ Children younger than 2 years old ♦ People with HIV/AIDS who are taking antiviral agents ♦ People who are presumed to have been infected with INH- or RIF-resistant *M. tuberculosis* ♦ Pregnant women or women expecting to be pregnant within the 12-week regimen	3 months	Once weekly	12
Rifampin (RIF) ♦ For persons who cannot tolerate INH or are exposed to INH-resistant TB ♦ Should not be used with certain combinations of anti-retroviral (ARV) therapy	4 months	Daily	120
Isoniazid (INH) and Rifampin (RIF)	3 months	Daily	90
Isoniazid (INH)	6 months	Daily	180
		Twice weekly*	52
	9 months	Daily	270
		Twice weekly*	76

*Use DOT

Reprinted from *Treatment for latent TB infection*, by the Centers for Disease Control and Prevention, 2020. Retrieved from https://www.cdc.gov/tb/topic/treatment/ltbi.htm

- Drug-resistant TB should be managed by or in close consultation with an expert in the disease.
- DOT should always be used in treating drug-resistant TB to ensure adherence.

Special Considerations

- Geriatric patients often have atypical presentation of disease.
- INH major adverse reactions are hepatotoxicity, peripheral neuropathy (vitamin B6 daily to decrease neuropathy and central nervous system [CNS] effects), and interactions with other drugs. Monitor closely.

TABLE 7–7.
BASIC TB DISEASE TREATMENT REGIMENS

PREFERRED REGIMEN	ALTERNATIVE REGIMEN	ALTERNATIVE REGIMEN
Initial phase: Daily INH (5 mg/kg), RIF (10 mg/kg), PZA (15–30 mg/kg), and ethambutol (EMB)* (15–20 mg/kg); for 56 doses (8 weeks)	Initial phase: Daily INH/RIF/PZA/EMB* for 14 doses (2 weeks)+, then twice weekly for 12 doses (6 weeks)	Initial phase: INH/RIF/PZA/EMB* 3 times weekly for 24 doses (8 weeks)
Continuation phase: Daily INH/RIF for 18 weeks or INH/RIF 3–5 times weekly for 18 weeks	Continuation phase: INH/RIF 2 times weekly for 36 doses (18 weeks)	Continuation phase: INH/RIF 3 times weekly for 54 doses (18 weeks)

*EMB can be discontinued if drug susceptibility studies demonstrate susceptibility to first-line drugs.

+Twice-weekly regimen should not be used in HIV-positive patients or patients.

Adapted from Treatment for TB disease, by the Centers for Disease Control and Prevention, 2022. Retrieved from https://www.cdc.gov/tb/topic/treatment/tbdisease.htm#Treatment-Regimen

- Pregnancy: PZA given along with INH; streptomycin contraindicated
- Lactation: Small doses of antituberculosis drugs are found in breast milk; however, do not discourage breastfeeding.
- Pharmacotherapy may cause interactions with other drugs.
- HIV-infected patients should be treated for 9 months.

When to Consult, Refer, Hospitalize

- All suspected or confirmed cases should be reported to local and state health departments.
- Refer all patients with active disease to specialist for treatment.
- Hospitalize patients if incapable of self-care, or if patient is likely to expose new susceptible persons.
- Some states may incarcerate noncompliant patients to ensure they take medication.

Follow-Up

Expected Course

- Baseline monitoring is not routinely indicated. Baseline monitoring of ALT is recommended for those persons who chronically consume alcohol, take concomitant hepatotoxic drugs, have viral hepatitis or other liver disease, and who are pregnant or within 3 months postpartum, and who are HIV-infected. Some experts recommend monitoring for patients older than 35 years. Treatment should be interrupted and generally modified for those with ALT 3 times the upper limit of normal (ULN) in the presence of hepatitis symptoms and/or jaundice, or 5 times ULN in the absence of symptoms.
- Patients should be evaluated at least monthly during therapy for adverse reactions, adherence to regimen, and signs and symptoms of TB disease. Bacteriologic examination of patient's sputum or other specimens should be done monthly until culture results are negative.
- If culture is positive after 2 months of therapy, reassess drug sensitivity and initiate DOT.
- Typically there are few complications and there is full resolution of infection when medications are taken as prescribed for full course.

Complications

- Drug-induced hepatitis, particularly in patient younger than 35 years, frequent monitoring of liver function indicated; drug induced neuropathy
- Treatment failure most often due to noncompliance
- Cavitary lesions can become secondarily infected.
- Drug resistance high if HIV-positive, treatment taken improperly, or from an area with high incidence of resistance
- Hemoptysis, pneumothorax, bronchiectasis, extensive pulmonary destruction, malignancy, and chronic pulmonary aspergillosis

Chronic Conditions

ASTHMA

Description

- Chronic, reversible inflammatory airway disease
- Episodes are variable and recurring with airflow obstruction, bronchial hyperresponsiveness, and underlying inflammation.
- Classified into four groups based on severity; see Table 7–8 and Table 7–9:
    - Intermittent, mild persistent, moderate persistent, and severe persistent

Etiology

- Inflammation and bronchospasm caused by allergic and nonallergic triggers
- Allergy triggers:
    - Seasonal or environmental allergens: pollens, feathers, warm-blooded pet epithelia, dust mite and cockroach excrement, molds, food additives/preservatives such as sulfites (rare)
- Nonallergic triggers:
    - Exercise-induced asthma, occurring 5 to 10 minutes following onset of strenuous activity; related to bronchial heat or water loss
    - Occupational asthma: triggers in workplace such as fumes, dyes, and chemicals
    - Diseases or infections such as bronchitis, gastroesophageal reflux, rhinitis/sinusitis, viral respiratory infections (especially RSV infections during infancy, rhinovirus in children younger than 2 years of age)
    - Drug induced: aspirin, nonsteroidal anti-inflammatory drugs (NSAIDs), indomethacin, beta blockers
    - Smoke and pollutants

Incidence and Demographics

- Affects people of all ages
- More than 25 million people affected in United States; about 5 million children affected
- Children, females, and Black and Puerto Rican people are more likely to have asthma.

- People with lower annual household income and residents of the Midwest and Northeast are more likely to have asthma.

Risk Factors

- Environmental exposure: dust mites, cats/dogs, cockroaches, RSV, fungus/molds, secondhand smoke, air pollution, grass/trees/weed pollen
- Occupational exposure: formaldehyde, fragrances, fumes
- Genetic characteristics: atopy, eczema, allergic rhinitis

Prevention and Screening

- Avoid allergens, tobacco smoke, aspirin, and NSAIDs if sensitive.
- Avoid exercise in cold temperatures and during high pollution/pollen levels.
- Reduce exposure to triggers by use of air filters and air conditioners, removal of rugs, stuffed animals, pets, perfumes, air fresheners, scented cleaning products, etc.
- Consider allergy immunotherapy when indicated.
- Treat upper respiratory infections, rhinitis, and gastroesophageal reflux when present.
- Recommend influenza vaccination annually.
- Carry EpiPen if at risk for anaphylaxis.

Assessment

History

- Characteristic symptoms: episodic wheezing (absent in severe exacerbation), chest tightness, dyspnea, chronic dry or spasmodic cough; symptoms worse at night, with exercise, exposure to cold temperatures, smoke, allergens
- Symptoms of emotional stress, upper respiratory infection, rhinitis/sinusitis, eczema/atopic dermatitis, nasal polyps
- Family history of asthma, allergies, or atopy
- Severity of symptoms (see Table 7–8 and Table 7–9)

TABLE 7–8.
ASTHMA CLASSIFICATION AND STEPWISE APPROACH FOR TREATMENT

ASTHMA CLASSIFICATION	INTERMITTENT	MILD	MODERATE	SEVERE		
	Step 1	Step 2	Step3	Step 4	Step 5	Step 6
Daytime symptoms	2 or fewer days/week	more than 2 but fewer than 7 days/week	Daily	All day		
Nocturnal awakenings	2 or fewer/ month	3 to 4 nights/ month	more than 1/week	Nightly		
Lung Function FEV1 (% preferred)	Normal FEV1	Normal FEV1	FEV1 60 to 80% predicted	FEV1 less than 60% predicted		
Interference with normal activity	None	Minor limitation	Some limitation	Extreme limitation		
Asthma exacerbations	1 or fewer/year	2 or more /year	≥2 or more /year	2 or more/year		
Preferred Treatment	SABA as needed	Low-dose ICS daily with SABA as needed or Low-dose ICS plus SABA, at the same time, as needed	Combination low-dose ICS-formoterol daily as a controller and 1–2 inhalations as needed for reliever therapy	Combination medium dose ICS-formoterol daily as a controller and 1–2 inhalations as needed for reliever therapy	Medium to high-dose ICS-LABA plus LAMA daily and SABA as needed	High-dose ICS-LABA daily; consider LAMA as substitute for LABA or as add-on therapy if not done previously Oral glucocorticoids, titrated

Alternative Treatment		Daily LTRA and SABA as needed	Medium-dose ICS daily and SABA as needed or Low-dose ICS-LABA combination daily or low-dose ICS plus LAMA daily or low-dose ICS plus LTRA daily and SABA as needed or Low-dose ICS daily plus zileuton and SABA as needed	Medium-dose ICS-LABA daily or medium-dose ICS plus LAMA daily and SABA as needed or Medium-dose ICS daily plus LTRA or zileuton and SABA as needed	Medium-high dose ICS-LABA daily or high-dose ICS + LTRA daily and SABA as needed	

TABLE 7–9.
ASTHMA CLASSIFICATION AND STEPWISE APPROACH FOR TREATMENT (GINA, 2022)

ASTHMA CLASSIFICATION			N/A			
			STEP 1 Infrequent viral wheezing and no or few interval symptoms	**STEP 2** Symptoms not consistent with asthma and asthma symptoms not well controlled on SABA or use of SABA twice a week over a month indic	**STEP 3** Asthma diagnosis, and asthma symptoms not well controlled on low dose ICS	**STEP 4** Asthma symptoms not well controlled on double ICS
≤5 years of age		**Preferred Controller**		Daily low dose ICS	Double low dose ICS	Continue controller & refer to specialist
		Other Controller Options	Consider intermittent short course ICS at onset of viral illness	Daily LTRC, or intermittent short course ICS at onset of illness	Low dose ICS + LTRA; Consider referral	Add LTRA, or increase ICS frequency, or add intermittent ICS
		Reliever	As needed SABA			

ASTHMA CLASSIFICATION			MILD		MODERATE		SEVERE
			STEP 1 *Symptoms fewer than 2 times/month*	**STEP 2** *Symptoms 2 or more times/month*	**STEP 3** *Symptoms 4–5 days/week or waking due to symptoms 1 or more time/week*	**STEP 4** *Daily symptoms or waking with symptoms 1 or more time/week and low lung function*	**STEP 5**

6–11 years of age		**Preferred Controller**	Low-dose ICS when SABA is taken	Daily low-dose ICS	Low-dose ICS-LABA, OR medium-dose ICS, OR very low-dose*ICS-formoterol and reliever (MART)	Medium-dose ICS-LABA, OR low-dose ICS-formoterol maintenance and reliever therapy (MART) (short course of corticosteroids might also be needed)	Refer to phenotypic assessment ± higher dose ICS-LABA or add on therapy
		Other Controller Options^	Consider daily low-dose ICS	Daily LTRA, or low-dose ICS when SABA is taken	Low-dose ICS + LTRA	Add tiotropium or add TRA	Add on anti-IL5 or, as last resort, consider add-on OCS, but consider side effects
		Reliever	As needed SABA (or low dose ICS-formoterol reliever for MART as above)				
			STEPS 1–2 *Symptoms* *Less than 4–5 days per week*		**STEP 3** *Symptoms 4–5 days/week or waking due to symptoms 1 or more time/week*	**STEP 4** *Daily symptoms or waking with symptoms 1 or more time/week and low lung function*	**STEP 5**
≥ 12 years of age	**TRACK 1***	**Controller** *(give with preferred reliever)*	Low-dose ICS-formoterol as needed		Low-dose ICS-formoterol maintenance	Medium-dose maintenance ICS-formoterol (may need to add short-course OCS)	Add-on LAMA; Referral; Consider high-dose maintenance ICS-formoterol ± anti-IgE, anti-IL5/5R, anti-IL4R, anti-TSLP

Continued

TABLE 7–9.
(CONTINUED)

ASTHMA CLASSIFICATION			MILD		MODERATE		SEVERE
		Preferred Reliever	As needed low-dose ICS formoterol				
			STEP 1 *Symptoms fewer than 2 times per month*	**STEP 2** *Symptoms 2 or more times/month, but less than 4–5 times days a week*	**STEP 3** *Symptoms most days or waking with asthma 1 or more time/week*	**STEP 4** *Daily symptoms or waking with symptoms 1 or more time/week and low lung function*	**STEP 5**
	TRACK 2⁺	**Controller**	ICS when SABA is taken	Low-dose maintenance ICS	Low-dose maintenance ICS-LABA	Medium-/high-dose maintenance ICS-LABA (may need to add short-course OCS)	Add-on LAMA; referral; consider high-dose maintenance ICS-formoterol ± anti-IgE, anti-IL5/5R, anti-IL4R, anti-TSLP
		Preferred Reliever	As needed SABA				

-Preferred Controller—to prevent exacerbations and control symptoms

-Reliever—quick-relief of acute asthma symptoms

*Preferred if the patient is less likely to be compliant with daily controller. ICS-containing therapy is recommended even if symptoms are not frequent as it reduces the risk of severe exacerbations and need for OCS.

⁺For use if unable to use preferred treatment, or if patient is stable, compliant with controller use, and no exacerbations on current therapy.

^Limited indications, or less evidence for efficacy or safety

Source: Global Initiative for Asthma (GINA). Global Strategy for Asthma Management and Prevention. (2022). Retrieved from https://ginasthma.org/wp-content/uploads/2022/05/GINA-Main-Report-2022-FINAL-22-05-03-WMS.pdf

1. National Heart, Lung, and Blood Institute. (2012). Expert panel report 3 (EPR 3): Asthma care quick reference diagnosing and managing asthma. Retrieved from https://www.nhlbi.nih.gov/sites/default/files/media/docs/asthsumm.pdf

2. National Heart, Lung, and Blood Institute. (2020). 2020 Focused Updates to the Asthma Management Guidelines: A Report from the National Asthma Education and Prevention Program Coordinating Committee Expert Panel Working Group. Retrieved from https://www.nhlbi.nih.gov/health-topics/all-publications-and-resources/2020-focused-updates-asthma-management-guidelines

Physical Exam

- Findings may be normal, vary with severity of attack
- Vital signs, with particular attention to respiratory rate
- General appearance: signs of respiratory distress (use of accessory muscles)
- Skin: atopic dermatitis/eczema
- Upper respiratory tract: rhinitis, nasal polyps, swollen nasal turbinates
- Lower respiratory tract: tachypnea, prolonged expiration phase, audible wheezing (may be absent in severe attacks due to decreased breath sounds)

Diagnostic Studies

- Blood test not routinely required; may find eosinophilia or elevated serum IgE levels
- Spirometry: measures forced expiratory volumo in 1 socond (FEV1) and forced vital capacity (FVC) in patients younger than 5 years of age. Baseline measurements are essential for diagnosis, then periodic monitoring.
- Bronchoprovocation testing: confirms diagnosis; used in patients with atypical presentation (normal baseline spirometry, no variable airflow limitation with spirometry or peak flow)
  - Inhaled methacholine, histamine, cold dry air, or exercise challenge test induces symptoms
- Peak expiratory flow (PEF) used for monitoring lung status, not to confirm diagnosis.
- Values vary with height, age, gender. Patient determines "personal best" or average of three readings on optimal day's PEF; less than 200 mL indicates severe obstruction.
  - 80% to 100% of patient's "personal best": good control, maintain treatment
  - 50% to 79%: acute exacerbation, adjust treatment
  - Less than 50%: severe asthma exacerbation, emergency treatment

- Chest X-ray: almost always normal; routinely recommended in severe asthma and in patients with comorbid conditions and/or with atypical symptoms; shows hyperinflation in uncomplicated episodes also used to evaluate patients for complicating cardiopulmonary processes
- Skin testing to determine allergic triggers

Differential Diagnosis

All Ages

- Foreign body aspiration
- Acute infections, viral, pneumonia, bronchitis, TB
- GERD
- Aspiration
- AIDS
- Psychogenic cough
- Neuromuscular weakness
- Vocal cord dysfunction

Adults

- COPD
- CHF
- Pulmonary embolism
- Bronchogenic carcinoma
- Cough secondary to ACE inhibitors
- Alpha antitrypsin deficiency

Children

- Allergic rhinitis
- Sinusitis
- Bronchiolitis (RSV)

- Laryngotracheobronchitis (croup)
- Cystic fibrosis
- Bronchopulmonary dysplasia
- Tracheoesophageal fistula
- Congenital heart disease

Management

Goals of therapy

- Reduce impairment:
  - Prevent chronic and troublesome symptoms.
  - Require infrequent use of inhaled short-acting beta$_2$ agonists (SABA).
  - Maintain near-normal pulmonary function.
  - Maintain normal activity levels.
  - Meet patient and family expectations of satisfaction with asthma care.
- Reduce risk:
  - Prevent recurrent exacerbations and minimize emergency department (ED) visits/hospitalization.
  - Prevent loss of lung function or reduced lung growth in children.
  - Provide optimal pharmacotherapy with minimal or no adverse effects of therapy.

Nonpharmacologic Treatment

- Develop written asthma action plan with patient/family.
- Identify and avoid factors that trigger asthma; control environmental triggers.
- Allergy skin testing to determine allergens.
- Maintain hydration; increase fluids during exacerbation.
- Address family, school, and/or day care issues; provide education, support, and counseling.
- Establish a patient/provider partnership with a detailed asthma action plan.
- Delivery of inhaled agents via "spacer" or holding chamber provides increased efficacy.

- Educate patients to rinse mouth out with water immediately after use of inhaler to avoid thrush
- No smoking

Pharmacologic Treatment

See Table 7.10.

- Guidelines for medication selection is based on age, severity, patient preference, and practical issues.
- Long-acting beta agonists (LABAs) should never be used alone due to the increased risk of death related to asthma or other respiratory conditions. The U.S. Food and Drug Administration (FDA) has a mandated "black box" warning applied to salmeterol-containing products.

How Long to Treat

- Dependent on the severity of the attacks; goal is to gain control as quickly as possible and decrease treatment gradually to least amount of medication needed to maintain control

Special Considerations

- Pregnancy:
  - Check asthma control at all prenatal visits. Asthma can improve or worsen during pregnancy; adjust medications as needed.
  - Most inhaled corticosteroid (ICS) agents are category C, except budesonide, montelukast, and zafirlukast, which are category B.
  - Remind patients to avoid exposure to tobacco smoke.
  - Treating asthma with medications is safer for mother and fetus than having poorly controlled asthma.
  - Maintaining lung function is essential for good fetal outcome.

TABLE 7–10.
ASTHMA MEDICATIONS

MEDICATION	PREPARATION	DOSAGE		COMMENTS
		ADOLESCENTS & ADULT ≥12 YEARS OF AGE (UNLESS OTHERWISE NOTED BELOW)	CHILDREN ≤5 YEARS OF AGE	
Short-acting beta-agonist (SABA)				
Albuterol MDI (Proventil HFA, Ventolin HFA)	90 μg/inhalation	2 inhalations every 4 to 6 hours as needed		
Albuterol Nebulizer Solution	0.083% (2.5 mg/3 mL) 0.5% (2.5 mg/0.5 mL) concentrate; must be diluted in 2.5 mL saline	2.5 mg every 4 to 6 hours as needed		
Levalbuterol MDI (Xopenex HFA)	45 μg/inhalation	1–2 inhalations every 4 to 6 hours prn		
Levalbuterol Nebulizer Solution	0.63 mg/3 mL 1.25 mg/3 mL 1.25 mg/0.5 mL concentrate; must be diluted in 2.5 mL saline	Administer 0.63 to 1.25 mg every 6 to 8 hours, as needed	Up to 3 doses per 24 hours	
Ipratropium SMI (Atrovent)	Ipratropium 20 μg and albuterol 100 μg/inhalation	2 inhalations every 6 hours, as needed		
Ipratropium SMI (Atrovent)	Ipratropium 0.5 mg and albuterol 2.5 mg per 3 mL/vial	Administer 1 vial (3 mL) every 4 to 6 hours, as needed		

Continued

TABLE 7–10.
(CONTINUED)

MEDICATION	PREPARATION	DOSAGE		COMMENTS
		ADOLESCENTS & ADULT ≥12 YEARS OF AGE (UNLESS OTHERWISE NOTED BELOW)	CHILDREN ≤5 YEARS OF AGE	
Inhaled Corticosteroids (ICS)				
Beclomethasone propionate HFA (QVAR)		Adults: 40–320 μg twice daily	Children 5–11 years: 40–80 μg twice daily	
Budesonide DPI (Pulmicort)	90–180 μg		1 to 2 inhalations twice per day	
Budesonide nebulization suspension	0.25 mg/2 mL 0.5 mg/2 mL 1 mg/2 mL		Once daily or as two divided doses	
Ciclesonide HFA (Alvesco)	80 or 160 μg/puff			
Fluticasone propionate HFA (Flovent)	44, 110, or 220 μg/puff	Dose varies	Dose varies	For patients ≥ 4 years of age
Fluticasone propionate DPI (Flovent diskus, Armonair Digihaler)	50, 100, or 250 μg/inhalation	1-2 inhalations twice daily	Dose varies	
Mometasone DPI	110 or 220 μg/inhalation		Dose varies	
Mometasone HFA MDI	50, 100, or 200 μg/puff	2 puffs twice daily		

		Systemic Glucocorticoids		
Methylprednisolone			0 to 11 years: 0.25 to 2 mg/kg orally per day or every other day	Given in the morning
Prednisolone				Titrate to the lowest acceptable dose that maintains control. Only used rarely for long-term control due to toxic effects
	Inhaled Corticosteroid plus Long-acting Beta-agonist (ICS-LABA Combinations)			
Budesonide-formoterol HFA (Symbicort)	80 μg/4.5 μg 160 μg/4.5 μg	2 inhalations twice a day		For patients 5 years or older
Fluticasone furoate-vilanterol DPI (Brand name: Breo Ellipta)	100 μg/25 μg 200 μg/25 μg	1 inhalation once daily		
Fluticasone propionate-salmeterol DPI (Advair Diskus)	100 μg/50 μg 250 μg/50 μg 500 μg/50 μg	1 inhalation twice a day		For patients 5 years or older
Fluticasone propionate-salmeterol HFA (Advair HFA)	45 μg/21 μg 115 μg/21 μg 230 μg/21 μg	2 inhalations twice a day		
Fluticasone propionate-salmeterol DPI (AirDuo RespiClick, AirDuo Digihaler)	55 μg/14 μg 113 μg/14 μg 232 μg/14 μg	1 inhalation twice a day		
Mometasone-formoterol HFA (Dulera)	100 μg/5 μg 200 μg/5 μg	2 inhalations twice a day		For patients age 12 years and older only

Continued

TABLE 7–10.
(CONTINUED)

MEDICATION	PREPARATION	DOSAGE		COMMENTS
		ADOLESCENTS & ADULT ≥12 YEARS OF AGE (UNLESS OTHERWISE NOTED BELOW)	CHILDREN ≤5 YEARS OF AGE	
Fluticasone-salmeterol DPI	100 μg/50 μg		5 to 11 years: 1 inhalation twice per day	
Fluticasone-salmeterol MDI	45 μg/21 μg		5 to 11 years: 2 puffs twice per day	
Mometasone-formoterol HFA MDI	50 μg/5 μg		5 to 11 years: 2 puffs twice per day	
ICS-LAMA-LABA Combinations				
Luticasone furoate-umeclidinium-vilanterol DPI (Trelegy Ellipta)	100 μg/62.5 μg/25 μg 200 mc/62.5 μg/25 μg	1 inhalation once daily		
Leukotriene Receptor Antagonists (LTRAs)				
Montelukast	4 mg or 5 mg chewable tablet 4 mg granule packets		1 to 5 years of age: 4 mg once daily 6 to 14 years of age: 5 mg once daily	Take at bedtime
Zafirlukast	10 mg tablet		5 to 11 years: 10 mg twice per day	Take on empty stomach

Long-acting Anticholinergic Agents				
Tiotropium SMI	Soft-mist inhaler 1.25 μg/ actuation		2 inhalations once daily.	Avoid in patients ≤4 years of age
Cromones				
Cromolyn sodium	20 mg/ampule for nebulization		20 mg 4 times per day	May cause bronchospasm Avoid in patients younger than 2 years of age
Methylxanthines				
Theophylline	Starting dose for approximately 10 mg/kg per day (max initial dose 300 mg/day)		Dose dependent on preparation	Monitor serum concentration levels Significant drug–drug interactions Used infrequently

SABA: short-acting beta agonist; ICS: inhaled glucocorticoid (inhaled corticosteroid); LABA: long-acting beta agonist; LAMA: long-acting muscarinic antagonist; LTRAs: leukotriene receptor antagonists;

HFA: metered dose inhaler with hydrofluoroalkane propellant; MDI: metered-dose inhaler; DPI: dry-powder inhaler; SMI: soft mist inhaler

Global Initiative for Asthma (GINA; 2022) GENERAL PRINCIPLES FOR STEPWISE APPROACH FOR ASTHMA TREATMENT IN PATIENTS

See Table 7–9.

- Traditionally, SABAs are used for reliever (rescue) therapy. The Global Initiative for Asthma (GINA) 2022 recommends ICS-formoterol (LABA), with a SABA as an alternative, for reliever therapy.
- Initial therapy is described below. If patient presents with acute exacerbation, a higher level of initial therapy may be needed; use of oral glucocorticoids may be necessary.
- At follow-up visits, check adherence, inhaler technique, environmental factors, and comorbid conditions.
- Stepdown if symptoms well controlled, lung function has been stable for at least 3 months
- Step up 1 or 2 steps if asthma is not well controlled or is very poorly controlled.
  - Before stepping up, check inhaler technique, poor adherence, environmental exposures; confirm symptom are a result of asthma.
- Refer to asthma specialist if step 4 or higher is required.
- For postmenopausal women using inhaled corticosteroids, consider calcium supplements (1,000–1,500 mg a day) and vitamin D (800 units a day).
- Bone mineral density testing if on long-term inhaled or oral corticosteroids to monitor osteoporosis
- Periodic ophthalmology exam if on oral corticosteroids
- Most medications are secreted in breast milk.
- Assess for ACE inhibitor use.
- Avoid ipratropium in patients with allergies to peanuts or soy; it contains soya lecithin and may precipitate an allergic reaction.
- In children, monitor growth if using steroids to manage asthma.
- Withhold varicella vaccine if child is receiving 2 mg/kg or more or 20 mg/day of oral prednisone.

When to Consult, Refer, Hospitalize

- When diagnosis is unclear
- Additional asthma education needed

- Specialized testing (bronchoprovocation, skin testing)
- Specialized treatments (immunotherapy, anti-IgE therapy)
- Moderate-to-severe persistent asthma in adults
- Moderate-to-persistent asthma in children
- Comorbidities: rhinitis, GERD, sinusitis, obstructive sleep apnea, COPD
- Poorly controlled asthma: frequent ED visits and hospitalizations for asthma
- Hospitalization: based on duration and severity of symptoms, severity of airflow obstruction, response to emergency department treatment, course and severity of prior exacerbations, access to medical care and medication, and adequacy of home condition

Follow-Up

Expected Course

- Follow-up depends on symptom severity, symptom control, knowledge level, social support, and other resources.
  - Every 2 to 6 weeks while gaining control
  - Every 1 to 6 months to monitor control
  - Every 3 months if step down in therapy is anticipated
- New asthmatics require frequent monitoring and patient education.
- Children need more frequent monitoring during growth spurts.
- Patients should monitor peak flow rates twice daily to establish baseline and then regularly.
- For acute exacerbation, follow-up in 24 hours, then 3 to 5 days, then weekly until symptoms are controlled and peak flow consistently 80% of predicted, and then monthly.
- Monitor theophylline levels 2 weeks after initiation of therapy and then every 4 months.

Complications

- Atelectasis, pneumonia, air leak syndromes (pneumomediastinum, pneumothorax), medication-specific side effects/interactions, respiratory failure, death (~50% of asthma deaths occur in adults 65 years and older)

CHRONIC OBSTRUCTIVE PULMONARY DISEASE (COPD)

Description

Chronic obstructive pulmonary disease (COPD) is a disease that is common and preventable, characterized by persistent respiratory symptoms and airflow limitation that is not fully reversible, due to airway and/or alveolar abnormalities caused by significant exposure to noxious irritants. Includes chronic bronchitis, emphysema, and—in some cases—asthma

- Chronic bronchitis: presence of increased mucus production and recurrent cough most days for at least 3 months of a year, for 2 consecutive years, without other underlying disease to explain the cough
- Emphysema: destruction of interalveolar septa within the distal or terminal bronchiole involving both airways and lung parenchyma

Patients with asthma whose airflow obstruction is not completely reversible are considered to have COPD. The etiology and pathogenesis of the COPD in these patients may vary from those who have chronic bronchitis or emphysema.

Associated with an increased risk of ICU admission, invasive ventilation, or death in patients with COVID-19.

Etiology

- Cigarette and/or cannabis smoking
- Air pollution
- Antiprotease deficiency (alpha-1 antitrypsin deficiency)
- Occupational exposure (firefighters)
- Infection (bacterial or viral)
- Occupational pollutants (cadmium, silica)

Incidence and Demographics

- COPD affects more than 15 million people in the United States.
- Seen more in women than men
- Onset in middle-aged or older adults
- Fourth leading cause of death in the United States

Risk Factors

- Tobacco smoking (most common risk factor)
- Passive smoking
- Cannabis use (1 joint equivalent to 2½–5 cigarettes)
- Severe viral pneumonia early in life
- Female sex
- Aging
- Alcohol consumption
- Airway hyperactivity
- Pollution: indoor or outdoor (dust, fumes, coal miners, metal molders, grain handlers)
- Periodontal disease

Prevention and Screening

- Smoking cessation and reduction of exposure to secondhand smoke
- Early detection through pulmonary function tests (PFTs) in high-risk groups
- Avoid outdoor activities when air pollutant concentrations are high.

Assessment

History

- Duration and characteristics of "classic symptoms:" chronic cough, chronic and progressive dyspnea, chronic sputum production
- Exercise/activity tolerance, dyspnea on exertion or at rest
- Chills/fever, weight gain/loss, edema, fatigue, angina
- Environmental/occupational history
- Asthma history
- Sleep habits (number of pillows used)
- Increase in sputum production or purulence along with dyspnea signals exacerbation
- Family history of COPD

- Smoking history (age at initiation, pack-year history since initiation, date when stopped smoking or current smoker)
- History of risk factors
  - Host factors—genetics, congenital/developmental anomalies
  - Tobacco smoking (including popular preparations)
  - Exposure to smoke from home cooking and heating fuels
  - Exposure to noxious particles and gases
- Impact on quality of life, activities of daily living, socioeconomic status
- Risk of exacerbations, history of previous treated events (two or more per year)
- Other comorbidities: cardiovascular diseases, osteoporosis, depression, anxiety, skeletal muscle dysfunction, metabolic syndrome, and lung cancer increase morbidity and hospitalizations. Assess and manage diseases appropriately.

Physical Exam

- Rarely diagnostic for COPD; physical findings usually present with severe disease
- Early disease: normal exam or may have prolonged expiration or wheezes on forced exhalation
- Progression of disease: exam may show hyperinflation, decreased breath sounds, wheezes, crackles at lung bases, or distant heart sounds; "barreled chest" may be present
- End-stage COPD: unusual positions to relieve dyspnea at rest (leaning forward with arms outstretched and weight supported on palms or elbow), use of accessory respiratory muscles of neck and shoulder girdle, pursed lip breathing, paradoxical retractions with inspiration, cyanosis, asterixis due to severe hypercapnia, enlarged tender liver, neck vein distention, yellow stains on fingers
- Chronic bronchitis: cyanosis, wheezing, weight gain, diminished breath sounds, distant heart sounds
- Emphysema: barrel chest (increased anteroposterior [AP] diameter), minimal wheezing, accessory muscles used, pursed lip breathing, cyanosis slight or absent, breath sounds diminished
- COPD symptoms are classified using the GOLD staging system based on degree of airflow limitation severity measured during PFTs. See Table 7–11.

TABLE 7–11.
CLASSIFICATION OF SEVERITY OF AIRFLOW LIMITATION IN COPD

CLASSIFICATION OF AIRFLOW LIMITATION SEVERITY IN COPD. (BASED ON POST-BRONCHODILATOR FEV1) IN PATIENTS WITH FEV1/FVC <0.70:		
GOLD 1	Mild	FEV1 ≥ 80% predicted
GOLD 2	Moderate	$50\% \leq FEV_1 < 80\%$ predicted
GOLD 3	Severe	$30\% \leq FEV_1 < 50\%$ predicted
GOLD 4	Very Severe	FEV1 < 30% predicted

Adapted from "Global Strategy for Diagnosis, Management and Prevention of Chronic Obstructive Pulmonary Disease", page 31, at www.goldcopd.org by Global Initiative for Chronic Obstructive Lung Disease (GOLD). Copyright 2024 by Global Initiative for Chronic Obstructive Lung Disease

- Comprehensive symptom assessment using validated questionnaires: COPD Assessment Test (CAT) and Clinical COPD Questionnaire (CCQ) are recommended. Medical Research Council (mMRC) scale used only to assess breathlessness.
- Patient's symptoms, risk of exacerbations, severity of spirometric abnormality, and other comorbid conditions are important to assess in the diagnosis of COPD. Although spirometry is required to diagnose COPD, patients with the following symptoms should also be considered for diagnosis:
  - Chronic cough, dyspnea, sputum production, exposure to risk factors.
- A person's respiratory symptoms and history of exacerbations should be used to assign ABCD categories. See the 2019 Global Initiative for Chronic Obstructive Lung Disease Pocket Guide at: https://goldcopd.org/gold-reports/ (Figure 2.4). The Refined ABCD Assessment Tool.

Diagnostic Studies

- PFT (spirometry): Reduced FEV1 determines severity of airflow limitation, whereas decreased FEV1/FVC ratio determines airflow limitation. FEV1/FVC less than 0.70 with use of post-bronchodilator is diagnostic for COPD
- Chest X-rays in emphysema: small heart, hyperinflation, possible bullous changes; flattened diaphragm; chronic bronchitis: increased bronchovascular markings, and cardiomegaly

- Consider pulse oximetry during acute exacerbations or in those patients who may be considered for long-term oxygen therapy.
- Arterial blood gases (ABGs) unnecessary unless FEV1 is less than 40% of predicted, hypoxia, or hypercapnia suspected; no abnormalities in early COPD; hypoxemia in advanced chronic bronchitis; compensated respiratory acidosis with chronic respiratory failure in chronic bronchitis
- Alpha-1 antitrypsin level to look for deficiency if COPD occurs before 45 years of age or family history of genetic disease
- Increased hemoglobin/hematocrit may be present with chronic bronchitis but not with emphysema.
- Chest CT may show diffuse bullous changes or upper lobe predominance; is not needed for diagnosis of COPD.

Differential Diagnosis

- Chronic obstructive asthma
- Chronic bronchitis with normal spirometry
- Bronchiectasis
- Bronchiolitis
- Congestive heart failure
- Tuberculosis
- Lung cancer
- GERD
- Sleep apnea
- Acute viral infection
- Normal aging of lungs
- Chronic pulmonary embolism

Management

Goal: relieve symptoms, improve exercise tolerance and health status, prevent disease progression, prevent and treat exacerbations, and reduce mortality

Nonpharmacologic Treatment

- Initiate and support smoking cessation.
- Reduce other risk factors: avoid exposure to colds and influenza; avoid respiratory irritants (secondhand smoke, dust, other air pollutants)
- Vaccinations: influenza and pneumococcal vaccines
- Oxygen therapy for patients with chronic hypoxemia
- Pulmonary rehabilitation decreases symptoms, improves quality of life, and promotes physical and emotional involvement in daily activities.
- Maintain ideal body weight, high protein/caloric diet, and regular daily exercise; rest often.
- Increase fluids and humidification.
- Breathing exercises with manual incentive spirometer; effective cough techniques
- Lung reduction surgery or lung transplantation in selected cases
- Palliative care, end-of life care, and hospice care for advanced COPD

Pharmacologic Treatment

- See Table 7–12 for pharmacologic therapy for stable COPD based on GOLD recommendations.
- Short-acting beta2-agonist (SABA): levalbuterol (Xopenex) MDI (metered dose inhaler) or solution for nebulizer every 6–8 hours; salbutamol (Albuterol) MDI, DPI (dry powder inhaler), or solution for nebulizer every 4–6 hours.
- Long-acting beta-agonist (LABA): salmeterol (Serevent) MDI, DPI every 12 hours; formoterol (Foradil) MDI or DPI or (Perforomist) nebulized every 12 hours; arformoterol (Brovana) solution for nebulizer, indacaterol (Arcapta Neohaler) DPI once daily.
- Short-acting anticholinergic (SAMA): ipratropium bromide (Atrovent) MDI or solution for nebulizer every 6–8 hours.
- Long-acting anticholinergic (LAMA): aclidinium bromide (Tudorza Pressair) DPI every 12 hours; tiatropium (Spiriva) DPI every 24 hours; umedidnium (Incruse Ellipta) DPI every 24 hours.
- Combination short-acting beta2-agonist plus anticholinergic inhaler (SABA/SAMA): fenoterol/ipratropium (Respimat) SMI or nebulized solution (Duovent) every 6–8 hours; salbutamol/ipratropium MDI (Combivent) or nebulized solution (DuoNeb) every 6–8 hours.

TABLE 7–12.
INITIAL PHARMACOLOGIC THERAPY FOR STABLE COPD

2 or more moderate exacerbations or 1 or more leading to hospitalization	**Group C** LAMA	**Group D** LAMA or LAMA + LABA* or ICS + LABA^ *Consider if highly symptomatic (e.g., at more than20) ^Consider if eos is 300 or higher
0 or 1 moderate exacerbations (not leading to hospital admission)	**Group A** A bronchodilator	**Group B** A long-acting bronchodilator (LABA or LAMA)
	mMRC 0–1, CAT above 10	**MMRC 2 or above, CAT 10 or above**

^eos: blood eosinophil count in cells per microliter, mMRC: modified Medical Research Council dyspnea questionnaire; CAT™ COPD Assessment Test™

Adapted from "Global Strategy for Diagnosis, Management and Prevention of Chronic Obstructive Pulmonary Disease," page 48, Figure 3.7 at goldcopd.org by Global Initiative for Chronic Obstructive Lung Disease (GOLD). Copyright 2024 by Global Initiative for Chronic Obstructive Lung Disease.

- Combination long-acting beta2-agonist plus anticholinergic (LABA/LAMA): undacaterol/gylcopyrronium (Utibron Neohaler) DPI every 12 hours; olodaterol/tiatropium (Rispimat) SMI every 24 hours.
- Phosphodiesterase-4 inhibitor (PDE-4): roflumilast (Daliresp) 500 mμ by mouth daily. Used as maintenance therapy to prevent exacerbations; decreases inflammation. Contraindications: moderate-to-severe liver impairment.
- Inhaled corticosteroids (ICS): beclomethasone (QVAR), budesonide (Pulmicort) inhaler; fluticasone (Flovent); flunisolide (Aerospan); mometasone (Asmanex). For moderate or severe disease and frequent exacerbation when long-acting bronchodilators are inadequate. Increase risk of pneumonia and fractures if used long term.
- Combined long-acting beta2-agonist plus inhaled corticosteroids (LABA/ICS): formeterol/budesonide (Symbicort); salmeterol/fluticasone (Advair); vilamerol/fluticasone (Breo Ellipta) MDI and/or DPI.
- Systemic corticosteroids: Prednisone (Deltasone) 40–60 mg by mouth daily or methylprednisolone 30–40 mg/day for 5–7 days for moderate or severe COPD exacerbations. Long-term therapy is not recommended.

- Methylxanthines: Aminophylline pill, syrup, or suppository. Theophylline: short-acting or long-acting pills. Up to 800 mg/day; monitor carefully; decrease dose used in renal impairment, liver dysfunction, CHF, or age 55 years and older; must monitor serum level, maintain therapeutic range. Use only if other bronchodilators are unaffordable or unavailable.
- Other medications:
  - Mucolytic agent: *N*-acetylcysteine (Mucomyst) nebulizer solution improves secretion.
  - Low-dose macrolides: decrease inflammation (clarithromycin, azithromycin, or erythromycin)
  - Antibiotics for severe exacerbation or presence of purulent sputum
    - Most common organisms: *H. influenzae, S. pneumoniae, M. catarrhalis;* may be due to viral infection, pneumonia
    - Choice of antibiotic is based on local bacterial resistance pattern
    - Trimethoprim-sulfamethoxazole (Bactrim DS): 160/800 mg every 12 hours
    - Amoxicillin-clavulanate (Augmentin): 875/125 mg every 12 hours or 500/125 mg three times daily.
    - Doxycycline (Vibramycin): 100 mg twice daily.
    - May use a fluoroquinolone such as levofloxacin (Levaquin), moxifloxacin (Avelox); azithromycin, cephalosporins
    - Antibiotics not indicated in younger patients with mild symptoms and infrequent exacerbation
    - Consider use in patients under 65 years of age with mild–moderate impairment of lung function (FEV1 50% or more predicted value with fewer than four exacerbations per year), or patients 65 years or older with FEV1 less than 50%, more than four exacerbations/year, or use of antibiotic within the last 3 months
- Home oxygen therapy: may improve survival in hypoxemia and cor pulmonale; initiate early if oxygen level is less than 88% on room air.
- Noninvasive positive-pressure ventilation if acute respiratory acidosis is present
- Alpha-1 antitrypsin if deficient: 60 mg/kg/week to maintain level over 80 mg/dL

Follow-up Treatment Principles

- Review symptoms and exacerbation risk
- Assess inhaler technique, adherence, and effect of non-pharmacologic interventions
- Adjust pharmacologic treatment, if needed.

How Long to Treat

- Chronic condition requiring ongoing therapeutic treatments and monitoring
- Antibiotic use in COPD exacerbation is controversial. However, it is recommended in patients with increased dyspnea, sputum volume, and sputum purulence or in patients requiring mechanical ventilation. Length of antibiotic therapy is usually 5–10 days.

Special Considerations

- Use caution with beta blockers, cough suppressants, antihistamines, or sedatives.
- Discuss advance directives and end-of-life decisions.

When to Consult, Refer, Hospitalize

- Consult: severe exacerbation, frequent hospitalizations, age younger than 40 years, rapid progression, weight loss, severe disease, comorbidities, or surgical evaluation
- Refer: to pulmonary rehabilitation program
- Hospitalize: acute decompensation (sudden development of resting dyspnea); severe underlying COPD; new physical signs (cyanosis, peripheral edema); response failure to initial medical management; frequent exacerbations; older age; insufficient home support; need for mechanical ventilation; serious comorbidities (decompensated CHF, new arrhythmias)

Follow-Up

Expected Course

- Routine follow-up is essential. Use the following principles to guide follow-up treatment:
  - Review symptoms and exacerbation risk
  - Assess inhaler technique, adherence, and effect of non-pharmacologic interventions
  - Adjust pharmacologic treatment, if needed.
- Monitor disease progression, development of complications, comorbidities, smoking status

Complications

- Malnutrition, cor pulmonale, hypercapnia, and pulse higher than 100 indicate poor prognosis.
- Poor sleep quality, infections, secondary polycythemia
- Acute or chronic respiratory failure, bullous lung disease, pneumothorax, lung cancer
- Arrhythmias, pulmonary hypertension, cardiovascular disease
- Osteoporosis, anxiety/depression, metabolic syndrome, diabetes

CASE STUDIES

CASE 1

A 40-year-old woman, on vacation visiting family in Florida, presents to the clinic for the first time with complaints of nonproductive cough and shortness of breath with wheezing for the past 4 days. She reports having similar symptoms in the past and was prescribed an albuterol inhaler, which relieved the symptoms. Today, she reports chest tightness and difficulties catching her breath, especially with activity.

Past Medical History (PMH): Seasonal allergic rhinitis, hypertension, GERD, obese

Medications: Norethindrone/ethinyl estradiol (Loestrin), albuterol inhaler AS NEEDED, lisinopril 10 mg daily by mouth, omeprazole (Prilosec) 20 mg daily by mouth

Social History: Married, has one daughter age 13 years; lives on ranch with family; has pets, livestock, and horses; is a social worker assisting immigrant population; reports tobacco use of one-half pack of cigarettes per day since she was 18 years old.

1. What additional history would you like to obtain?

   Exam: Temp 99.6°F, pulse 88 bpm, resp 22, blood pressure 128/78 mmHg, and resting oxygen saturation of 92%. She appears to be mildly uncomfortable but is able to speak in sentences. Skin: pink, warm, dry, intact without bruising or rash. Nose: clear sinus drainage, no sinus tenderness, mild turbinate inflammation. Mouth: pink, moist mucous membranes with postnasal drainage noted in posterior pharynx. Chest: mild wheezing that is worse with forced expiration and no other adventitious sounds audible on auscultation. Heart: regular sinus rate and rhythm without murmurs, gallops, clicks.

2. What are the possible diagnoses?
3. What diagnostic tests would you initially order?
4. Your working diagnosis is asthma. What is your treatment plan?
5. On follow-up, patient is doing much better; however, her tuberculin skin test came back positive with induration greater than 10 mm. What is your course of action now?

CASE 2

A 64-year-old woman presents to the clinic with complaints of cough for past 8 days. States she was seen in the clinic last week and has been using OTC antihistamines and cough syrup; however, the symptoms appear to be worsening. She reports feeling warm, no energy, with cough productive of green sputum. She states that her blood sugars have been higher than normal (220 mg/dL) the past 3 days. She states that her four grandchildren, who live with her, were sick 2 weeks ago with URI but are fine now.

PMH: Diabetes

Medications: Metformin 1,000 mg by mouth twice a day, lisinopril 10 mg by mouth once daily, ASA 81 mg by mouth once daily, atorvastatin (Lipitor) 10 mg by mouth once daily.

Social History: Single, lives in a two-bedroom home with four grandchildren under the age of 10 years; has no running water in home; denies tobacco, alcohol, or drug use.

1. What additional history would you obtain?

   Exam: Temp 102°F, pulse 110 bpm, resp 28, blood pressure 102/78 mmHg, oxygen saturation is 98% on room air. Alert, appears ill, fatigued, with continuous coughing throughout exam. HEENT: unremarkable other than clear sinus drainage and mild congestion. Neck: supple without adenopathy or thyromegaly. Chest: rhonchi and decreased breath sounds, bilateral dullness to bases with percussion. Heart: sinus tachycardia without murmurs. Extremities: without signs of cyanosis or edema. Remainder of her examination is normal. Laboratory results include: complete blood count (CBC) with elevated white blood cell (WBC) count of 18,000 cells/mm3, with a differential of 85% neutrophils and 20% lymphocytes; basic metabolic panel (BMP) with glucose elevated at 196 mg/dL, creatinine 1.3 mg/dL, BUN 30 mg/dL, and normal electrolytes.

2. What are the most likely differential diagnoses?
3. What other diagnostic tests would you order?
4. What is your treatment plan?
5. What are potential complications to this condition?

CASE 3

A 45-year-old man presents to the clinic with complaints of sinus congestion and pain with intermittent nosebleeds for the past 4 weeks. States he has tried OTC antihistamines and saline nasal spray with some relief. However, today, he states he is just not feeling good. He reports fatigue, body aches, low-grade fever, and night sweats for the past 5 days. This morning he reports having a productive cough of white sputum tinged with nickel-sized blood clots. He also complains of pleuritic chest pains but no shortness of breath.

PMH: Unremarkable; denies cardiac or pulmonary disease

Social History: Divorced, construction worker, has smoked a pack of cigarettes per day since he was 15; occasionally consumes alcohol (six-pack of beer every month).

1. What additional history would you like to obtain?

   Exam: Temp 97.4°F, pulse 88, resp 18, blood pressure 126/72 mmHg, oxygen saturation is 98% on room air. He is alert, oriented, fatigued. HEENT: unremarkable other than dry blood in nares. Chest: lungs clear bilaterally without wheezing, rhonchi, rales. Heart: regular sinus rate and rhythm without murmurs, clicks, or gallops.

2. What are the most likely differential diagnoses?
3. Which initial test is most appropriate?
4. What are the major causes of hemoptysis?
5. Your working diagnosis is bronchitis. What is your treatment plan?
6. What is your diagnosis and treatment plan in a patient who expectorates a large amount of blood over a 24-hour period?

CASE STUDIES DISCUSSION

CASE 1

1. What additional history would you like to obtain?

   Characteristic symptoms of asthma: episodic wheezing (absent in severe exacerbation), chest tightness, dyspnea, chronic dry or spasmodic cough; symptoms worse at night, with exercise, and exposure to cold temperatures, smoke, allergens. History of emotional stress, upper respiratory infection, rhinitis/sinusitis, eczema/atopic dermatitis, heartburn, acid reflux, nasal polyps. Any family history of asthma, allergies, or atopy? Severity of symptoms?

2. What are the possible diagnoses?

   COPD, CHF, pulmonary embolism, bronchogenic carcinoma, acute infections, viral, pneumonia, bronchitis, TB, GERD, psychogenic cough, lung cancer, AIDS, vocal cord dysfunction, neuromuscular weakness

3. What diagnostic tests would you initially order?

   Blood test is not routinely required in the diagnosis of asthma. PPD to rule out TB. Spirometry: measures forced expiratory volume in 1 second (FEV1) and forced vital capacity (FVC) in patients younger than 5 years of age. Baseline measurements are essential for diagnosis, and then periodic monitoring. Bronchoprovocation testing: confirms diagnosis; used in patients with atypical presentation (normal baseline spirometry, no variable airflow limitation with spirometry or peak flow). Peak expiratory flow (PEF) used for monitoring lung status, not to confirm diagnosis. Chest X-ray: almost always normal; routinely recommended in severe asthma and in patients with comorbid conditions and/or with atypical symptoms. Skin testing to determine allergic triggers. CT scan to rule out pulmonary embolism may be warranted.

4. Your working diagnosis is asthma. What is your treatment plan?

   Education. Develop written asthma action plan with patient/family. Identify and avoid factors that trigger asthma; control environmental triggers. Allergy skin testing to determine allergens, if needed. Maintain hydration; increase fluids during exacerbation. Establish a patient/provider partnership with a detailed asthma action plan. Educate patients to rinse mouth out with water immediately after use of inhaler to avoid thrush. Smoking cessation/no smoking. Low-dose ICS-formoterol for maintenance and as needed for quick relief of acute symptoms and prevention of exercised-induced bronchospasm. A low-dose maintenance ICS-LABA with an as-needed SABA is another option.

5. On follow-up, patient is doing much better; however, her tuberculin skin test came back positive with induration greater than 10 mm. What is your course of action now?

   Patient has latent TB. Education and counseling regarding the importance of adherence. Education on the symptoms caused by adverse reactions of the TB treatment medications (no appetite, nausea, vomiting, jaundice, fever longer than 3 days, abdominal pain, neuropathy of fingers and toes, skin rash, easy bleeding, aching joints, dizziness, easy bruising, blurred or changed vision, ringing in ears, hearing loss, tingling/numbness around mouth). If symptom(s) present, stop medication and contact health care provider immediately. There are four different treatment plans for latent TB: isoniazid (INH) for 9 months or 6 months' duration (depending on patient's age and or health status), rifapentine (RPT), or rifampin (RIF). Treatment must be modified if the patient is a contact of an individual with drug-resistant TB disease. Consultation with a TB expert is advised if the known source of TB infection has drug-resistant TB.

CASE 2

1. What additional history would you obtain?

   Onset either abrupt, insidious, or current or recent stay at health care–related facility. Recent or concurrent URI, fever, cough (productive or nonproductive), dyspnea, chills, sweats, rigors, fatigue, malaise, myalgias, chest discomfort, headache, anorexia, abdominal pain; pleuritic chest pain; patients generally feel unwell. Older adults: often present with weakness and mental status change. History of chronic obstructive pulmonary disease or human immunodeficiency virus infection. Occupation, animal exposures, and sexual history helpful to identify the specific infectious agent. Recent travel history (within 2 weeks) may help identify *Legionella* pneumonia (seen on cruise ships and hotel stays). Influenza suggested with typical symptoms during peak influenza season. ICU admission, mechanical ventilation, or aspiration history.

2. What are the most likely differential diagnoses?

   Pulmonary edema, asthma exacerbation, atelectasis, acute bronchitis, bronchiolitis, bronchiectasis, COPD, COVID-19, foreign body aspiration, fungal pneumonia, lung abscess, respiratory failure, viral pneumonia, *Pneumocystis jirovecii* pneumonia, pulmonary tuberculosis, lung cancer

3. What other diagnostic tests would you order?

   COVID-19 test: negative confirmed. Chest X-ray: infiltrates confirmed. Routine laboratory testing usually unnecessary to establish an etiology in outpatients with community-acquired pneumonia (CAP). Suctioned or expectorated sputum gram stain. Nasopharyngeal washings for RSV enzyme immunoassay (children). CBC, two sets of blood cultures (usually reserved for hospitalized patients), CRP, procalcitonin levels,

CMP. WBC count elevated (may be low in older adults or immunocompromised patients). Legionella urine antigen test if *Legionella* suspected. Bronchoalveolar lavage or protected specimen brush with quantitative cultures. Serial chest X-rays or chest CT scan if health care–associated pneumonia

4. What is your treatment plan?

   Hydration, high humidity, rest, smoking cessation, avoidance of secondhand smoke, chest physiotherapy for bacterial pneumonia, oxygen if needed, semi-upright or upright positioning, noninvasive ventilation using continuous positive airway pressure (CPAP) or bilevel positive airway pressure (BiPAP) with endotracheal intubation, incentive spirometry to help prevent postoperative pneumonia.

   Empiric treatment is often necessary because often not able to identify pathogen. Adult CAP outpatient (previously healthy, no antibiotics in past 3 months): Macrolide: azithromycin (Zithromax): over 12 years old: 500 mg (two 250 mg tablets) initially, then 250 mg (one tablet) daily x 4 days or 500 mg by mouthdaily x 3 days; or clarithromycin (Biaxin): adults: 500 mg (one tablet) twice a day x 5 days; clarithromycin XL: two 500 mg tablets (1,000 mg) once daily PO x 5 days or erythromycin (Erythrocin) 500 mg by mouth BID x 10 days (not generally used due to side effects); or tetracycline: Doxycycline 100 mg by mouth twice a day x 10 days

5. What are potential complications to this condition?

   Necrotizing pneumonia, respiratory failure, empyema, abscesses, cavitation, broncho-pleural fistula, sepsis

CASE 3

1. What additional history would you like to obtain?

   Smoking and travel history. Onset and duration of symptoms; amount, frequency, and characteristics of sputum; is there white or purulent phlegm mixed with blood? Determine if nonpulmonary source of bleeding: vomiting, expectoration from naso-pharynx, anticoagulant drug use, substance use, chest trauma. Associated symptoms: weight loss, night sweats, dyspnea, fever, fatigue, bruising, hematuria, rash, joint pain or swelling. TB exposure, dates of last TB test, and chest X-ray. Past cardiac, pulmo-nary, hematological, or immunological history. Environmental exposure, asbestos

2. What are the most likely differential diagnoses?

   Acute and chronic bronchitis, pneumonia, tuberculosis (TB), and lung cancer

3. Which initial test is most appropriate?

   Directed by history and physical findings. Tuberculin skin test (PPD), unless positive in the past. Chest X-ray. CBC with differential and platelets. Gram stain of sputum:

infection; acid-fast stain: TB. Sputum cytologic exam: malignancy. Renal function, urinalysis, liver function tests, brain natriuretic peptide (BNP). Serologic testing: antinuclear antibodies, antineutrophil cytoplasmic antibodies, antiglomerular basement membrane antibodies, anticardiolipin antibodies. Coagulation studies: PT, PTT, bleeding time if bleeding present in more than one site. Bronchoscopy for patients at risk of cancer, TB. High-resolution chest CT: complementary to bronchoscopy (test of choice for suspected small peripheral malignancies). Ventilation-perfusion scan/ angiography: pulmonary embolism.

4. What are the major causes of hemoptysis?

   Acute and chronic bronchitis, pneumonia, tuberculosis (TB), and lung cancer. Inflammation of tracheobronchial mucosa due to minor erosion from bronchiectasis, sarcoidosis, Wegener's granulomatosis, lupus pneumonitis. Bronchovascular fistula, injury to pulmonary vasculature due to lung abscess, aspergillomas, or pulmonary emboli causing pulmonary infarction; trauma; foreign body. Increased pulmonary capillary pressure due to pulmonary edema, mitral stenosis, AV malformations, or granuloma formation. Bleeding disorders or anticoagulant therapy. Nonpulmonary sources: nose or gastrointestinal tract. Cryptogenic hemoptysis: negative workup; etiology unknown in 30% to 40% of patients, 90% resolve in 6 months. Cocaine and tobacco use are risk factors.

5. Your working diagnosis is bronchitis. What is your treatment plan?

   Rest, adequate hydration, steam inhalations, vaporizers, smoking cessation or avoid smoke, treat associated illnesses. Antibiotic treatment is not recommended. Consider antivirals if influenza is suspected.

6. What is your diagnosis and treatment plan in a patient who expectorates a large amount of blood over a 24-hour period?

   Hemoptysis. Admit to hospital for further evaluation and management for massive blood loss (200 mL/day or more).

REFERENCES

American Cancer Society. (2022a). *Key statistics for lung cancer.* Retrieved from https://www.cancer.org/cancer/lung-cancer/about/key-statistics.html#:~:text=Lung%20cancer%20mainly%20occurs%20in,when%20diagnosed%20is%20about%2070

American Cancer Society. (2022b). *What is lung cancer?* Retrieved from https://www.cancer.org/cancer/lung-cancer/about/what-is.html

Asthma and Allergy Foundation of America. (2021a). *Asthma disparities in America.* Retrieved from https://www.aafa.org/asthma-disparities-burden-on-minorities.aspx

Asthma and Allergy Foundation of America (2021b). *Asthma facts and figures.* Retrieved from https://www.aafa.org/asthma-facts/

Centers for Disease Control and Prevention. (2016). *Interferon-gamma release assays (IGRAs)—Blood tests for TB infection.* Retrieved from https://www.cdc.gov/tb/publications/factsheets/testing/igra.htm

Centers for Disease Control and Prevention. (2018). Update on recommendations for use of once-weekly isoniazid-rifapentine regimen to treat latent Mycobacterium tuberculosis infection. *Morbidity and Mortality Weekly Report (MMRW), 67*(25), 723–726. Retrieved from https://www.cdc.gov/mmwr/volumes/67/wr/mm6725a5.htm?s_cid=mm6725a5_w

Centers for Disease Control and Prevention. (2019). *Tuberculosis—United States, 2018. Morbidity and Mortality Weekly Report (MMRW), 68*(11), 257–262. Retrieved from https://www.cdc.gov/mmwr/volumes/68/wr/mm6811a2.htm

Centers for Disease Control and Prevention. (2020a). *Tuberculin skin testing.* Retrieved from https://www.cdc.gov/tb/publications/factsheets/testing/skintesting.htm

Centers for Disease Control and Prevention. (2020b). *Treatment regimens for latent TB infection.* Retrieved from https://www.cdc.gov/tb/topic/treatment/ltbi.htm

Centers for Disease Control and Prevention. (2021). *TB in children.* Retrieved from https://www.cdc.gov/tb/topic/populations/TBinChildren/default.htm

Centers for Disease Control and Prevention. (2022). *Treatment of TB disease.* Retrieved from https://www.cdc.gov/tb/topic/treatment/tbdisease.htm#Treatment-Regimen

Domino, F. J. (2022). *The 5-minute clinical consult, 2021* (30th ed.). Philadelphia, PA: Lippincott, Williams & Wilkins.

Deutsch-Feldman, M., Pratt, R. H., Price, S. F., Tsang, C. A., & Self, J. L. (2021). *Tuberculosis—United States, 2020. Morbidity and Mortality Weekly Report (MMWR), 70,* 409–414. DOI: http://dx.doi.org/10.15585/mmwr.mm7012a1

Freeman, A. M., & Leigh, T. R. (2021). *Viral pneumonia.* In: *StatPearls.* Treasure Island, FL: StatPearls Publishing. Retrieved from https://www.ncbi.nlm.nih.gov/books/NBK513286/

Gilbert, D. N., Chambers, H.F., Saag, M. S., Pavia, A. T. He, & Boucher, H. W. (2021). *Sanford guide to antimicrobial therapy.* Sperryville, VA: Antimicrobial Therapy, Inc.

Global Initiative For Chronic Obstructive Lung Disease (GOLD). (2022). *Global strategy for the diagnosis, management, and prevention of chronic obstructive pulmonary disease: 2022 report.* Retrieved from https://goldcopd.org/2022-gold-reports/

Global Initiative for Asthma (GINA). Global Strategy for Asthma Management and Prevention. (2022). Retrieved from https://ginasthma.org/wp-content/uploads/2022/05/GINA-Main-Report-2022-FINAL-22-05-03-WMS.pdf

Hay Jr. W. W., Levin M. J., Abzug M. J., & Bunik M. (2020). Current diagnosis & treatment: Pediatrics. (25th ed.). New York, NY: McGraw Hill. Retrieved from https://accessmedicine.mhmedical.com/content.aspx?bookid=2815&sectionid=244254196

Kathuria, H., Hollingsworth, H. M., Vilvendhan, R., & Reardon, C. (2020). Management of life-threatening hemoptysis. *Journal of Intensive Care, 8*(23). Retrieved from https://doi.org/10.1186/s40560-020-00441-8

Kimberlin, D. W., Barnett, E. D., Lynfield, R., & Sawyer, M. (2021). *Red book: 2021–2024 report of the committee on infectious disease* (32nd ed.). Itaska, IL: American Academy of Pediatrics.

Kinkade, S., & Long, N. A., (2016). Acute bronchitis. *American Academy of Family Physicians, 94*(7), 560–565.

Metlay, J. P., Waterer, G. W., Long, A. C., Anzueto, A., Brozek, J., Crothers, K., Cooley, L. A., Dean, N. C., Fine, M. J., Flanders, S. A., Griffin, M. R., Metersky, M. L., Musher, D. M., Restrepo, M. I., & Whitney, C. G. (2019). Diagnosis and treatment of adults with community-acquired pneumonia: An official clinical practice guideline of the American Thoracic Society and Critical Care Medicine. *American Journal of Respiratory Critical Care Medicine, 200*(7), e45–e67. https://doi.org/10.1164/rccm.201908-1581ST

Musher, D. M., & Thorner, A. R. (2014). Community-acquired pneumonia. *New England Journal of Medicine, 371*(17), 1619–1628.

National Cancer Institute. (2022a). *Non–small cell lung cancer treatment (PDQ)—Health professionals version.* Retrieved from https://www.cancer.gov/types/lung/hp/non-small-cell-lung-treatment-pdq

National Cancer Institute. (2022). *Small cell lung cancer treatment (PDQ)—Health professionals' version.* https://www.cancer.gov/types/lung/hp/small-cell-lung-treatment-pdq

National Heart, Lung, and Blood Institute. (2020). *2020 Focused updates to the asthma management guidelines: A Report from the National Asthma Education and Prevention Program Coordinating Committee Expert Panel Working Group.* Retrieved from https://www.nhlbi.nih.gov/health-topics/all-publications-and-resources/2020-focused-updates-asthma-management-guidelines

National Lung Screening Trial Research Team. (2011). Reduced lung-cancer mortality with low-dose computed tomographic screening. *New England Journal of Medicine, 365*(5), 395–409.

Pahal, P., Rajasurya, V., & Sharma, S. (2021). Typical bacterial pneumonia. In *StatPearls.* StatPearls Publishing. https://www.ncbi.nlm.nih.gov/books/NBK534295/

Papadakis M. A., & McPhee S. J., & Rabow M. W., & McQuaid K. R. (2022). *Current medical diagnosis & treatment 2022.* McGraw Hill. https://accessmedicine.mhmedical.com/content.aspx?bookid=3081&sectionid=258579269

Piedro, P. A., & Stark, A. R. (2022). Bronchiolitis in infants and children: Clinical features and diagnosis. *UpToDate.* Retrieved from https://www.uptodate.com/contents/bronchiolitis-in-infants-and-children-clinical-features-and diagnosis?search=bronchiolitis%20incidence&source=search_result&selectedTitle=1~150&usage_type=default&display_rank=1

Ralston, S. L., Lieberthal, A. S., Meissner, H. C., Alverson, B. K., Baley, J.E., Gadomski, A. M., Johnson, D. W., Light, M. J., Maraqa, N. F., Mendonca, E. A., Phelan, K. J., Zorc, J. J., Stanko-Lopp, D., Brown, M. A., Nathanson, I., Rosenblum, E., Sayles, S., & Hernandez-Cancio, S. (2014.) Clinical practice guideline: The diagnosis, management, and prevention of bronchiolitis. *American Academy of Pediatrics, 134*(5):e1474.

Rodriguez-Molinero, A., Narvaiza, L., Ruiz, J., & Galvez-Barron, C. (2013). Normal respiratory rate and peripheral blood oxygen saturation in the older adult population. *Journal of the American Geriatrics Society, 61*(12), 2238–2240.

Sattar, S. B., & Sharma, S. (2021). *Bacterial pneumonia.* In *StatPearls.* StatPearls Publishing; https://www.ncbi.nlm.nih.gov/books/NBK513321/

Sung H., Ferlay J., Siegel R. L., Laversanne M., Soerjomataram I., Jemal A., & Bray F. (2021). Global cancer statistics 2020: GLOBOCAN estimates of incidence and mortality worldwide for 36 cancers in 185 countries. *Cancer Journal for Clinicians, 71*(3), 209–249.

Woods, C. R. (2022). Croup: Clinical features, evaluation, and diagnosis. *UpToDate.* Retrieved from https://www.uptodate.com/contents/croup-clinical-features-evaluation-and-diagnosis?search=croup&source=search_result&selectedTitle=2~78&usage_type=default&display_rank=2#H4

World Health Organization (WHO). (2018). *Global tuberculosis report 2018.* Retrieved from https://www.who.int/tb/publications/global_report/en/

CHAPTER 8

CARDIOVASCULAR DISORDERS

Mary Elizabeth Duffy, DNP, RN, FNP-BC, ACNP-BC, DCC

General Approach

- Heart disease and stroke continue to be the leading causes of death in the United States for both men and women.
- Heart disease was the cause of death for 647,457 people, 23% overall deaths, in 2017 (NHANES, 2019)
- Primary and secondary prevention strategies are essential to reduce the risk of heart disease and stroke. Identification of high-risk patients through screening is critical to provide preventive education, early treatment, and appropriate referral.
- Clinicians should refer to evidence-based national guidelines for risk assessment, screening, and goal-directed cardiac therapy at the ACC (American College of Cardiology) https://www.acc.org/guidelines#/tab1 and AHA (American Heart Association) https://www.heart.org/en/news/guidelines-resource-center
- Clinicians should use evidence-based tools such as the Atherosclerotic Cardiovascular Disease (ASCVD) Risk Estimator Plus Calculator at https://tools.acc.org/ASCVD-Risk-Estimator-Plus/#!/calculate/estimate/ to identify patients at elevated risk who might benefit from treatment.
- Patients should be assessed according to risk stratification and treated to obtain optimal risk reduction with individualized drug therapy guided by each patient's clinical profile.
- Evidence-based blood pressure recommendations from the ACC/AHA can be found at https://www.acc.org/latest-in-cardiology/ten-points-to-remember/2017/11/09/11/41/2017-guideline-for-high-blood-pressure-in-adults https://www.acc.org/~/media/Non-Clinical/Files-PDFs-Excel-MS-Word-etc/Guidelines/2017/Guidelines_Made_Simple_2017_HBP.pdf
- For managing blood cholesterol, clinicians should refer to the 2018 AHA/ACC/AACVPR/AAPA/ABC/ACPM/ADA/AGS/APhA/ASPC/NLA/PCNA Guideline on the Management of Blood Cholesterol: A Report of the American College of Cardiology/American Heart Association Task Force on Clinical Practice Guidelines at https://www.ahajournals.org/doi/10.1161/CIR.0000000000000625

- Clinicians must assess each patient with chest pain and determine whether the condition is life-threatening or safe to manage on an outpatient basis.
- Nonpharmacologic measures are often effective; educate patients to modify lifestyle risk factors.
- Adherence can be a major problem because of health beliefs, cost of medications, side effects, dosing regimens, and difficulty making lifestyle changes; assess individual reported challenges to personalize and simplify treatment plans.
- Providers reduce health disparities and the risk of heart disease by increasing cultural sensitivity and awareness of implicit bias. For more information see the ACC guidelines for implicit bias (Ross, 2020).
- Providers stay up to date on stroke management guidelines at https://professional.heart.org/en/guidelines-and-statements (see Chapter 15: Neurologic Disorders)
- Clinicians should consider cardiovascular disease potential in children and apply the 2011 Integrated Guidelines for Cardiovascular Health and Risk Reduction in Children and Adolescents, which are found here: https://www.nhlbi.nih.gov/health-topics/integrated-guidelines-for-cardiovascular-health-and-risk-reduction-in-children-and-adolescents https://pubmed.ncbi.nlm.nih.gov/30798614/
- High-risk pediatric patients require risk reduction by specialists (de Ferranti et al, 2019).

Red Flags

- *Chest pain* should be triaged and evaluated promptly to exclude any life-threatening conditions. An immediate brief history will include age; past medical history focused on cardiac and pulmonary problems; and onset, location, radiation, quality, intensity, and duration of pain. Determine associated symptoms, relieving and aggravating factors, pattern of pain, risk factors for cardiac disease, and family history of hypertension or cardiac disease. Assess vital signs and heart and lung sounds, obtain 12-lead electrocardiography (ECG) and pulse oximetry, and integrate assessment findings and risk factors to determine the best management plan. Refer for emergent care if indicated.
- If patient has right-sided ECG changes, severe anemia, or hypersensitivity, *do not* give nitroglycerin.
- Nitroglycerin should not be given to someone who has recently received a phosphodiesterase-5 (PDE-5) inhibitor (i.e., sildenafil, vardenafil, or tadalafil)
- Patients with myocardial infarction (MI) may present with
  - ◊ severe ischemic pain lasting more than 20–30 minutes;
  - ◊ pain is not relieved with nitroglycerin; and

- ◊ may be accompanied by nausea, vomiting, anxiety, diaphoresis, pre-syncope, syncope, and dyspnea. (MI patients may also have atypical presentation with pain in the arm, jaw, neck, or back without chest pain. Atypical presentation in women includes fatigue without pain.)

- ♦ If there is an acute episode of chest pain, administer oxygen and nitroglycerin (if no contraindication), call 911, and transport to emergency facility. For nonacute episodes, consult with a physician, refer to a cardiologist, or pursue workup based on history and physical.

- ♦ Sudden, spontaneous tachycardia of 140–220 beats per minute is known as *paroxysmal atrial tachycardia* (PAT) and may occur in healthy individuals, older adults, those with chronic obstructive pulmonary disease (COPD), and as a sign of digitalis toxicity.
  - ◊ Patients may report that the tachycardia starts and ends abruptly, lasts minutes to several hours, and may be accompanied by anxiety, dizziness, mild chest pain, and shortness of breath.
  - ◊ Rhythm is regular and ECG shows P waves characteristically different from before it started. If asymptomatic and nonrecurrent in healthy individuals, it does not need treatment.
  - ◊ If of long duration and symptomatic, patient should be referred to the emergency department (ED) for treatment. If recurrent, refer to a cardiologist.

- ♦ Signs and symptoms associated with pneumothorax or pulmonary emboli include sudden onset of chest pain, hypotension, syncope, dyspnea, tachypnea, and tachycardia. If patient has a risk for thrombophlebitis (recent surgery, immobility, oral contraceptive use, or a recent fracture), consider pulmonary emboli. Some patients with pulmonary emboli may be asymptomatic. Acute presentation requires transfer to an emergency facility.

- ♦ A hypertensive patient with sudden onset of knife-like or tearing pain in the chest or upper abdomen may have a dissecting aneurysm. Initiate emergency transport system immediately. ***Do not*** give aspirin if you suspect dissecting aneurysm.

- ♦ When using statin medications and fibric acids, be alert for signs and symptoms of rhabdomyolysis (muscle pain or weakness) that can lead to renal failure.

- ♦ Metabolic syndrome, with its constellation of hypertension, diabetes mellitus, hyperlipidemia, and abdominal obesity, is associated with increased risk for heart disease and stroke.

HEART SOUNDS

- ♦ Evaluation of heart sounds is a vital part of the assessment of any patient with a cardiovascular problem.

- Bell of stethoscope: low tones, that is: S3, S4, mitral stenosis heard best
- Diaphragm of stethoscope: mid- to high-pitched tones heard best, that is: mitral regurgitation, aortic stenosis
- S_1 = (Systole), "lub"
  - closure of the tricuspid and mitral valves (atrioventricular [AV] valves);
  - heard best at the apex, left fifth intercostal space (ICS), midclavicular line at the left lower sternal border (LLSB)
- S_2 = (Diastole) "dub"
  - closure of the aortic and pulmonary valves (semilunar valves);
  - best heard at the second left ICS close to the sternal border
  - Normal splitting of S_2 during inspiration is due to a greater negative pressure in the thoracic cavity = increased systemic venous return = increased blood volume in the right ventricle (RV) = delayed closure of the pulmonary valve
  - Abnormal splitting of S_2 (wide splitting, narrow splitting, or single S_2) is seen in conditions where the RV ejection time is prolonged, that is: atrial septal defect (ASD), pulmonary stenosis (PS), right bundle branch block [RBBB]), and the pulmonary valve closes early (pulmonary hypertension), or where only one semilunar valve is present (pulmonary atresia, aortic atresia, truncus arteriosus)
- S_3 = low-frequency sound heard early in diastole; related to the rapid filling of the ventricles
  - Heard best at apex or LLSB using the bell, as it is a low-pitched sound
  - With tachycardia, forms a "Kentucky" ventricular gallop
  - May be normal in children and during pregnancy and in some athletes (over 35 years of age)
  - S_3 age 40 or older, a loud S_3 is abnormal (usually audible in conditions with dilated ventricles and decreased compliance)
- S_4 = low-frequency sound heard late in diastole
  - Rare in infants and children
  - Always pathological; seen in conditions with decreased ventricular compliance, with left ventricular hypertrophy (LVH)
  - Best heard at the apex using the bell as it is a low-pitched sound
  - With tachycardia, forms a "Tennessee" gallop

Common Cardiovascular Disorders

HYPERTENSION

Description

In 2017, Hypertension is defined by the American College of Cardiology/American Heart Association (ACC/AHA) as blood pressure (BP) above 130/80 mmHg (see Table 8–1). Majority (90%–95%) have primary (or essential) hypertension, whereas 5%–10% have secondary hypertension. Correct BP measurement requires:

- Avoid smoking or caffeine for more than 30 minutes prior to BP measurement.
- Do not cross legs.
- Initial visit measure BP in both arms
- Have patient seated comfortably with back supported, feet on the floor and arm supported in horizontal position.
- Rest 5 minutes prior to BP measurement.
- Take 2 or more measurements per visit, more than 2 minutes apart
- BP cuff placed at heart level
- Use appropriate cuff size
- Use an average of more than 2 readings taken on more than 2 occasions to estimate BP level

Etiology

- Hypertension is due to an increase in peripheral arterial resistance.
- Theories of causation include impaired renin-angiotensin cascade, sympathetic nervous system hyperactivity, defect in natriuresis (sodium excretion), and elevated intracellular calcium (excess arterial constriction).
- Primary hypertension is usually idiopathic or may be due to renal retention of salt and water, increased endogenous pressure activity, or both. Essential hypertension accounts for 90%–95% of high blood pressure (HBP).
- Secondary hypertension is caused by renovascular disease, vascular problems such as aortic coarctation or renal artery stenosis, endocrine dysfunction such as in Cushing's syndrome and pheochromocytoma, neurologic disorders, and certain medications (oral contraceptives, corticosteroids, sympathomimetics).

TABLE 8–1.
ACC/AHA 2017 CLASSIFICATION OF BLOOD PRESSURE FOR ADULTS AND RECOMMENDATIONS FOR TREATMENT FOR HYPERTENSION

BP CLASSIFICATION	RECOMMENDATIONS
Normal Less than 120/80	Promote healthy lifestyle, reassess BP every year
Elevated 120–129/ less than 80	Lifestyle modification Reassess BP in 3–6 months
Stage 1 SBP 130–139 or DBP 80–89	LOW RISK; No ASCVD and 10-year CVD risk less than 10%, Lifestyle modification follow-up BP in 3–6 months, if remains elevated consider initiating drug therapy HIGH RISK; ASCVD or 10-year CVD risk greater than10%, Lifestyle modification and initiate drug therapy, reassess BP in 1 month and if at goal, reassess in 3–6 months, if not at goal consider adding another BP lowering medication Thiazide-type diuretic for most; may consider ACEI, ARB, BB, CCB or combination
Stage 2* SBP 140+ or DBP 90+	Lifestyle modification and medications (usually thiazide-type diuretic and ACEI, ARB, BB, or CCB) Reassess BP in 1 month. If at goal, reassess every 3–6 months, and if not, verify adherence to medication regimen and consider increasing medication therapy
Hypertensive Urgency SBP above 180+ and/or DBP above 120 ***without*** end-organ damage	May be due to noncompliance with medications for hypertension. Restart or escalate hypertension medication therapy Reassess BP in 48–72 hours
Hypertensive Emergency SBP above 180+ and/or DBP above 120 ***with*** end-organ damage	Refer immediately, admit to ICU See (Whelton, 2017) for IV antihypertensive recommendations Reduce BP by maximum 25% over first hour; then to 160/100 mmHg over following 2—6 hours, then to normal over 24–48 hours

*If there is a disparity in category between the systolic and diastolic pressures, the higher value determines the stage.

ACEI = angiotensin-converting enzyme (ACE) inhibitor, ARB = angiotensin II receptor blocker, BB = beta-blocker, CCB = calcium channel blocker, DBP = diastolic blood pressure, ICU = intensive care unit, SBP, systolic blood pressure.

Avoid combining ACEI with ARB.

Adapted from Whelton, P., Carey, R., & Aronow, W., et al. (2017). 2017 ACC/AHA/AAPA/ABC/ACPM/AGS/APhA/ASH/ASPC/NMA/PCNA Guideline for the Prevention, Detection, Evaluation, and Management of High Blood Pressure in Adults: Executive Summary. *Journal of the American College of Cardiology, 71*(*19*), 2199–2269. https://doi.org/10.1016/j.jacc.2017.11.005

Incidence and Demographics (CDC, 2020)

- Hypertension is a risk factor for heart disease and stroke, the leading causes of death in the United States.
- Essential hypertension was the primary diagnosis for 33.6 million visits to physician offices and 1.1 million visits to emergency departments.
- Hypertension was the primary or contributing cause in more than 670,000 deaths in the United States (CDC, 2020)
- Approximately 47% of persons, or 116 million people, in the United States have hypertension.
- Approximately 24% of persons with hypertension have their condition under control.
- About 37 million adults (45%) in the United States with uncontrolled hypertension have a BP of 140/90 mmHg or higher.
- The cost to the United States of high blood pressure is about $131 billion each year.
- Incidence of high blood pressure in the United States adult population
    1. Men (50%) versus women (44%).
    2. Non-Hispanic Black adults (56%),
    3. non-Hispanic White adults (48%),
    4. non-Hispanic Asian adults (46%),
    5. Hispanic adults (39%).

Risk Factors

- *Modifiable Risk Factors*
- Cigarette smoking and/or secondhand smoke
- Dyslipidemia—high levels of low-density lipoprotein (LDL) or triglycerides, low levels of high-density lipoprotein (HDL)
- Diabetes mellitus
- Overweight/obese
- Unhealthy diet
- Sedentary lifestyle, physical inactivity
- *Relatively Fixed Risk Factors*
- Chronic kidney disease (CKD)

- Male sex
- Increased age
- Family history
- Obstructive sleep apnea
- Psychosocial stress
- Low socioeconomic/educational status

Prevention and Screening

- Patient education for prevention of risk factors, lifestyle modification recommendations
- Per the National Heart, Lung, and Blood Institute (NHLBI, 2013) routine BP screening should begin at age 3
- Screening every 3–5 years for low-risk adults 18–39 years of age with normal blood pressure
- If have risk factors for hypertension, screen at least twice a year
- Use the Atherosclerotic Cardiovascular Risk Screening (ASCVD) tool to calculate 10-year risk estimate for cardiovascular disease and treatment guidelines at https://tools.acc.org/ASCVD-Risk-Estimator-Plus/#!/calculate/estimate/

Assessment

History

- Usually asymptomatic in essential hypertension; "silent killer"
- Occipital headaches can occur upon awakening with severe hypertension, dizziness, rarely epistaxis
- Somnolence, confusion, visual disturbances, nausea, vomiting (hypertensive encephalopathy)
- Personal history for risk factors; family history of hypertension
- Past medical history for comorbid conditions such as gout or sexual dysfunction, or for effects on target organs

Physical Exam

- Elevated blood pressure (usually the only sign)
- Body mass index (BMI) may be over 30; children may be obese or thin with failure to thrive
- Abdominal obesity is defined as waist circumference
  - greater than 40 inches (102 cm) in men, South Asian male greater than 35 inches (90 cm) and
  - greater than 35 inches (88 cm) in women, South Asian female greater than 31 inches (80 cm)
- S_4 gallop, possible displaced point of maximal intensity (PMI) because of ventricular hypertrophy
- Renal artery bruit, carotid bruit, hepatosplenomegaly, edema, decreased peripheral pulses, funduscopic changes (such as AV nicking) with secondary hypertension; or target organ damage—angina/MI, transient ischemic attack (TIA), stroke, peripheral arterial disease

Diagnostic Studies

- Laboratory tests:
  - Urinalysis
  - Complete blood count (CBC), blood urea nitrogen (BUN)
  - Creatinine, calcium
  - Lipid profile
  - Serum electrolytes
  - Estimated glomerular filtration rate (eGFR)
  - Glucose
  - Thyroid-stimulating hormone (TSH)
  - ECG
- Treatment resistant hypertension, young age, acromegaly, kidney disease, sleep apnea may indicate secondary hypertension
- For secondary hypertension clinicians test for underlying cause (see Table 8–2 for specific tests).

TABLE 8–2.
DIAGNOSTIC SCREENING TESTS FOR CAUSES OF SECONDARY HYPERTENSION

SUSPECTED HYPERTENSION CAUSE	TEST
Renal Parenchymal disease	Renal ultrasound, estimated glomerular filtration rate (eGFR)
Coarctation of the aorta	Echocardiogram
Cushing's syndrome and other glucocorticoid excess states including chronic steroid therapy	Dexamethasone suppression test
Drug or alcohol induced	Urinary drug screening
Pheochromocytoma	24-hour urinary metanephrines or plasma metanephrines
Primary aldosteronism and other mineralocorticoid excess states	Plasma aldosterone/renin ratio with correction of hypokalemia and withdrawal of aldosterone antagonists for at least 4–6 weeks
Renovascular disease	Doppler flow study; magnetic resonance angiography, abdominal computerized tomography (CT)
Obstructive sleep apnea	Berlin questionnaire, Epworth Sleepiness Score, Sleep study with overnight oximetry
Thyroid/parathyroid disease	Thyroid-stimulating hormone (TSH), free thyroxine, calcium, serum parathyroid hormone (PTH)

Adapted from Whelton, P., Carey, R., & Aronow, W., et al. (2017) 2017 ACC/AHA/AAPA/ABC/ACPM/AGS/APhA/ASH/ASPC/NMA/PCNA Guideline for the Prevention, Detection, Evaluation, and Management of High Blood Pressure in Adults. *Journal of American College of Cardiology, 71*(19) e127–e248. https://doi.org/10.1016/j.jacc.2017.11.006

Differential Diagnosis

Essential versus secondary causes of hypertension

- Pregnancy
- Renal artery stenosis
- Renal failure
- Renal parenchymal disease (polycystic or dysplastic kidneys)

- Coarctation of aorta
- Patent ductus arteriosus
- Pheochromocytoma
- Cushing's disease
- Hyperaldosteronism
- Thyroid disease
- Increased intracranial pressure
- Hypervolemia

Management

Nonpharmacologic Treatment

- Nonpharmacologic lifestyle interventions recommended for all stages of hypertension (see Box 8–1)
- Avoid oral contraceptives in at-risk individuals.
- DASH diet
- Avoid stimulant-containing decongestants.
- Adequate sleep, recommended adults sleep 7 to 9 hours/night
- Monitor for target organ damage (TOD).
- Advise 150 minutes/week of moderate aerobic activity, that is: brisk walking, jogging, swimming, cycling
- Adults with Stage 1 hypertension who are at low risk (ASCVD 10-year risk is less than 10%), lifestyle modification is recommended with repeat BP in 3 to 6 months

Pharmacologic Treatment

(see TABLE 8–3)

- Children (refer to specialist for treatment)
- Adults with Stage 1 hypertension who are at high risk (ASCVD 10-year risk is 10% or higher), lifestyle modification plus medication treatment is recommended with repeat BP in 1 month after initial diagnosis

BOX 8–1. ACC/AHA NONPHARMACOLOGICAL INTERVENTIONS/LIFESTYLE RECOMMENDATIONS FOR HTN TREATMENT AND PREVENTION

- Stop smoking.
- Lose weight if overweight or obese and maintain ideal body weight (body mass index 18.5 to 24.9 kg/m2)
- Reduce intake of dietary saturated fat and cholesterol
- Limit alcohol intake to no more than:
    - men <2 drinks daily (28 g of pure alcohol), women <1 drink daily (14 g of pure alcohol)
    - a standard drink is approximately 14 g of pure alcohol, which is equivalent to
        - either one 12 oz beer (5% alcohol) or
        - 5 oz wine (approximately 12% alcohol) or
        - 1.5 oz of distilled spirits (approximately 40% alcohol)
- Moderate to vigorous aerobic activity 150 minutes per week. Aerobic physical activity such as brisk walking 30 minutes per day
- DASH (Dietary Approaches to Stop Hypertension) diet, reduce sodium intake to <1,500 mg sodium. If recommended goals for sodium are not attainable, reduce intake by at least 1,000 mg/day, which lowers BP and reduces CVD by approximately 30%.
- Maintain adequate intake of dietary potassium (approximately 3,500–5,000 mg/per day), calcium (approximately 1,000 mg per day), and magnesium (300 mg per day).

- ♦ Pharmacologic treatment is recommended in Stage 1 hypertension () for
    - ◊ high-risk adults with Stage 1 hypertension who have preexisting CVD or an estimated 10-year ASCVD risk of at least 10%,
    - ◊ The BP threshold for drug treatment in Stage 1 hypertension for high-risk adults is BP of 130/80 mmHg or higher
- ♦ Pharmacologic therapy is NOT recommended in Stage 1 hypertension for
    - ◊ lower-risk adults without preexisting CVD and an estimated 10-year ASCVD risk less than 10%
    - ◊ The BP threshold for drug treatment in Stage 1 hypertension for lower-risk adults without preexisting CVD and an estimated 10-year ASCVD risk less than 10%, is 140/90 mmHg or higher.

TABLE 8–3.
EVIDENCE-BASED ANTIHYPERTENSIVE MEDICATIONS AND DOSING FOR HIGH-RISK ADULTS WITH STAGE 1 HYPERTENSION AND ADULTS WITH STAGE 2 HYPERTENSION

DRUG	DAILY DOSAGE	COMMENTS	SIDE EFFECTS
Primary Agents			
THIAZIDE (TYPE) DIURETICS			
Hydrochlorothiazide (HCTZ) ChlorthalidoneIndapamide (Lozol) Metolazone	25–50 mg once daily 12.5–25 mg once daily 1.25–2.5 mg once daily 2.5–5 mg once daily	Chlorthalidone preferred due to trial supporting decrease CVD Use these agents with caution in persons with gout	Anorexia, nausea, vomiting, cramping due to potassium and possibly sodium depletion; increased glucose, uric acid levels, chlorthalidone may cause gynecomastia
ACE INHIBITORS (ACEIs)			
Lisinopril (Prinivil, Zestril) Benazepril Fosinopril Quinapril Captopril (Capoten) Enalapril (Vasotec) Moexipril Perindopril Ramipril Trandolapril	10–40 mg once daily 10–40 mg 1–2 times/day 10–40 mg once daily 10–80 mg 1–2 times/day 12.5–150 mg 2–three times/day 5–40 mg 1–2 times/day 7.5–30 mg 1–2 times/day 4–16 mg once daily 2.5–20 mg 1–2 times/day 1–4 mg once daily	DO NOT use in combination with direct renin inhibitors or ARBs AVOID in pregnancy DO NOT use if history of angioedema on ACEI Persons with severe renal artery stenosis (RAS) at increased risk for acute renal failure	Hyperkalemia, especially if have CKD or taking potassium supplements

Continued

TABLE 8–3.
(CONTINUED)

DRUG	DAILY DOSAGE	COMMENTS	SIDE EFFECTS
ANGIOTENSIN RECEPTOR BLOCKERS			
Eprosartan (Teveten) Azilsartan Candesartan (Atacand) Irbesartan (Avapro) Losartan (Cozaar) Olmesartan Telmisartan Valsartan (Diovan)	600–800 mg 1–2 times/day 40–80 mg once daily 8–32 mg once daily 150–300 mg once daily 50–100 mg 1–2 times/day 20–40 mg once daily 20–80 mg once daily 80–320 mg once daily	Do not use in combination with ACEI or direct renin inhibitor Avoid in pregnancy If patient has angioedema from ACEI, may start an ARB 6 weeks after ACEI was discontinued	Hyperkalemia increased risk if patient has CKD, or takes potassium supplements or is on potassium-sparing medications Severe bilateral renal artery stenosis increases risk of acute kidney failure
CALCIUM CHANNEL BLOCKERS *Dihydropyridines*			
Amlodipine (Norvasc) Felodipine Isradipine Nicardipine SR Nifedipine LA Nisoldipine	2.5–10 mg once daily 2.5–10 mg once daily 5–10 mg 2 times/day 60–120 mg 2 times/day 30–90 mg once daily 17–34 mg once daily	Avoid use in persons with heart failure with reduced ejection fraction (HFrEF); but if necessary, may use amlodipine or felodipine	Peripheral edema (more common in women), nausea, headache, constipation
CALCIUM CHANNEL BLOCKERS *Non-dihydropyridines*			
Diltiazem ER (Cardizem) Verapamil IRVerapamil SR Verapamil delayed onset ER	120–360 mg once daily 120–360 mg three times/day 120–360 mg 1–2 times/day 100–300 mg once daily	DO NOT use if person has HFrEF Monitor for drug reactions with diltiazem and verapamil (cytochrome P450 3A4 [CYP3A4] major substrate and moderate inhibitor)	Avoid using with beta blockers as increases risk for heart block and bradycardia

Secondary Agents			
LOOP DIURETICS			
Bumetanide Furosemide Torsemide	0.5–2 mg 2 times/day 20–80 mg 2 times/day 5–10 mg once daily	Preferred diuretic for persons with moderate to severe CKD (GFR less than 30 mL/min) and/or symptomatic heart failure	Hypovolemia, hypokalemia, dehydration, hyperuricemia
POTASSIUM SPARING DIURETICS			
Amiloride Triamterene	5–10 mg 1–2 times/day 50–100 mg 1–2 times/day	Minimally effective antihypertensive monotherapy agents Avoid in person with severe CKD (eGFR less than 45 mL/min) In patients on thiazide monotherapy with hypokalemia, consider adding a potassium-sparing diuretic in combination with a thiazide Side effects: hypokalemia, hyponatremia, dehydration	
ALDOSTERONE ANTAGONIST DIURETICS			
Eplerenone Spironolactone	50–100 mg 1–2 times/day 25–100 mg once daily	Preferred agents in primary aldosteronism and resistant hypertension. Spironolactone is associated with greater risk of gynecomastia and impotence as compared with eplerenone. This is common add-on therapy in resistant hypertension. Avoid use with potassium supplements, other potassium-sparing diuretics, or significant renal dysfunction. Eplerenone often requires daily dosing two times/day for adequate BP lowering. Side effects: hypokalemia, hyponatremia, dehydration	

Continued

TABLE 8–3.
(CONTINUED)

DRUG	DAILY DOSAGE	COMMENTS	SIDE EFFECTS
BETA BLOCKERS—CARDIOSELECTIVE			
Atenolol Betexolol Bisoprolol Metoprolol tartrate (Lopressor) Metoprolol succinate	25–100 mg twice/day 5–20 mg once daily 2.5–10 mg once daily 100–200 mg twice/day 50–200 mg once daily	Not first line agent; target pts with chronic heart failure (CHF), coronary artery disease (CAD), post MI. Possible side effects: bradycardia, depression, fatigue, exercise intolerance, asthma	
BETA BLOCKERS—CARDIOSELECTIVE AND VASODILATORY			
Nebivolol	4–40 mg once daily	Causes nitric oxide–induced vasodilation Avoid stopping abruptly	
BETA BLOCKERS—NON-CARDIOSELECTIVE			
Nadolol Propranolol IR Propranolol LA	40–120 mg once daily 80–160 mg twice/day 80–160 mg once daily	Avoid in persons with reactive airway disease. Avoid stopping abruptly	
BETA BLOCKERS—INTRINSIC SYMPATHOMIMETIC ACTIVITY			
Acebutolol Penbutolol Pindolol	200–800 mg twice/day 10–40 mg once daily 10–60 mg twice/day	Avoid, especially in persons with heart failure or ischemic heart disease Avoid stopping abruptly	
BETA BLOCKERS—COMBINED ALPHA- AND BETA-RECEPTOR			
Carvedilol Carvedilol phosphate Labetolol	12.5–50 mg twice/day 20–80 mg once daily 200–800 mg twice/day	Avoid stopping abruptly In persons with HFrEF, Carvedilol is preferred	

DIRECT RENIN INHIBITOR			
Aliskiren	150–300 mg once daily	DO NOT use in combination with ARBs, ACEIs. Avoid in pregnancy. May cause hyperkalemia in those on potassium-sparing diuretics, potassium supplements, or with CKD. May cause ARF in those with bilateral renal artery stenosis	
ALPHA-1 BLOCKERS			
Doxazosin Prazosin Terazosin	1–16 mg once daily 2–20 mg 2–three times/day 1–20 mg 1–twice/day	May cause orthostatic hypotension especially in older adults. In those with benign prostatic hypertrophy (BPH) may consider as second-line agent	
CENTRAL ALPHA$_2$ AGONIST AND OTHER CENTRALLY ACTING DRUGS			
Clonidine oral Clonidine patch Methyldopa Guanfacine	0.1–0.8 mg twice/day 0.1–0.3 mg once weekly 250–1,000 mg twice/day 0.5–2 mg once daily	Due to significant CNS adverse effects used as last line, especially in older adults Avoid abrupt cessation of clonidine and taper to avoid rebound hypertension	
DIRECT VASODILATORS			
Hydralazine Minoxidil	100–200 mg 2–three times/day 5–100 mg 1–three times/day	May cause reflex tachycardia and fluid retention; use with a beta blocker and diuretic.	

ACEIs = angiotensin-converting enzyme inhibitors

Adapted from Whelton, P., Carey, R., & Aronow, W., et al. (2018). 2017 ACC/AHA/AAPA/ABC/ACPM/AGS/APhA/ASH/ASPC/NMA/PCNA Guideline for the Prevention, Detection, Evaluation, and Management of High Blood Pressure in Adults. *Journal of the American College of Cardiology, 71*(19) e127–e248. https://doi.org/10.1016/j.jacc.2017.11.006

- Recommended drug classes for compelling indications as listed below include:
  - Diabetes: ARB, thiazide diuretics, dihydropyridine CCB
  - CKD (eGFR less than 60 mL/min): ACEI, ARB
  - Heart failure with reduced ejection fraction (EF): diuretics, ARNI, ACEI, ARB, BB
  - Post-acute myocardial infarction: BB, ACEI, aldosterone
  - Thiazides or CCBs may be more effective for African Americans, even with diabetes mellitus

How Long to Treat

- Treatment is usually lifelong

Special Considerations

- Start with low doses for geriatric patients to avoid serious side effects. Consider starting initial monotherapy with low dose thiazide diuretic, an ACEI or ARB, or a dihydropyridine CCB.
- Older adults are at high risk for orthostatic hypotension; monitor BP in supine and standing before and after initiation of medication therapy, assess for polypharmacy
- Pregnancy: can continue drug(s) used before pregnancy, except ACEIs, ARBs, and direct renin inhibitors; beta-blockers may cause growth retardation in early pregnancy; if hypertension develops during pregnancy (after the first 20 weeks of pregnancy), use or transition to labetolol, nifedipine, or methyldopa (Whelton, 2017).
- ACEI causes dry cough in approximately 5% to 20% of persons and is more common in women

When to Consult, Refer, Hospitalize

- Consult with a physician or specialist when initiating drug treatment for a child with hypertension.
- Refer as needed for evaluation and treatment of secondary causes of hypertension.
- Refer to a specialist (nephrologist, cardiologist, ophthalmologist) for end-organ damage.
- Consult physician when no response to first-line therapy, escalating hypertension.
- Refer immediately for hospital admission in hypertension emergency (hypertensive encephalopathy, severe preeclampsia/eclampsia, cerebral hemorrhage, dissecting aortic aneurysm, unstable angina, MI, pulmonary embolism (PE), severe heart failure).

Follow-Up

- Frequent initial follow-up until normotensive, then routine visits every 3–6 months depending on patient clinical situation; for BP above 180 systolic or 110 diastolic, follow-up in 48 to 72 hours
- Improve adherence by keeping treatment simple and inexpensive; educate patient and family about hypertension; encourage lifestyle modification along with drug treatment.

Expected Course

- Usually requires lifelong treatment; progression depends on ability to control the disease

Complications

- TOD includes stroke, coronary heart disease, LVH, congestive heart failure, kidney failure, aortic dissection, retinopathy

DYSLIPIDEMIA

Description

- General term used to describe a variety of lipid abnormalities, including low-density lipoprotein cholesterol (LDL-C), high-density lipoprotein cholesterol (HDL-C), and triglycerides (TGs) that deviate from normal ranges and increase the risk of cardiovascular disease. Elevation in blood lipids is often due to abnormal lipid metabolism (see Table 8–4).

Etiology

- Hyperlipidemias (also called dyslipidemias) are either primary (some genetic forms) or secondary (related to fat, calorie, and alcohol intake; medication use; or caused by metabolic diseases such as hypothyroidism, diabetes mellitus, liver disease, obesity, and nephrosis).
- Serum cholesterol and its lipoprotein carriers (LDL-C, very low-density lipoprotein [VLDL], and HDL-C) are known to be a risk factor for ASCVD.
- The combination of LDL-C and VLDL-C is called non–HDL-C and is more atherogenic than either lipoprotein alone.

TABLE 8–4.
ACC/AHA CLASSIFICATION OF LIPOPROTEINS IN ADULTS

TYPE	LEVEL	RECOMMENDATION
Low-Density Lipoprotein Cholesterol (mg/dL)	<100	Optimal
	<130	Low risk, fewer than 2 risk factors
	<70	If patient has heart disease or diabetes
Total Cholesterol (mg/dL)	<200	Desirable, normal
	201–239	Borderline high
	>240	High
High-Density Lipoprotein Cholesterol (mg/dL)	>40	Men
	>50	Women
	<40	Associated with increased risk CVD, often genetic cause
	>60	Associated with decreased risk CVD
Triglycerides (mg/dL)	<150	Normal
Recommended lifestyle modifications: decrease simple carbohydrates and sugars, avoid alcohol, eat low-fat diet, fish with omega-3 (i.e., sardines, salmon) twice a week, maintain recommended BMI for height/weight, increase aerobic activity	>150	Increased CVD risk, can be due to genetic primary cause (familial hypertriglyceridemia) and/or secondary acquired disorders, i.e., metabolic syndrome, diabetes, alcohol abuse, hyperthyroidism, kidney disease, medications—anabolic steroids, isotretinoin, diuretics, second-generation antipsychotics, oral estrogens., antiretrovirals, tamoxifen, nonselective beta blockers (propranolol)—lifestyle modifications
	>500	Identify cause, no alcohol due to risk of pancreatitis Treat with fibrates, i.e., fenofibrate (Tricor), gemfibrozil (Lopid), and bezafibrate (Bezalip) High-dose statins (atorvastatin, rosuvastatin) can decrease TG level approximately 33%–50% Niacin (vitamin B3) can decrease TG level up to 40% and raise HDL up to 40% in high doses; may take with aspirin to decrease risk of niacin "flush"; take after meal start low does, and increase slowly; lifestyle modifications
	>1000	High risk of acute pancreatitis

Adapted from Grundy, S. M., et al., (2019). 2018 AHA/ACC/AACVPR/AAPA/ABC/ACPM/ADA/AGS/APhA/ASPC/NLA/PCNA Guideline on the Management of Blood Cholesterol: Executive Summary: A Report of the American College of Cardiology/American Heart Association Task Force on Clinical Practice Guidelines. *Circulation*, *139*(25), e1046–e1081. https://doi.org/10.1161/CIR.0000000000000624

- The main protein embedded in LDL-C and VLDL-C is apolipoprotein B (apoB), and like non–HDL-C, apoB is a stronger indicator of atherogenicity than LDL-C alone.
- Familial or genetic syndromes include familial hypercholesterolemia, polygenic hypercholesterolemia, familial defective apolipoprotein B-100, familial hypertriglyceridemia, familial combined hyperlipidemia, and familial hyperchylomicronemia with marked increase in triglycerides.
- Total cholesterol (TC) is influenced by 4 major classes of lipoproteins: chylomicrons, VLDL, LDL, and HDL.
  - HDL carries fat away from blood vessels and prevents or delays atherosclerosis.
  - LDL facilitates forming of cholesterol deposits in the blood vessels.
  - Isolated elevated LDL may be seen in familial hypercholesterolemia.
- Other causes include thyroid disease, Cushing's disease, hepatic disease, malignancy, and pancreatitis.

Incidence and Demographics

- During 2015 and 2018, approximately 12% of adults age 20 and older hadTC higher than 240 mg/dL, and an estimated 17% had HDL below 40 mg/dL
- Nearly 94 million adults age 20 or older in the United States haveTC levels higher than 200 mg/dL and
- Approximately 28 million adults age 20 or older in the United States haveTC levels higher than 240 mg/dL
- Almost 7% of children and adolescents in the United States have elevatedTC levels
- High cholesterol has no symptoms
- High cholesterol levels can increase a person's risk for atherosclerotic cardiovascular disease
- Incidence of high cholesterol in the United States adult population
  - non-Hispanic Asian adults (males 13%, females 10.3%),
  - Hispanic adults (males 12.4%, females 9.2%),
  - non-Hispanic White adults (males 10.1%, females 13.1%),
  - Non-Hispanic Black adults (males 9.2%, females 10.5%).
- CDC (2022) https://www.cdc.gov/cholesterol/facts.htm#:~:text=High%20total%20cholesterol%20in%20the%20United%20States&text=Nearly%2094%20million%20U.S.%20adults,levels%20above%20240%20mg%2FdL.&text=Nearly%207%25%20of%20U.S.%20children,19%20have%20high%20total%20cholesterol

Prevention and Screening

- 2018 ACC/AHA Guidelines recommend that health care providers conduct an ASCVD 10-year risk assessment (static.heart.org/riskcalc/app/index.html#!/baseline-risk) to discuss risks and treatment options with patients. The ASCVD risk calculator combines all major risk factors (high blood pressure, abnormal cholesterol, diabetes, age, race) to estimate a patient's probability for developing ASCVD
- Screen for above risk factors.
- Heart healthy lifestyle throughout the lifespan (see Box 8–2) decreases overall ASCVD risk (smoking cessation, hypertension management, weight management, increasing physical activity, and DASH, Mediterranean, or vegetarian diet).
- Treat comorbid conditions.
- Measure BP in all adults at least every 2.5 years.
- Assess dietary intake with routine evaluations.
- Measure lipid profile in adults 20 years of age and older at least every 5 years.
- Universal screening for children without risk once at age 9–11 years and again between 17 and 21 years.

Assessment

History

- Obtain history for other coronary heart disease (CHD) risk factors, family history of hyperlipidemia, dietary and alcohol intake, exercise.
- Dyslipidemia rarely produces symptoms unless there are symptoms of related diseases, reactions to medications.
- Medications such as thiazide diuretics, treatment for acute pancreatitis, hepatitis, renal disease

Physical Exam

- Xanthomas: in familial hypercholesterolemia—papules, plaques, or nodules in the tendons, eyelids, buttocks, knees, and skin folds
- Corneal arcus before age 50–60 years, and in young White people
- Obesity

BOX 8–2.

Risk-Enhancing Factors for ASCVD

- Family history of early ASCVD (men younger than 55 years, women younger than 65 years of age)
- Current high cholesterol (LDL-C 160–189 mg/dL; non-HDL-C 190–219 mg/dL)
- Persistently elevated triglyceride level (higher than 175 mg/dL)
- Metabolic syndrome
- Chronic kidney disease
- Chronic inflammatory conditions (i.e., rheumatoid arthritis, HIV, psoriasis)
- History of early menopause
- History of pre-eclampsia
- High-sensitivity C-reactive protein higher than 2.0 mg/dL
- Elevated lipoprotein A 50 mg/dL or higher or 125 nmol/L or higher
- Elevated apolipoprotein B 130 mg/dL or higher
- Ankle brachial index (ABI) below 0.9

Risk Enhancers Specific for Diabetes Mellitus

- Diabetes mellitus type 2 for more than 10 years or type 1 for more than 20 years
- Albuminuria greater than 30 µg of albumin/mg creatinine
- eGFR less than 60 mL/min/1.73 m^2
- Retinopathy
- Neuropathy
- ABI less than 0.9

Adapted from Grundy, S. M., et al., (2019). 2018 AHA/ACC/AACVPR/AAPA/ABC/ACPM/ADA/AGS/APhA/ASPC/NLA/PCNA Guideline on the Management of Blood Cholesterol: Executive Summary: A Report of the American College of Cardiology/American Heart Association Task Force on Clinical Practice Guidelines. *Circulation, 139*(25), e1046–e1081. https://doi.org/10.1161/CIR.0000000000000624

Diagnostic Studies

- Fasting fractionated lipid profile to include total cholesterol, triglycerides, HDL, LDL, VLDL, apoB
- Comprehensive metabolic panel to detect other metabolic abnormalities
- Urinalysis to detect kidney disease
- Thyroid screening: TSH, free T4 (FT4)
- Liver function tests to rule out liver disease and before starting medication
- Baseline ECG

Differential Diagnosis

- Nephrotic syndrome
- Chronic renal failure
- Diabetes mellitus
- Hypothyroidism
- Cushing's syndrome
- Chronic liver disease
- Excessive alcohol intake
- Pancreatitis
- Obesity
- Hyperuricemia
- Medications
- Pregnancy

Management

See Table 8–5

TABLE 8–5.
ACC/AHA 2018 TREATMENT GUIDELINES FOR HYPERCHOLESTEROLEMIA

RISK ASSESSMENT	LDL GOAL	TREATMENT	IF TARGET LDL NOT REACHED
VERY HIGH History of multiple major ASCVD events* or 1 major ASCVD event and multiple high-risk conditions** (10-year risk greater than 20%)	<70 mg/dL	High-intensity statin	If LDL-C level remains ≥70 mg/dL (≥1.8 mmol/L) on high-intensity statin, may add ezetimibe to maximally dosed (tolerated) statin therapy. If after adding ezetimibe to statin and LDL greater than 70, may add a PCSK9 inhibitor
HIGH RISK Severe primary hypercholesterolemia LDL-C level ≥190 mg/dL (≥4.9 mmol/L]), without calculating 10-year ASCVD risk	<100 mg/dL	High-intensity statin	If LDL-C level remains ≥100 mg/dL (≥2.6 mmol/L) on high-intensity statin, may add ezetimibe If LDL-C level on statin plus ezetimibe remains ≥100 mg/dL (≥2.6 mmol/L) and patient has multiple factors that increase subsequent risk of ASCVD events, consider adding a PCSK9 inhibitor
Adults age 40 to 75 years of age with diabetes mellitus and LDL-C ≥70 mg/dL (≥1.8 mmol/L),	<70 mg/dL	Moderate-intensity statin	
Adults with diabetes mellitus at higher risk, i.e., multiple risk factors or age 50 to 75 years,	<70mg/dL	High intensity statin	Reasonable to use a high-intensity statin to reduce the LDL-C level by ≥50%.
Adults age 40 to 75 years, NO diabetes mellitus, with LDL-C levels ≥70 mg/dL (≥1.8 mmol/L), with a 10-year ASCVD risk of ≥7.5% OR (same as above) with 10-year ASCVD risk of ≥20%	<70mg/dL	Moderate-intensity statin High-intensity statin	May consider coronary artery calcium (CAC) prior to initiating statin therapy if uncertain

Continued

TABLE 8–5.
(CONTINUED)

RISK ASSESSMENT	LDL GOAL	TREATMENT	IF TARGET LDL NOT REACHED
INTERMEDIATE RISK Adults 40 to 75 years of age NO diabetes mellitus, LDL-C levels ≥70 mg/dL to 189 mg/dL (≥1.8–4.9 mmol/L), 10-year risk of 7.5% to 19.9%, with +risk-enhancing factors favor	<160 mg/dL	Moderate-intensity statin	♦ Consider CAC if uncertain about starting statin therapy ♦ If CAC is zero, may withhold or delay treatment with statin therapy, except in cigarette smokers, those with diabetes mellitus, and those with a strong family history of premature ASCVD. ♦ CAC score of 1 to 99 favors statin therapy, especially if ≥55 years of age. ♦ CAC score ≥100 Agatston units or ≥75th percentile, statin therapy is indicated unless risk outweighs benefit

*Major ASCVD Events are considered:

- ◊ Recent ACS (within the past 12 months)
- ◊ History of MI (other than recent ACS event listed above)
- ◊ History of ischemic stroke
- ◊ Symptomatic peripheral arterial disease (history of claudication with ankle brachial index (ABI) <0.85, or previous revascularization or amputation)

**High-Risk Conditions are considered

- ◊ Age ≥65 years
- ◊ Heterozygous familial hypercholesterolemia
- ◊ History of prior coronary artery bypass surgery or percutaneous coronary intervention outside of the major ASCVD event(s)
- ◊ Diabetes mellitus
- ◊ Hypertension
- ◊ CKD (eGFR 15–59 mL/min/1.73 m^2)
- ◊ Current smoking
- ◊ Persistently elevated LDL-C (LDL-C ≥100 mg/dL [≥2.6 mmol/L]) despite maximally tolerated statin therapy and ezetimibe

Adapted from Grundy, S. M., et al., (2019). 2018 AHA/ACC/AACVPR/AAPA/ABC/ACPM/ADA/AGS/APhA/ASPC/NLA/PCNA Guideline on the Management of Blood Cholesterol: Executive Summary: A Report of the American College of Cardiology/American Heart Association Task Force on Clinical Practice Guidelines. *Circulation, 139*(25), e1046–e1081. https://doi.org/10.1161/CIR.0000000000000624

Nonpharmacologic Treatment

(see Box 8–1)

- Lifestyle modifications (see Box 8–1): smoking cessation, increased physical activity, moderation of alcohol intake (no alcohol with hypertriglyceridemia), Mediterranean diet recommended
- LDL is primary indicator for treatment.

Pharmacologic Treatment

(see Table 8–6)

- The enzyme 3-hydroxy-3-methylglutaryl coenzyme A (HMG-CoA) reductase inhibitors (statins) are the drug of choice for most patients with hypercholesterolemia.
- Statin side effects include myalgias with normal creatine kinase (CK) and severe adverse reactions, although rarely can include myositis/myopathy with weakness and symptoms and an upper limit of normal CK, rhabdomyolysis with a CK more than 10 times normal with renal injury, statin-associated autoimmune myopathy, new onset of diabetes mellitus in persons at risk, that is, metabolic syndrome, BMI 30 or higher, hemoglobin A1c (HbA1c) above 6%; three times upper limit of normal liver transaminase, hepatic failure, decreased memory/cognition
    - Lowers LDL, increases HDL
    - Atorvastatin (Lipitor), simvastatin (Zocor): metabolized by cytochrome P450 (CYP)3A4
    - Drug/food interactions: cyclosporine, erythromycin, itraconazole, ketoconazole, fibric acid, diltiazem, verapamil, fluoxetine, nefazodone
    - Contraindicated in liver disease, pregnancy, lactation
    - Rhabdomyolysis may develop if fibrate used in patient with renal dysfunction
    - Monitor liver function tests
- Ezetimibe (Zetia) is the most used nonstatin agent.
    - Decreases cholesterol absorption in the intestine
    - Lowers LDL-C levels by 13% to 20%
    - Metabolized in the liver and the small intestine
    - No dose adjustment needed in patients with renal insufficiency or mild hepatic dysfunction.
    - Low incidence of side effects: headache, diarrhea

TABLE 8–6.
GUIDELINE STATIN TREATMENT AND PERCENT REDUCTION IN LDL-C

	HIGH-INTENSITY	MODERATE-INTENSITY	LOW-INTENSITY STATIN
LDL-C Lowering	50% or higher	30%–49%	less than 30%
Clinical Use	Clinical ASCVD Severe primary hypercholesteremia with LDL above 190 mg/dL Very high-risk ASCVD: ♦ one major ASCVD event with multiple high-risk conditions or ♦ multiple major ASCVD events Diabetes ages 50–75 years with LDL above 70 mg/dL	Patients with diabetes ages 40–75 years with LDL above 70 mg/dL Age 40–75 years with ASCVD 10-year risk above 7.5% with risk-enhancing factors Age 40–75 years with ASCVD 10-year risk 7.5%–19.9% with risk-enhancing factors	
Statins	Atorvastatin (40 mg) 80 mg Rosuvastatin 20 (40 mg)	Atorvastatin 10 mg (20 mg) Rosuvastatin (5 mg) 10 mg Simvastatin 20–40 mg* Pravastatin 40 mg (80 mg) Lovastatin 40 mg (80 mg) Fluvastatin XL 80 mg Fluvastatin 40 mg BID Pitavastatin 1–4 mg	Simvastatin 10 mg Pravastatin 10–20 mg Lovastatin 20 mg Fluvastatin 20–40 mg
Additional Agents:	Ezetimibe is the most used nonstatin agent. It lowers LDL-C levels by 13% to 20% and has a low incidence of side effects.	Bile acid sequestrants reduce LDL-C levels by 15% to 30% depending on the dose. Bile acid sequestrants are not absorbed and do not cause systemic side effects, but they are associated with gastrointestinal complaints (e.g., constipation) and can cause severe hypertriglyceridemia when fasting	

Continued

TABLE 8–6. (CONTINUED)

	HIGH-INTENSITY	MODERATE-INTENSITY	LOW-INTENSITY STATIN
		triglycerides are ≥300 mg/dL (≥3.4 mmol/L). PCSK9 inhibitors are powerful LDL-lowering drugs. They generally are well tolerated, but long-term safety remains to be proven	

*Although simvastatin 80 mg was evaluated in randomized controlled trials (RCTs), it is not recommended by the U.S. Food and Drug Administration (FDA) due to increased risk of myopathy, including rhabdomyolysis

Adapted from Grundy, S. M., et al., (2019). 2018 AHA/ACC/AACVPR/AAPA/ABC/ACPM/ADA/AGS/APhA/ASPC/NLA/PCNA Guideline on the Management of Blood Cholesterol: Executive Summary: A Report of the American College of Cardiology/American Heart Association Task Force on Clinical Practice Guidelines. *Circulation, 139*(25), e1046–e1081. https://doi.org/10.1161/CIR.0000000000000624

- Bile acid sequestrants reduce LDL-C levels by 15% to 30% depending on the dose.
  - Bile acid sequestrants are not absorbed and do not cause systemic side effects, but they are associated with gastrointestinal complaints (e.g., constipation) and can cause severe hypertriglyceridemia when fasting triglycerides are ≥300 mg/dL (≥3.4 mmol/L).
  - May safely be used in combination with other lipid-lowering medications
  - Interference with other drugs, (to be taken 1 hour before other medication or 4 hours after) and fat-soluble vitamins
  - Cholestyramine (Questran) maintenance dose 2–4 packs a day
  - Colestipol (Colestid) maintenance dose 5 g given once a day or twice a day
- PCSK9 inhibitors are powerful LDL-lowering drugs. They generally are well tolerated, but long-term safety remains to be proven.

How Long to Treat

- Treatment is usually lifelong.

Special Considerations

- In women, using conjugated estrogens reduces LDL approximately 15% and increases HDL approximately 15%; use as adjunct, not as replacement to cholesterol-lowering agents.
- Total cholesterol and LDL levels are not measured before 2 years of age; no treatment recommended before that age.
- Pregnancy and lactation: levels normally elevated, usually do not test
- Older adults: treatment controversial in adults 90 and older, insufficient studies for this age group.
- It may be reasonable to stop statin therapy when physical or cognitive functional decline, multiple comorbidities, frailty, or reduced life-expectancy limits the potential benefits of statin therapy in adults 75 years of age or older.
- It may be reasonable to measure CAC in adults 76 to 80 years of age with an LDL-C level of 70 to 189 mg/dL (1.7 to 4.8 mmol/L), to avoid having to start a statin if the CAC score is zero.

When to Consult, Refer, Hospitalize

- Refer all pediatric and adult patients who are not controlled with therapy to a cardiologist and endocrinologist.
- Refer if patient is pregnant or has comorbid conditions.
- Refer to a dietitian, especially if dietary compliance is poor.
- Start immediate treatment for triglycerides over 1,000 mg/dL; patient may need to be hospitalized.

Follow-Up

- Repeat cholesterol levels 4 to 12 weeks after initiating a statin or after dose adjustment; repeat every 3 to 12 months as needed.
- Assess responses to lifestyle and statin therapy by the percentage of reduction in LDL-C levels compared with baseline. For ASCVD patients at very high risk, with LDL-C levels ≥70 mg/dL (≥1.8 mmol/L) on maximal statin therapy, add nonstatin therapy.
- Every 1–2 years with lipid profile for patients not requiring drug therapy

- Visits for patients requiring drug therapy should include tolerance of medication (myalgias), diet assessment, compliance with exercise routine, 24-hour recall of diet, and appropriate lab tests.
- Inquire about new medications; many medications affect lipid parameters.
- For patients on drug therapy, monitor lipids and liver function tests every 6 weeks until goal is reached.
- Visits every 4–8 weeks initially, until lipid control is achieved, and then every 6 months; with comorbid conditions, visits every 3–4 months.

Expected Course

- Dependent on etiology, CAD
- Usually lifelong

Complications

- CAD progression, stroke, MI
- Peripheral vascular disease
- Rhabdomyolysis, liver dysfunction secondary to drug treatment
- Pancreatitis (with triglycerides higher than 1,000 mg/dL)

HYPERLIPIDEMIA TREATMENT FOR CHILDREN, ADOLESCENTS, AND YOUNG ADULTS

(see Tables 8–7 through 8–10)

Epidemiology

Obesity combined with a moderate to severe elevation in triglycerides (TG), normal to mild elevation in LDL-C, and reduced high-density lipoprotein cholesterol (HDL-C) are patterns that have been shown to be associated with the beginning and progression of atherosclerotic plaque in children and adolescents as seen on pathology and imaging studies.

TABLE 8–7. SCREENING FOR HYPERLIPIDEMIA IN CHILDREN AND YOUNG ADULTS

AGE	RECOMMENDATION	GRADE RECOMMENDATION*
Birth to 24 Months	No lipid screening	Grade C Recommend
2 to 8 Years	No routine lipid screening EXCEPT: If	Grade B Recommend
	♦ Parent, grandparent, aunt/uncle, or sibling with MI, angina, stroke, coronary artery bypass graft (CABG)/stent/angioplasty at younger than 55 years in males, younger than 65 years in females	Strongly Recommend
	♦ Parent with TC 240 mg/dL or higher or known dyslipidemia	Strongly Recommend
	♦ Child has diabetes, hypertension, BMI 95th percentile or higher, or cigarette smoker, or	Strongly Recommend
	♦ Child has moderate- or high-risk medical condition	Strongly Recommend
	Recommend measuring fasting lipid profile (FLP) × 2 and average results (second one to be measured after 2 weeks, and within 3 months of initial lipid profile);	
9 to 11 Years	Universal Screening ♦ Non-FLP: Calculate non-HDL-C: Non-HDL-C = TC – HDL-C. (disregard TG and LDL-C in nonfasting sample) IF ♦ Non-HDL 145 mg/dL or higher or HDL lower than 40 mg/dL *Then* Measure FLP × 2, *OR* ♦ FLP: LDL-C ≥130 mg/dL, non-HDL-C ≥145 mg/dL HDL-C <40 mg/dL, TG ≥100 mg/dL if older than 10 years old, ≥130 mg/dL if ≥10 years → Repeat FLP after 2 weeks but within 3 months.	Grade B Strongly Recommend

Continued

TABLE 8–7.
(CONTINUED)

AGE	RECOMMENDATION	GRADE RECOMMENDATION*
12 to 16 Years	No Routine Screening EXCEPT, do measure FLP x 2 (second to be measured between 2 weeks and 3 months), average results of both tests, IF new knowledge of	Grade B Recommend
	♦ Parent, grandparent, aunt/uncle or sibling with MI, angina, stroke, CABG/stent/angioplasty, sudden death younger than 55 years old in males, and 65 years old in females	Strongly Recommend
	♦ Parent with TC 240 mg/dL or higher or known dyslipidemia	Strongly Recommend
	♦ Patient has diabetes, hypertension, BMI 85th percentile or greater, or smokes cigarettes	Strongly Recommend
	♦ Patient has moderate- or high-risk medical condition (see below)	Strongly Recommend
	Routine lipid screening is not recommended in ages 12–16 years due to very low sensitivity and specificity for predicting adult LDL–C levels and very high false-negative results in this age group. Selective screening recommended as stated above	
17 to 21 years	Universal Screening once during this time frame Non-FLP: Calculate non-HDL-C: Non-HDL-C = TC − HDL-C* **17–19 years**: Non-HDL-C ≥145 mg/dL, HDL-C <40 mg/dL FLP × 2 OR FLP: LDL-C ≥130 mg/dL, non-HDL-C ≥145 mg/dL HDL-C <40 mg/dL, TG ≥130 mg/dL Repeat FLP after 2 weeks but within 3 months **20–21 years**: Non-HDL-C ≥190 mg/dL, HDL-C <40 mg/dL (disregard TG and LDL in non-FLP)	

Continued

TABLE 8–7. (CONTINUED)

AGE	RECOMMENDATION	GRADE RECOMMENDATION*
	FLP × 2, average results and use Adult Treatment Panel III (ATP III) management algorithm OR FLP: LDL-C ≥160 mg/dL, non-HDL-C ≥190 mg/dL HDL-C <40 mg/dL, TG ≥150 mg/dL Repeat FLP after 2 weeks but within 3 months, average results ATP III management algorithm	Grade B Recommend

*Grades reflect the findings of the evidence review.

Adapted from *Expert Panel on Integrated Guidelines for Cardiovascular Health and Risk Reduction in Children and Adolescents Full Report.* NIH Publication No. 12–7486, October 2012, pp. 98–99. Retrieved from https://www.nhlbi.nih.gov/files/docs/guidelines/peds_guidelines_full.pdf

TABLE 8–8. LIPID RANGES FOR CHILDREN, ADOLESCENTS, AND YOUNG ADULTS*

CATEGORY	ACCEPTABLE	BORDERLINE HIGH	HIGH
Total Cholesterol	<170 (<190)	170–199 (190–224)	≥200 (≥225)
LDL-C	<110 (<120)	110–129 (120–159)	≥130 (≥160)
Non-HDL-C	<120 (<150)	120–144 (150–189)	≥145 (≥190)
Apolipoprotein B (ApoB)	<90	90–109	≥110
TRIGLYCERIDES			
0–9 years	<75	75–99	≥100
10–19 years	<90	90–129	≥130
(Young Adult)	(<115)	(115–149)	(≥150)
HDL-C	>45 (>45)	40–45 (40–45)	<40 (<40)
Apolipoprotein A-1 (ApoA-1)	>120	115–120	<115

*Young Adult recommendations are in parentheses.

Adapted from *Expert Panel on Integrated Guidelines for Cardiovascular Health and Risk Reduction in Children and Adolescents Summary Report.* NIH Publication No. 12–7486, October 2012, pp. 98–99. Retrieved from https://www.nhlbi.nih.gov/files/docs/guidelines/ peds_guidelines_full.pdf

TABLE 8–9.
AGE AND EVIDENCE-BASED RECOMMENDATIONS FOR PHARMACOLOGIC TREATMENT OF CHILDREN WITH DYSLIPIDEMIA

AGE	RECOMMENDATION	EVIDENCE GRADE
Birth to 10 Years	Medications by lipid specialist only Pharmacologic treatment is limited to children with severe primary hyperlipidemia (homozygous familial hypercholesterolemia, primary hypertriglyceridemia with TG 500 mg/dL or higher), or a high-risk condition or evident cardiovascular disease	Grade C Recommend
11 to 21 Years	Detailed family history and risk factor (RF) assessment required before start of drug therapy.* High- to moderate- level RFs and risk conditions (RCs).	Grade C Strongly Recommend
	LDL-C: If average LDL-C 250 mg/dL or higher, consult lipid specialist	Grade B Strongly Recommend
	If average LDL-C 130–250 mg/dL or higher, or non-HDL greater than 145 mg/dL: Refer to dietitian for medical nutrition therapy with Cardiovascular Health Integrated Lifestyle Diet (CHILD 1)	Grade A Strongly Recommend
	CHILD 2-LDL × 6 months, repeat fasting lipid panel (FLP) Repeat FLP: LDL-C lower than 130 mg/dL, continue CHILD 2-LDL, reevaluate in 12 months	Grade A Strongly Recommend
	LDL-C 190** mg/dL or higher, consider initiation of statin therapy	Grade A Strongly Recommend
	LDL-C 130–189 mg/dL or higher, negative family history, no other RF or RC, continue CHILD 2-LDL, reevaluate every 6 months	Grade B Recommend
	LDL-C 160–189 mg/dL with positive family history positive OR at least 1 high-level RF/RC OR at least 2 moderate-level RFs/RCs, consider statin therapy	Grade B Recommend
	LDL-C 130–159 mg/dL or higher + at least 2 high-level RFs/RCs OR 1 high-level + 2 moderate-level RFs/RCs, consider statin therapy	Grade B Recommend
	Children on statin therapy should be counseled and carefully monitored	Grade A Strongly Recommend
	Detailed FH and RF/RC assessment required before initiation of drug therapy***	Grade C Strongly Recommend

Continued

TABLE 8–9. (CONTINUED)

AGE	RECOMMENDATION	EVIDENCE GRADE
	TG: If average TG 500 mg/dL or higher, consult lipid specialist.	Grade B Recommend
	If average TG 100 mg/dL or higher in a child under 10 years old, or 130 mg/dL or higher in a child age 10 to 19 years, or lower than 500 mg/dL or higher: Refer to dietitian for medical nutrition therapy with CHILD 1 and then CHILD 2-TG for 6 months.	Grade B Strongly Recommend
	Repeat fasting lipid profile: ♦ TG lower than 100 (130) mg/dL, continue CHILD 2-TG, monitor every 6 to 12 months	Grade B Strongly Recommend
	TG 100 (130) mg/dL or higher, reconsult dietitian for intensified CHILD-2TG diet counseling.	Grade C Recommend
	TG 200–499 mg/dL or higher, non-HDL 145 mg/dL or higher, consider fish oil, consult lipid specialist	Grade D Recommend
	NON-HDL-C: Children 10 years or older with non-HDL-C 145 mg/dL or higher after LDL-C goal achieved may be considered for additional treatment with statins, fibrates, or niacin in conjunction with a lipid specialist consultation.	Grade D Optional

*Consideration of drug therapy based on the average of 2 FLPs or higher, obtained at least 2 weeks but no more than 3 months apart.

**If average LDL-C 190 mg/dL or higher after CHILD 2-LDL and child is age 8 to 9 years with +FH *OR* at least 1 high-level RF/RC *OR* at least 2 moderate-level RFs/RCs, statin therapy may be considered.

***Consideration of drug therapy based on the average of 2 fasting lipid profiles obtained at least 2 weeks but no more than 3 months apart.

Note: If child is obese, nutrition therapy should include caloric restriction and increased activity beyond that recommended for all children.

Adapted from *National, Heart, Lung and Blood Institute, Expert Panel on Integrated Guidelines for Cardiovascular Health and Risk Reduction in Children and Adolescents Full Report.* NIH Publication No. 12–7486, October 2012, pp. 126–128. Retrieved from https://www.nhlbi.nih.gov/files/docs/guidelines/ peds_guidelines_full.pdf

TABLE 8–10.
MEDICATIONS FOR MANAGING HYPERLIPIDEMIA IN CHILDREN AND YOUNG ADULTS

TYPE OF MEDICATION	MECHANISM OF ACTION	MAJOR EFFECTS	MEDICATION/DOSE/AGE INDICATION	ADVERSE REACTIONS	FDA APPROVAL IN YOUTH
HMG-CoA reductase inhibitors (statins)	Inhibits cholesterol synthesis in hepatic cells, decreases cholesterol pool, resulting in upregulation of LDL receptors	Mainly lowers LDL-C; some decrease in TG and modest increase in HDL-C	Atorvastatin ♦ Age 10–17 years 10–20 mg orally daily (HeFH) ♦ Age 10 years or older 10–80 mg orally daily (HoFH) Fluvastatin ♦ Age 10–16 years 20–80 mg orally daily (HeFH) Lovastatin ♦ Age 10–17 years 10–40 mg orally daily (HeFH) Pravastatin ♦ Age 8–13 years 20 mg orally daily (HeFH) ♦ Age 14–18 years 40 mg orally daily (HeFH) Rosuvastatin ♦ Age 8–9 years 5–10 mg orally daily (HeFH) ♦ Age 10–17 years 5–20 mg orally daily (HeFH) Simvastatin ♦ Age 10–17 years 10–40 mg orally daily (HeFH)	Increased hepatic enzymes, increased creatine kinase, myopathy possibly progressing to rhabdomyolysis	All statins listed approved as an adjunct to diet to lower LDL-C in adolescent boys and postmenarchal girls ages 10–18 years (8+ years for pravastatin) with HeFH and LDL-C ≥190 mg/dL, or ≥160 mg/dL with family history of premature CVD and 2+ CVD risk factors in pediatric patients

Continued

TABLE 8–10.
(CONTINUED)

TYPE OF MEDICATION	MECHANISM OF ACTION	MAJOR EFFECTS	MEDICATION/DOSE/AGE INDICATION	ADVERSE REACTIONS	FDA APPROVAL IN YOUTH
Bile acid sequestrants	Binds intestinal bile acids interrupting enterohepatic recirculation, more cholesterol converted into bile acids, decreases hepatic cholesterol pool, upregulates LDL receptors	Lowers LDL-C; small increase in HDL; raises TG	Cholestyramine ♦ Age 6–12 years 80 mg/kg orally three times a day. (maximum daily dose [MDD] 8 g/day) (hypercholesterolemia) ♦ Adolescents 4 g orally twice a day (MDD 8 g/day) (hypercholesterolemia) Colesevelam ♦ Age 10–17 years 3,750 mg orally daily (HeFH)	Limited to gastrointestinal tract: gas, bloating constipation, cramps	No pediatric indication listed for cholestyramine or colestipol; colesevelam indicated as monotherapy or with statin for LDL-C reduction in boys and postmenarchal girls ages 10–17 years with positive family history after diet trial if LDL-C ≥190 mg/dL or if LDL-C ≥160 mg/dL with Family history premature CVD or 2+ more CVD risk factors in the pediatric patient
Cholesterol absorption inhibitors	Inhibits intestinal absorption of cholesterol and plant sterols, decreases hepatic cholesterol pool, upregulates LDL receptors	Mainly lowers LDL-C; some decrease in TG and small increase in HDL-C	Ezetimibe ♦ Age 10–17 years 10 mg orally daily (HeFH)	Myopathy, gastrointestinal upset, headache	No

Adapted from *National, Heart, Lung and Blood Institute, Expert Panel on Integrated Guidelines for Cardiovascular Health and Risk Reduction in Children and Adolescents Full Report.* NIH Publication No. 12–7486, October 2012, pp. 126–128. Retrieved from https://www.nhlbi.nih.gov/files/docs/guidelines/ peds_guidelines_full.pdf

According to the National Health and Nutrition Examination Survey (NHANES), approximately 20% of children 12 to 19 years of age have lipid disorders. Mixed dyslipidemia occurs in up to 42% of children with obesity. The prevalence of dyslipidemia in the pediatric age group is as follows:

- Decreased HDL (to 40 g/dL or lower) approximately 12.1%
- Elevated TG (to 130 mg/dL or higher) approximately 10.2%
- Elevated TC (to 200 mg/dL or higher) approximately 7.1%
- Elevated LDL-C (to 130 mg/dL or higher) approximately 6.4%
- Elevated non-HDL-C (to 145 mg/dL or higher) approximately 6.4%

Risk factors that contribute to dyslipidemia include: diet, level of physical activity, BMI, medications, predisposition, and medical conditions. According to NHANES data, the prevalence of dyslipidemia was 14% in children in the normal weight category, 22% in the overweight category (BMI greater than 85 percentile), and 43% in children with obesity (BMI greater than 95percentile; Gujral, 2022).

DEFINITIONS OF RISK FACTORS (RFS) FOR DYSLIPIDEMIA ALGORITHMS

Risk factors for ASCVD progress from childhood to adulthood. Adopting a healthy lifestyle at an early age is the best preventative strategy for those without genetic dyslipidemias.

- (+) Family history: myocardial infarction; angina; coronary artery bypass graft/stent/angioplasty; sudden cardiac death in parent, grandparent, aunt, or uncle; male younger than 55 years old, female younger than 65 years old
- High-Level RFs: Hypertension requiring medication therapy (BP 99th percentile [+5 mm Hg])
  - Current cigarette smoker
  - BMI 97th percentile
  - Presence of high-risk conditions
  - Diabetes mellitus is also a high-level risk factor and considered a high-risk condition, CVD equivalent by the *Adult Treatment Panel III* recommendations for adults.
- Moderate-Level RFs: Hypertension not requiring drug therapy
  - BMI above 95th and below 97th percentile
  - HDL-C lower than 40 mg/dL
  - Presence of moderate-risk condition

Special Risk Conditions

- High Risk:
  - Diabetes, type 1 and type 2
  - CKD/end-stage renal disease/post–renal transplant
  - Post orthotopic heart transplant
  - Kawasaki disease with current aneurysms
- Moderate Risk:
  - Kawasaki disease with regressed coronary aneurysms
  - Chronic inflammatory disease (systemic lupus erythematosus, juvenile rheumatoid arthritis)
  - HIV infection
  - Nephrotic syndrome

PRIMARY DYSLIPIDEMIA

Familial Hypercholesterolemia (FH)

Autosomal dominant genetic disorder of cholesterol metabolism, characterized by very high levels of LDL-C from birth.

- Premature ASCVD may occur in 1 of 200 individuals with heterozygous FH (and up to 1 in 100 persons of French Canadian, South African, Dutch Afrikaner, South Asian India, and Ashkenazi Jewish descent with heterozygous FH due to decreased genetic diversity).
- Those with heterozygous FH are usually asymptomatic with LDL-C range 155 to 500 mg/dL. They may exhibit tendon xanthomas and premature corneal arcus.
- The homozygote FH is rarer, with a prevalence of 1 per million. LDL-C in homozygous FH is usually above 500 mg/dL. Tuberous, planar, and tendon xanthomas, aortic stenosis; and corneal arcus may be seen in homozygote FH.

Hereditary Hypertriglyceridemia

Secondary causes of hypertriglyceridemia are much more prevalent than genetic causes.

- Prevention of acute pancreatitis is a priority in severe cases.
- Genetic causes should be considered if TG level is above 500 mg/dL.
- Familial hypertriglyceridemia occurs in approximately 1% of the population.

Secondary Causes of Dyslipidemia

- Exogenous: alcohol, isotretinoin, beta-blockers, some oral contraceptives, some antiretroviral agents
- Endocrine: obesity, hypothyroidism, hypopituitarism, type 2 diabetes, pregnancy, polycystic ovarian syndrome, lipodystrophy
- Renal: CKD, nephrotic syndrome
- Infectious: acute viral or bacterial infection, HIV, hepatitis, hepatic obstructive liver disease/cholestatic conditions, biliary cirrhosis
- Inflammatory diseases: systemic lupus erythematosus, juvenile rheumatoid arthritis
- Other: Kawasaki disease, anorexia nervosa, solid organ transplantation, childhood cancer survivor

Adapted from *National, Heart, Lung and Blood Institute, Expert Panel on Integrated Guidelines for Cardiovascular Health and Risk Reduction in Children and Adolescents Full Report.* NIH Publication No. 12–7486, October 2012, pp. 126–128. Retrieved from https://www.nhlbi.nih.gov/files/docs/guidelines/ peds_guidelines_full.pdf

Recommendations for Use of HMG-COA Reductase Inhibitors (Statins) in Children and Adolescents

Patient Selection

- Use algorithm and risk-factor categories to select statin therapy for patients.
- Include preferences of patient and family in decision making.
- In general, do not start treatment with statins before age 10 years. (Patients with high-risk family history, high-risk conditions, or multiple risk factors might be considered for medication initiation at age 10 years or younger.)
- Precaution/contraindication with potentially interactive medications (cyclosporine, niacin, fibric acid derivatives, erythromycin, azole antifungals, nefazodone, many HIV protease inhibitors).

Check for potential interaction with all current medications at baseline.

- Obtain baseline hepatic panel and creatine kinase (CK) before initiating treatment.

Initiation and Titration

- Choice of particular statin is a matter of preference. Providers are encouraged to develop familiarity and experience with one of the statins, including dosage regimen and potential drug–drug interactions.
- Start with the lowest dose, once daily, usually at bedtime. Atorvastatin and rosuvastatin can be taken in the morning or evening because of their long half-lives.
- Measure baseline CK, alanine aminotransferase (ALT), and aspartate aminotransferase (AST).
- Instruct the patient to report all potential adverse effects, especially muscle cramps, weakness, asthenia, and more diffuse symptoms suggestive of myopathy.
- Advise female patients about concerns with pregnancy and the need for appropriate contraception.
- Advise about potential future medication interactions, especially cyclosporine, niacin, fibric acid derivatives, erythromycin, azole antifungals, nefazodone, and HIV protease inhibitors. Check for potential interaction whenever any new medication is initiated.
- Whenever potential myopathy symptoms present, stop medication and assess CK; determine relation to recent physical activity. A CK level that is 10 times above the upper limit of reported normal requires assessment for rhabdomyolysis. is cause for concern, considering the impact of physical activity. Monitor the patient for resolution of myopathy symptoms and any associated increase in CK. Consideration can be given to restarting the medication once symptoms and laboratory abnormalities have resolved.
- After 4 weeks, measure fasting lipid profile (FLP), ALT, and AST.
- The threshold for worrisome levels of ALT or AST is more than 3 times the upper limit of reported normal.
- Target levels for LDL-C: Minimal lower than 130 mg/dL; Ideal lower than 110 mg/dL
    - If target LDL-C levels are reached and there are no myopathy symptoms or laboratory abnormalities, continue therapy and recheck FLP, ALT, and AST in 8 weeks and then 3 months.
    - If laboratory abnormalities are seen or symptoms are reported, temporarily withhold the medication and repeat the blood work in 2 weeks. If and when abnormalities resolve, the medication may be restarted with close monitoring.
    - If target LDL-C levels are not achieved, increase the dose by one increment (usually 10 mg) and repeat the blood work in 4 weeks. If target LDL-C levels are still not achieved, dose may be further increased by one increment or another agent (bile acid sequestrant or cholesterol absorption inhibitor) may be added under the direction of a lipid specialist.

Maintenance Monitoring

- Monitor growth (height, weight, and BMI relative to normal growth charts), sexual maturation, and development.
- Whenever potential myopathy symptoms present, stop medication and assess CK.
- Monitor fasting lipoprotein profile, ALT, and AST every 3–4 months in the first year, every 6 months in the second year and beyond, and whenever clinically indicated.
- Monitor and encourage compliance with lipid-lowering dietary and medication therapy. Serially assess and counsel for other risk factors, such as weight gain, smoking, and inactivity.

Special Considerations

- Risk factors for ASCVD progress from childhood to adulthood
- Counsel adolescent females about statin contraindications in pregnancy and the need for abstinence or use of appropriate contraceptive measures.
- Use of oral contraceptives is not contraindicated if medically appropriate. Seek referral to an adolescent medicine or gynecologic specialist as appropriate.

When to Consult, Refer, Hospitalize

- Refer all pediatric and adolescent patients with LDL-C levels of 250 mg/dL or greater and/or TG levels of 500 mg/dL or greater to a lipid specialist.

Follow-Up

- As per age guideline in Table 8–7
- Repeat cholesterol levels 4 to 12 weeks after initiating a statin or after dose adjustment; repeat every 3 to 12 months as needed.

Cardiovascular Disease/ Coronary Artery Disease (Cad)

ANGINA PECTORIS/STABLE ANGINA

Description

- Coronary artery disease may develop over years as a result of atherosclerotic lesions that decrease the arterial lumen. Over time, blood flow to the heart may be reduced, producing cardiac ischemic disease.
- Angina is a clinical manifestation of ischemic heart disease, occurring when blood flow to an artery is compromised sufficiently to decrease myocardial oxygen and produce subsequent chest discomfort. Stable angina is characterized by chest discomfort or anginal equivalent symptom, onset with exertion, and alleviated at rest or with nitroglycerin (maximum of 3 sublingual (SL) nitroglycerin (NTG) tablets 5 minutes apart).
  - Angina is often one of the first symptoms or warning signs of underlying CAD.
- It is vital to recognize the signs and symptoms of angina and to appropriately risk stratify and manage these individuals.
  - Classic: substernal pressure or heaviness associated with exertion or anxiety, resolves with rest and/or SL NTG
  - Women younger than age 50 with angina frequently awaken from sleep with chest pain.
  - Types include:
    - Stable: pain duration less than 15 minutes; no change in frequency, severity, or duration of anginal symptoms during the preceding 6 weeks
    - Unstable: recent change in characteristic angina symptoms and may occur at rest; see Acute Coronary Syndrome (ACS)
    - Variant (Prinzmetal): transient ST-segment elevation at rest, with angina symptoms related to coronary spasm usually involving right coronary artery

Etiology

- The mechanism behind stable angina is the result of oxygen supply–demand mismatch. The myocardial oxygen demand exceeds the myocardial oxygen supply, which often leads to the manifestation of symptoms.
  - Several factors contribute to stable angina; the most common etiology is coronary artery stenosis due to atherosclerotic plaque. The stenosis prevents adequate supply of oxygen to the myocardium during times of increased demand, that is, exercise, stress, illness.

  - ◊ The four factors that contribute to myocardial oxygenation are heart rate, perfusion pressure, collateral blood flow, and coronary artery diameter and tone.
- Endothelial cells that line the coronary arteries are responsible for regulating vascular tone and preventing intravascular thrombosis. If the endothelial cells or these functions are impaired in any way, it may result in the development of CHD.
  - ◊ Mechanisms such as stress, hypertension, hypercholesterolemia, viruses, bacteria, and immune complexes can all impair or injure the endothelial lining. When endothelial injury occurs, it produces an immune response, which leads to fibrous tissue formation.
  - ◊ Smooth muscle remodeling forming fibrous caps can lead to coronary artery stenosis, causing angina or acute coronary syndrome (Gillen, 2021).
- Plaques formed on the intimal lining of artery are composed of lipoproteins, cellular components, and extracellular matrix molecules. Plaque accumulation causes the inner lining of the blood vessels to thicken and blood vessels to lose elasticity.
- Atherosclerosis first appears as a fatty streak, which progresses for about 30 years.
- Foam cells are macrophages that ingest LDLs, and the fatty deposits (LDL) cause them to have a foamy appearance—hence the name foam cells. Early in atherosclerosis, foam cells congregate on the fatty lipids on artery walls and plaque begins to form and then develops into a multilayered plaque with a stabilizing fibrous cap.
  - ◊ As early as the fourth decade, the plaque becomes unstable and the foam cells necrose and rupture underneath the fibrous cap.
  - ◊ With progression, the fibrous cap tears and bleeds to produce a thrombus, which occludes the blood vessel either completely or partially and causes decreased blood flow and ischemia or necrosis (MI).
  - ◊ The process of atherosclerosis is accelerated by tobacco use, hypertension, diabetes mellitus, hyperlipidemia, genetics, coronary artery vasospasm, aortic stenosis, and aortic insufficiency.

Incidence and Demographics

- Heart disease is the leading cause of death in the United States.
- Angina affects approximately 10 million people in the United States.
- Rates for US 2020
  - ◊ 1 of every 5 deaths; approximately 697,000 people died from heart disease.
  - ◊ CAD is the most common type of heart disease; approximately 382,820 people died.
  - ◊ Approximately 2 in 10 deaths due to CAD happened in adults younger than 65 years of age.

- At age 40 years, the lifetime risk of developing coronary disease is estimated at 49% for men and 32% for women.
- The cost of heart disease in the United States between 2017 and 2018 was approximately $229 billion each year.
- Nearly 20.1 million adults in the United States 20 years and older have CAD—approximately 7.2% of the population.
- Every 40 seconds in the United States someone has a heart attack.
- Approximately 1 of 5 heart attacks are silent; the person is unaware of the occurrence or the damage.
  - (CDC, 2022) https://www.cdc.gov/heartdisease/facts.htm

Risk Factors

- Male, hypertension, hyperlipidemia, diabetes mellitus, tobacco use, familial history of premature cardiac death (males before age 55, females before age 65); menopausal women without estrogen replacement. (Estrogen treatment for postmenopausal women increases risk of ovarian cancer; however, lack of estrogen increases the risk for CAD.)
- Excessive alcohol consumption
- Cocaine
- Advancing age
- Obesity
- Physical inactivity
- Poor dietary intake
- Metabolic syndrome is a risk factor for CVD; it is defined based on the National Cholesterol Education Program's Adult Treatment Panel III as having at least 3 of the following:
  - waist circumference greater than 102 cm in men or 88 cm in women,
  - triglyceride level greater than 150 mg/dL,
  - high-density lipoprotein cholesterol lower than 40 mg/dL in men or lower than 50 mg/dL in women,
  - systolic blood pressure at least 130 mm Hg or diastolic blood pressure at least 85 mm Hg or
  - taking hypertension medications, or

- ◇ fasting plasma glucose level at least 100 mg/dL or
- ◇ taking diabetes medications.

Prevention and Screening

- Modifiable lifestyle changes associated with coronary risk factors
- Treatment of comorbid conditions: CAD, hypertension, diabetes mellitus, hyperlipidemia
- Low-fat and low-sodium diet
- Regular aerobic exercise
- Avoidance of excessive alcohol intake; smoking cessation

Assessment

History

- It is important to conduct a thorough history, examination, laboratory studies, diagnostic tests, imaging workup, and evaluation to determine the cause of angina in each individual, to risk stratify, and to provide optimal medical treatment and management of risk factors.
- Classic presentation of substernal pressure or heaviness associated with exertion or anxiety and relieved with rest or NTG
  - ◇ Arm, back, neck, jaw, or upper stomach pain or discomfort
  - ◇ Each patient has typical pattern: subjective description of tightness, squeezing, burning, pressure, heaviness.
  - ◇ Change in patient's typical pattern indicative of unstable angina
  - ◇ Women may present with atypical signs and symptoms such as shortness of breath, nausea or vomiting (N/V), palpitations, fatigue, and gastrointestinal reflux disease (GERD)-like symptoms

Physical Exam

- Vital signs: elevation in BP, pulse, and respirations
- Holosystolic murmur may be present
- Transient S3 or S4

- Mitral valve prolapse; intermittent claudication may be present
- Sparse hair growth on distal extremities with associated peripheral vascular disease

Diagnostic Studies

- ECG at the time of the pain may show changes; between episodes, ECG may be normal.
- ECG normal in 25%–50% patients during angina episode; may find evidence of prior MI (Q waves)
- ECG unreliable in patients with bundle branch block, Wolf-Parkinson-White syndrome
- Chest X-ray: assess heart size, look for pulmonary edema, pleural effusions, and aortic aneurysm
- Exercise stress test: S-T segment depression (less accurate in women)
- Exercise thallium imaging: hypoperfusion found in areas with diminished uptake
  - Used for clarification with ECG abnormalities, often in women and with digoxin and beta-blocker use
- CBC, electrolytes, cardiac enzymes, pulse oximetry as indicated
- Radionuclide ventriculography: left ventricle imaging to differentiate infarction from ischemia
- Technetium: tagged red blood cells (RBCs), highly sensitive for CAD (nonspecific)
- Coronary angiography: definitive for diagnosis of CAD
- Rapid sequence MRI: calcified coronary arteries (not sensitive to coronary lesions)

Differential Diagnosis

Management

Nonpharmacologic Treatment

- Modification of risk factors (see Box 8–1): maintain ideal body weight, stop smoking, decrease stress, increase aerobic activity to moderate level 150 minutes/week, decrease cholesterol levels (LDL-C, VLDL), diet low in saturated fat and sodium
- Cardiac rehabilitation as indicated

TABLE 8–11.
CHEST PAIN DIFFERENTIAL DIAGNOSIS BY SYSTEM

SYSTEM	DIFFERENTIAL DIAGNOSIS
Cardiac	Pericarditis
	Aortic dissection
	Acute Coronary Syndrome (ACS)/MI
	Heart failure (HF)
Gastrointestinal	Gastroesophageal reflux disease (GERD)
	Cholecystitis
	Esophageal spasm
	Peptic ulcer
Respiratory	Costochondral pain
	Pneumothorax
	Pneumonia
	Pleurisy
	Asthma
	Pulmonary emboli
Musculoskeletal	Chest wall syndrome
	Shoulder arthropathy
Psychological	Anxiety
	Panic disorders
	Depression

Pharmacologic Treatment

- Optimal management of comorbid conditions: hyperlipidemia, diabetes, CHF, hypertension, arrhythmias
- New guidelines suggest treatment in patients with symptomatic chronic stable angina to prevent MI or death and to reduce symptoms. Use ASCVD 10-year risk assessment tool to assess risk and treatment.
  - ◊ High-risk individuals with known CVD should be prescribed daily low-dose aspirin or clopidogrel when aspirin is absolutely contraindicated.
  - ◊ HMG-CoA reductase inhibitor, a statin should be initiated for LDL-lowering therapy (see Tables 8–5 and 8–6)

- ◇ ACEIs or ARBs: May be used in primary prevention to assist in BP control, recommended for high-risk individuals or those with known CVD. The use of ACEIs or ARBs in high-risk individuals has been shown to reduce the risk of cardiovascular and all-cause mortality (Gillen, 2021).

- ♦ Medications for symptom management include
  - ◇ Beta-blockers: decrease anginal symptoms by decreasing heart rate, BP, and contractility, which decreases anginal symptoms by decreasing myocardial oxygen demand
  - ◇ Nitrates: causes relaxation of vascular smooth muscle, resulting in dilation of veins; this decreases cardiac preload and myocardial oxygen demand and relieves anginal symptoms
  - ◇ SL NTG or NTG spray are prescribed for immediate relief of angina in patients with chronic stable angina.
  - ◇ Ranolazine: FDA approved for stable angina symptom control; mechanism of action is unknown

Drug-Specific

- ♦ Nitroglycerin: 0.3 to 0.6 mg SL 5 minutes before any activity likely to produce angina, up to 1.5 mg daily as needed
- ♦ Nitrates (long-acting): used to promote coronary vasodilation
  - ◇ Patient education regarding storage and use of NTG so it will remain effective; when and how to take it; when to go for medical help
  - ◇ Monitor for hypotension with NTG use
  - ◇ Drug tolerance develops rapidly in patients taking NTG; patient should have a planned drug-free interval of 10–14 hours on a scheduled basis
  - ◇ Isosorbide dinitrate: 10–40 mg orally three times a day.
  - ◇ Isosorbide mononitrate: 10–40 mg orally twice or sustained release 30–120 mg daily (MDD 240 mg).
  - ◇ Nitro-Dur skin patch 0.2–0.8 mg/hour, on for 12 hours then off for 12 hours
- ♦ Aspirin: 81–325 mg daily
- ♦ Hyperlipidemic medication: decrease LDL to 100 or lower; see preceding section on Hyperlipidemia (see Table 8–5 and 8–6)
- ♦ Beta-blockers: decrease heart rate, contractility, and oxygen requirements
  - ◇ Monitor bradycardia, fatigue, depression, CHF, asthma
  - ◇ Metoprolol 25–200 mg twice a day, atenolol 25–200 mg once a day

- Calcium channel blockers: coronary vasodilation with reduction myocardial oxygen
  - Best drug for vasospasm
  - Monitor headache, pedal edema, constipation
  - Avoid verapamil and diltiazem in patients with arrhythmias
  - Coronary spasm: nifedipine XL (Procardia) 30–120 mg once a day; verapamil (Calan) 120–320 mg once a day; diltiazem (Cardizem) 120–480 mg once a day.
  - Avoid short-acting calcium channel blockers.

How Long to Treat

- Depends on etiology
- Often until revascularization

Special Considerations

- Women often have atypical symptoms.
- Geriatric patients: use low therapeutic doses to avoid side effects, monitor closely
- Pregnancy: exclude other diagnoses, cardiologist to follow-up

When to Consult, Refer, Hospitalize

- Consult with a physician on new and uncontrolled cases.
- Refer to cardiologist for invasive procedures; coronary revascularization, intolerable symptoms and medication failure; known stenosis of left main artery more than 50% with or without angina; left ventricular dysfunction and three-vessel damage; unstable angina with ischemia on exercise stress test; or post-infarction continuing angina or ischemia.
- Transfer to the nearest ED and hospitalize for acute angina unrelieved with pharmacologic therapy; patient should crush non-enteric-coated, chewable aspirin 325 mg and swallow en route to medical facility.

Follow-Up

- Individualized follow-up is dependent on symptoms and condition; minimum every 3 months.

Complications

- MI, cardiac arrest, CHF, death

ACUTE CORONARY SYNDROME (ACS)

Description

Refers to a group of diseases, including non-ST elevation myocardial infarction (NSTEMI) and ST elevation myocardial infarction (STEMI), which lead to decreased myocardial blood flow and myocardial tissue death (necrosis) resulting from myocardial oxygen demand severely compromised by thrombus formation, leading to subsequent reduction in coronary blood flow with total coronary occlusion.

(Q-wave transmural infarction or STEMI or nonocclusion (non-Q-wave nontransmural infarction or NSTEMI)).

Etiology

- CAD: coronary thrombosis secondary to ruptured atherosclerotic plaque
- Coronary spasm

Incidence and Demographics

- Some 805,000 people in the United States have heart attacks each year (CDC, 2020).
- Global incidence with mortality 30%–40%
- Male preponderance fourth through sixth decade, equal by age 70

Risk Factors

- It is important to identify risk factors to risk-stratify management and treatment
- See CAD risk factors: smoking, male sex, diabetes, hypertension, hyperlipidemia, physical inactivity, obesity, poor nutrition, +family history of early ASCVD (women younger than 65, men younger than 55 years of age), cocaine use may cause vasospasm causing ACS

Prevention and Screening

- Calculate 10-year ASCVD risk to assess the need for primary prevention strategies.

History

- Presentation in older adults is often nonspecific.
- Women may have nonstandard presentation; frequently awakened at night with pain, shortness of breath, palpitations, nausea or vomiting, fatigue
- Older adult patients may have no symptoms "silent MI."
- Shortness of breath, CHF
- Pain radiation at rest or minimal activity
- Classic: oppressive retrosternal chest pain, may radiate to left arm or jaw, not relieved by NTG; nausea or vomiting; diaphoresis

Physical Exam

- High incidence of mortality within first hour following cardiac event
- May have obvious pain; usually reduced sensitivity to pain in older adults—"silent MI"
- Nonspecific presentation, delirium, syncope, weakness
- Vital signs: hypotension, tachycardia, dyspnea
- General appearance: apprehensive, appears ill, ashen color
- Respiratory: shortness of breath, crackles
- Heart: S3, S4, new mitral regurgitation murmur, arrhythmia

Diagnostic Studies

- ECG diagnostic in 85% of cases with ST-segment elevation, Q waves, inverted T waves
- Subendocardial infarction: note ST-segment depression (may be the only finding)
- Cardiac enzymes (see Table 8–14)
- Cardiac catheterization or angiography to evaluate for coronary artery occlusion or disease
- Myocardial perfusion imaging (MPI)

TABLE 8–12.
CARDIAC ENZYMES IN THE DIAGNOSIS OF MI

LAB	ONSET	COMMENT
Creatine kinase-myocardial band (CK: MB) 1 and 2	3–4 hours	Sensitive, not specific
Troponin I and T	2–3.5 hours	Highly specific
Lactate dehydrogenase (LDH) 1 and 2	24 hours	Sensitive, not specific

TABLE 8–13.
NY HEART ASSOCIATION FUNCTIONAL CLASSIFICATION OF HEART FAILURE

CLASS	FUNCTIONAL CAPACITY: HOW A PATIENT WITH CARDIAC DISEASE FEELS DURING PHYSICAL EXERTION
I	Patients with cardiac disease but resulting in no limitation of physical activity. Ordinary physical activity does not cause undue fatigue, palpitation, dyspnea, or anginal pain.
II	Patients with cardiac disease resulting in slight limitation of physical activity. They are comfortable at rest. Ordinary physical activity results in fatigue, palpitation, dyspnea, or anginal pain.
III	Patients with cardiac disease resulting in marked limitation of physical activity. They are comfortable at rest. Less than ordinary activity causes fatigue, palpitation, dyspnea, or anginal pain.
IV	Patients with cardiac disease resulting in inability to carry on any physical activity without discomfort. Symptoms of heart failure or the anginal syndrome may be present even at rest. If any physical activity is undertaken, discomfort increases.

Adapted from Heidenreich, P., Bozkurt, B., & Aguilar, D., et al. (2022). 2022 AHA/ACC/HFSA Guideline for the Management of Heart Failure. *Journal of the American College of Cardiology, 79*(17) e263–e421. https://doi.org/10.1016/j.jacc.2021.12.012*

Differential Diagnosis

- Unstable angina
- Aortic dissection
- Aortic stenosis
- Pericarditis
- PE

TABLE 8–14.
2022 ACC/AHA/HFSA CLASSIFICATION OF HEART FAILURE BY LEFT VENTRICULAR EJECTION FRACTION (LVEF)

HF TYPE BY EF	LVEF CRITERIA
HF with reduced EF (HFrEF)	LVEF less than 40%
HF with improved EF (HFimpEF)	Previous LVEF less than 40% and follow-up LVEF 40% or higher
HF with mildly reduced EF (HFmrEF)	LVEF 41%–49% with Evidence of provokable and or spontaneously increased LV filling pressures as seen in elevated natriuretic peptide, and on invasive and noninvasive hemodynamic measurements
HF with preserved EF (HFpEF)	LVEF above 50% Evidence of provokable and or spontaneously increased LV filling pressures as seen in elevated natriuretic peptide, and on invasive and noninvasive hemodynamic measurements

Adapted from Heidenreich, P., Bozkurt, B., & Aguilar, D., et al. (2022). 2022 AHA/ACC/HFSA Guideline for the Management of Heart Failure. *Journal of the American College of Cardiology,* 2022 May, *79*(17) e263–e421. https://doi.org/10.1016/j.jacc.2021.12.012

- Esophageal spasm
- Biliary tract disease
- GERD
- Pancreatitis
- Chest wall muscle spasm
- Hypertensive emergency

Management

Nonpharmacologic Treatment Recommendations

- See lifestyle modification (Box 8–1)
- Acute: immediate referral to emergency department for evaluation and stabilization

- Post-MI:
  - diet low in saturated fat and sodium; caloric restriction if appropriate
  - treat underlying risk factors (hypertension, hyperlipidemia)

Pharmacologic Treatment

Acute

- NTG SL 0.3–0.6 mg every 5 minutes, total 3 doses
- Unrelieved chest pain: transport to nearest ED or chest pain center with Primary percutaneous coronary intervention (PCI) capability.
- PCI is the recommended triage strategy for patients with STEMI and ischemic symptoms occurring for less than 12 hours
- Goal of door to balloon time is less than 90 minutes
- Aspirin 325 mg chewable
- Oxygen via nasal cannula at 2 L, if available
- Thrombolytic therapy may confer benefit if initiated within 3–12 hours after onset of pain if PCI unavailable

Postinfarction

- Smoking cessation, lifestyle modifications (see Box 8–1)
- Antiplatelet agent
  - aspirin 81–325 mg once a day unless contraindicated, is usually prescribed with one of the following antiplatelet agents; however, if patient is unable to tolerate aspirin, one of the agents below may be prescribed alone and vice versa
  - clopidogrel (Plavix) 75 mg po daily,
  - prasugrel (Effient),
  - ticagrelor (Brilinta)
- Beta-blockers improve survival rates and should be started within first 24 hours.
  - Exception, do not give to patient with marked CHF, cardiogenic shock or bronchospasm
  - Monitor bradycardia, fatigue, depression
  - Metoprolol 25–200 mg twice a day, or Lopressor, or Toprol XL
  - Atenolol 25–200 mg once a day

- Calcium channel blockers are not effective and are indicated for secondary prevention.
- ACEI/ARBs are the cornerstone of therapy; prevent progression of left ventricular dysfunction.
  - In patients with left ventricular dysfunction, reduce morbidity
  - Most effective for patients with diabetes, hypertension
  - Monitor cough and renal function, including hyperkalemia.
  - Rare: life-threatening angioedema caused by drug
  - Lisinopril 2.5–10 mg once a day; start with small dose, titrate up
- Statin—high dose
  - atorvastatin (Lipitor) 80 mg orally daily
  - Monitor for myalgias, LFTs
- Glycosides: consider use in CHF
- Nitrates (isosorbide dinitrate, Isordil; NTG patch, pills, or spray)
  - Effective for residual ischemia and coronary atherosclerosis, dilates coronary vessels
  - Monitor for hypotension

Special Considerations

- ACEI should be considered for all patients.

When to Consult, Refer, Hospitalize

- Patients with symptoms of ACS (chest discomfort with or without radiation to the arm[s], back, neck, jaw, or epigastrium; shortness of breath; weakness; diaphoresis; nausea; lightheadedness) should be instructed to call 911 and be transported to the hospital by ambulance rather than by friends or relatives.
- Patients with symptoms that may represent ACS should not be evaluated solely over the telephone but should be instructed to call 911 and be transported to the hospital by ambulance.
- Initial post-MI care and evaluation by cardiologist

Follow-Up

- Long-term management; visits at least every 3 months

Expected Course

- ACS is associated with very high morbidity and mortality and is best managed by an interprofessional team that includes the ED physician, cardiologist, internist, pharmacist, and primary caregivers.
- The condition is managed primarily by the cardiologist but the prevention is managed by the primary care provider or nurse practitioner.
- The patient should be urged to stop smoking, maintain a healthy body weight, exercise regularly, and remain compliant with the medications. The outlook for patients who are treated promptly is good but those with severe disease and noncompliance have high morbidity, including premature death.
- https://www.ncbi.nlm.nih.gov/books/NBK459269/

Complications

- Death
- Chronic heart failure
- Ventricular tachycardia or ventricular fibrillation in first 24 hours
- Atrial fibrillation (AF) and flutter, bradycardia, heart block
- Deep vein thrombosis
- Pulmonary embolism
- Mitral regurgitation
- Cardiogenic shock

HEART FAILURE (HF)

Description

- A complex clinical syndrome characterized by insufficient cardiac output to meet the metabolic demands of the body, due to decreased contractility (systolic failure) or decreased ventricular filling (diastolic failure); any structural or functional impairment of ventricular ejection of blood (systole) or filling (diastole).
- It is a progressive disease and advanced stages are associated with decreased survival.

Etiology

- Most common cause in children is congenital heart disease with volume or pressure overload.
- Acquired causes are metabolic abnormalities, severe hypoxia, acidosis, viral infection, myocarditis, acute rheumatic carditis, rheumatic valvular heart disease, cardiomyopathy, prolonged supraventricular tachycardia, complete heart block, severe anemia, acute hypertension, and bronchopulmonary dysplasia.
- *Left-sided failure:* An acute process causes abrupt decrease in the output of a previously healthy heart. This might include acute MI, acute papillary muscle rupture, acute dysrhythmia, acute valvular regurgitation, or drug toxicity.
- *Right-sided failure:* Chronic strain on compensatory mechanisms finally produces a hypertrophied heart that cannot keep up with metabolic demands. Chronic strain may be caused by chronic hypertension; hypertrophic or restrictive cardiomyopathy; chronic, subclinical sympathetic nervous system stimulation; chronic valvular stenosis/regurgitation causing higher pressure; and drug toxicity.

Incidence and Demographics

- Occurs in infants through old age
- Male preponderance until age 75; then equal occurrence
- Most frequent hospital admitting diagnosis

Risk Factors

- Factors precipitating HF in patients with underlying heart disease include:
  - Nonadherence to medications
  - Excess salt intake, stress, obesity, pulmonary infection
  - Uncontrolled hypertension
  - Dyslipidemia
  - Inadequate medical therapy for cardiac risk factor (e.g., hypertension, hyperlipidemia, and so on)
  - Progression or complications of underlying disorder such as arrhythmias and cardiac muscle damage
  - Increased or decreased volume, anemia, electrolyte imbalance
  - Chronic or overuse of drugs such as nonsteroidal anti-inflammatory drugs (NSAIDs), acetaminophen, beta-blockers, steroids; digitalis toxicity; alcohol

Prevention and Screening

- Control of underlying disorder
- Monitoring for and treatment of risk factors
- Genetic screening is recommended for first-degree relatives of individuals with genetic or inherited cardiomyopathies

Assessment

History

- (see Tables 8–15 for HF Classification and Table 8–16 for stages of HF)
- Dyspnea on exertion, diminished exercise capacity, weakness
- Nocturia, orthopnea, paroxysmal nocturnal dyspnea, nocturnal cough
- Edema
- Anorexia
- Infants present with poor feeding, poor weight gain, tachypnea that worsens during feeding, cold sweat
- Older children may complain of shortness of breath (especially with activity), puffy eyelids, swollen feet, exercise intolerance

Physical Exam

- Overall appearance, noting whether short of breath on walking or sitting
- Basilar rales, wheezes, S_3 gallop rhythm, displaced point of maximal impulse (PMI)
- Cool extremities, cyanosis, pallor or grayish blue color
- Change in mental status
- Ascites, hepatomegaly
- Hypotension, pulsus alternans, tachycardia, tachypnea
- Frothy pink sputum
- Edema, rapid weight gain
- Jugular venous distention

TABLE 8–15.
AHA/ACC STAGES OF HEART FAILURE

STAGES	DEFINITION AND CRITERIA
A	**NO Symptoms,** but **at risk for Heart Failure (HF)**, may have ♦ structural heart disease or cardiac biomarkers of stretch or injury (e.g., people with hypertension, atherosclerotic CVD, diabetes, metabolic syndrome and obesity, genetic variant for cardiomyopathy, exposure to cardiotoxic agents, or positive family history of cardiomyopathy
B	**Pre-HF**, No symptoms or signs of HF and evidence of one of the following: ♦ *Structural heart disease* Reduced left or right ventricular systolic function Reduced ejection fraction, reduced strain Ventricular hypertrophy Chamber enlargement Wall-motion abnormalities Valvular heart disease ♦ *Evidence for increased filling pressures** By invasive hemodynamic measurements By noninvasive imaging suggesting elevated filling pressures (e.g., Doppler echocardiography) ♦ *Patients with risk factors and increased levels of B-type natriuretic peptide (BNP) or* *Persistently elevated cardiac troponin* in the absence of competing diagnoses resulting in such biomarker elevations such as acute coronary syndrome, CKD, pulmonary embolus, or myopericarditis
C	**Symptomatic HF** ♦ structural heart disease with current or previous symptoms of HF.
D	**Advanced HF** ♦ Refractory HF, marked HF symptoms that interfere with daily life and with recurrent hospitalizations despite attempts to optimize goal-directed medical therapy (GDMT)

Adapted from Heidenreich, P., Bozkurt, B., & Aguilar, D., et al. (2002). 2022 AHA/ACC/HFSA Guideline for the Management of Heart Failure. *Journal of the American College of Cardiology, 79*(17) e263–e421. https://doi.org/10.1016/j.jacc.2021.12.012

TABLE 8–16.
DRUG TREATMENT FOR ADULTS WITH CHRONIC HEART FAILURE

DRUGS	TREATMENT REGIMEN	COMMON SIDE EFFECTS
BETA-BLOCKERS		
Bisoprolol	1.25 mg orally once daily, titrate *slowly* to target 10 mg orally once daily	Bradycardia, depression, fatigue
Carvedilol (Coreg)	3.125 mg orally twice daily, titrate *slowly* to 25 mg twice daily for weight less than 85 kg and 50 mg orally twice daily for 85 kg or higher:	Bradycardia, depression, fatigue
Metoprolol succinate	12.5 mg to 25 mg daily, titrate to target 200 mg once daily	Same as above
ARNIS		
Sacubitril/ valsartan (Entresto)	Initial dose 24/26 mg to 49/51 mg twice daily to target 97/103 mg twice daily	Contraindicated with concomitant ACEI. If switching from ACEI to ARNI sacubitril/ valsartan, allow 36-hour washout period between administration of each drug Hypotension, hyperkalemia, cough, dizziness, orthostasis Monitor for drug–drug interactions
ANGIOTENSIN-CONVERTING ENZYME INHIBITORS (ACEIS)		
Captopril (Capoten)	6.25 mg orally three times daily to target 50 mg orally three times daily	Angioedema, hypotension cough—may be significant Hyperkalemia—use with caution in renal impairment
Enalapril (Vasotec)	2.5 mg orally twice daily, titrate to target 10 mg to 20 mg orally twice daily	Same as above
Lisinopril (Zestril)	2.5 mg to 5 mg orally daily to target 20 mg to 40 mg orally daily	Same as above
Ramipril	1.25 mg orally daily to target 10 mg orally daily	Same as above

Continued

TABLE 8–16.
(CONTINUED)

DRUGS	TREATMENT REGIMEN	COMMON SIDE EFFECTS
ANGIOTENSIN II RECEPTOR BLOCKERS (ARBS)		
Candesartan (Atacand)	4 mg to 8 mg orally daily to target 32 mg orally daily.	Angioedema, severe hypotension, hyperkalemia, renal impairment
Losartan (Cozaar)	25–50 mg orally daily to target max 150 mg orally daily	Same as above
Valsartan (Diovan)	40 mg orally twice daily, titrate to 160 mg orally twice daily	Same as above
ALDOSTERONE ANTAGONISTS		
Eplerenone	25 mg orally once daily, titrate to target 50 mg orally once daily	Stomach pain, chest/arm/back or jaw pain, SHORTNESS OF BREATH, tachycardiac, hive like swelling
Spironolactone	12.5 mg to 25 mg orally daily to target 25 mg to 50 mg orally daily	Dizzy, fatigue, muscle cramps, vomiting, diarrhea, stomach pain
SGLT2 Inhibitors		
Dapagliflozin	10 mg orally daily	Contraindicated in type 1 diabetes. Hold for "sick day;" genital mycotic infections highest in women (10%–15%), 15% temporary reduction in eGFR resolves in 1–3 months
Empagliflozin	10 mg orally daily	Contraindicated in type 1 diabetes Hold for "sick day;" genital mycotic infections highest in women (10%–15%), 15% temporary reduction in eGFR resolves in 1–3 months
VASODILATORS		
Hydralazine (Apresoline)	25 mg orally 3x/day to target 75 mg orally three times/day	Headache, flushing, upset stomach, vomiting
Isosorbide dinitrate (Isordil)	20 mg orally three times/day to target 40 mg orally three times/day	Nausea, worsening chest pain, rash, hives, itching

Continued

TABLE 8–16. (CONTINUED)

DRUGS	TREATMENT REGIMEN	COMMON SIDE EFFECTS
Fixed-dose combination isosorbide dinitrate/ hydralazine	20mg/37.5mg (1 tablet) po three times/daily to target 2 tablets po three times/daily	Headache, dizziness, lightheadedness, weakness, nausea or vomiting, tachycardia, ankle edema
IVABRADINE		
Ivabradine	2.5 mg to 5 mg orally twice daily Titrate to HR 50–60 bpm MDD 7.5 mg orally twice daily	Blurred vision, chest pain, fast or irregular heart rate, lightheadedness, dizziness or fainting, fatigue
LOOP DIURETICS		
Furosemide (Lasix)	20 mg up to 80 mg orally daily, may increase by 20–40 mg every 6–8 hours, not to exceed MDD: 600 mg orally daily in severe edematous states	Hyponatremia, hypokalemia, dehydration
Torsemide (Demadex)	10 mg to 100 mg orally daily, increase slowly as needed	Same as above
Bumetanide	0.5 mg to 5 mg orally daily, increase slowly as needed	Same as above
LOOP DIURETICS		
Furosemide (Lasix)	20 mg up to 80 mg orally daily, may increase by 20–40 mg q 6–8 hours, not to exceed MDD: 600 mg orally daily in severe edematous states	Dehydration, blurred vision, headache, fever, ringing in the ears, hearing loss, frequent urination
Torsemide (Demadex)	10 mg to 100 mg orally daily, increase slowly as needed	Frequent urination, cough, constipation, weight loss, vomiting, headache, sore throat
Bumetanide	0.5 mg to 5 mg orally daily, increase slowly as needed	Frequent urination, dizziness, upset stomach, diarrhea, ringing in ears, hearing loss

Adapted from Heidenreich, P., Bozkurt, B., & Aguilar, D., et al. (2022). 2022 AHA/ACC/HFSA Guideline for the Management of Heart Failure. *Journal of the American College of Cardiology, 79*(17) e263–e421. https://doi.org/10.1016/j.jacc.2021.12.012*

- Framingham classification states diagnosis of heart failure is based on the presence of either 2 major or 1 major and 2 minor of the following criteria
    - ◊ Major criteria:
        - Paroxysmal nocturnal dyspnea (PND)
        - Neck vein distension
        - Rales
        - Acute pulmonary edema
        - Cardiomegaly on radiographic imaging
        - Pulmonary edema
        - Weight loss of 4.5 kg or more in 5 days in response to treatment
        - S3 gallop
        - Hepatojugular reflux
        - Central venous pressure (CVP) above16 cm water
        - Circulation time of 25 seconds or more
    - ◊ Minor criteria:
        - Dyspnea on exertion with routine exertion
        - Nocturnal cough
        - Pleural effusion
        - Tachycardia higher than120 bpm
        - Hepatomegaly
        - Bilateral ankle edema
        - Vital capacity decreases one-third of maximal recorded value
- Although elements of both left- and right-sided failure often exist in a patient, it is often possible to identify the etiology of the problem by sorting symptoms into these two categories:
- *Left-sided failure* produces signs and symptoms of acute low cardiac output and high pulmonary pressures: dyspnea at rest, anxiety, chest discomfort/heaviness, pale skin, murmur of mitral regurgitation, S_3 gallop, crackles through most of the lung field bilaterally, frothy cough.
- *Right-sided failure* produces symptoms of compensated chronic fluid retention/overload: dyspnea with exertion, easily fatigued, paroxysmal nocturnal dyspnea, orthopnea, anorexia, basilar rales, abdominal fullness, jugular venous distention, lower extremity edema, hepatosplenomegaly, hepatic/splenic hum, pulsatile chest wall heave, displaced point of maximal impulse, single or multiple murmurs of stenosis or regurgitation.

Diagnostic Studies

- HF is a clinical diagnosis and diagnostic tests are used only to assist in identifying the cause and to determine severity and identify complications.
- Chest X-ray (anterior/posterior views): to assess for pleural effusions, pulmonary edema, cardiomegaly, and to exclude pneumonia
- 12-lead electrocardiogram: identify arrhythmias, type of heart disease, ischemia, infarction
- 2D echocardiogram: ejection fraction (EF) determines severity; assists in determining the cause of HF (type of heart defect, enlarged chambers, decreased left ventricular function), may perform an alternative imaging to assess LVEF such as: cardiac magnetic resonance imaging (CMRI), cardiac computed tomography (CCT), and radionuclide imaging
- Maximal exercise testing with and without respiratory gas exchange and/or blood oxygen saturation should be done to assess cardiac and pulmonary function with activity; more severe disease is indicated when there is an inability to walk more than short distances and with decreased oxygen consumption.
- In individuals with HF and CAD who may be candidates for revascularization it is recommended to perform noninvasive stress imaging such as stress echocardiography, single-photon emission CT (SPECT), CMRI, or positron emission tomography (PET) to detect myocardial ischemia.
- Cardiac catheterization: not routine (important for primary etiology)
- Endomyocardial biopsy: useful only for myocarditis or infiltrative disease and in rapidly progressive and unexplained cardiomyopathy

Laboratory Studies

- CBC may indicate anemia or infection as a potential cause for HF
- Electrolytes, BUN, creatinine, LFTs, cardiac enzymes, urinalysis, arterial blood gases, pulse oximetry
- B-type natriuretic peptide (BNP) and N-terminal pro-B-type (NT-proBNP) levels increase in HF and are useful to risk stratify in acute decompensation
- TSH may indicate thyroid cause for HF
- If suspect ACS draw cardiac enzymes troponin I orT

Other Studies

- Hemochromatosis screening as iron overload affects cardiac function
- Screen for sleep apnea or sleep-disturbed breathing which affects neurohormonal activation
- Screen for HIV as HF may be due to infectious process or treatment medications causing CAD
- Test for rheumatologic diseases such as pheochromocytoma, amyloidosis, which may cause cardiomyopathy
- Blood and urine electrophoresis for light chain disease
- Holter monitoring may reveal arrhythmias
- Genetic screening and counseling for at-risk individuals with a first-degree relative with cardiomyopathy

Differential Diagnosis

- Renal disease
- Failure to thrive
- COPD
- Nephrotic syndrome
- Cirrhosis
- Pulmonary emboli
- Acute MI
- Pneumonia
- Asthma
- Bacterial endocarditis
- Chronic venous insufficiency

Management

- The severity of the HF dictates the course of medical/surgical management; the goal is to improve quality of life by reducing symptoms.

Nonpharmacologic Treatment

- Identify and treat underlying disease and control precipitating factors.
- Control leg edema with elastic pressure stockings and elevation of legs.
- Daily weight assessment
- See lifestyle modification (Box 8–1)
- Aerobic exercise over the long term may reverse LV remodeling in persons with clinically stable HF, whereas isometric exercise has not been shown to have this effect.
- Dietary sodium restriction to 2–3 g/day, DASH diet
- Fluid restriction to 2 L/day if evidence of hyponatremia (Na less than 130 mEq/dL) and for those whose fluid status is difficult to control despite use of high-dose diuretics and sodium restriction.
- Caloric supplementation is recommended for patients with evidence of cardiac cachexia.
- Patient education, cardiac rehabilitation: goal is to balance activity with metabolic restriction.
- Oxygen as needed
- Other options: surgical—valve replacement and cardiac transplantation

Pharmacologic Treatment

- see Table 8–16
- Pediatric patients requiring medications should be managed by cardiologists.
- Patients frequently need a 3–4 drug regimen to control symptoms of cardiac impairment.
- Diuretics reduce preload and left ventricular filling.
- ACEIs are the cornerstone of therapy; prevent progression of left ventricular dysfunction.
- Beta-blockers improve ventricular function and reduce postinfarction mortality.
- Glycoside improves contractility in systolic failure.
- Vasodilators reduce afterload.
- Anticoagulants prevent thrombus formation; generally used when EF less than 20%.
- In normal kidney function,
  - furosemide 40 mg is approximately equal to bumetanide 1 mg and torsemide 20 mg.

- In patients with impaired kidney function,
  - the normal dose ratio of furosemide-to-bumetanide falls from 40:1 to approximately 20:1 because of an increase in extrarenal bumetanide clearance in such patients.
- The 2022 ACC/AHA/HFSA guidelines recommend the following medications to treat
  - Stage A (at risk for HF) (class I recommendations): treat hypotensive individuals with goal-directed medical therapy (GDMT) per ACC/AHA guidelines, use sodium-glucose cotransporter-2 inhibitors (SGLT2Is) in patients with type 2 diabetes and patients with CVS or at high risk for CVD to prevent hospitalization
  - Stage B (pre-HF) (class I recommendations):
    - LVEF 40% or less:
      - use an ACEI (decreases mortality, prevents symptomatic HF) or
      - BB (prevents symptomatic HF)
    - LVEF 40% or less and recent or remote history of ACS/MI:
      - statins to prevent adverse CV events and prevent symptomatic HF,
      - use evidence-based BB to decrease mortality
    - LVEF 40% or less and recent ACS/MI and unable to tolerate ACEI, use an ARB
    - LVEF less than 30% with minimum of 40 days post-MI with NewYork Heart Association (NYHA) class I symptoms while on GDMT and with life expectancy above1 year, ACC/AHA recommends implantable cardioverter-defibrillator (ICD) as primary prevention of sudden death
  - HFrEF (NYHA class II–IV, HFrEF [LVEF 40% or less]) to reduce risk of HF, hospitalization, and death
    - ACEI, magnetic resonance angiography (MRA), or dapagliflozin or empagliflozin for HFrEF
    - BB for stable HFrEF
    - Angiotensin receptor-neprilysin inhibitor (ARNI) sacubitril/valsartan as ACEI replacement
    - ARB if unable to tolerate ACEI or ARNI (should also get BB and an MRA)
    - Loop diuretic if signs and symptoms of congestion
    - Renin-angiotensin-aldosterone system (RAAS) inhibition with ACEI or ARB or ARNI (class 1 recommendations)
      - Patients with HFrEF and NYHA class II–III symptoms: Use ARNI for reduction of morbidity/mortality
      - Patients with previous/current symptoms of chronic HFrEF: When ARNI is not feasible, ACEI is of benefit for reduction of morbidity/mortality

- Patients with previous/current symptoms of chronic HFrEF and intolerant of ACEI due to cough or angioedema and when ARNI is infeasible: Use ARB for reduction of morbidity/mortality
- Patients with chronic symptomatic HFrEF NYHA class II–III tolerant of ACEI/ARB: Replace with an ARNI for further reduction of morbidity/mortality

◇ HFmrEF (NYHA class II–IV, HFmrEF)

- Diuretics if patient has congestion
- ACEI, ARB, BB, MRA, or ARNI sacubitril/valsartan may be considered to decrease risk of HF, hospitalization, and death

◇ HFpEF

- Diuretics if patient has congestion

How Long to Treat

- Acute episodes: until resolution and stabilization of symptoms
- Chronic condition: indefinitely

Special Considerations

- Geriatric patients: special attention to dosage requirements
- Lactation: multiple drug regimen is of concern
- Pharmacologic therapy for heart failure (HF) includes but is not limited to the following
  - ◇ Hydralazine and nitrates to improve symptoms, ventricular function, exercise capacity, and survival in patients who cannot tolerate an ACEI/ARB or as an add-on therapy to ACEI/ARB and beta-blockers in the Black population for survival benefit
  - ◇ Digoxin, which can lead to a small increase in cardiac output, improvement in heart failure symptoms, and decreased rate of heart failure hospitalizations
  - ◇ Anticoagulants to decrease the risk of thromboembolism
  - ◇ Selective sodium-glucose cotransporter-2 (SGLT2) inhibitors to reduce the risk of cardiovascular death

When to Consult, Refer, Hospitalize

- Consult with a cardiologist for initial diagnosis with management plan.
- Consult with palliative care for interdisciplinary team management and goal setting with shared decision-making.

- Refer all pediatric patients and pregnant and lactating women with HF to a cardiologist for treatment.
- Refer if complications or exacerbation does not respond to treatment.

Follow-Up

- Every 3 months if stable
- Patient education about diet, activity, medication, self-monitoring, what symptoms to report

Expected Course

- Chronic: poor prognosis if EF less than 20% or steady decline after diagnosis
- Acute: generally responsive to initial treatment

Complications

- Electrolyte disturbances, arrhythmias, digitalis toxicity

SYNCOPE

Description

- Temporary loss of consciousness, accompanied by fainting; loss of muscle tone; and possibly brief tonic contractions of the face, extremities, and trunk

Etiology

- Systemic hypotension leads to brief cerebral ischemia, causing loss of function.
- Simple syncope usually is a vasovagal event, triggered by fear, pain, excitement, or extended periods of standing still, especially in warm environments.
- Cough syncope is seen predominantly in asthmatic children.
- Syncope is classified as due to orthostatic hypotension, neurally mediated (reflux) and cardiac

- ◇ Neurally mediated syncope affecting blood flow and vascular tone; this is the most common type, occurring in approximately 45% of occurrences. It may be due to
  - vasovagal (neurocardiogenic),
  - situational (cough, defecation, micturition, postprandial, deglutition), or
  - secondary to carotid sinus hypersensitivity
  - Orthostatic hypotension, which may be due to medications, peripheral neuropathy, decreased blood flow, autonomic failure
  - Pathophysiology involves interaction between autonomic systems paradoxically favoring parasympathetic or vagal tone, which causes bradycardia and hypotension.
- ◇ Cerebrovascular causes
  - Neurologic disorders, vertebrobasilar insufficiency, TIAs, or migraines are rare
- ◇ Cardiac, approximately 20% of syncope presentations are related to cardiac causes, most often caused by arrhythmias, conduction, hemodynamic, or structural abnormalities:
  - Arrhythmia (both tachycardia and bradycardia),
  - Long QT syndrome is usually characterized by a loss of consciousness during exercise or emotional stress and is accompanied by cardiac rhythm abnormalities, and
  - less frequently caused by a structural cardiac abnormality such as hypertropic obstructive cardiomyopathy (HOCM), myocardial infarction, PE, or valvular abnormalities
- ◇ Approximately 10% of syncopal presentations are due to orthostatic hypotension characterized by postural hypotension, frequently related to impaired increase in systemic vascular resistance. Other factors may include effects of medication, hypovolemia, dehydration, acute blood loss, and autonomic dysfunction. Postural tachycardia syndrome is the most common form of orthostatic syncope; it affects approximately 500,000 people in the United States. It is more prevalent in younger adults, predominantly women.
- ◇ Pathophysiology related to reflex-mediated vasomotor instability; decreased cardiac output or blood flow obstruction; metabolic disruptions (hypoglycemia, hypoxia, hyperventilation); neurologic events (seizures, cerebrovascular diseases)
- ◇ Other symptoms that may mimic syncope
  - Seizures
  - Metabolic causes such as hypoglycemia, symptomatic anemia, hypoxia
  - Psychogenic issues such as panic attacks, anxiety, depression, conversion disorder

Incidence and Demographics

- Syncope accounts for 1% to 1.5% of all emergency department visits, 250,000 annual hospital admissions, at a median hospital cost of $8,500.
- Approximately 40% of adults will experience at least one episode of syncope (Runser, 2017).
- Vasomotor syncope or "fainting" is common in young women and associated with stress or pain.
- A diagnosis can be made in 45%–50% of cases.
- Syncopal events occur in 10%–15% of all adolescents.
- Simple syncope is uncommon before age 10–12 and occurs more frequently in girls.

Risk Factors

- Cardiac disease, diabetes
- Vasodilators, diuretics, adrenergic-blocking agents
- Age, family history of sudden death
- Prolonged QT syndromes
- Asthma and cough

Prevention and Screening

- Adequate hydration

Assessment

History

- Detailed, including symptoms before and after event (position changes, prolonged standing, exposure to warm environment)
- Lightheadedness, diaphoresis, nausea, visual changes before event
- Length of loss of consciousness, seizure activity, height of fall, any injuries including to tongue
- Confusion or drowsiness after event

- Associated cardiac or neurological symptoms: chest pain, diaphoresis, palpitations, headache, diplopia, aphasia, unilateral motor weakness, paresthesia
- Incontinence of bladder or bowel
- Past medical history: cardiac, neurologic; family history of heart disease, seizures
- Medications: vasodilators, beta-blockers, diuretics, anticholinergics
- Recent drug or medication use
- Interview family member or witness

Physical Exam

- Vital signs including orthostatic changes
- Cardiovascular: arrhythmia, murmurs, displaced PMI (cardiomegaly), bruits, difference in blood pressure between arms including orthostatic pressures
- Neurologic exam for focal deficits

Diagnostic Studies

- ECG for arrhythmia and other cardiac disease
- Chest X-ray if associated coughing
- CBC and electrolytes to rule out anemia, metabolic abnormalities
- Fasting blood glucose, thyroid function tests
- Pregnancy testing in women of childbearing age
- Echocardiography to rule out valvular disease, particularly if murmur
- If exertional syncope, stress testing to rule out ischemia
- Holter or event monitoring to rule out arrhythmia
- Tilt table to evaluate autonomic dysfunction
- Electrophysiologic studies if recurrent event and still no known etiology
- Electroencephalography if seizure history or seizures suspected
- Brain imaging if focal neurologic signs (CT or MRI)
- Carotid or transcranial Doppler studies if bruits or to rule out vertebrobasilar insufficiency

Differential Diagnosis

- Vasomotor syncope
- Orthostatic hypotension
- Acute myocardial infarction
- Sick sinus syndrome
- Drug reaction
- Cough or micturition
- Conduction disorders (AV block)
- Arrhythmias
- Aortic stenosis
- Pulmonary stenosis or hypertension
- Congenital anomalies with right–left shunting
- Seizure
- Vertebrobasilar TIA
- Psychogenic cause (hyperventilation)
- Metabolic abnormality

Management

Nonpharmacologic Treatment

- In cases of benign syncope (vasomotor), explain etiology to patient and advise lying down when prodromal symptoms occur.
- Simple syncope can be managed by avoiding triggers, pushing fluids, and salt loading during hot weather.
- The patient also can be taught to contract the calf muscles repeatedly while sitting or standing still.
- Long QT syndrome can sometimes be managed by the implantation of a cardiac pacemaker.
- Occasionally a left cervicothoracic sympathectomy is necessary.

Pharmacologic Treatment

- Medical management depends on etiology.
- Use the smallest doses of antihypertensive medications and eliminate any unnecessary drugs.
- Use beta-adrenergic blocking agents for recurrent episodes of simple syncope or prolonged QT syndrome.
- Improve management of asthma episodes.

Special Considerations

- Further evaluation is necessary in the presence of known heart disease, arrhythmias, pathological murmurs, and exertional syncope.
- With geriatric patients, increased risk secondary to comorbidities, polypharmacy, autonomic neuropathy, and dehydration due to decreased fluid intake.
- Syncope common in third trimester of pregnancy due to aortocaval compression by the enlarged uterus in the supine position; try left-side lying position.

When to Consult, Refer, Hospitalize

- Hospitalize for ventricular tachycardia, sustained supraventricular tachycardia, suspected myocardial infarction, medication that can cause malignant arrhythmias (torsades de pointes with quinidine), or any other high risk for cardiac syncope.
- Hospitalize for acute focal neurologic signs.
- Hospitalize older people who cannot be safely managed in their present living environments.
- Refer to cardiology if prolonged QT syndrome is suspected or if simple syncope is hard to control.
- Refer to neurology for new-onset seizures.
- Refer for mental health evaluation if psychogenic origin is suspected.

Follow-Up

Expected Course

- Depends on etiology; pediatric patient may outgrow simple syncope by young adulthood.

Complications

- Depends on etiology
- Increased risk of complications with heart disease, advanced age, and polypharmacy

MURMURS

Description

- Sounds created when there is turbulent forward blood flow because of partial obstruction of a stenotic heart valve or turbulent backward flow through an incompetent valve due to faulty valve closure (regurgitation) that produces an abnormal sound distinguishable from other heart sounds
- Innocent (functional, physiologic, benign) murmurs: turbulent flow as blood is ejected from a chamber or from increased or vigorous flow across a valve; associated with no structural abnormality

Etiology

- Organic: congenital or acquired (atherosclerosis)
- Functional: resulting from another medical condition such as anemia, fever, thyrotoxicosis, pregnancy
- Innocent murmurs: no evidence of cardiac pathology
- Rheumatic fever is a potential contributor to all murmurs.
- Infective endocarditis: regurgitation murmurs
- Other contributing factors include:
  - Aortic stenosis: congenital and senile calcifications
  - Aortic regurgitation: high blood pressure, aortic dissection, syphilis, collagen vascular disease
  - Mitral regurgitation: ruptured chordae tendineae, CAD, mitral valve prolapse
  - Tricuspid regurgitation: right ventricular failure, right ventricular infarction

Incidence and Demographics

- Murmurs are common and can occur in all ages.
- Eighty percent of children have innocent murmurs sometime during childhood, usually beginning at age 3.
- An innocent murmur is a frequent finding in the third trimester of pregnancy.
- Older adults often have a II/VI systolic ejection murmur because of decreased compliance of the heart.

Risk Factors

- Age: children and older adults have the most murmurs.
- Physiologic states of increased metabolic demand: fever, anemia, pregnancy, hyperthyroidism
- Heart disease

Prevention and Screening

- Prevention through treatment of streptococcal pharyngitis to prevent rheumatic fever
- Screening through periodic routine examinations

Assessment

History

- Symptoms such as shortness of breath, syncope, chest pain, palpitations, and exercise intolerance indicate pathologic murmur
- Family history of heart disease; prenatal and perinatal history
- Signs or history of infections and illness
- Activity level and endurance; feeding; crying; cyanosis

Physical Exam

- Skin color and moisture; nail clubbing
- Vital signs; pulses; posture
- Neck for distended veins, bruits, and thyromegaly

- Lungs for adventitious sounds
- Chest for asymmetry, precordial bulge, thrill, heave, and PMI
- Abdomen for organomegaly
- Extremities for edema
- Assessment of murmurs
  - Grading of intensity (see Table 8–17)
  - Location: area with greatest intensity
  - Radiation: heard in direction of blood flow
  - Pitch: high, medium, low
  - Quality: soft, harsh, rumbling
  - Timing: within the cardiac cycle (systolic between S_1/S_2; diastolic between S_2/S_1)
  - Once auscultated, a murmur must be identified as systolic or diastolic.
  - S_1 is mitral and tricuspid valve closure.
  - S_2 is aortic and pulmonic valve closure.
  - The period between S1 and S2 is systole.
  - The period between S2 and S1 is diastole.
- Murmurs that occur after S_1 and before S_2 are systolic.
  - Mitral and tricuspid regurgitation (backflow through an incompetent valve)
  - Aortic and pulmonic stenosis (turbulent flow through a tight opening)
- Murmurs that occur after S_2 and before S_1 are diastolic.
  - Aortic and pulmonic regurgitation (backflow through an incompetent valve)
  - Mitral and tricuspid stenosis (turbulent flow through a tight opening)

TABLE 8–17.
GRADING OF MURMURS

GRADE	CHARACTERISTICS
I/VI	Very faint, may not be heard in all positions
II/VI	Quiet but heard immediately upon placing the stethoscope on the chest
III/VI	Moderately loud
IV/VI	Loud accompanied by palpable thrill
V/VI	Very loud, heard with a stethoscope partly off the chest; accompanied by palpable thrill
VI/VI	Heard with the stethoscope entirely off the chest and accompanied by palpable thrill

- Once murmurs are identified as systolic or diastolic, the likely valve of origin must be identified by location (see Figure 8–1 and Table 8–18).
- Murmurs loudest at the second ICS, right sternal border (RSB), are likely aortic.
- Murmurs loudest at the second ICS, LSB, are likely pulmonic.
- Murmurs loudest at the fourth ICS, LSB, are likely tricuspid.
- Murmurs loudest at the fifth ICS, midclavicular line (MCL), are likely mitral.
    - *Systolic regurgitant murmur:* begins with S1 and usually lasts throughout systole (pansystolic or holosystolic); caused by blood flow from a chamber that is at a higher pressure throughout systole than the receiving chamber (associated *only* with ventricular septal defect [VSD], mitral and tricuspid regurgitation [MR and TR])
    - *Diastolic:* early diastolic (caused by the incompetence of the aortic or pulmonary valve); mid-diastolic (caused by turbulence of the tricuspid or mitral valve); or presystolic (caused by flow through the AV valves during ventricular diastole—tricuspid or mitral stenosis [TS or MS])

TABLE 8–18.
HEART SOUNDS AND RELATED HEART VALUES POSITIONS

DIASTOLE	SYSTOLE	DIASTOLE	SYSTOLE
S2	S1	S2	S1
A/P close	M/T close	A/P close	M/T close
M/T open	A/P open	M/T open	A/P open

FIGURE 8–1.
STANDARD CHEST AUSCULTATORY POINTS

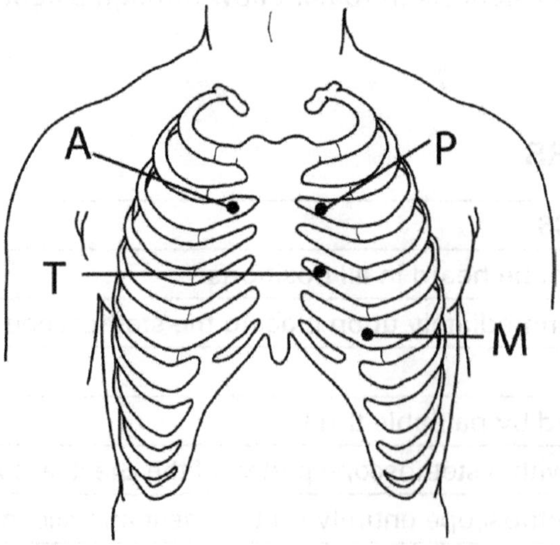

- Continuous murmur: S_1 through S_2; conditions such as patent ductus arteriosus (PDA)
- Innocent heart murmurs ((functional, physiologic, benign); see Tables 8–19 and 8–20)
- LSB, 2nd through 4th left intercostal spaces and apex
- Grade I–II/VI; low pitch; soft, short, nonradiating, midsystolic
- Variable loudness; heard best in supine position, diminishes with upright position
- Interpretation of murmurs
- Once timing and placement are identified, the valvular disorder is evident.
- A systolic murmur at the second ICS, RSB, is an aortic murmur occurring when the aortic valve is open—aortic stenosis.

TABLE 8–19. TYPES OF MURMURS

TYPE OF MURMUR	CHARACTERISTICS OF THE MURMUR
Systolic murmur	Occurs between S1 and S2 Systolic ejection murmur: interval between S_1 and onset of murmur (also referred to as crescendo-decrescendo); caused by blood flow through stenotic or deformed semilunar valves or by increased blood flow through normal semilunar valves (causing AS, PS) Systolic regurgitant murmur: begins with S_1 and usually lasts throughout systole (pansystolic or holosystolic); caused by blood flow from a chamber at a higher pressure throughout systole than receiving chamber (associated only with VSD, MR, and TR)
Diastolic murmur	Occurs between S2 and S1 Classified as early diastolic and caused by the incompetence of the aortic or pulmonary valve, atrial and pulmonic regurgitation (AR, PR); mid-diastolic, caused by turbulence of the tricuspid or mitral valve; or presystolic, caused by flow through the atrioventricular valves during ventricular diastole (tricuspid or mitral stenosis [TS, MS])
Continuous murmur	Occurs with S_1 and continues through the S_2 into diastole Seen with conditions such as patent ductus arteriosus (PDA), pulmonary artery (PA) stenosis, Blalock-Taussig shunt
Innocent heart murmurs	Arise from cardiovascular structures in absence of anatomic (functional) murmur abnormalities (80% of children have innocent murmurs sometimes during childhood, usually beginning at 3 years old); also referred to as functional, benign, or physiological murmurs. (See also Table 8–20.)

TABLE 8–20. CLASSIFICATION OF INNOCENT MURMURS IN CHILDREN

TYPE OF MURMUR	CHARACTERISTICS OF THE MURMUR
Vibratory murmur (Still's murmur)	Usually detected at 3–6 years of age; uncommon before 2 years of age Described as a musical, buzzing, "twanging string," or vibratory sound Heard best at middle left sternal border (MLSB) or between left lower sternal border (LLSB) and apex when patient is in supine position; diminishes when patient is upright or does Valsalva maneuver Midsystolic and grade II–III/VI in intensity; not accompanied by a thrill Intensity may increase with anemia, fever, or exercise; ECG and chest -X-ray are normal
Pulmonary ejection murmur	Usually detected at 8–14 years of age; heard best at the left upper sternal border (LUSB) Early to mid-systolic; grade I–III/VI in intensity; not accompanied by a thrill; soft and blowing ECG and chest X-ray are normal
Pulmonary flow murmur of the newborn	Blood flow through sharply angulated right and left pulmonary arteries at birth; usually detected in newborns, especially those with low birth weights, and disappears by 3–6 months of age Heard best at the ULSB Mid-systolic and grade I–II/VI in intensity; not accompanied by a thrill Transmits well to the right and left chest, back, and both axillae Normal ECG and chest X-ray
Venous hum	Originates from turbulence in the jugular venous system; usually detected at 3–6 years old Heard best at the infraclavicular and supraclavicular areas (disappears when the patient is supine or when the neck veins are gently occluded) Continuous humming murmur Normal ECG and chest X-ray
Carotid bruit	Originates from turbulence in the carotid arteries; detected at any age; systolic ejection murmur; grade II–III/VI in intensity Rarely, a thrill is palpable over the carotid artery Normal ECG and chest X-ray

SYSTOLIC MURMURS

Aortic Stenosis

- Second ICS right of sternum, with patient sitting and leaning forward
- Valve is open when stenotic murmur occurs and is caused by forward flow through stenotic valve
- Begins after S_1 and is a crescendo-decrescendo or diamond-shaped ejection murmur
- Radiation into neck from aortic area
- Medium pitch with variable intensity
- Harsh, loudest at base; musical at apex
- Mid-systolic
- Systolic thrill may be present
- Seen frequently in older adults and associated with a diminished S_2

Tricuspid Regurgitation

- Lower LSB
- Begins with S_1; high-pitched, smooth, blowing quality
- Pansystolic regurgitant murmur, increases in intensity with inspiration
- Right ventricular lift
- Always associated with pathology, usually diseased right ventricle from rheumatic heart disease

Ventricular Septal Defect

- LSB (3rd to 5th ICS)
- Radiation wide over precordium but not into axilla
- Loud (particularly base), harsh, pansystolic regurgitant murmur with thrill

Hypertrophic Obstructive Cardiomyopathy

- LSB
- No radiation
- Murmur increases with Valsalva maneuver, decreases with patient squatting
- Mid-systolic

Pulmonic Stenosis

- LSB 2nd or 3rd ICS, pulmonary area
- Generally, no radiation unless loud, then toward left neck
- Variable intensity, medium pitch
- Mid-systolic: begins after S_1 with crescendo-decrescendo contour
- Associated with thrill if significant pathology; usually congenital cause

Mitral Regurgitation

- A systolic murmur at the fifth ICS, MCL, occurring when the mitral valve is closed
- Location: apex; frequently radiates to wide area of chest and to left axilla
- Intensity variable, often loud; does not increase with inspiration
- Pitch is high with blowing quality
- S_3 usually also heard
- Pansystolic regurgitant murmur frequently accompanied with thrill
- Begins with S_1 (which may be decreased)
- Valve closed when the murmur occurs; noise caused from backflow through incompetent valve
- Always pathologic

Diastolic Murmurs

- Always pathologic, indicative of heart disease
- Often heard best with the bell of the stethoscope

Mitral Stenosis

- Listen with patient in left lateral decubitus position, also with exercise.
- Diastolic rumbling murmur that begins after a short period of silence after S_2
- Low in pitch, heard best with bell of stethoscope in light skin contact
- No radiation
- Loudest at apex; best heard after mild exercise
- A diastolic murmur occurring at the fifth ICS, MCL, is a mitral murmur occurring when the mitral valve is open

Aortic Regurgitation

- Heard at LSB with patient leaning forward and listening with diaphragm of stethoscope pressed firmly on the chest
- Early diastolic murmur that begins immediately after S_2 and diminishes in intensity
- Blowing, high-pitched, decrescendo
- Heard with rheumatic heart disease or syphilis
- A diastolic murmur at the second ICS, RSB, an aortic murmur occurring when the aortic valve is closed

Pulmonary Valve Insufficiency

- LSB 2nd ICS
- Radiates mid-right sternal border
- High-pitched, loudest base, decrescendo murmur

Continuous Murmurs (Quality Often Varies When Patient Changes Position)

- Patent ductus arteriosus
- Coarctation of the aorta
- Peripheral pulmonary stenosis

Diagnostic Studies

- ECG to detect underlying heart disease
- CBC to look for signs of infection, anemia
- Chest X-ray to evaluate heart failure, size of heart
- Echocardiography for valve pathology and systolic/diastolic function
- Angiography for more thorough evaluation
- Fluoroscopy to show calcified aortic valve

Differential Diagnosis

- See preceding descriptions of systolic and diastolic murmurs.

Management

Nonpharmacologic Treatment

- Patient education on disease entity and lifestyle modifications for underlying disorder
- Valvular surgical repair

Pharmacologic Treatment

- Stabilize hemodynamic deficiencies.
- Antibiotics for endocarditis prophylaxis as indicated

How Long to Treat

- Often a chronic condition

Special Considerations

- Geriatric patients: aortic stenosis common
- Pregnancy: monitor throughout pregnancy with intervention and cardiac consultation for any change in objective findings

When to Consult, Refer, Hospitalize

- Consult or refer if symptomatic (signs of heart failure, growth failure, syncope, cyanosis); diastolic murmur; systolic murmur that is loud (grade III/IV or with a thrill), long in duration, and transmits well to other parts of the body; abnormally strong or weak pulses; abnormal cardiac size or silhouette or pulmonary vasculature on chest X-ray.
- Refer to pediatric cardiologist for murmur in conjunction with chromosomal abnormalities (especially trisomy 13, trisomy 18, and trisomy 21).
- If abnormal ECG and symptomatic, hospitalization may be necessary

Follow-Up

- Asymptomatic patients should be assessed at least annually and at every visit.
- Innocent murmurs: none necessary
- Monitor murmurs associated with pregnancy; if they worsen, refer to cardiology.

Complications

- Chronic heart failure
- Poor activity tolerance; growth and development problems
- Progression of mitral stenosis—potential for thrombus formation and hypoxia
- Progression of mitral regurgitation—associated with dyspnea and orthopnea
- Atrial fibrillation with mitral stenosis and mitral regurgitation
- Stroke or TIA
- Bacterial endocarditis

MITRAL VALVE PROLAPSE (MVP)

Description

- Condition characterized by decreased ventricular load, resulting in prolapse of valve leaflets during systole
- Produces a mid-systolic click and late-systolic murmur

Etiology

- Strong familial pattern, associated with a connective tissue disorder such as Marfan syndrome and Ehlers-Danlos syndrome (nearly all patients with Marfan syndrome have MVP); systemic lupus erythematosus (SLE)
- One-third of patients have congenital heart disease (atrial septum defect, ventricular septum defect, or Ebstein's anomaly).
- May be caused by rheumatic endocarditis or ruptured chordae tendineae post-MI
- May be idiopathic; 50% of cases are in children
- Pathology involves abnormal valvular collagen leading to degeneration. Excessive tissue increases orifice size. Function of the papillary muscle and chordae apparatus is abnormal. MVP is the most common cause of mitral regurgitation.

Incidence and Demographics

- Adolescents and young adults; more common in females and thin patients; may be comorbid with minor chest wall deformities
- 3% of the general population; 5% of pediatric population; 75% without morbidity/mortality

Risk Factors

- Familial history
- Connective tissue disorders
- Mitral regurgitation

Prevention and Screening

- Proper dental care and prophylaxis to prevent endocarditis
- Anticoagulation to prevent thrombus/embolus for patients with risk factors
- Screening through periodic routine exams

Assessment

History

- Frequently asymptomatic
- Palpitations, lightheadedness, dyspnea, fatigue, syncope
- Anxiety, panic attacks
- Possible chest pain, usually mild

Physical Exam

- Murmur and clinical findings may vary from visit to visit.
- Late systolic murmur: begins in mid or late systole and can continue through S_2
- Mid- and late-systolic clicks may be audible.
- Positional murmur changes: When patient is standing, lying on left side, or with Valsalva, click is closer to the first heart sound (S_1); with squatting, click is farther from first heart sound (S_1).
- The MVP murmur increases with the handgrip maneuver, versus hypertrophic cardiomyopathy murmur, which decreases with hand grip. The handgrip maneuver also decreases the duration of the murmur and delays the timing of the mid-systolic click in MVP.
- Body build: thin, tall in some cases
- Autonomic abnormalities: orthostatic hypotension
- Mitral regurgitation (MR): holosystolic murmur, radiation to axilla, frequent thrill
- A high incidence of thoracic skeletal anomalies (80%) are seen in association with MVP:
  - Pectus excavatum (50%)
  - Straight back (20%)
  - Scoliosis (10%)

Diagnostic Studies

- Echocardiogram: diagnostic, should be repeated with significant change in murmur or accompanying clinical findings; will detect and quantify MR
- ECG: usually normal; possible atrial or ventricular arrhythmias; left atrial/ventricular enlargement

- Chest X-ray: normal
- Tilt table test to identify autonomic dysfunction
- Holter monitor to identify arrhythmia

Differential Diagnosis

- Stenotic mitral or tricuspid valve
- Pericarditis
- Tricuspid valve prolapse
- Papillary muscle dysfunction
- Hypertrophic cardiomyopathy

Management

Nonpharmacologic Treatment

- No treatment or activity restrictions in patients with asymptomatic MVP (about 75%)
- Patients who are symptomatic (palpitations, lightheadedness, syncope) or have arrhythmias should undergo treadmill exercise testing, ambulatory ECG monitoring, or both.
- Surgery: mitral valve replacement

Pharmacologic Treatment

- It is NOT recommended to give prophylactic antibiotics with invasive procedure and dental cleaning to prevent endocarditis in asymptomatic mitral valve prolapse unless patient has a history of endocarditis or mitral regurgitation is present.
- Beta-blockers such as atenolol 25–50 mg if patient has exercise-induced arrhythmias, palpitations, and panic attacks except with asthma. Propranolol (Inderal) for pediatrics
- Digoxin is effective in preventing fatigue, chest pain, and with SVT
- Anticoagulation for atrial fibrillation and mitral regurgitation: warfarin (Coumadin) to maintain international normalized ratio (INR) of 2.0–3.0
- Consider antiplatelet therapy with low-dose aspirin, or anticoagulant therapy with coumadin in those with MVP and thromboembolic episodes
- ACEIs if significant mitral regurgitation is present

How Long to Treat

- Lifelong monitoring and treatment unless patient undergoes surgical valve replacement

Special Considerations

- Males over 50 have higher incidence of complications.
- Pregnancy may improve symptoms of MVP.

When to Consult, Refer, Hospitalize

- Referral to a cardiologist for initial diagnosis, symptomatic patients, arrhythmias, heart failure, and complications

Follow-Up

- Monitor for MR with echocardiogram annually for problems; every 2–3 years for mild/moderate murmur with regurgitation; every 5 years for click only.

Expected Course

- Most have stable lifetime function.
- Approximately 5%–10% have progression to severe mitral regurgitation (MR).
- Patients younger than 50 years old with normal left ventricular function and no symptoms tend to have excellent survival with medical treatment, even those with severe MR.
- High-risk patients (i.e., those with moderate-to-severe MR and reduced left ventricular systolic function) have increased cardiac morbidity and mortality rates.

Complications

- Uncommon, usually relate to underlying heart disease
- Stroke or TIA from embolus
- Progression to or worsening mitral regurgitation

- CHF, arrhythmia
- Infective endocarditis
- Sudden death

ATRIAL FIBRILLATION

Description

- Most common arrhythmia, acute or chronic, characterized by nonsynchronized irregular atrial and ventricular activity
- Untreated rates from atria 200–600/minute with ventricular rate 80–180/minute
- Difference between apical rate and pulse rate is pulse deficit
- Non–life threatening by itself; however, comes with major risk of thromboembolism
- The 2019 AHA guideline updates recommend that only patients with moderate to severe mitral stenosis or mechanical heart valves are to be excluded from the use of direct-acting oral anticoagulants (DOACs)
- Terms used are valvular atrial fibrillation and nonvalvular were previously used to determine anticoagulation with warfarin vs. a DOAC

Etiology

- Extra-cardiac causes include pulmonary embolus, surgery, alcohol intoxication and withdrawal, hyperthyroidism
- May be preceded by premature atrial contraction
- May be idiopathic or have a variety of cardiac causes, including rheumatic heart disease, cardiomyopathy, atrial septal defect, MVP, sick sinus syndrome, acute myocardial infarction, heart failure, and pericarditis
- Chaotic electrical activity within the atria; AV node continuously stimulated by atrial impulses, so ventricular rate is irregular and usually rapid
- Ineffective atrial emptying results in hemodynamic instability, poor cardiac output, and stasis of blood.

Incidence and Demographics

- According to the CDC (2019), in the United States, it is estimated that 12.1 million people will have atrial fibrillation in 2030
- Increases with aging
- High blood pressure accounts for approximately 1 in 5 cases
- In the United States, atrial fibrillation is the primary diagnosis for more than 454,000 hospitalizations and contributes to approximately 158,00 deaths each year
- High recurrence of episodes
- Atrial fibrillation is the cause for approximately 1 of 7 strokes (CDC, 2019) and is associated with about a five time increase in ischemic stroke https://www.cdc.gov/heartdisease/atrial_fibrillation.htm

Risk Factors

- Conditions that increase the risk for atrial fibrillation include: advancing age, hyperthyroidism, high blood pressure, obesity, chronic kidney disease, ischemic heart disease, moderate to heavy alcohol use, enlarged heart chambers, heart failure, diabetes, European ancestry

Prevention and Screening

- Patient should avoid excessive alcohol, caffeine, and nicotine.
- Treat comorbid conditions.
- Assess and aggressively respond to triggers that compromise hemodynamic stability: acute MI, CHF, or pulmonary embolus.

Assessment

History

- Variable symptoms, from asymptomatic to severe
- Initial presentation may be with paroxysmal rhythm
- Palpitations, angina, fatigue, decline in activity level, marked dyspnea, dizziness, syncope
- Review of systems (ROS) for symptoms of hyperthyroidism, underlying cardiac disease, alcohol use

Physical Exam

- Tachycardia, irregular pulse—marked deficit between apical rate and radial pulse
- Pallor, orthostatic blood pressure changes
- Peripheral edema, jugular venous distention
- Tachypnea
- CNS disturbance: decreased mental acuity

Diagnostic Studies

- ECG: confirmatory with absent P waves, irregular ventricular rate, and rhythm 100–160 beats
- Cardiac event monitor
- Transthoracic or transesophageal echocardiography to assess underlying cardiac dysfunction and valvular disease
- Thyroid function tests, electrolytes (calcium, magnesium, sodium, potassium),
- BNP—assess for heart failure, troponin—assess for MI, digoxin level if on this medication
- Chest CT if pulmonary embolus is suspected (shortness of breath, chest pain)

Differential Diagnosis

- Hyperthyroidism
- Hypertension
- Pulmonary embolus
- Atrial flutter
- Sinus tachycardia
- Alcoholism

Management

Nonpharmacologic Treatment

- Treat underlying disorders.
- Lifestyle: avoid caffeine, decongestants, alcohol, nicotine, stimulants

- Refer for invasive therapy for refractory cases: cardioversion, radiofrequency catheter ablation of AV node, percutaneous left atrial appendage occlusion procedures
- Pacemaker implantation

Pharmacologic Treatment

- Medical management by a cardiologist

Acute

- Hospital setting under care of cardiologist for cardioversion and possible anticoagulation
- IV beta-blockers, IV non-dihydropyridine calcium channel blockers, IV digoxin, or IV amiodarone can be administered to slow ventricular rate; consider electrocardioversion for unstable atrial rhythm

Chronic (rate control)

- Digitalis glycosides
    - Digoxin: loading dose 0.25 mg IV with repeat dosing to a maximum of 1.5 mg over 24 hours, or start at maintenance dose; maintenance 0.125–0.25 mg daily
    - Check drug levels 6–8 hours after last dose or before dose.
    - Monitor toxicity: fatigue, anorexia, weakness, and nausea.
    - Digoxin ventricular response control is less effective with activity.
- Beta-blockers (side effects: constipation, dizziness, headaches)
    - Metoprolol tartrate 25–100 mg orally twice daily
    - Metoprolol XL 50–400 mg orally once daily
    - Atenolol 25–100 mg orally once daily
    - Propranolol 10–40 mg orally three or four times a day.
    - Nadolol 10–240 mg orally daily
    - Carvedilol 3.125–25 mg orally twice daily
    - Bisoprolol 2.5–10 mg orally daily
    - Use caution with medications; some have a depressing effect on the AV node.

- Nondihydropyridine calcium channel blocker
  - Do NOT use nondihydropyridine calcium channel blockers in patients with decompensated heart failure.
  - Nondihydropyridine calcium channel blockers:
    - verapamil ER 180–480 mg orally daily
    - diltiazem 120–360 mg orally daily
- Other: amiodarone (Cordarone) 100–200mg orally daily is also used but has a black box warning of hepatic injury, pulmonary toxicity, thyroid disease (hyper- or hypothyroidism), peripheral neuropathy, visual impairment, and worsening arrhythmia
- Arrhythmia more than 48 hours: anticoagulation therapy maintained 3–4 weeks before cardioversion (see anticoagulation treatment below)

How Long to Treat

- Anticoagulation therapy is indefinite unless situations arise that would contraindicate therapy.
- The CHA2DS2-VASc tool is extensively employed to guide decision making for anticoagulation in patients with atrial fibrillation at risk of stroke. (see Table 8–21).
  - *CHA_2DS_2-VASc score of 0:* No antithrombotic therapy. Do not offer anticoagulation for persons younger than 65 years of age with no other risk factor than gender (i.e., woman with score 1—no anticoagulation).
  - *CHA_2DS_2-VASc score of 1:* Oral anticoagulation or aspirin antiplatelet therapy is recommended but oral anticoagulation is preferable.
  - *CHA_2DS_2-VASc score ≥2:* Oral anticoagulation is recommended
- See Table 8–21 for assessment of stroke risk using CHA_2DS_2-VASc score and Table 8–22 the acronym for hypertension, abnormal liver/renal function, stroke history, bleeding history, labile INR, older adult, drug/alcohol usage (HAS-BLED) bleeding risk for patients with atrial fibrillation on anticoagulation.

Antiplatelet or Anticoagulant Agents to decrease stroke risk:

- *Antiplatelet Agent for Atrial Fibrillation*
  - Aspirin
- *Anticoagulants for Atrial Fibrillation with a mechanical valve or moderate to severe mitral stenosis*
  - Warfarin (Coumadin)—vitamin K antagonist, recommended for atrial fibrillation with moderate-to-severe mitral stenosis or a mechanical heart valve and endstage kidney disease

TABLE 8–21.
ASSESSMENT OF STROKE RISK USING CHA2DS2-VASC SCORE AND BLEEDING RISK FOR PATIENTS WITH ATRIAL FIBRILLATION ON ANTICOAGULATION

CHA2DS2-VASC	SCORE
Chronic heart failure	1
Hypertension	1
Age 75 *years* or older	2
Diabetes mellitus	1
Stroke/transient ischemic attack (TIA)/thromboembolism (TE)	2
Vascular disease (prior MI, PAD, or aortic plaque)	1
Age 65–74 years old	1
Sex, female (only add if another risk factor is present)	1
Maximum Score	**9**

CHA2DS2-VASC SCORE	ADJUSTED STROKE RISK (%)
0	0
1.	1.3
2	2.2
3	3.2
4	4.0
5	6.7
6	9.8
7	9.6
8	6.7
9	15.2

◊ Warfarin requires INR target 2.5 monitoring, activated partial thromboplastin time (aPTT), CBC, platelet count, LFTs, creatinine monitoring.

◊ Initial dose is 5 mg; start at 2.5 mg orally daily for older adult, frail persons over 70 years of age.

◊ Check INR every 2–3 days for first two checks (INR 2–3, or check with cardiologist for target INR goal) then weekly; once stable check every 4 weeks.

◊ Education includes: monitor for bleeding, avoid over-the-counter NSAIDs (including aspirin), avoid foods and drinks rich in vitamin K (cranberry, grapefruit juice, kale, spinach, Brussels sprouts, green leafy vegetables)

TABLE 8–22
BLED-SCORE TO ASSESS THEIR RISK FOR BLEEDING

HAS-BLED	SCORE
Hypertension (systolic blood pressure higher than160 mmHg	1
Abnormal renal and liver function (1 point each)	1 or 2
Stroke	1
Bleeding tendency	1
Labile international normalized ratios (INRs) if on Coumadin (warfarin)	1
Older adults (65 years and older)	1
Drugs or alcohol (1 point each)	1 or 2
Maximum Score	**9**

- *Anticoagulants for Nonvalvular Atrial Fibrillation*—patients without a mechanical valve or moderate to severe mitral stenosis
  - ◇ Non–vitamin K oral anticoagulants (NOACs) (see below) also known as direct-acting oral anticoagulants (or DOACs) are preferred over warfarin to decrease stroke risk in patients who DO NOT have moderate to severe mitral stenosis or a mechanical heart valve. Prior to starting these agents, hepatic and renal function tests should be performed and followed up annually. Do not require INR monitoring
  - ◇ Dabigatran (Pradaxa): a direct thrombin inhibitor, NOT recommended in end-stage kidney disease or dialysis; decrease dosing if moderate to severe CKD with creatinine clearance (CrCl) 15 to 30 mL/min, reversal agent idarucizumab for life-threatening bleeding; dosing below
    - 150 mg orally twice daily (CrCl above 30 mL/min)
    - 75 mg orally twice daily (CrCl 15–30 mL/min)
    - Not recommended for CrCl less than 15 mL/min
  - ◇ Rivaroxaban (Xarelto): Factor Xa inhibitor, NOT recommended in end-stage kidney disease or dialysis; decrease dosing if moderate to severe CKD with CrCl 50 mL/min or lower, reversal agent andexanet alfa (Andexxa, a recombinant factor Xa) may be used for life-threatening bleeding; dosing below
    - 20 mg orally daily with evening meal (CrCl above 50 mL/min)
    - 15 mg orally daily with evening meal (CrCl 15–50 mL/min)
    - Not recommended for CrCl less than 15 mL/min
  - ◇ Apixaban (Eliquis): Factor Xa inhibitor, reversal agent andexanet alfa (Andexxa, a recombinant factor Xa) may be used for life-threatening bleeding; decrease dosing if moderate to severe CKD with serum creatinine 1.5 mg/dL or above; dosing below
    - 5 or 2.5 mg orally twice daily (CrCl above 30 mL/min)
    - No recommendations for CrCl less than 30 mL/min

◊ Edoxaban (Savaysa): Factor Xa inhibitor; NOT recommended in end-stage kidney disease or dialysis; decrease dosing if moderate to severe CKD with CrCl 15 to 30 mL/min: dosing below
  - 60 mg orally daily (CrCl above 30 mL/min)
  - 30 mg orally daily (CrCl 15–50 mL/min)
  - Not recommended for CrCl less than 15 mL/min

◊ When patients are on anticoagulant therapy, use the HAS BLED score to assess their risk for bleeding (see Table 8–22).

Special Considerations

♦ Geriatric patients: prevalent problem

♦ Patients at risk for bleeding with history of coronary artery stenting, in lieu of triple therapy, may be on double therapy with clopidogrel and low-dose rivaroxaban (15 mg orally daily) or dabigatran (150 mg orally twice daily) to decrease bleeding risk; refer to cardiologist.

♦ Pregnancy (rare): digoxin safe; cardioversion does not affect fetus; anticoagulation may result in spontaneous abortion, although heparin does not cross placenta.

◊ Recommendations for IV heparin during first trimester; oral warfarin second and third trimester

When to Consult, Refer, Hospitalize

♦ Initially, refer all patients to cardiologist for evaluation and management plan; refer pregnant women for management; and refer patients who are not controlled back to cardiologist for evaluation.

♦ Percutaneous left atrial appendage

Follow-Up

♦ At least monthly for INR if on warfarin (target 2.5)

Expected Course

♦ Prognosis is dependent on underlying cause.

♦ Exercise and activity levels may be limited because of hemodynamic instability.

Complications

- Heart failure
- Stroke, peripheral arterial embolism
- Bradycardia, torsades de pointes with drug treatment
- Bleeding with anticoagulants

Congenital Heart Defects

PATENT DUCTUS ARTERIOSUS (PDA)

Description

- The ductus arteriosus is a normal fetal structure between the left pulmonary artery and the descending aorta.
- Functional closure of the ductus arteriosus usually occurs within 48 hours after birth.
- Anatomic closure is completed by 2–3 weeks of age.
- PDA becomes clinically significant if it persists past the neonatal period; it is unlikely to close spontaneously after that time and may produce signs and symptoms of pulmonary overcirculation.

Etiology

- Idiopathic
- High altitude
- Maternal exposure to rubella during first trimester
- Genetic or familial

Incidence and Demographics

- Full-term infants: 0.02 to 0.006% of live births in the United States; at high altitudes (above 4,500 feet), 15 per 1,000 live births
- Premature infants: 20% of premature infants more than 32 weeks of gestation, up to 60% in infants less than 28 weeks of gestation, prevalence in infants with birth weight less than 2500 g, 30%; less than 1200 grams birth weight, 80% (Kim, 2018)

- As an isolated lesion, PDA occurs in approximately 0.008% of live premature births (Kim, 2018)
- According to Kim (2018), the mortality rate for patent ductus arteriosus (PDA) left untreated is estimated at 20% by age 20 years, 42% by age 45 years, and 60% mortality rate by age 60 years. Approximately, 0.6% of those with PDA undergoes spontaneous closure every year.

Risk Factors

- Environmental triggers such as viruses and drugs
- Prematurity, neonatal respiratory distress syndrome, genetic disorders, that is, hypoplastic left heart syndrome, transposition of the great vessels, and pulmonary stenosis
- More prevalent in females vs. males: ratio 2:1 (except if rubella exposure, then risk is equal)

Assessment

History

- Symptoms dependent on volume of pulmonary blood flow; patients are usually asymptomatic with a small PDA
- A moderate to large shunt may cause symptoms of CHF (tachypnea, sweating, poor feeding/poor weight gain), irritability, and lower respiratory tract infections.

Physical Exam

- Classic finding is a "machinery" murmur with continuous systolic and diastolic components, heard best at the ULSB and left infraclavicular area; none may be heard with severe left ventricular failure
- Patients with small PDAs usually have normal physical growth and normal pulses/pulse pressure.
- Tachycardia, tachypnea, crackles in cases of pulmonary overcirculation
- Hyperdynamic precordium

Diagnostic Studies

- ECG: normal or left ventricular, atrial hypertrophy depending on amount of the shunt
- Chest X-ray: normal with a small PDA. Varying degrees of cardiomegaly with enlargement of left atrium, left ventricle, and ascending aorta. Increased pulmonary vascular markings are proportionate to the amount of left-to-right shunting.
- Echocardiography: Doppler studies can provide functional information. Dimensions of the left atrium and ventricle can indirectly assess the amount of left-to-right shunting; the greater the dilation of these chambers, the larger the shunt.
- Cardiac catheterization: not necessary for diagnostic evaluation

Differential Diagnosis

- Arteriovenous malformations (systemic, pulmonary, or coronary)
- Venous hum
- Ventricular septal defect with aortic regurgitation
- Mitral regurgitation
- Pulmonary atresia
- Persistent truncus arteriosus
- Aortopulmonary septal defect (AP window)
- Peripheral pulmonary stenosis
- Total anomalous venous connection
- Collaterals in coarctation of the aorta in tetralogy of Fallot/pulmonary atresia
- Anomalous origin of the left coronary artery from the pulmonary artery
- Ruptured sinus of Valsalva aneurysm

Management

Pharmacologic Treatment

- Indomethacin (Indocin; a prostaglandin synthetase inhibitor) or IV ibuprofen during the first 10 to 14 days of life
  - Contraindications to the use of indomethacin: BUN greater than 25 mg/dL or creatinine greater than 1.8 mg/dL, platelet count lower than 80,000/mm^3,

necrotizing enterocolitis, hyperbilirubinemia, and bleeding tendency (including intracranial hemorrhage)

Surgical Treatment

- Premature infants
  - If medical therapy is unsuccessful or indomethacin is contraindicated after 2–3 attempts, surgical repair is indicated.
  - Percutaneous coil embolization is performed in the cardiac catheterization laboratory. Percutaneous closure is not currently available for very small or preterm infants; new devices under study may make it feasible to close even large PDAs or PDAs in small infants.
  - Surgical ligation performed by thoracoscopy with minimal surgical incision is the currently used procedure.
  - The existence of a PDA, regardless of size, is an indication for surgery because of the risk of endocarditis, heart failure, and eventual pulmonary hypertension
  - A PDA ligation is performed between 6 months and 2 years of age; PDAs in asymptomatic infants may be closed electively at a time chosen by the family and surgeon.
  - Surgical mortality is less than 1%.
  - Complications are rare and include injury to the laryngeal nerve (hoarseness), left phrenic nerve (left hemidiaphragm paralysis), or thoracic duct (chylothorax).

Special Considerations

- None

When to Consult, Refer, Hospitalize

- Refer all infants, children, adults with PDA-type murmurs to a pediatric cardiologist.

Follow-Up

- No activity restrictions unless pulmonary hypertension is present
- Infective endocarditis prophylaxis for 6 months after surgery/coil embolization
- Controversy exists about in children silent PDAs detected by ultrasound but not clinically significant, should be repaired at all

Complications

- Complications post surgery are unusual; may include infective endocarditis, CHF, recurrent pneumonia, pulmonary vascular obstructive disease (PVOD), pulmonary hypertension, and pulmonary or systemic emboli
- Rarely, aneurysm of the PDA may occur.

ATRIAL SEPTAL DEFECT (ASD)

Description

- Defect (opening) in the atrial septum
- Four types: primum (30%), secundum (50%–70%), sinus venosus (less than 10%), coronary sinus septal (less than 10%)

Etiology

- No known genetic cause; most are sporadic; primum ASDs associated with trisomy 21

Incidence and Demographics

- Isolated cases (those not associated with other cyanotic heart lesions) occur in 0.5–1/1,000 live births (5%–10% of all congenital heart disease cases).
- ASDs account for less than 10% of congenital heart disease in infants, but more than 30% of cases are diagnosed in adults because findings may be subtle and not detected earlier.
- A 2019 study using data from birth-defect tracking systems across the United States estimates that 2,118 babies in the United States are born with an ASD, or every year, 1 in every 1,859 babies born in the United States are born with an ASD. (CDC, 2019)

Risk Factors

- Genetic predisposition with environmental triggers such as viruses and drugs
- Prematurity

Assessment

History

- Even with moderate to large ASDs, infants and children are usually asymptomatic.
- Children with significant defects may be small, but true failure to thrive is rare.
- The physiologic impact of the left-to-right shunt increases with age, initially manifests as exercise intolerance, and can lead to overt CHF.
- Progressive increase in symptoms in second and third decades of life

Physical Exam

- In large defects, height and weight may be slightly below normal.
- Heart rate is usually normal; patient may have mild tachycardia; blood pressure is normal.
- A prominent precordial bulge or right ventricular heave may be present.
- Classic finding is wide, split S_2; may have split S_1 with loud second component.
- Grade II–III/VI medium-pitched systolic ejection murmur heard best at ULSB or LMSB secondary to pulmonary valve stenosis
- Mid-diastolic rumble at LLSB due to increased flow across the tricuspid valve may be heard with large left-to-right shunts.

Diagnostic Studies

- ECG: usually normal sinus rhythm. Right axis deviation and mild right ventricular hypertrophy or RBBB and an rSR′ pattern in lead V1 may be seen.
- Chest X-ray: may be normal or show cardiomegaly with right atrial enlargement or right ventricular enlargement, prominent main pulmonary artery, increased pulmonary vascular markings. Large pulmonary artery is best seen on lateral view.
- Echocardiography: transthoracic or transesophageal technique, can identify location of ASD and demonstrate pulmonary venous return
- Cardiac catheterization: not necessary for diagnostic evaluation; performed if defect can be closed using an atrial occlusion device

Differential Diagnosis

- Pulmonary stenosis
- Innocent murmur
- Physiologic "flow" murmur (e.g., anemia, fever)
- Tricuspid stenosis

Management

- Patients with an isolated defect 3–8 mm in size have a spontaneous closure rate of 80% by 18 months of age.
- Patients with an isolated defect less than 3 mm diagnosed by 3 months of age have a spontaneous closure rate of 100% by 18 months of age.
- ASDs larger than 8 mm rarely close spontaneously.
- Infective endocarditis does not occur in patients with isolated ASDs.

Nonpharmacologic Treatment

- Exercise restriction unnecessary

Pharmacologic Treatment

- No treatment for ASD, but if signs and symptoms of CHF develop, treatment with digoxin and diuretics are indicated
- Infective endocarditis prophylaxis unnecessary unless there are associated cardiac lesions

Surgical

- High pulmonary vascular resistance (PVR) is contraindication for surgery.
- Surgery may be postponed until 3–4 years of age due to high incidence of spontaneous closure; however, if heart failure develops that does not respond to medical management, then surgery would be performed earlier, in infancy
- Surgical closure of the ASD

- Direct closure of the defect with a patch or stitch closure
- Incision made through median sternotomy
- Performed under cardiopulmonary bypass through atrial approach or hemisternotomy, limited thoracotomy, or partial or full submammary skin incision
- Surgical mortality is less than 1%; mortality rate is higher during infancy and in patients with high PVR.
- Complications include postoperative arrhythmias (7%–20%) and cerebrovascular accident.
- Placement of atrial occlusion devices to close the ASD (done in the cardiac catheterization laboratory) may be possible for secundum defects.

Special Considerations

- None

When to Consult, Refer, Hospitalize

- Refer all patients with ASD-type murmurs to a cardiologist.

Follow-Up

- Patients without chronic heart failure are managed conservatively.
- If patient is asymptomatic with small ASD after first year of life, see every 1–2 years to monitor for spontaneous closure of the ASD.

Postoperative Follow-Up

- Congenital cardiology visit within 1 week after discharge and thereafter per cardiologist instructions
- No activity restrictions unless complications from surgery have occurred
- No infective endocarditis prophylaxis for an isolated ASD
- Long-term follow-up required for patients with postoperative arrhythmias
- Aspirin with or without clopidogrel for 6 months post catheter or surgical closure to decrease risk of thrombus

Complications

- Chronic heart failure and pulmonary hypertension (in third to fourth decades of life)
- Atrial arrhythmias (flutter/fibrillation) risk is long term
- Holt-Oram syndrome: tricuspid or mitral insufficiency
- Risk of bacterial endocarditis up to 6 months post-surgery
- Rarely, cerebrovascular accident

VENTRICULAR SEPTAL DEFECT (VSD)

Description

- Defect (opening) in the ventricular septum
- VSDs are classified as membranous or muscular, depending on location of defect.
- Varied in size, from tiny openings with no hemodynamic compromise to large openings with accompanying pulmonary hypertension and chronic heart failure
- VSDs may be isolated or found with coarctation of the aorta, sub-aortic stenosis, tetralogy of Fallot, and transposition of the great vessels.

Etiology

- The etiology of VSD is primarily unknown; however, several genetic factors including chromosomal, single gene, and polygenic inheritance have been identified as causing VSD (Dakkak, 2022). Maternal infection (febrile illness, influenza, rubella), maternal diabetes mellitus, phenylketonuria, and toxin exposures (cocaine, marijuana, alcohol) and medications, that is, ibuprofen and metronidazole, have been linked to VSD (Dakkak, 2022).

Incidence and Demographics

- VSD is the most common form of congenital heart disease, usually detected by a murmur heard between 2 and 6 weeks.
- Isolated cases (those not associated with other cyanotic heart lesions) occur in 0.3% of newborns (37% of all CHD cases); up to 90% may close spontaneously (Dakkak, 2022)

- 3% of children with a VSD have a parent with a VSD.
- 30%–50% of VSDs close in the first 2 years of life.

Risk Factors

- Genetic predisposition with environmental triggers such as viruses and drugs
- Prematurity

Prevention and Screening

- Early referral to a congenital cardiologist

Assessment

History

- Patients with small VSDs are usually asymptomatic with normal growth and development.
- Symptoms vary with the size of the VSD and the degree of left-to-right shunting.
  - ◇ Patients with moderate to large shunts show delayed growth and development, increased incidence of respiratory infections, decreased exercise tolerance, and signs and symptoms of chronic heart failure (CHF).
  - ◇ CHF usually does not occur until 6–8 weeks of life, after the decrease in pulmonary vascular resistance and pulmonary artery pressure.
- Infants may have severe dyspnea, feeding difficulties, profuse perspiration, and duskiness with crying or infection.

Physical Exam

Small VSDs

- Patients are acyanotic and well developed.
- Precordial activity is normal; thrill is typically not palpable.
- Normal physiologic splitting of S_2
- Grade II–VI/VI harsh systolic regurgitant murmur heard best at LLSB

Moderate to Large VSDs

- Infants may have failure to thrive, show signs of CHF (usually by 2 months of age).
- Hepatomegaly may be present.
- Tachycardia
- Increased intensity of the precordial impulse
- S_2 is narrowly split.
- Harsh pansystolic murmur heard best at the LLSB; may obscure 1st and 2nd heart sounds
- Handgrip increases murmur due to increased afterload
- Apical diastolic rumble
- Eisenmenger syndrome presents with cyanosis, dyspnea, syncope, secondary erythrocytosis, desaturation, clubbing

Diagnostic Studies

- *ECG*: Normal with small VSDs. LVH and occasional left atrial enlargement may be seen with moderate VSDs. Combined ventricular hypertrophy with or without left atrial enlargement with large VSDs. Monitor for possible pulmonary hypertension or pulmonic stenosis, which results in right ventricular hypertrophy.
- *Chest X-ray*: Normal with small VSDs; with moderate to large shunt VSDs, cardiomegaly of varying degrees that involves the LA, LV, and sometimes the RV. Pulmonary vascular markings (PVMs) increased. The degree of cardiomegaly and increased PVMs is directly proportional to the amount of left-to-right shunting.
- *Echocardiography*: Two-dimensional echocardiography can determine the anatomic location, size, and number of VSDs. Doppler studies can provide visualization of the shunt and are also used to screen for the development of left ventricular outflow tract disease and spontaneous closure
- *Cardiac MRI and CT*: Useful in cases that are difficult to visualize on echocardiography
- *Cardiac catheterization*: Strongly recommended for critically ill children before surgery. Provides detailed information about the anatomic location of the VSD, hemodynamics, quantitative measurements of shunting, and level of pulmonary vascular resistance.
- *Selective left ventriculography*: shows "gooseneck" deformity of left ventricular outflow tract

Differential Diagnosis

- Tricuspid regurgitation
- Mitral regurgitation
- Patent ductus arteriosus
- Atrial septal defect
- Subaortic membrane

Management

- Small defects close spontaneously up to 85% to 90% of the time during the first year of life (Dakkak, 2022); moderate defects close up to 30%–50%; large defects will decrease in size as the patient grows but have a low spontaneous closure rate. Muscular defects have a higher spontaneous closure rate than membranous defects.

Nonpharmacologic Treatment

- Observation only for small to moderate VSDs
- Frequent feedings of high-caloric formula, orally or through a nasogastric tube, may help address growth failure in children with moderate to large VSDs.

Pharmacologic Treatment

- Infective endocarditis prophylaxis, as long as VSD is present and until 6 months after surgical correction
- If signs and symptoms of CHF develop, treatment includes digoxin and diuretics.
- Anemia should be corrected by oral iron therapy.

Surgical Treatment

- If growth failure cannot be improved with medical management, the VSD should be closed surgically within the first 6 months of life. For infants who respond to medical therapy, surgery should be postponed to allow time for spontaneous closure.
- Surgical closure of a VSD
- Direct closure of the defect with a patch or stitch closure through a median sternotomy

- Surgical mortality is 2%–5% after the age of 6 months, higher in patients younger than 2 months of age and those with multiple VSDs or associated defects.
- Complications include residual VSD shunt (20% of patients), RBBB (10% of patients), complete heart block (less than 5% of patients), rarely, cerebrovascular accident.
- VSD closure by percutaneous device is high risk in surgical candidates due to severe PAH, multiple comorbidities, and those who had prior cardiothoracic surgery such as residual or recurrent VSD (Dakkak, 2022).

Special Considerations

- None

When to Consult, Refer, Hospitalize

- Refer all patients with VSD-type murmurs to a cardiologist.

Follow-Up

- Patients without CHF or pulmonary hypertension are managed conservatively, with close monitoring of growth.
- Patients younger than 6 months with CHF and growth failure should be seen monthly.

Postoperative Follow-Up

- Cardiology follow-up as directed by surgery
- No activity restrictions unless complications from surgery have occurred
- Infective endocarditis prophylaxis may be discontinued 6 months after surgery; however, for residual VSD, continue infective endocarditis prophylaxis indefinitely.
- Long-term follow-up required for patients who had transient heart block postoperatively

Complications

- Subacute bacterial endocarditis
- Pulmonary over circulation/pulmonary hypertension

- Left ventricular volume overload
- Aortic insufficiency
- Eisenmenger syndrome
- Acquired left ventricular outflow tract obstruction
- Aneurysm of the interventricular septum
- Mitral regurgitation leading to valve replacement
- Heart block requiring pacemaker placement

COARCTATION OF THE AORTA (COA)

Description

- Discrete narrowing of the aorta, most often just distal to the subclavian artery
- Two distinct presentations
  - ◊ Neonatal period: coarctation is usually severe; associated with closing of ductus arteriosus; presents at 4–10 days of life
  - ◊ Infancy, childhood: typically no symptoms; coarctation is less severe; may have good collateral flow to descending aorta

Etiology

- Cause unknown

Incidence and Demographics

- Occurs in 0.06% to 0.08% of the general population, 6%–8% of all CHD cases (Law, 2022)

Risk Factors

- Other cardiac defects such as aortic hypoplasia, bicuspid aortic valve (85%), PDA (60%), VSD (50%), mitral valve abnormalities, and Shone's syndrome (multiple left-sided obstruction lesions including mitral stenosis, subaortic membrane, valvular aortic stenosis) are often associated with COA.
- Turner syndrome (XO): 30%–35% have COA, karyotype screening recommended for all females with COA

Prevention and Screening

- Early referral

Assessment

History

Symptomatic Infants

- Poor feeding and weight gain
- Dyspnea
- Signs of chronic heart failure
- Circulatory shock
- Normal newborn discharge examination (if PDA did not close and was supplying blood flow to descending aorta)

Asymptomatic Children

- Majority of children asymptomatic until late childhood
- Occasionally, complaints of pain or weakness in the legs following exercise; headache secondary to hypertension

Physical Exam

Symptomatic Infants

- Hallmark is absent or weak femoral pulses
- Pale, varying degrees of respiratory distress
- Oliguria or anuria
- General circulatory shock with severe acidosis
- Differential cyanosis (lower part of body appears cyanotic because of right-to-left ductal shunting)
- Decreased or absent lower-extremity pulses; qualitative difference between brachial and femoral pulse

- Blood pressure discrepancy between the upper and lower extremities (higher in the arms)
- Loud single S_2; a gallop usually present.
- Nonspecific systolic ejection murmur, although 50% of affected infants do not have murmur

Asymptomatic Children

- Normal growth and development
- Decreased or absent lower-extremity pulses
- Hypertension in upper extremities (normally thigh or calf systolic pressure higher than arm)
- Systolic thrill may be present in suprasternal notch.
- Accentuated A2, normally split S_2
- II–IV/VI systolic ejection murmur heard best at the URSB, MLSB, or LLSB, which radiates to the left interscapular region posteriorly
- Ejection click frequently audible

Diagnostic Studies

- ECG: Usually normal. RVH or RBBB may be present in infants; LVH can be seen in older children with longstanding COA.
- Chest X-ray: Marked pulmonary edema and cardiomegaly are seen in symptomatic infants. In older children, the heart size is normal or slightly enlarged. A "3 sign" on an overpenetrated chest X-ray (due to a double aortic curve/abnormal contour of the arch) or an E-shaped indentation on a barium-filled esophagus may be seen. Rib notching between the 4th and 8th ribs may be present in older children but is rare before the age of 5 years. Rib notching is erosion of the ribs caused by dilated intercostal collateral vessels.
- Echocardiography: Two-dimensional echocardiography and color flow Doppler studies can show the site and extent of coarctation and provide information about left ventricular function and other left-sided lesions.
- Cardiac catheterization allows measurement of pressure above and below coarctation.
- MRI can be used to further define the location and severity of the COA and provide data about collateral vessels.

Differential Diagnosis

- Aortic stenosis
- Pulmonary stenosis
- Patent ductus arteriosus

Management

Nonpharmacologic Treatment

Symptomatic Infants

- Oxygen
- Surgical intervention to follow

Asymptomatic Children

- Patients with mild COA should be followed closely for the development of hypertension or systolic pressure differences between the arms and legs

Pharmacologic Treatment

Symptomatic Infants

- Prostaglandin E1 infusion to reopen the ductus arteriosus (0.5 µg/kg/min)
- Correction of acidosis and metabolic disturbances
- Inotropic agents (dopamine or dobutamine)
- Diuretics

Asymptomatic Children

- Patients with mild COA should be followed closely for the development of hypertension or systolic pressure differences between the arms and legs. Occasionally these children will require chronic antihypertensive therapy, usually with beta-blockers or ACEI, most commonly if the repair is performed before the patient is 5 years of age.

Surgical Treatment

Symptomatic Infants

- Surgery to repair the COA should be performed urgently on infants with CHF.
- Surgical correction of COA
- Surgery is performed without bypass through a left posterolateral thoracotomy.
- Types of repair include:
  - End-to-end anastomosis (area of coarctation resected, distal and proximal aorta anastomosed end-to-end)
  - Patch aortoplasty (area of coarctation incised, elliptical Dacron patch sutured in place to widen diameter)
  - Subclavian flap aortoplasty (distal subclavian artery divided, flap of proximal portion of vessel used to expand the coarcted area)
- Ductus is always ligated with these surgical techniques.
- Surgical mortality is less than 5%.
- Complications include residual obstruction or recoarctation (6%–33%) and postoperative renal failure.
- Balloon angioplasty may be performed if coarctation recurs.

Asymptomatic Children

- Upper-extremity hypertension or a systolic gradient of ≥20 mmHg between upper and lower extremities is an indication for elective repair of a COA in children 2–4 years old; mortality less than 1%.
- Older children should be operated on as soon as the diagnosis of COA is made.
- Surgical correction of COA
- Surgery performed without bypass through a left posterolateral thoracotomy.
- Types of repair are the same as in symptomatic infants.
  - End-to-end is the repair of choice for discrete COA in older children.
  - Complications include spinal cord paralysis producing paraplegia due to limited collateral circulation during cross-clamping of aorta (0.4%), postoperative rebound hypertension, and post-coarctectomy (reperfusion) syndrome.
  - Balloon angioplasty of native COA (no history of surgical intervention) is controversial; may be performed if coarctation recurs.

Special Considerations

- None

When to Consult, Refer, Hospitalize

- Refer all patients with a COA-type murmur to a cardiologist.
- Refer patients with hypertension to a cardiologist if other causes have been ruled out.

Follow-Up

- Symptomatic infants should be followed every 6–12 months to evaluate for recoarctation.
- Asymptomatic children can be seen annually to assess for persistent hypertension, recoarctation, subaortic stenosis, and persistent myocardial dysfunction.
- Require infective endocarditis prophylaxis indefinitely, because of associated bicuspid aortic valve and recoarctation.

Cyanotic Congenital Heart Defects

TETRALOGY OF FALLOT (TOF)

Description

- Syndrome of congenital heart defects with four components:
  - Large VSD in the membranous region of the ventricular septum
  - Pulmonary stenosis
  - Overriding aorta
  - Obstructive right ventricular hypertrophy

Etiology

- Cause unknown but it has been associated with
  - Microdeletions of chromosome 22q11 and Alagille syndrome with *JAG1/NOTCH2* mutations

- ◇ Mutations in methylenetetrahydrofolate reductase polymorphism, transcription factor NKX2.5, and mutations in *TBX1* and *ZFPM2*
- ◇ Maternal diabetes, maternal intake of retinoic acid, phenylketonuria (Diaz-Frias, 2022)

Incidence and Demographics

- Occurs in 3 to 5 of every 1,000 live births (7% to 10% of all CHD cases); most common cyanotic CHD beyond 1 week of age (Diaz-Frias, 2022)

Risk Factors

- Genetic predisposition with environmental triggers such as viruses and drugs
- Prematurity

Assessment

History

- Heart murmur audible in the newborn period
- Most patients symptomatic with cyanosis present at birth
- History of hypoxic spells, especially with crying or exercise
- Parents may describe child as squatting while walking.
- Patients with acyanotic (pink)TOF asymptomatic
- Hypoxic spells ("tet" spells)
- Spells usually occur after crying, feeding, or defecation
- Spells usually consist of rapid and deep breathing, irritability and prolonged crying, increased cyanosis, and decrease in intensity of murmur.
- Severe hypoxic spell may lead to limpness, convulsion, cerebral vascular accident (CVA), or even death

Physical Exam

- Varying degrees of cyanosis, with hypercyanosis occurring later in infancy
- Growth retardation if cyanosis is severe

- Tachypnea
- Clubbing may be present if cyanosis has been longstanding (usually more than 6 months).
- Normal S_1 and single S_2 (because aorta is located more anteriorly than normal)
- Active precordium, grade III–IV/VI systolic ejection murmur heard best at middle and upper left sternal border (caused by right ventricular outflow tract obstruction); the greater the obstruction, the softer the murmur
- Continuous murmur representing PDA shunt may be audible in patients with TOF and pulmonary atresia.

Diagnostic Studies

- *ECG:* Normal QRS axis with acyanotic TOF and right axis deviation with cyanotic TOF. Right ventricular hypertrophy and right atrial hypertrophy are usually present. Combined ventricular hypertrophy (CVH) may be seen in acyanotic TOF.
- *Chest X-ray:* Findings in patients with acyanotic TOF are the same as in those with a small to moderate VSD. With cyanotic TOF, heart size ≤ normal. PVMs are decreased.

Heart may appear "boot-shaped" because of a concave main pulmonary artery with an upturned apex. Right aortic arch (25%) and right atrial enlargement (25%) may be present.

- *Echocardiography:* Two-dimensional echo can determine the anatomical location, size, and number of VSDs; assess the anatomy of the right ventricular outflow tract (RVOT), pulmonary valve, and pulmonary arteries; and image the coronary arteries. Doppler studies can visualize the VSD shunt and estimate a pressure gradient across the RVOT obstruction.
- Up to 50% are diagnosed by fetal echocardiogram antenatally.
- *Cardiac catheterization:* Recommended before surgical repair of TOF

Differential Diagnosis

- Aortic stenosis
- Bronchiolitis
- Pneumonia
- Pneumothorax

Management

- Treatment of cyanotic spells includes knee-chest positioning, oxygen, intravenous fluid bolus, sodium bicarbonate to treat acidosis, morphine sulfate to calm child, vasoconstrictors (epinephrine [Adrenalin] or phenylephrine) to increase systemic vascular resistance, and beta-blockers (Inderal) to cause RVOT relaxation.

Pharmacologic Treatment

- Treat iron-deficiency anemia, since anemic children are more likely to have a CVA.
- Provide infective endocarditis prophylaxis.

Surgical Treatment

- Asymptomatic and acyanotic children are repaired at 6–12 months of age.
- Asymptomatic and minimally cyanotic children are repaired at 3–24 months of age, depending on the amount of pulmonary artery hypoplasia.
- Mildly cyanotic infants who have had a palliative shunt procedure may have a complete repair 1–2 years after the shunt procedure.
- Symptomatic infants with a favorable RVOT and pulmonary arteries are repaired at 3–4 months of age.
- Surgical repair of TOF
- Patch closure of VSD and reconstruction of the RVOT by resection of the infundibular tissue and placement of a transannular patch
- Incision is made through a median sternotomy under cardiopulmonary bypass.
- Surgical mortality is 2%–5% during the first 2 years of life; higher in patients under 3 months of age and older than 4 years of age and those with severe pulmonary hypoplasia and associated defects
- Complications include bleeding during the postoperative period, pulmonary valve regurgitation, residual RVOT obstruction, RV dysfunction, residual VSD, RBBB, and, rarely, complete heart block or ventricular arrhythmias.

Special Considerations

- None

When to Consult, Refer, Hospitalize

- Refer all patients with a TOF-type murmur to a cardiologist.

Follow-Up

- Symptomatic infants should be seen monthly until surgical repair. Asymptomatic children can be seen every 3–6 months until surgical repair.

Postoperative Follow-Up

- Cardiology
- Varying levels of activity restrictions
- Infective endocarditis prophylaxis indefinitely
- Required long term for patients who had sinus node dysfunction, surgical heart block, or ventricular arrhythmias postoperatively, whether or not pacemaker was placed

Complications

- Hypoxic spells ("tet" spells)
- Right ventricular dysfunction
- Ventricular arrhythmias
- Rarely, brain abscess and cerebrovascular accident
- Infective endocarditis
- Polycythemia

Peripheral Vascular Disorders

PERIPHERAL ARTERIAL DISEASE

Description

- Chronic or acute entity consisting of obstruction or narrowing of the major arteries, commonly affecting the lower extremities and most frequently a result of atherosclerosis

Etiology

- Acute thrombus leading to embolus
- Chronic atherosclerotic lesions
- Inflammatory component in thromboangiitis obliterans (Buerger's disease), giant cell (temporal) arteritis
- May also be caused by trauma or entrapment (thoracic, popliteal)

Incidence and Demographics

- Older adults
- Male preponderance

Risk Factors

- Age 40 years and older
- Tobacco use
- Hyperlipidemia, hypertension, atherosclerosis
- Diabetes mellitus or fasting serum glucose greater than 110 mg/dL
- Obesity

Prevention and Screening

- Lifestyle modification
- Identification and treatment of comorbid conditions

Assessment

History

- Acute: pain, paresthesia, paralysis, pallor, pulselessness
- Chronic: lower extremity aching, fatigue occurring with activity and relieved by cessation of activity (intermittent claudication); pain develops at rest as disease progresses

- Aorta: back or abdominal pain; femoral; hip, buttock, calf pain
- See Table 8–23 for classification of peripheral vascular disease.

Physical Exam

- Pale, cool, diminished, or absent pulses in extremity; bruit of femoral artery possible
- Severity determined by the amount of time required for venous filling and return of color
- Absent or decreased hair and nail growth of the lower extremities
- Waxy pallor of affected extremity, or dependent rubor with hyperemia due to compensatory reflex vasodilation of the microvasculature causing bright red distal extremity

Diagnostic Studies

- Diagnosis is clinical but Doppler ultrasound is used to determine severity.
- Angiography for acute or surgical candidates

Differential Diagnosis

- Musculoskeletal strains
- Osteoarthritis
- Acute arterial spasm
- Deep vein thrombosis (DVT)
- Acute embolic conditions
- Thromboangiitis obliterans (Buerger's disease)

TABLE 8–23.
FONTAINE CLASSIFICATION OF PERIPHERAL VASCULAR DISEASE

STAGE	CLINICAL FEATURE
1	Silent
2	Intermittent claudication
3	Rest ischemia
4	Ulceration or gangrene

Management

Nonpharmacologic Treatment

- Acute arterial occlusion: Avoid elevating affected extremity; protect extremity and refer for heparin therapy immediately.
- Smoking cessation
- Control/treat comorbid diseases: hyperlipidemia, diabetes mellitus, hypertension
- Initiate prescribed exercise program: preferably walking to point of pain to develop collateral circulation
- Educate patient about signs and symptoms that require immediate attention.
- Stage 3: diagnostic testing for possible surgery

Pharmacologic Treatment

- Acute: heparin IV, possible embolectomy
- Chronic: pentoxifylline (Trental) 400 mg three times a day.; aspirin or cilostazol (Pletal) 100 mg twice a day to decrease platelet aggregation
- Aspirin 81–324 mg/day for all patients

Special Considerations

- Risk of arterial occlusion increases with age

When to Consult, Refer, Hospitalize

- Refer to vascular surgeon for new-onset, severe, and stage 3 or greater symptoms; acute arterial occlusion; or arteriosclerosis obliterans (proliferation of the intima leads to occlusion of lumen of the arteries).

Follow-Up

- Every 3 months if stable
- Patient education about medications, care of feet

Expected Course

- Chronic: symptoms differ, with slow progression to rapid deterioration

Complications

- Gangrene
- Amputation

VENOUS THROMBOSIS

Description

- Deep vein thrombosis (DVT): acute blood clot formation in the deep lower extremity or pelvic veins with ambiguous presenting signs or symptoms
- Superficial: acute inflammation and clot formation with associated redness and tenderness along superficial vein

Etiology

- Thrombosis consists of red blood cells, platelets, and fibrin attached to part of the inflamed vessel wall.
- DVT caused by:
  - Immobilization secondary to surgery, prolonged bed rest, prolonged travel by plane or car
  - Venous incompetence, vascular wall injury
  - Chronic heart failure
  - Hypercoagulable states: inherited coagulation deficits, malignancy, and estrogen use
- Superficial thrombosis (saphenous vein frequently involved) caused by:
  - IV therapy, trauma
  - Bacterial infection

Incidence and Demographics

- Common; with an incidence of 1.6 per 1000 people annually (Waheed, 2022)
- Yearly incidence of DVT is approximately 80 cases per 100,000, with a prevalence of lower limb DVT of 1 case per 1000 population. More than 200,000 people a year in the United States develop venous thrombosis and approximately 50,000 of those cases are complicated by PE (Waheed, 2022).
- Female preponderance
- High incidence with total hip replacement

Risk Factors

- Increased coagulation risk due to: genetic deficiencies (antithrombin III deficiency, factor V Leiden mutation, anticoagulation proteins C and S)
- Acquired risks for coagulation: sepsis, cancer, MI, vasculitis, heart failure, SLE, inflammatory bowel disease, nephrotic syndrome, smoking, diabetes, hypertension, burns, oral estrogens
- DVT
  - Obesity
  - Orthopedic surgery, immobility, trauma
  - Pregnancy, oral contraceptives
  - Malignancy, coagulation defects (see above)
  - Venous catheters
  - Rheumatoid disease, lupus
  - High altitude elevations, polycythemia vera
- Superficial
  - Aseptic procedures

Prevention and Screening

- Limit period of immobility
- Prophylactic anticoagulation for associated risk factors
- Avoidance of estrogen-containing oral contraceptives, or use low dose
- Postsurgical mechanical leg compression

Assessment

History

- DVT frequently asymptomatic
- Possible unilateral leg pain or tenderness of calf, swelling, and discoloration
- With superficial thrombosis: acute episode with definite timeframe, local redness, tender cord, swelling, dull pain over inflamed vein, fever

Physical Exam

- DVT: reproducible tenderness with calf compression (Homan's sign), leg circumference greater than uninvolved leg because of swelling; cool extremity with weak distal pulses; however, signs often unreliable
- Superficial thrombosis: isolated induration, redness, and tenderness along vein, but no significant swelling of the extremity

Diagnostic Studies

- Coagulation profile: platelets, prothrombin time (PT), PTT, CBC, LFTs, occult blood; monitor platelets daily with heparin treatment
- D-Dimer
- B-mode ultrasound combined with Doppler flow detection: highly sensitive and specific for popliteal and femoral thrombi
- Impedance plethysmography: more accurate than duplex ultrasound, which is less precise in the detection of calf vein thrombi
- Nuclear scanning: iodine 125–labeled fibrinogen detects active clot formation
- Contrast venography: the most sensitive and specific contrast venography; most effective
- Clinical decision rules such as the Pulmonary Embolism Rule-Out Criteria (PERC) and the Wells Criteria should be used when evaluating a possible DVT (Waheed, 2022)

Differential Diagnosis

- Cellulitis
- Musculoskeletal strain

- Lymphedema
- Acute arterial occlusion
- Ruptured Baker's cyst

Management

Nonpharmacologic Treatment

- DVT
  - Initially hospitalize with bed rest and leg elevation, anticoagulation
  - After stabilization, prompt mobilization
  - Intermittent pneumatic compression followed by graded pressure stockings
  - Calf DVT as outpatient
  - Compression stockings: Below-knee graduated compression stockings with an ankle pressure greater than 23 mmHg for 2 years if no contraindications
  - Inferior vena cava filters: If anticoagulation is contraindicated or if emboli are occurring despite adequate anticoagulation
- Superficial
  - Bed rest with leg (or extremity) elevated, local heat
  - If sepsis, hospitalization often required

Pharmacologic Treatment

- Anticoagulation therapy for proximal DVT and those with PE, as acute treatment and prophylaxis
- DVT treatment according to cause:
  - Cancer-associated DVT
  - Low-molecular-weight heparin (LMWH) and factor Xa inhibitors, including rivaroxaban
  - Consider higher levels of anticoagulation if recent cancer diagnosis, adverse effects of cancer treatments such as vomiting, extensive venous thromboembolism (VTE) circumstances
  - When once-daily oral therapy is preferred management, may use rivaroxaban, edoxaban, and vitamin-K antagonist (VKA)
  - DVT, with liver disease, treat with LMWH. Direct-acting oral anticoagulants (DOACs) are contraindicated with elevated INR levels.

- ◊ DVT with renal disease and CrCl less than 30 mL/min, VKAs are recommended. DOACs and LMWH should NOT be given in patients with end-stage renal disease.
- ◊ DVT with history of CAD, it is recommended to start one of the following: VKA, rivaroxaban, apixaban, or edoxaban.
- ◊ DVT with any history of GI bleeding, VKA and apixaban are preferred treatments. DOACs, (dabigatran), factor Xa inhibitors, (rivaroxaban), and selective factor Xa inhibitors (edoxaban) should be avoided; may be associated with higher rates of GI bleeding.
- ◊ Poor compliance with DVT, VKA is preferred.
- ◊ If thrombolytic therapy is indicated, unfractionated heparin is warranted
- ◊ In patients who may need reversal of thrombolytic therapy, note that reversal agents are not available for all DOACs.
- ◊ Pregnancy: LMWH is anticoagulation therapy. (Most anticoagulants have the potential to cross the placenta.)

♦ Guidelines for duration of treatment.

- ◊ LMWH or fondaparinux for 5 days or until INR is above 2 for 24 hours (in renal failure patients or in patients with increased risk of bleeding, use unfractionated heparin)
- ◊ VKAs for 3 months
- ◊ In patients with cancer, consider anticoagulation with LMWH for 6 months.
- ◊ In patients with unprovoked DVT, consider VKAs more than 3 months.
- ◊ Rivaroxaban is an oral factor Xa inhibitor recently approved by the FDA and does not require regular INR monitoring.
- ◊ Monitor platelet count and if drops to less than 75,000, change from heparin to fondaparinux, as it is not associated with heparin-induced thrombocytopenia.

♦ Thrombolysis: The indications for the use of thrombolytics include:

- ◊ Symptomatic iliofemoral DVT
- ◊ Symptoms lasting fewer than 14 days
- ◊ Good functional status
- ◊ A life expectancy of 1 year or more
- ◊ Low bleeding risk

♦ **Thrombolytic treatment can result in an intracranial bleeding; careful patient selection is imperative.

♦ The duration of DVT treatment is 3 to 6 months, but those with recurrent episodes, those undergoing cancer treatment, may require at least 12 months of treatment or more.

♦ Inferior vena cava filters (IVC) are not recommended in acute DVT. There are both permanent and temporary inferior vena cava filters available. These devices may decrease the rate of recurrent DVT but do not affect survival. Today, only patients with contraindications to anticoagulation can be treated with the insertion of an IVC filter.

(Waheed, 2022)

How Long to Treat

- Treat single-episode DVT for 3 to 6 months, longer if recurrent, associated with pulmonary embolus
- Aseptic inflammation of superficial thrombosis subsides in 1–2 weeks

Special Considerations

- Geriatric patients: common because of predisposing factors, age-related coagulation deficiencies
- Pregnancy: Use heparin LMWH; warfarin is a teratogen.
- Lactation: unknown if heparin and warfarin are secreted in breast milk
- Oncology patients—risk of hemorrhage with heparin
- Rivaroxaban, apixaban, dabigatran, edoxaban, and betrixaban are newer factor Xa inhibitors approved for prophylaxis of DVT.
- In patients who may need reversal of thrombolytic therapy, note reversal agents are not available for all DOACs.

When to Consult, Refer, Hospitalize

- Consult with physician for evaluation and management, and possible hospitalization.
- Refer to vascular specialist for recurrences or complications.

Follow-Up

- Monitor oral anticoagulation and for signs of recurrence.
- Provide patient education about wearing support hose, warfarin complications, DOAC complications, and symptoms of PE.

Expected Course

- Prognosis is good once the danger of PE has passed.

Complications

- PE
- Chronic venous insufficiency
- Septic thrombophlebitis, osteomyelitis with superficial thrombosis

VENOUS INSUFFICIENCY

Description

- Chronic condition characterized by noninflammatory incompetence of the venous backflow valves in the veins of the lower extremities. Blood is regurgitated through the valves, resulting in engorgement and secondary edema of the lower leg.

Etiology

- Venous valves become incompetent, unable to maintain efficient flow of blood back to heart
- May be caused by leg trauma, prior thrombophlebitis, or conditions that cause abnormally high venous pressure

Incidence and Demographics

- Female predominance
- Onset in late adulthood
- An estimated 6 to 7 million have chronic venous insufficiency (Patel, 2022).

Risk Factors

- Trauma, obesity, pregnancy, history of thrombophlebitis
- Prolonged immobility, particularly standing
- Familial tendency, increases with age

Prevention and Screening

- Early aggressive treatment of thrombophlebitis
- Avoidance of prolonged standing and immobility
- Weight loss if appropriate
- Avoidance of restrictive lower-extremity garments

Assessment

History

- Pain varies from minimal discomfort to marked pain with ulcers.
- Lower-extremity edema worsens with prolonged standing.
- Mild pruritus of lower extremity, scratching
- Recurrent stasis ulcers, weeping, crust formation
- Previous history of thrombophlebitis at site
- Bilateral aching, cramping in the lower extremities—typically worse at night
- Bilateral lower-extremity edema with prolonged standing; relieved when legs are elevated
- Fatigue

Physical Exam

- Hyperpigmentation of distal extremity; appears brown or reddish; brawny, hyperpigmented thick skin
- Wet ulceration may be present distally, often over the medial aspect of the lower leg.

- Dependent pitting edema of lower extremity
- Varicosities may be present.
- Check femoral, popliteal, dorsalis pedis, and posterior tibial pulses.

Diagnostic Studies

- Stasis ulcer: culture and sensitivity
- Venous reflux testing
- Duplex ultrasonography
- Doppler studies: assess vascular status

Differential Diagnosis

- Cellulitis
- Stasis dermatitis
- Lymphedema
- Acute phlebitis
- Fungal infection
- Atopic dermatitis
- Severe contact dermatitis
- Varicose veins

Management

Nonpharmacologic Treatment

- Elastic stockings before ambulation
- Elevation of foot of bed
- Avoid prolonged positions or inactivity.
- Weight reduction for obese patients, exercise

- Refer for wound debridement and management.
- Treat ulcers with bandages, antimicrobial dressing, or Unna boot.

Pharmacologic Treatment

- No oral medications recommended
- Oral antibiotic for positive wound culture

How Long to Treat

- Chronic condition
- Treat exacerbations until resolution

Special Considerations

- Control edema; venous ulcer will not heal or remain healed with edema.

When to Consult, Refer, Hospitalize

- Refer to vascular specialist or wound care center for refractory ulcers.

Follow-Up

- Depends on clinical situation; usually every 3 months if stable
- Patient education about use of support hose, weight loss, sitting whenever possible

Expected Course

- Chronic, recurrent with frequent exacerbation if adherence with preventive measures is poor

Complications

- Bacterial infection
- Stasis ulcers
- Thrombus
- DVT
- PE

VARICOSE VEINS

Description

- Superficial, dilated, tortuous veins arising from incompetent valves and high venous pressure in the lower extremities, usually distant and involving the saphenous vein

Etiology

- Congenitally incompetent valves
- Prior thrombophlebitis
- Pregnancy, obesity, ascites
- Idiopathic, may have familial tendencies

Incidence and Demographics

- Female preponderance
- 23% of adult U.S. population (Weiss, 2020)

Risk Factors

- Prolonged weight bearing, standing
- Pregnancy, obesity, age
- Clothing that causes vasoconstriction of lower extremities

Prevention and Screening

- Weight control
- Elevation of lower extremities
- Elastic support when ambulatory
- Avoidance of restrictive clothing

Assessment

History

- Fatigue, aching, heaviness, and cramping, primarily of lower extremities
- Menses may be a precipitating factor.

Physical Exam

- Dilated and tortuous veins
- Standing: gravitational advantage to visualize veins
- Hyperpigmentation of distal leg
- Veins palpable

Differential Diagnosis

- Chronic venous insufficiency
- Peripheral neuropathy
- Nerve root compression
- Osteoarthritis—hip
- Arterial insufficiency
- Lymphedema
- Post-phlebitic syndrome

Diagnostic Studies

- Not indicated unless unusual presentation or complications such as DVT

Management

Nonpharmacologic Treatment

- Elastic compression stockings up to the knee before ambulation
- Patient should avoid prolonged weight-bearing and standing and not cross legs when sitting.
- Weight loss; elevation of leg when sitting
- Avoidance of restrictive garments
- Low-sodium diet in salt-sensitive persons
- Sclerotherapy, laser surgery, or ligation and stripping of saphenous vein for severe, refractory cases

Pharmacologic Treatment

- No oral medication available to treat varicosities

How Long to Treat

- Chronic problem

Special Considerations

- Pregnancy: frequent problem

When to Consult, Refer, Hospitalize

- Referral to surgeon if severe and refractory

Follow-Up

- If symptomatic

Expected Course

- Improvement with surgery
- Usually worsens with dependent positions such as standing

Complications

- Thrombophlebitis, varicose ulcers
- Secondary fungal and bacterial infection
- Eczema
- Neuritis from scarring secondary to stripping surgery

CASE STUDIES

CASE 1

Lori is a 44-year-old White female who presents to the clinic for a well-woman exam. She works as a telephone operator in a busy law firm office. Lori voices no complaints today. Diet recall indicates high-fat meals, including junk foods. She states that she loves cheese.

Past Medical History (PMH): Smokes 2 packs per day for 15 years; past medical history significant for hypertension; drinks 3 beers daily

Medications: hydrochlorothiazide 50 mg once a day

1. What additional history would you ask regarding her cardiovascular status?

   Exam: vital signs: BP 128/84; weight, 133 pounds; height, 64 inches; eyes, yellow-orange raised lesions on eyelids; remainder of exam is unremarkable

2. Would you order any diagnostic test on this patient?
3. If your suspicions are correct, what actions would be required?
4. When Lori returns to the clinic 6 months later with total cholesterol 252, HDL 30, and LDL 170, how will you intervene?
5. What complications can occur with this problem and the treatment regimens?

CASE 2

Baby Joe is 1 month old and presents to the clinic because he is not feeding well and his mother states he is losing weight. Baby Joe was delivered vaginally at 36 weeks of gestation. His birth weight was 4 lb, 9 oz. The baby is taking 2 oz of formula over a 55-minute period.

Medications: None

1. Are there any other history questions you would like to ask?

   Exam: vital signs: temp: 98.0° F/ear, weight: 5 lb, 2 oz. Crying and irritable, sweating; systolic thrill, II/VI continuous murmur at the upper LSB, heart rate 180; respiratory rate 60 with bilateral crackles; hepatomegaly noted.

2. What are your differential diagnoses?
3. What is your management plan?

Case 3

Mr. Jones is 56 years old and presents to the clinic complaining of decreased appetite, shortness of breath, and swelling in his feet. He is unable to perform normal activities without becoming winded and has a productive cough.

PMH: 6 lb weight gain in the past 7 days. Past medical history significant for hypertension, hyperlipidemia, and MI.

Medications: atorvastatin 20 mg/day, lisinopril 40 mg/day

1. What additional history would you ask?

   Exam: vital signs: blood pressure 90/40; pulse 120; resp 24; skin: cyanotic; CV: S3 gallop, jugular distention; lungs: basilar rales and wheezing; abdomen: hepatomegaly, ascites; extremities: 3+ pedal edema bilaterally

2. What diagnostic studies would you order?
3. What is your differential diagnosis?
4. What is your management plan?

CASE STUDIES DISCUSSION

CASE 1

1. What additional history would you ask regarding her cardiovascular status?

   Personal and family history of CHD, diabetes mellitus, hyperlipidemia; any previous lipid evaluation; history of activity/exercise; comprehensive health maintenance history; previous attempt at smoking/alcohol cessation; history of psychosocial stressors; any comorbid disease; abdominal pain; rheumatic disorders; medication history including OTCs, pregnancies

2. Would you order any diagnostic test on this patient?

   Baseline ECG; fasting lipid profile (total cholesterol, triglycerides, HDL, LDL, VLDL, risk ratio); apolipoprotein B; comprehensive metabolic panel, U/A, TSH, free T4; possibly chest X-ray, CBC with differential, CMP

3. If your suspicions are correct, what actions would be required?

   Step 2 diet and exercise program; referral to nutritionist for diet counseling; tobacco and alcohol cessation program; counseling for stress reduction

4. When Lori returns to the clinic 6 months later with total cholesterol 252, HDL 30, and LDL 170, how will you intervene?

   Reinforce Step 2 diet and exercise. Start on a statin such as atorvastatin (Lipitor) 10 mg/day; plan on monitoring hepatic function panel every 4–6 weeks after starting therapy x 3 months and again with any dose

5. What complications can occur with this problem and the treatment regimens?

   Hyperlipidemia: CAD progression, stroke, peripheral vascular disease. Drug treatment: pancreatitis, rhabdomyolysis, hepatic dysfunction

CASE 2

1. Are there any other history questions you would like to ask?

   Weight history since birth; prenatal/delivery history; voiding/stooling history in past 24 hours; 24-hour intake history; feeding behavior, sleep pattern

2. What are your differential diagnoses?

   Patent ductus arteriosus, arteriovenous malformations, venous hum, ventricular septal defect with aortic regurgitation, pulmonary atresia, persistent truncus arteriosus, aortopulmonary septal defect, peripheral pulmonary stenosis, total anomalous venous connection, tetralogy of Fallot.

3. What is your management plan?

   Refer child to emergency room for admission and evaluation with cardiologist.

CASE 3

1. What additional history would you ask?

   Characteristics of cough and sputum; need for additional pillows to sleep—orthopnea; fever; detailed history on comorbid diseases.

2. What diagnostic studies would you order?

   Chest X-ray, ECG, echocardiogram, electrolytes, U/A, pulse oximetry, cardiac enzymes, BUN, arterial blood gases.

3. What is your differential diagnosis?

   CHF, renal disease, COPD, nephrotic syndrome, cirrhosis, pulmonary emboli, MI, pneumonia, asthma, chronic venous insufficiency.

4. What is your management plan?

   Give O_2 and consult with physician to plan hospital admission to stabilize; identify and treat underlying disease. At follow-up, educate about sodium and fluid restriction, control leg edema with elastic pressure stockings and elevation of legs, record daily weights; multiple medications needed to treat—diuretics, ACEI, beta-blocker, glycoside, vasodilators, and anticoagulants.

REFERENCES

Amsterdam, E. A., Wenger, N. K., Brindis, R. G., Casey, D. E., Ganiats, T. G., Holmes, D. R., Jaffe, A. S., Jneid, H., Kelly, R. F., Kontos, M. C., Levine, G. N., Liebson, P. R., Mukherjee, D., Peterson, E. D., Sabatine, M. S., Smalling, R. W., & Zieman, S. J. (2014). 2014 AHA/ACC Guideline for the management of patients with non–ST-elevation acute coronary syndromes. *Journal of the American College of Cardiology, 64*(24), e139–e228. https://doi.org/10.1016/j.jacc.2014.09.017

ASCVD Risk Estimator Plus App. https://tools.acc.org/ASCVD-Risk-Estimator-Plus/#!/calculate/estimate/

Boudi, F. B., & Ali, Y. S. (2014). *Risk factors for coronary artery disease.* Retrieved from http://emedicine.medscape.com/article/164163-overview

Brunton, S. (2021). Updates in the management of peripheral arterial disease: Focus on reduction of atherothrombotic risk. *The Journal of Family Practice, 70*(8 Suppl). https://doi.org/10.12788/jfp.0290

Congenital Heart Defects—Facts about Atrial Septal Defects | CDC. (2019, November 19). Centers for Disease Control and Prevention. https://www.cdc.gov/ncbddd/heartdefects/atrialseptaldefect.html

Chen J. Y., Zhang A. D., Lu H. Y., Guo J., Wang F. F., & Li Z. C. (2013). $CHADS_2$ versus CHA_2DS_2-VASc score in assessing the stroke and thromboembolism risk stratification in patients with atrial fibrillation: A systematic review and meta-analysis. *Journal of Geriatric Cardiology,* (10), 258–66.

Classes of Heart Failure. (2022, June 2). www.heart.org. Retrieved from https://www.heart.org/en/health-topics/heart-failure/what-is-heart-failure/classes-of-heart-failure

Dakkak, W., & Oliver, T.I. *Ventricular septal defect.* [Updated 2022 May 10]. In: StatPearls [Internet]. Treasure Island (FL): StatPearls Publishing; 2022 Jan-. Available from: https://www.ncbi.nlm.nih.gov/books/NBK470330/

Data and Statistics on Congenital Heart Defects | CDC. (2020, December 9). Centers for Disease Control and Prevention. https://www.cdc.gov/ncbddd/heartdefects/data.html

de Ferranti, S. D., Steinberger, J., Ameduri, R., Baker, A., Gooding, H., Kelly, A. S., Mietus-Snyder, M., Mitsnefes, M. M., Peterson, A. L., St-Pierre, J., Urbina, E. M., Zachariah, J. P., & Zaidi, A. N. (2019). Cardiovascular risk reduction in high-risk pediatric patients: A scientific statement from the American Heart Association. *Circulation, 139*(13). Retrieved at https://doi.org/10.1161/cir.0000000000000618

Diaz-Frias, J., Guillaume, M. Tetralogy of Fallot. [Updated 2022 Jan 18]. In: StatPearls [Internet]. Treasure Island (FL): StatPearls Publishing; 2022 Jan-. Available from: https://www.ncbi.nlm.nih.gov/books/NBK513288/

Dobrowolski, P., Prejbisz, A., Kuryłowicz, A., Baska, A., Burchardt, P., Chlebus, K., Dzida, G., Jankowski, P., Jaroszewicz, J., Jaworski, P., Kamiński, K., Kapłon-Cieślicka, A., Klocek, M., Kukla, M., Mamcarz, A., Mastalerz-Migas, A., Narkiewicz, K., Ostrowska, L., Śliż, D., Tarnowski, W., . . . Bogdański, P. (2022). Metabolic syndrome—a new definition and management guidelines: A joint position paper by the Polish Society of Hypertension, Polish Society for the Treatment of Obesity, Polish Lipid Association, Polish Association for Study of Liver, Polish Society of Family Medicine, Polish Society of Lifestyle Medicine, Division of Prevention and Epidemiology Polish Cardiac Society, "Club 30" Polish Cardiac Society, and Division of Metabolic and Bariatric Surgery Society of Polish Surgeons. *Archives of Medical Science: AMS, 18*(5), 1133–1156. https://doi.org/10.5114/aoms/152921

Dumitru, I., MD. (2022, July 8). *Heart Failure: Practice Essentials, Background, Pathophysiology*. https://emedicine.medscape.com/article/163062-overview

Eisen, A., Giugliano, R. P., & Braunwald, E. (2016). Updates on acute coronary syndrome. *JAMA Cardiology, 1*(6), 718. https://doi.org/10.1001/jamacardio.2016.2049

Expert Panel on Integrated Guidelines for Cardiovascular Health and Risk Reduction in Children and Adolescents (2012). Retrieved at https://www.nhlbi.nih.gov/files/docs/guidelines/peds_guidelines_full.pdf

Framingham Heart Study. (2013). *Atrial fibrillation*. Retrieved from http://www.framinghamheart-study.org/risk/atrial.html

Gerhard-Herman, M. D., Gornik, H. L., Barrett, C., Barshes, N. R., Corriere, M. A., Drachman, D. E., Fleisher, L. A., Fowkes, F. G. R., Hamburg, N. M., Kinlay, S., Lookstein, R., Misra, S., Mureebe, L., Olin, J. W., Patel, R. A. G., Regensteiner, J. G., Schanzer, A., Shishehbor, M. H., Stewart, K. J., & Treat-Jacobson, D. (2017). 2016 AHA/ACC Guideline on the Management of Patients with Lower Extremity Peripheral Artery Disease: A Report of the American College of Cardiology/American Heart Association Task Force on Clinical Practice Guidelines. *Circulation, 135*(12), e726–e779. https://doi.org/10.1161/CIR.0000000000000471

Grundy, S. M., Stone, N. J., Bailey, A. L., Beam, C., Birtcher, K. K., Blumenthal, R. S., Braun, L. T., de Ferranti, S., Faiella-Tommasino, J., Forman, D. E., Goldberg, R., Heidenreich, P. A., Hlatky, M. A., Jones, D. W., Lloyd-Jones, D., Lopez-Pajares, N., Ndumele, C. E., Orringer, C. E., Peralta, C. A., . . . Yeboah, J. (2019). 2018 AHA/ACC/AACVPR/AAPA/ABC/ACPM/ADA/AGS/APHA/ASPC/NLA/PCNA guideline on the management of blood cholesterol: A report of the American College of Cardiology/American Heart Association Task Force on Clinical Practice Guidelines. *Circulation, 139*(25). https://doi.org/10.1161/cir.0000000000000625

Gulati, M., Levy, P. D., Mukherjee, D., Amsterdam, E., Bhatt, D. L., Birtcher, K. K., Blankstein, R., Boyd, J., Bullock-Palmer, R. P., Conejo, T., Diercks, D. B., Gentile, F., Greenwood, J. P., Hess, E. P., Hollenberg, S. M., Jaber, W. A., Jneid, H., Joglar, J. A., Morrow, D. A., & O'Connor, R. E. (2021). 2021 AHA/ACC/ASE/CHEST/SAEM/SCCT/SCMR Guideline for the Evaluation and Diagnosis of Chest Pain: Executive Summary. *Journal of the American College of Cardiology, 78*(22), 2218–2261. https://doi.org/10.1016/j.jacc.2021.07.052

Gujral, J., & Gupta, J. *Pediatric dyslipidemia.* [Updated 2022 Jul 28]. In: StatPearls [Internet]. Treasure Island (FL): StatPearls Publishing; 2022 Jan-. Available from: https://www.ncbi.nlm.nih.gov/books/NBK585106/

Flynn, J. T., Kaelber, D. C., Baker-Smith, C. M., Blowey, D., Carroll, A. E., Daniels, S. R., de Ferranti, S. D., Dionne, J. M., Falkner, B., Flinn, S. K., Gidding, S. S., Goodwin, C., Leu, M. G., Powers, M. E., Rea, C., Samuels, J., Simasek, M., Thaker, V. V., & Urbina, E. M. (2017). Clinical practice guideline for screening and management of high blood pressure in children and adolescents. *Pediatrics,* 140(3). https://doi.org/10.1542/peds. 2017-1904

Gillen, C., Goyal, A. Stable Angina. [Updated 2021 Dec 21]. In: StatPearls [Internet]. Treasure Island (FL): StatPearls Publishing; 2022 Jan-. Available from: https://www.ncbi.nlm.nih.gov/books/NBK559016/

Heidenreich, P., Bozkurt, B., Aguilar, D., et al. (2022). 2022 AHA/ACC/HFSA Guideline for the Management of Heart Failure. *Journal of the American College of Cardiology, 79*(17) e263–e421. https://doi.org/10.1016/j.jacc.2021.12.012

Heidenreich, P. A., Bozkurt, B., Aguilar, D., Allen, L. A., Byun, J. J., Colvin, M. M., Deswal, A., Drazner, M. H., Dunlay, S. M., Evers, L. R., Fang, J. C., Fedson, S. E., Fonarow, G. C., Hayek, S. S., Hernandez, A. F., Khazanie, P., Kittleson, M. M., Lee, C. S., Link, M. S., Milano, C. A., . . . Yancy, C. W. (2022). 2022 AHA/ACC/HFSA Guideline for the Management of Heart Failure: A Report of the American College of Cardiology/American Heart Association Joint Committee on Clinical Practice Guidelines. *Circulation, 145*(18), e895–e1032. https://doi.org/10.1161/CIR.0000000000001063

Jagadish, P. S., & Kabra, R. (2019). Stroke risk in atrial fibrillation: Beyond the CHA2DS2-VASc score. *Current Cardiology Reports, 21*(9). https://doi.org/10.1007/s11886-019-1189-6

January, C. T., Wann, L. S., Calkins, H., Chen, L. Y., Cigarroa, J. E., Cleveland, J. C., Ellinor, P. T., Ezekowitz, M. D., Field, M. E., Furie, K. L., Heidenreich, P. A., Murray, K. T., Shea, J. B., Tracy, C. M., & Yancy, C. W. (2019). 2019 AHA/ACC/HRS focused update of the 2014 AHA/ACC/HRS guideline for the management of patients with atrial fibrillation. *Journal of the American College of Cardiology, 74*(1). https://doi.org/10.1016/j.jacc.2019.01.011

Jauch, E. C. (2022, December 6). *Ischemic stroke: Practice essentials, background, anatomy.* https://emedicine.medscape.com/article/1916852-overview

Kelly, A. S., Barlow, S. E., Rao, G., Inge, T. H., Hayman, L. L., Steinberger, J., Urbina, E. M., Ewing, L. J., & Daniels, S. R. (2013, September 9). *Severe obesity in children and adolescents: Identification, associated health risks, and treatment approaches.* Circulation. Retrieved November 29, 2022, from https://www.ahajournals.org/doi/10.1161/CIR.0b013e3182a5cfb3

Kim, L. (2022, July 8). *Patent ductus arteriosus (PDA).* Background, anatomy, pathophysiology. Retrieved January 9, 2023, from https://emedicine.medscape.com/article/891096-

Kim, K. H., Kerndt, C. C., Adnan, G., et al. Nitroglycerin. [Updated 2022 Sep 27]. In: StatPearls [Internet]. Treasure Island (FL): StatPearls Publishing; 2022 Jan-. Available from: https://www.ncbi.nlm.nih.gov/books/NBK482382/

Kleindorfer, D. O., Towfighi, A., Chaturvedi, S., Cockroft, K. M., Gutierrez, J., Lombardi-Hill, D., Kamel, H., Kernan, W. N., Kittner, S. J., Leira, E. C., Lennon, O., Meschia, J. F., Nguyen, T. N., Pollak, P. M., Santangeli, P., Sharrief, A. Z., Smith, S. C., Turan, T. N., & Williams, L. S. (2021). 2021 guideline for the prevention of stroke in patients with stroke and transient ischemic attack: A guideline from the american heart association/american stroke association. *Stroke, 52*(7). P. e364–e467. https://doi.org/10.1161/str.0000000000000375

Law, M. A., & Tivakaran, V.S. *Coarctation of the aorta.* [Updated 2022 Aug 8]. In: StatPearls [Internet]. Treasure Island (FL): StatPearls Publishing; 2022 Jan-. Available from: https://www.ncbi.nlm.nih.gov/books/NBK430913/

Lawton, J. S., Tamis-Holland, J. E., Bangalore, S., Bates, E. R., Beckie, T. M., Bischoff, J. M., Bittl, J. A., Cohen, M. G., DiMaio, J. M., Don, C. W., Fremes, S. E., Gaudino, M. F., Goldberger, Z. D., Grant, M. C., Jaswal, J. B., Kurlansky, P. A., Mehran, R., Metkus, T. S., Nnacheta, L. C., & Rao, S. V. (2021). 2021 ACC/AHA/SCAI Guideline for coronary artery revascularization. *Journal of the American College of Cardiology, 79*(2). https://doi.org/10.1016/j.jacc.2021.09.006

Lee, P. M., & Gerriets, V. *Nitrates.* [Updated 2022 Jul 11]. In: StatPearls [Internet]. Treasure Island (FL): StatPearls 5877. 77yy77y7y6Publishing; 2022 Jan-. Available from: https://www.ncbi.nlm.nih.gov/books/NBK545149/

National Heart, Lung, and Blood Institute. (2012). Expert Panel on Integrated Guidelines for Cardiovascular Health and Risk Reduction in Children and Adolescents summary report. Retrieved from https://www.nhlbi.nih.gov/files/docs/peds_guidelines_sum.pdf

National Heart, Lung, and Blood Institute. (2013). *Integrated guidelines for cardiovascular health and risk reduction in children and adolescents—2011.* Retrieved from http://www.nhlbi.nih.gov/health-pro/guidelines/current/cardiovascular-health-pediatric-guidelines

Patel, S. K., & Surowiec, S. M. *Venous insufficiency.* [Updated 2022 Aug 1]. In: StatPearls [Internet]. Treasure Island (FL): StatPearls Publishing; 2022 Jan-. Available from: https://www.ncbi.nlm.nih.gov/books/NBK430975/

Poothirikovil Venugopalan, M. B. B. S. (2022, March 15). *Pediatric mitral valve prolapse medication.* Beta-adrenergic blocking agents, Antiplatelet agents, Diuretics, ACE inhibitors, Cardiac glycoside. Retrieved January 12, 2023, from https://emedicine.medscape.com/article/890425-medication#2

Powers, W. J., Rabinstein, A. A., Ackerson, T., Adeoye, O. M., Bambakidis, N. C., Becker, K., Biller, J., Brown, M., Demaerschalk, B. M., Hoh, B., Jauch, E. C., Kidwell, C. S., Leslie-Mazwi, T. M., Ovbiagele, B., Scott, P. A., Sheth, K. N., Southerland, A. M., Summers, D. V., & Tirschwell, D. L. (2019b). Guidelines for the early management of patients with acute ischemic stroke: 2019 update to the 2018 guidelines for the early management of acute ischemic stroke: A Guideline for healthcare professionals from the american heart association/american stroke association. *Stroke, 50*(12). https://doi.org/10.1161/str.0000000000000211

Qurat-ul-ain Jelani, M. D. (2022, September 6). *Mitral Valve Prolapse Treatment & Management.* Medical Care, Surgical Care. Retrieved January 12, 2023, from https://emedicine.medscape.com/article/155494-treatment#d8

Ross, H. (2020, January 24). Implicit bias: Recognizing the unconscious barriers to quality care and diversity in medicine. *Cardiology Magazine, 49*(1), 22–25. https://www.acc.org/latest-in-cardiology/articles/2020/01/01/24/42/cover-story-implicit-bias-recognizing-the-unconscious-barriers-to-quality-care-and-diversity-in-medicine

Scirica, B., et al. (2010). Acute coronary syndrome. *Journal of the American College of Cardiology, 55*(14), 1403–1415. https://doi.org/10.1016/j.jacc.2009.09.071

Shah, S. N., Gangwani, M. K., & Oliver, T. I. (2022). *Mitral valve prolapse.* [Updated 2022 Aug 1]. In: StatPearls [Internet]. Treasure Island (FL): StatPearls Publishing.. Available from: https://www.ncbi.nlm.nih.gov/books/NBK470288/

Singh, A., Museedi, A. S., & Grossman, S. A. (2022). *Acute coronary syndrome.* [Updated 2022 Jul 11]. In: StatPearls [Internet]. Treasure Island (FL): StatPearls Publishing. Available from: https://www.ncbi.nlm.nih.gov/books/NBK459157/

Stephens, E., & Schrage, E. D. (2020). Peripheral vascular disease: Background, pathophysiology, prognosis. *EMedicine.* https://emedicine.medscape.com/article/761556-overview

Tarek Ajam, M. D. (2022, November 9). *CHADS2 score for stroke risk assessment in atrial fibrillation.* CHADS2 and CHA2DS2-VASc Score for Stroke Risk Assessment in Atrial Fibrillation. Retrieved January 12, 2023, from https://emedicine.medscape.com/article/2172597-overview

Tsao, C. W., Aday, A. W., Almarzooq, Z. I., Alonso, A., Beaton, A. Z., Bittencourt, M. S., Boehme, A. K., Buxton, A. E., Carson, A. P., Commodore-Mensah, Y., Elkind, M. S. V., Evenson, K. R., Eze-Nliam, C., Ferguson, J. F., Generoso, G., Ho, J. E., Kalani, R., Khan, S. S., Kissela, B. M., & Knutson, K. L. (2022). Heart Disease and Stroke Statistics—2022 Update: A Report From the American Heart Association. *Circulation, 145*(8). https://doi.org/10.1161/cir.0000000000001052

Waheed, S. M., Kudaravalli, P., & Hotwagner, D. T. *Deep vein thrombosis.* [Updated 2022 Nov 23]. In: StatPearls [Internet]. Treasure Island (FL): StatPearls Publishing; 2022 Jan-. Available from: https://www.ncbi.nlm.nih.gov/books/NBK507708/

Wang, S. S., & Ali, Y. S. (2019, November 10). *Metabolic syndrome: Practice essentials, background, pathophysiology.* Medscape.com. https://emedicine.medscape.com/article/165124-overview

Weiss, R. (2022, January 11). *Varicose veins and spider veins.* Practice essentials, background, pathophysiology. Retrieved January 8, 2023, from https://emedicine.medscape.com/article/1085530-overview

Whelton, P. K., Carey, R. M., Aronow, W., et al. (2018). 2017 ACC/AHA/AAPA/ABC/ACPM/AGS/APhA/ASH/ASPC/NMA/PCNA Guideline for the Prevention, Detection, Evaluation, and Management of High Blood Pressure in Adults. *Journal of the American College of Cardiology, 71*(19), e127–e248. https://doi.org/10.1016/j.jacc.2017.11.006

Whelton, P., Carey, R., Aronow, W., et al. (2018). 2017 ACC/AHA/AAPA/ABC/ACPM/AGS/APhA/ASH/ASPC/NMA/PCNA Guideline for the Prevention, Detection, Evaluation, and Management of High Blood Pressure in Adults: Executive Summary. *Journal of the American College of Cardiology, 71*(19) 2199–2269. https://doi.org/10.1016/j.jacc.2017.11.005

Wilson, P. W. F., Polonsky, T. S., Miedema, M. D., Khera, A., Kosinski, A. S., & Kuvin, J. T. (2019). Systematic review for the 2018 AHA/ACC/AACVPR/AAPA/ABC/ACPM/ADA/AGS/APHA/ASPC/NLA/PCNA guideline on the management of blood cholesterol. *Journal of the American College of Cardiology, 73*(24), 3210–3227. https://doi.org/10.1016/j.jacc.2018.11.004

Yancy, C. W., Jessup, M., Bozkurt, B., Butler, J., Casey, D. E., Drazner, M. H., Fonarow, G. C., Geraci, S. A., Horwich, T., Januzzi, J. L., Johnson, M. R., Kasper, E. K., Levy, W. C., Masoudi, F. A., McBride, P. E., McMurray, J. J., Mitchell, J. E., Peterson, P. N., Riegel, B., . . . Wilkoff, B. L. (2013). 2013 ACCF/AHA Guideline for the Management of Heart Failure. *Journal of the American College of Cardiology, 62*(16), e147–e239. https://doi.org/10.1016/j.jacc.2013.05.019

Yancy, C. W., Januzzi, J. L. Jr, Allen, L. A., et al. (2018). 2017 ACC Expert Consensus Decision Pathway for Optimization of Heart Failure Treatment: Answers to 10 Pivotal Issues About Heart Failure with Reduced Ejection Fraction: A Report of the American College of Cardiology Task Force on Expert Consensus Decision Pathways. *Journal of the American College of Cardiology, 71,* 201.

CHAPTER 9

GASTROINTESTINAL DISORDERS

Kara Ventura, DNP, FNP-BC, CPNP, DCC

General Approach

- Older adults are less likely to feel pain with abdominal conditions and do not always present with classic symptoms or lab findings, are more likely to have vague diffuse pain, and tend to have a less acute presentation than younger patients.
- Iron-deficiency anemia in a male, postmenopausal female, or older adult patient always warrants an upper and lower endoscopy to rule out a gastrointestinal source of bleeding or cancer.
- Antidiarrheal medications should never be given to patients younger than 5 years old or any patient with bloody diarrhea, fever, fecal leukocytes, or abdominal pain because of the possible development of a systemic infection from retained toxins. These patients require prompt evaluation and referral.
- Every tender, nonreducible hernia must be referred to a surgeon for prompt evaluation.
- Careful history-taking of most gastrointestinal (GI) problems will help to determine the location of the problem.
- Always repeat abdominal exam before discharging the patient to validate initial results or detect new findings; document assessment.
- Always examine the tender area last to avoid referred pain.

RED FLAGS

- A patient who presents with fever, chills, leukocytosis (elevated total white blood cell [WBC] count with increased neutrophils [polys] and bands on the differential), and rebound tenderness warrants rapid assessment and referral to an acute care facility for a surgical consultation.
- Abdominal pain lasting more than 6 hours or pain that awakens the patient at night requires evaluation and possible referral.
- New-onset constipation in patients age 50 years and over is a warning sign.

Gastrointestinal Signs and Symptoms

DYSPHAGIA

Description

- Difficulty in swallowing (oropharyngeal dysphagia) and having food pass from the mouth down the esophagus to the stomach (esophageal dysphagia); odynophagia—painful swallowing—is an alarm symptom that requires immediate evaluation to determine cause and treatment.
- Patients describe oropharyngeal dysphagia as a feeling of food getting stuck, indicative of upper esophageal or pharyngeal disease; may present as difficulty swallowing solids or liquids, described as trouble initiating a swallow; coughing; choking; nasal regurgitation (oropharyngeal dysplasia); sensation of food "sticking" after it is swallowed (esophageal dysphasia).
- May be a structural or neuromuscular problem caused by such conditions as gastroesophageal reflux disease (GERD), esophageal spasm, Barrett's esophagus, benign esophageal or peptic stricture, esophagitis, esophageal rings (also webs and diverticula), carcinoma, goiter, myasthenia gravis, multiple sclerosis, hypothyroidism, Parkinson's disease, achalasia, scleroderma, or polymyositis.
- May present as chest pain
- *Not* attributed to normal aging
- Diagnostic workup may include:
  - Complete blood count (CBC) and stool for occult blood to evaluate for bleeding (carcinoma)
  - Liver functions tests (LFTs) to evaluate for metastatic process
  - Blood urea nitrogen (BUN), albumin to evaluate nutritional status
  - Thyroid function tests to rule out hypothyroidism
  - Electrocardiography (ECG) and cardiac workup if chest pain is the presenting symptom
  - Endoscopy: standard test for diagnosis and management of esophageal diseases because it allows for biopsy and definitive tissue diagnosis. It can identify a mechanical obstruction or an inflammatory process or provide evidence of an esophageal motor disorder
  - Barium swallow or upper GI series: Often done first to differentiate between mechanical lesions and esophageal motility problems. If a motility problem is suspected, barium swallow should be done first. If a mechanical lesion is suspected, an endoscopy is often done first.

  - ◊ Esophageal pH recording to evaluate for GERD if difficulty establishing diagnosis
  - ◊ Video esophagography—esophageal manometry (not a first-line test)
  - ◊ Outpatient treatment if patient not malnourished and not high risk for aspiration
- ♦ Treat identifiable condition.
- ♦ Goal is to treat underlying cause and maintain nutritional status during workup; consider liquid supplementation.
- ♦ Older adults may have poor-fitting dentures that contribute to the problem.
- ♦ Use thickened liquids for people with dysphagia to prevent aspiration.
- ♦ Refer any patient with new symptoms and no obvious treatable cause to a gastroenterologist—particularly the older patient, and those with weight loss, bleeding, iron-deficiency anemia, history of chronic GERD, or history of heavy alcohol and tobacco use.

ABNORMAL LIVER FUNCTION TESTS (LFTS)

Description

- ♦ Serum liver chemistries are useful in evaluating liver function and include: alanine aminotransferase (ALT) and aspartate aminotransferase (AST). ALT is highest in liver disease and AST is less specific; elevated in liver, cardiac, skeletal muscle, kidney, brain, pancreas, or lung disease. Evaluate hepatic cellular integrity; bilirubin (direct and indirect), alkaline phosphatase (ALP), and gamma-glutamyl transpeptidase (GGT). Assess hepatic excretion and prothrombin time (PT) and serum albumin. Evaluate hepatic protein synthesis.

Etiology

- ♦ The prevalence of mildly elevated transaminase levels is around 10%–20% in the general population. Elevated aminotransferases (ALT and AST) may be seen in conditions including biliary obstruction, viral hepatitis, cirrhosis, metastatic liver disease, autoimmune disease, and drug-induced liver injury.
- ♦ These enzymes are found in multiple tissues and are released into the plasma in response to cellular injury.
- ♦ ALT is found predominately in the liver, so it is more specific than AST for evaluating hepatocellular damage.

- AST is found in liver, cardiac, skeletal, kidney, and brain tissue; elevated levels alone may indicate tissue damage in any of those organ systems (e.g., myocardial ischemia or musculoskeletal injury).
- The highest levels of ALT and AST (usually over 500 U/L) occur with severe viral hepatitis, drug-induced liver injury (e.g., acetaminophen, phenytoin, rifampin), or ischemic hepatitis. Moderate elevations (usually less than300 U/L) are present in mild to acute viral hepatitis, chronic active hepatitis, cirrhosis, and liver metastases. Mild elevation may be present in biliary obstruction, with higher levels suggesting the development of cholangitis (causing hepatic cell necrosis), with also an elevation in ALP. In alcoholic liver disease, the AST/ALT ratio may be more than 2. A ratio of AST/ALT more than 1 may be seen with fatty liver as seen associated with pregnancy and metabolic syndrome.
- An elevated bilirubin (a degradation product of heme) should be fractionated to determine if it is predominantly conjugated (direct, processed by the liver) or unconjugated (indirect, not processed by the liver).
- Elevations in direct bilirubin are usually caused by impaired excretion of bilirubin from the liver because of hepatocellular disease, biliary tract obstruction, drugs, or sepsis.
- Indirect bilirubin elevation is caused by hemolysis or ineffective erythropoiesis (increased bilirubin production); neonatal jaundice, Gilbert's or Crigler-Najjar syndromes (impaired bilirubin conjugation because of enzyme deficiency); or when hepatic bilirubin uptake is decreased because of drugs, heart failure, or portosystemic shunting.
- Alkaline phosphatase (or ALP) is an enzyme found in various tissues, including the liver, bone, intestine, and placenta (more than 80% from liver and bone).
- Elevated ALP levels (in the absence of bone disease or pregnancy) usually represent impaired biliary tract function.
- Fractionation of an elevated serum ALP can be done to determine the source; however, elevation of other liver function tests is helpful in establishing a hepatic cause.
- Mild to moderate increases (usually one to two times normal) occur with hepatocellular disorders such as hepatitis or cirrhosis.
- High serum elevations (up to 10 times normal or greater) can occur with extrahepatic biliary tract obstruction (usually a gallstone blocking the common bile duct) or intrahepatic cholestasis (bile retention in the liver) as seen with drug-induced cholestasis and biliary cirrhosis.
- The ALP is usually mildly elevated in incomplete biliary tract obstruction and in metastatic and infiltrative liver disease (e.g., leukemia, lymphoma, and sarcoidosis).
- An elevated ALP is also present in nonhepatic disorders, with the most common being bone disease (Paget's disease and bone metastases).

- Elevated GGT in liver disease is useful in differentiating the origin of an elevated ALP (hepatic vs. bone), as they both tend to increase in similar hepatic diseases.
- GGT is also a highly sensitive indicator of acute alcohol ingestion and of other agents that stimulate the hepatic microsomal oxidase system, such as barbiturates and phenytoin.
- The GGT enzyme is also present in the pancreas, kidney, heart, and brain, and elevations may occur in disorders involving those organ systems.
- A prolonged PT is caused by impaired hepatic synthesis of coagulation factors seen in significant liver disease and/or with vitamin K deficiency that may occur with malnutrition, malabsorption (e.g., cholestasis, steatorrhea, pancreatic insufficiency), and warfarin use. If administration of vitamin K corrects the PT, a deficiency was present.
- Decreased serum albumin, the primary protein synthesized by the liver, may be caused by chronic liver disease, or by other nonhepatic factors such as malnutrition, hormonal factors, or excessive protein loss (nephrotic syndrome or protein-losing enteropathy).

Risk Factors

- Alcohol
- Drugs metabolized by liver, drug-induced liver injury
- Genetic predisposition
- Nonalcoholic fatty liver disease
- Viral hepatitis
- Hemochromatosis

Assessment

History

- Many patients are asymptomatic with mild, transient elevations.
- Generalized symptoms of fever, anorexia, malaise, weight loss, jaundice, arthralgias, myalgias, rash, and pruritus may be present.
- Gastrointestinal symptoms include anorexia, nausea, vomiting, abdominal pain, dark urine, and pale stools.
- Additional history is aimed at identifying potential risk factors: history of hepatitis exposure, gallstones, transfusions, previous surgery, medications (including vitamins

and herbs, over-the-counter [OTCs] medications,[especially acetaminophen]), alcohol and drug use, sexual practices, occupational exposure, and travel history.

Physical Exam

- Skin exam: jaundice (include sclera), spider angiomas, palmar erythema, gynecomastia, caput medusae (annular purple discoloration around umbilicus or ostomy), and ecchymosis
- Abdominal exam: ascites, tenderness (usually right upper quadrant), enlarged gallbladder, hepatomegaly, and splenomegaly; liver may be smaller than normal in advanced liver disease.
- Extremities: asterixis, temporal and proximal muscle wasting, and peripheral edema

Diagnostic Studies

- If the patient is asymptomatic, repeat LFTs before ordering any other tests. If normal, repeat testing in 3 to 6 months is suggested.
- If repeat testing results are abnormal, obtain hepatitis serologies to exclude viral hepatitis A, B, and C (see section on Viral Hepatitis).
- If the patient is symptomatic, further tests are guided by history and physical exam (see Table 9–1); consider:
    - Monospot and cytomegalovirus (CMV) immune globulin G (IgG), IgM titers
    - Abdominal ultrasound: best screening test to evaluate for gallstones; can also detect biliary tree dilation, biliary obstruction, cholecystitis, fatty liver, and liver parenchymal disease
    - Computerized tomography (CT) scan (with IV contrast): best test to evaluate liver parenchymal disease and space-occupying lesions (tumor or abscess); can also assess biliary tree dilation and identify obstructing lesion
    - Magnetic resonance imaging (MRI): similar to CT scan but can better visualize vessels without the use of IV contrast
    - Endoscopic retrograde cholangiopancreatography (ERCP) and percutaneous transhepatic cholangiography (PTC): usually done after screening with ultrasound, CT, or MRI to further assess cause, location, and extent of biliary tree abnormalities
    - Liver biopsy: definitive study to determine the cause and extent of hepatocellular and infiltrative liver disease; biopsy may be guided using ultrasound or CT

TABLE 9–1. INTERPRETING LIVER FUNCTION TESTS

LIVER FUNCTION TEST	ENZYME FOUND IN	CAUSE OF ELEVATION	CONDITIONS WHERE SEEN	COMMENTS
Bilirubin: direct (conjugated, processed by liver)	Liver, blood, urine	Impaired excretion of bilirubin from the liver	Hepatocellular disease, biliary tract obstruction, drugs, sepsis	
Bilirubin: indirect (unconjugated, not processed by the liver)	Liver, blood, urine	Hepatic bilirubin uptake is decreased	Hemolysis or portosystemic shunting, drugs, heart failure, ineffective erythropoiesis, neonatal jaundice	
Alkaline phosphatase	Bone, liver, intestine, placenta	Impaired biliary tract function (cholestasis), infiltrative liver disease or impaired hepatic excretion	*Mild*: hepatitis, cirrhosis, early cancer *High*: biliary tract obstruction, cholestasis	Increases with age, women more than men. Also elevated in bone disease, bony metastasis, and Paget's disease
GGT	Liver, pancreas, kidney, heart, brain	Hepatic excretion	Sensitive for acute alcohol ingestion, drugs such as barbiturates and phenytoin	Differentiates the origin of an elevated ALP between bone and liver
Transaminases	Many tissues	Acute hepatocellular injury—from necrosis or inflammation	*Mild*: biliary obstruction, mild viral chronic or active and alcoholic hepatitis, cirrhosis, and liver metastases	Do not indicate severity of liver injury; most common cause of elevation is alcoholic hepatitis
ALT	Predominantly liver, more specific test	Celiac disease	*High*: viral hepatitis, drug-induced liver injury	
AST	Liver, cardiac, skeletal, kidney, brain			AST twice as high as ALT is typical of alcoholic liver injury
Prothrombin time (PT)	Blood	Impaired hepatic synthesis of coagulation factors	Significant liver disease	If vitamin K corrects the PT, a deficiency was present
Albumin	Blood serum	Impaired hepatic protein synthesis, excess protein loss	Chronic liver disease	May decrease with age

Management

- Aimed at correcting underlying cause

Nonpharmacologic Treatment

- Avoid drugs and other agents that are hepatotoxic.
- Management will vary depending on etiology.

Special Considerations

- Geriatric patients: higher incidence of neoplasm in this age group
- Pregnancy: elevated ALP common because present in placental tissue; CT scans contraindicated

When to Consult, Refer, Hospitalize

- Consult with or refer to a physician or specialist when significantly abnormal LFT results persist without an identifiable cause, or for symptomatic patients in need of specialized diagnostic tests and management.

Follow-Up

- Recheck studies every 3 to 6 months.

CONSTIPATION

Description

- A symptom as well as a diagnosis where there is decrease in frequency of stools, excessive difficulty passing stools, leakage from rectum, and straining with defecation.

Etiology

- Most common cause: functional etiologies—poor dietary intake of fiber and fluids, behavioral habits such as change in environment with travel or schedule, sedentary lifestyle; occurs in children most often when cereal is first introduced to diet, during toilet training, or entry to school.
- Psychogenic; chronic constipation can begin in first year of life.
- Congenital disorders
- Medications: opiate analgesics, calcium channel blockers, anticholinergics, diuretics, aluminum-based antacids, calcium, and iron supplements, nonsteroidal anti-inflammatory drugs (NSAIDs), antihistamines, antipsychotics, anti-Parkinson's agents, laxative abuse

Prevention and Screening

- Exercise; increase daily fiber and fluid intake
- If possible, establish a time each day to defecate and do not ignore the urge to defecate.
- Provide anticipatory guidance regarding toilet-training techniques.

Assessment

- Rome III criteria must include at least two of the following for 12 weeks in the previous 6 months:
  - ◊ Fewer than three stools per week
  - ◊ Straining at least one-quarter of the time
  - ◊ Hard stools at least one-quarter of the time
  - ◊ Need for manual assist at least one-quarter of the time
  - ◊ Sense of incomplete evacuation at least one-quarter of the time

Physical Exam

- Abdominal and gynecological exam for masses, pain
- Rectal exam: sphincter tone, fissures, size of rectal vault, rectal prolapse, presence of stool and consistency, masses

- Neurologic exam
- In frail older adults, evaluate systemic signs of fever, delirium, urinary retention, arrhythmias, tachypnea.

Diagnostic Studies

- American Gastroenterological Association (AGA) guidelines suggest CBC, blood sugar, thyroid-stimulating hormone (TSH), calcium, and creatinine routinely
- Sigmoid/colonoscopy if red flags are present
- Flat plate and upright abdominal films to evaluate for obstruction
- Colonoscopy or barium enema if patient is anemic to evaluate for colorectal cancer; consider in any adult with new onset 50 years and older

Management

Nonpharmacologic Treatment

- Increase fiber in adults: 20–35 g/day.
- Increase fiber gradually, over a 2-week period.
- Increase fluid intake, particularly water, to 1.5–2 liters per day.

Pharmacologic Treatment

- First-line:
  - Hydrophilic colloids or bulk-forming agents: psyllium (Metamucil, Fiberall) 3.4 g one to three times daily; methylcellulose (Citrucel) 2 g one to three times daily; polycarbophil (FiberCon) 1 g one to three times daily; can be used on a long-term basis
  - Surfactants: used to soften stools; docusate sodium (Colace) 50–200 mg daily; used short term up to 2 weeks; may be used longer and do not induce dependency
  - Osmotic laxatives: used for acute constipation and should not be used long term; should result in a bowel movement in 0.5 to 3 hours or longer. Miralax (polyethylene glycol) 17 g daily, is found to be superior to others in category. Lactulose and sorbitol, 15–60 mL, at bedtime, are equally effective but tend to cause flatulence, bloating, and cramping. Magnesium hydroxide suspension (Milk of Magnesia) 30–60 mL × 1 dose (should not be given to patients with renal insufficiency).

- Second-line:
  - ◊ Stimulants: stimulate fluid secretion, colonic contraction; may cause cramping; use infrequently; include Senokot, Ex-Lax, Dulcolax, and Correctol; Peri-Colace acts as lubricant with mineral oil to coat stool
  - ◊ Lubiprostone (Amitiza) 24 μm twice a day is approved for chronic constipation in adults as well as irritable bowel syndrome (IBS).
- Constipation with fecal impaction
  - ◊ First removal of impaction by use of sodium phosphate enemas; two to three enemas over a 2-day period
  - ◊ Once impaction removed, begin long-term therapy
- Mineral oil: adults 60 mL/dose, max two doses/day; children 1 mL/kg/dose twice a day, max 90 mL/day *or*
- Lactulose: adults 15 mL twice a day; children 0.5 mL/kg/dose twice a day
- Treat for 3 to 6 months along with nonpharmacological treatments.

Special Consideration

- Evaluate diet, fluid intake, medications, activity in older adults.

When to Consult, Refer, Hospitalize

- Refer to a gastroenterologist if patient fails to respond to treatment; stool positive for occult blood, weight loss is present, and for individuals age 50 and over with sudden, unexplained change in bowel pattern.

Expected Course

- With treatment, constipation should resolve in several days if there is no significant underlying problem, such as bowel obstruction.
- With exercise, a daily bowel regimen and an increase in fiber and fluids, should, for the most part, resolve permanently.

DIARRHEA

Definition

- Increased frequency, looseness, and volume of stools; may be either acute or chronic condition; infants 6 to 24 months are at highest risk of morbidity and mortality

Etiology

- Produced by one or more of the following: abnormal intestinal motility, decreased water absorption, and/or increased fluid secretion
- *Acute:* most caused by infectious agents, viruses, bacterial toxins, or drug (see Table 9–2)
- *Chronic:* many causes but often from hardy agents that are difficult to treat and eradicate, spread by fecal–oral route

Incidence and Demographics

- Common worldwide; 11% of general population

Risk Factors

- Institutional settings such as day care, nursing homes, schools
- Travel to area with water and soil contamination
- Improper cooking and preparation methods, especially items from street vendors where constancy of temperature is issue
- Recent antibiotic use

Prevention and Screening

- Handwashing, particularly after using bathroom
- Avoid water supply while traveling to endemic areas, including water for toothbrushing, ice cubes
- Proper food preparation and cooking of cold salads and meats
- Rotavirus vaccine

Assessment

History

- Determine whether symptoms were sudden in onset or chronic.
- Anorexia, vomiting, malaise, headache, myalgias

TABLE 9–2.
COMMON CAUSES OF ACUTE DIARRHEA

ORGANISM	TRANSMISSION	INCUBATION	SIGNS AND SYMPTOMS	TYPE OF STOOLS	LAB DATA	SPECIAL NOTATIONS
VIRAL						
Rota and Norwalk (Noro)	Fecal–oral	24–72 hours	Nausea, vomiting, cramps, fever	Watery	No WBCs in stool	Most common causes: Rotavirus in children (6–24 months) More common in winter Norwalk in children older than 2 years, adolescents and adults. Vomiting most prominent symptom in children Diarrhea most prominent symptom in adults
Bacterial						
Staphylococcus aureus	Food: ham, poultry, creams, mayonnaise	30 minutes–6 hours	Nausea, vomiting, cramps	Soft, not watery	No WBCs in stool	Onset abrupt, others with symptoms, look for common source
Clostridium perfringens	Food: beef, ham, Mexican cuisine	8–12 hours	Nausea, vomiting, epigastric pain	Watery	No WBCs in stool	Onset not as abrupt as with *S. aureus*
Campylobacter jejuni	Food: chicken; Water, fecal material	1–7 days	Nausea, vomiting, abdominal pain, malaise, fever	Watery, gross and occult blood	WBCs in stool positive culture	Abdominal pain can mimic appendicitis

Continued

TABLE 9–2.
(CONTINUED)

ORGANISM	TRANSMISSION	INCUBATION	SIGNS AND SYMPTOMS	TYPE OF STOOLS	LAB DATA	SPECIAL NOTATIONS
Salmonella	Food: poultry, red meat, eggs, unpasteurized milk Water Contact with infected pets (turtles, reptiles) Fecal–oral	6–72 hours	Nausea, vomiting, abdominal cramps, fever	Watery, gross and occult blood	WBCs in stool Positive culture	Common in children younger than 5 and adults older than 70 years
Shigella	Food, water Fecal–oral	1–7 days	Abdominal pain Fever	Watery, occult blood, no gross blood	WBCs in stool Positive culture	Most common in 1- to 4-year-olds, common in childcare centers
Escherichia coli	Food, water contaminated with feces "Traveler's diarrhea"	8 hours—3 days	Abdominal cramps	Watery	Usually no WBCs Positive culture	History of recent travel
Protozoal						
Giardia lamblia	Fecal–oral	1–4 weeks	Abdominal	Soft, pale, watery,	Stool positive for ova & parasites	Acute presentation of diarrhea from drinking contaminate water or recreational water (pools)
Cryptosporidium	Water		Pain, flatulence, distension, anorexia	Foul-smelling	Stool positive for ova and parasites	Chronic or recurrent diarrhea

- Obtain medication history, including any recent courses of antibiotics plus laxative or antacid use.
- Inquire about sexual practices and risk of HIV infection.
- Obtain description of bowel pattern; contributing factors such as certain foods or stress, family history; and stool characteristics (bloody, watery, with mucus, fatty, foul-smelling).
- Weight loss
- Travel history: Incubation period is 2 to 4 days for many viruses.
- Surgical history; history of exposure to others with similar illness
- Symptoms of hyperthyroidism

Physical Exam

- Signs of dehydration: tachycardia, confusion, orthostatic hypotension, poor skin turgor, dry mucous membranes, depressed fontanel, eyes sunken, crying without tears, listless, decreased urine output; fever is variable and ranges from afebrile to significant elevations
- Abdominal exam may reveal hyperactive bowel sounds and generalized tenderness.
- Signs of peritonitis (rebound tenderness) may be seen with severe inflammatory diarrhea.
- Particularly in children, look for other possible causes of diarrhea such as otitis media and urinary tract infection (UTI).
- Based on presentation, severity, and duration, test if symptoms are severe or diarrhea lasts longer than 7 days
    - Stool cultures are now lower in importance in workup; use instead molecular testing (culture-independent diagnostic tests [CIDT]), ova and parasites, *Clostridium difficile* toxin, occult blood, fecal calprotectin
- CBC to look for anemia, leukocytosis, and eosinophilia (often seen in parasitic infections and inflammatory bowel diseases [IBDs])
- Electrolytes: evaluate for hypokalemia, hyponatremia
- BUN and creatinine: elevations may be indicative of dehydration
- Blood cultures if systemic infection is suspected: high fever, chills, leukocytosis
- In patients with diarrhea lasting more than 3 weeks:
    - Sigmoidoscopy or colonoscopy to diagnose colitis
    - Evaluate for malabsorption: vitamin B12, folate, vitamin D, albumin, cholesterol, iron, iron-binding capacity, prothrombin time, D-xylose absorption test, 24-hour fecal fat collection to diagnose steatorrhea.

Differential Diagnosis

- Appendicitis
- Volvulus
- Cystic fibrosis
- Intussusception
- Inflammatory bowel syndrome
- IBD
- IBS
- Meningitis
- Pancreatitis
- Pneumonia
- Lactose intolerance
- Colon cancer
- Diverticulitis
- Pseudomembranous colitis
- Fecal impaction
- Malabsorption
- Cholinergic drugs and magnesium laxative abuse

Management

Nonpharmacologic Treatment

- Adequate hydration with fluids containing electrolytes and carbohydrates
- In infants without signs of dehydration, continue with formula or breast milk but increase amount; may change to soy-based formula for diarrhea (Isomil/DF, Enfamil, ProSobee, or Lacto Free) while ill.
- Normal diet when patient able to tolerate; no longer recommending BRAT diet (bananas, rice, applesauce, toast) because not calorie dense and not enough fat and protein
- In children with signs of mild dehydration, give 50 mL/kg of oral replacement therapy (ORT) such as Pedialyte, plus 10 mL/kg for each stool over a 4-hour period; sports drinks may be used in children 3 years of age and older.

- If vomiting is present, start with small volumes: 5 mL every 2 to 3 minutes and increase gradually if vomiting subsides. Also increase ORT by estimated volume loss with emesis.

Pharmacologic Treatment

- Antidiarrheal agents: If no contraindications (fever, bloody stools), may consider using:
  - Loperamide (Imodium): adults: 4 mg initially followed by 2 mg after each loose stool for a maximum of 16 mg in 24 hours; not recommended in children
  - Bismuth subsalicylate (Pepto-Bismol): adults: two tablets or 30 mL every 30 to 60 minutes, max eight doses/day; children 6 to 9 years: 10 mL every 30 to 60 minutes, max eight doses/day . 9 to 12 years: 15 mL every 30 to 60 minutes, max eight doses/day
- In adults, empirical antibiotic treatment while awaiting stool culture results for patients with moderate to severe fever, bloody stools, tenesmus, or presence of fecal leukocytes
  - Fluoroquinolones: drugs of choice, as they provide good coverage for most invasive bacterial pathogens
  - Ciprofloxacin (Cipro) 500 mg twice a day *or* levofloxacin (Levaquin) 500 mg daily
- Alternative agents
  - Trimethoprim-sulfamethoxazole 160/800 (Bactrim DS) twice a day *or* erythromycin 250–500 mg four times a day
- If *Giardia* or *C. difficile* is suspected:
  - Metronidazole (Flagyl) 250 mg three times a day for 7 days (avoid alcohol use during and for 48 hours after); for *C. difficile*, 500 mg three times a day for 10 to 14 days
  - Option for *C. difficile*, oral vancomycin
- Generally, antibiotics are not used to treat children until the causative organism is known and then only:
  - *Campylobacter:* erythromycin 20–50 mg/kg/day divided into four doses for 5 to 7 days
  - *Shigella:* Bactrim 1 mL/kg/day divided into two doses for 5 days
  - *E. coli:* Bactrim 1 mL/kg/day divided into two doses for 3 days
  - *Giardia:* furazolidone 6 mg/kg/day divided into four doses for 7 to 10 days (Furox: 1 5 mg/kg/day in four divided doses)
  - Alinia: for *Giardia*; may be given orally; do not use in children younger than 12 months; suspension for ages 1 to 11 years; tablets only for 12 years and older
  - Replace lost fluids and electrolytes.
  - Probiotics in patients taking antibiotics to prevent diarrhea

How Long to Treat

- Depends on underlying cause; for acute diarrhea because of an infection, generally 5 to 7 days

Special Considerations

- For chronic diarrhea, treatment may vary according to underlying cause.
- Geriatric patients are at greater risk for dehydration and complications.
- Neonates are at greater risk for severe infection and should be referred immediately.
- Pregnancy and lactation: If antimicrobials are required, check safety profile for use.
- Other: Immunocompromised patients are at a greater risk for chronic diarrhea from an infectious process such as from *Cryptosporidium* (a common, self-limiting infection that people with an intact immune system can clear in a few days without treatment).

When to Consult, Refer, Hospitalize

- Consult with physician for any child with significant signs and symptoms of dehydration (more than 10% increased pulse rate, poor skin turgor, depressed fontanel, delayed capillary refill, less than 1 mg/kg/hour urine output).
- Consult for possible hospitalization for infants under 3 months with bacterial diarrhea.
- Any patient with bloody diarrhea, fever, acute abdominal pain, and leukocytosis should be referred and evaluated immediately in an acute-care setting.
- Any patient who has not had resolution of diarrhea within 3 weeks needs to be referred to a gastroenterologist for evaluation.

Follow-Up

- Depends on cause and severity; none may be necessary if hydration maintained

Expected Course

- Acute diarrhea should resolve in 24 to 48 hours.

ACUTE ABDOMINAL PAIN

Definition

- Can be caused by obstruction of hollow viscus, altered bowel motility, capsular distention, peritoneal irritation, mucosal ulceration, vascular insufficiency, nerve injury, abdominal wall injury, or pain referred from an extra-abdominal site

Assessment

History

- Determine the onset, progression, migration, character and intensity, and localization.
  - Onset: *sudden, rapid,* or *gradual*
- Sudden: patient able to relate time of onset to a precise moment
  - Most often associated with perforation of the gastrointestinal tract that may be caused by a duodenal or gastric ulcer, diverticulum, or foreign body
  - Other causes: ruptured ectopic pregnancy, ruptured aortic aneurysm, mesenteric infarction, embolism of the abdominal muscle
- Rapid: begins within a few seconds and increases in severity in a short period of time
  - Often associated with intestinal obstruction, ureteral stone, cholecystitis, pancreatitis, diverticulitis, appendicitis, penetrating duodenal or gastric ulcer
- Gradual: pain slowly becomes more severe over a course of hours or days
  - History of onset vague
  - Often associated with a chronic inflammatory process, neoplasm, or a large bowel obstruction
  - Progression
- Perforated bowel often presents as a sudden onset of pain that abates dramatically if the perforation seals off and there is no further leakage of bowel content or blood into the peritoneum.
- A small bowel obstruction may present as intermittent attacks of pain that progress into a steady constant pain suggestive of vascular compromise.
- Migration
  - Pain that changes from the original site of onset to another location
  - Acute appendicitis may begin as periumbilical or epigastric pain and then localize to the right lower quadrant.

- ◊ A perforated duodenal ulcer causes pain initially in the epigastrium (because of leakage of gastric contents) and can migrate to the lower quadrants where the gastric material localizes in the abdominal cavity.
- ◊ Cholecystitis often causes irritation of the phrenic nerve, resulting in diaphragmatic pain that can radiate to the right shoulder, right scapula, or between the shoulder blades (Kehr's sign).

- ♦ Character and intensity
  - ◊ Cramping, dull, or aching and either constant or intermittent
  - ◊ Cramping (or colicky) abdominal pain increases in intensity in short waves, with intermittent periods of complete absence of pain. Often associated with mechanical small bowel obstruction. Short pain-free intervals may indicate a more proximal bowel obstruction; longer pain-free intervals may indicate a more distal obstruction.
  - ◊ Dull or aching abdominal pain that is constant is often caused by distention or edema of the abdominal wall or bowel wall, or inflammation of an abdominal organ (such as the capsule of the liver or spleen).
- ♦ Localization
  - ◊ Visceral pain due to distension of a hollow viscus is often localized poorly and often perceived in the midline; epigastric, mid-abdominal, or lower abdominal area.
  - ◊ Patients with visceral pain frequently change positions in an attempt to alleviate the pain.
  - ◊ Somatic pain is due to peritoneal inflammation and is usually sharper and more localized to the diseased area.
  - ◊ Patients with peritonitis often lie still on one side with their knees and hips flexed.
  - ◊ Pain from peritonitis is intensified by jarring motions (bumping into the bed).
  - ◊ In children, the closer the pain is to the umbilicus, the less likely it is to be organic.
- ♦ Additional information:
  - ◊ Have the patient rate pain on a scale of 1 to 10.
  - ◊ Determine if pain interferes with sleep; factors that precipitate or relieve the pain; relationship of pain to meals, specific foods, menstrual cycle, urination, defecation, exertion, and inspiration.
  - ◊ Fever, chills, nausea, vomiting, diarrhea, constipation, or urogenital symptoms may be present.
  - ◊ Blood in the stool, urine, or emesis may be present.
  - ◊ Social history includes alcohol and intravenous drug use.

◇ Gynecological history: Evaluate for possible pregnancy or sexually transmitted disease (STD).

◇ In children, include questions regarding irritability, ability to console, fussiness with feedings, whether infant clenches fists or draws feet up when crying.

Physical Exam

- Assess for fever, tachycardia, orthostatic hypotension, pallor, jaundice, perspiration, restlessness, and body positioning.
- Abdominal exam: Perform with knees flexed if patient is in severe pain.
- Observe for any surgical scars, distention.
- Bowel sounds: High-pitched tinkling sounds suggest a dilated bowel with air and fluid under tension. Rushes of high-pitched sounds indicate intestinal obstruction. Absent bowel sounds indicate an ileus or peritonitis.
- Inspect and palpate for hernias: abdominal, inguinal, or umbilical.
- Palpate for localized tenderness, rigidity, guarding, and rebound tenderness (an indication of peritonitis). Check for costovertebral angle (CVA) tenderness (with pyelonephritis or urolithiasis). Evaluate for hepatosplenomegaly and fluid wave (ascites from liver disease).
- Assess for Rovsing's sign, psoas sign, obturator sign (see the Appendicitis section), and Murphy's sign (see the Cholecystitis section).
- Rectal exam: Rectal wall pain can be an indication of appendicitis or abscess.
- Pelvic exam: for all women with abdominal pain
- In children, assess growth parameters.
- Other systems for possible origin because of possibility of referred pain, based on history

Diagnostic Studies

- CBC with differential; may show leukocytosis or anemia
- Serum electrolytes, glucose, BUN, and creatinine
- LFTs may be abnormal with liver involvement (AST, ALT, ALP, bilirubin, PT, partial thromboplastin time [PTT]).

- Amylase and lipase may be elevated in pancreatic disease.
- Beta-human chorionic gonadotropin (beta-HCG): Always obtain in women of childbearing age.
- STD testing if appropriate
- Urinalysis to rule out infection and hematuria (children with appendicitis may have some red blood cells [RBCs] and WBCs in urine)
- Check stool for blood.
- Abdominal ultrasound or transvaginal ultrasound for possible tubo-ovarian pathology
- CT scan for possible appendicitis, abscess, diverticular disease, kidney stones, and enlarged pancreas
- Consider if diagnosis unclear
  - ECG: Rule out referred pain from cardiac etiology.
  - Chest X-ray to evaluate for heart, lung, and mediastinal disease
  - Flat-plate and upright abdominal film
  - Abdominal MRI
  - Upper and lower GI barium studies
  - Endoscopy, colonoscopy, sigmoidoscopy
  - ERCP
  - Hydroxy-iminodiacetic acid (HIDA) gallbladder scan

Differential Diagnosis

Diffuse Pain

- Generalized peritonitis
- Metabolic disturbances
- Psychogenic illness
- Abdominal aortic aneurysm (AAA)
- Gastroenteritis
- Pancreatitis

Right Upper Quadrant

- Cholecystitis
- Cholelithiasis
- Hepatitis
- Hepatic abscess
- Right lower lobe pneumonia
- Subphrenic abscess

Right Lower Quadrant

- Appendicitis
- Cecal diverticulitis
- Ectopic pregnancy
- Ovarian cyst/torsion
- Endometriosis
- Pelvic inflammatory disease
- Ureteral calculi
- Mittelschmerz (colicky pain associated with ovulation)

Left Upper Quadrant

- Splenic enlargement/hematoma
- Left lower lobe pneumonia
- Cardiac disease
- Pancreatitis

Left Lower Quadrant

- Diverticulitis
- Ectopic pregnancy
- Ovarian cyst/torsion

- Endometriosis
- Mittelschmerz
- Ureteral calculi
- Pelvic inflammatory disease

Epigastric or Midline

- Gastritis
- Cardiac disease
- Peptic ulcer disease
- Pancreatitis
- Abdominal aortic aneurysm

Management

- Varies depending on underlying cause of the abdominal pain (see specific GI problems discussed in this chapter)

Special Considerations

- Geriatric patients: Presentation may be subtle, without classic symptoms.

When to Consult, Refer, Hospitalize

- Refer for immediate surgical evaluation in cases of acute abdominal pain associated with high fever with leukocytosis, clinical findings suggestive of peritonitis, or evidence of bleeding.
- Consult with a physician or refer to specialist if diagnosis is unclear or patient is unstable.

Follow-Up

- Varies by etiology

Common Gastrointestinal Conditions

ACUTE GASTROENTERITIS (AGE)

Definition

- General term used for symptoms of nausea, vomiting, and/or diarrhea caused by inflammation from infection of the stomach and intestinal mucosa. Symptoms may be caused by cholinergic hyperactivity or by the gut as it attempts to rid itself of irritating contents.

Etiology

- The visceral afferent nerves of the GI tract and the chemoreceptors are stimulated and send messages to the cerebral cortex that induce vomiting.
- Diarrhea is produced from the increased fluid secretion caused by inflammation of the bowel lining, or by damage to bowel mucosa, or by abnormal intestinal motility.
- Most caused by a viral, bacterial, or protozoal/parasitic infection
- Also can occur from an allergic or chemical reaction, from swallowed inorganic materials, or emotional stress
- Gastric distress is one of the most common adverse reactions to medication.

Incidence and Demographics

- Very common worldwide

Risk Factors

- Foreign travel, ingesting contaminated food or water
- Exposure to others who have an infectious gastroenteritis
- Day care or institutional living
- Medication adverse effects
- Recent course of antibiotics
- Lactose intolerance

Prevention and Screening

- Careful food preparation, good handwashing, proper cleaning of fresh fruits and vegetables before eating; drinking bottled water and cooked foods when traveling to foreign countries; using bottled water for ice in drinks and tooth-brushing

Assessment

History

- Acute onset of nausea, vomiting, and/or diarrhea; usually multiple episodes; symptoms may vary from mild to severe
- Fever, abdominal pain, anorexia, malaise, myalgia, and headache may be present.
- Characteristics of diarrhea: watery, soft, with mucus or blood

Physical Exam

- With severe AGE, may see symptoms of dehydration and electrolyte imbalance including dry, flushed skin; dry mucous membranes; poor skin turgor; decreased urine output; rapid pulse; and orthostatic blood pressure
- Bowel sounds may be hyperactive.
- There may be diffuse abdominal tenderness and distention, or abdominal exam may be unremarkable.
- If significant localized rebound tenderness is present especially with a fever and an elevated WBC count, suspect acute surgical abdomen. Acute gastroenteritis does not present with significant rebound tenderness.

Diagnostic Studies

- Obtain laboratory work if no spontaneous resolution of symptoms within 72 hours; usually not necessary
- Stool for culture and ova and parasites to identify a causative organism if present:
- *Shigella, Salmonella, E. coli*
- Stool for *C. difficile*, especially if recent course of antibiotics
- Stool for leukocyte and occult blood to rule out bacterial infection

- CBC with differential to evaluate for leukocytosis and eosinophilia (increased number of eosinophils commonly seen in parasitic infections)
- Electrolytes to evaluate for dehydration and electrolyte abnormalities

Differential Diagnosis

- Acute appendicitis
- Cholecystitis
- Fecal impaction
- Ileus
- IBD
- IBS
- Bowel obstruction
- Pelvic inflammatory disease
- Diverticulitis

Management

Nonpharmacologic Treatment

- Often initial treatment is supportive: bed rest, fluid replacement (rapid intravenous rehydration may be required starting with isotonic fluids, saline, and then adding glucose), and advancing the diet as tolerated
- Clear liquid diet advance as tolerated using BRATY diet: bananas, rice, applesauce, toast, yogurt
- Children ages 5 years to adults: no solid foods; give clear liquids in small amounts (15 mL every 10 min) and gradually increase if no vomiting occurs. If no vomiting for 4 hours and tolerating 8 oz/hour, may begin small amount of regular foods as tolerated. If vomiting reoccurs at any point, let stomach rest (approximately 1 hour), then restart small amounts of clear liquids.
- In younger children 1 month to 5 years of age, give ORT at 50 mL/kg over 4 hours; start with sips and gradually increase; may continue formula or regular diet if tolerated.

Pharmacologic Treatment

- Antidiarrheal agents are controversial in AGE because the causative pathogen needs to be eliminated from the body. In mild to moderate diarrheal illness, antidiarrheal medications can be used with caution (but not if fever and with blood in stool).
- If vomiting continues despite slow intake of fluids, consider use of antiemetic.
- Chemoreceptor trigger zone suppressors will suppress vomiting; antihistamines are more effective for nausea than for acute vomiting; antimotility agents to suppress diarrhea prolong absorption time of water in the gut but also may cause retention of organism/toxin.
- Antibiotics are used only when an organism is isolated and symptoms are not resolved; when leukocytes or dysentery are present, for treatment of *Shigella*, when there are 8 to 10 stools per day, or if patient is immunocompromised, consider metronidazole (Flagyl), trimethoprim-sulfamethoxazole (Bactrim), fluoroquinolones (Cipro).

Special Considerations

- Geriatric and pediatric patients are at higher risk for dehydration
- Pregnancy and lactation: If antimicrobials are required, check safety profile before use.
- Hospitalization required with severe dehydration, electrolyte imbalance, and/or metabolic acidosis; in older adults or the immunocompromised; for severe abdominal pain, rebound tenderness, or neurological symptoms

Follow-Up

- None may be necessary if patient remains hydrated.

Expected Course

- Usually self-limiting with vomiting limited to 24 to 48 hours, diarrhea may last 3 to 5 days; inflammation of the bowel due to a drug reaction may last for several weeks.

GASTROESOPHAGEAL REFLUX DISEASE (GERD)

- Symptomatic condition characterized by reflux or retrograde passage of low pH gastroduodenal contents into the esophagus, larynx, or lungs causing pain, irritability, or vomiting; in children—poor weight gain, respiratory disorders

- In infants, regurgitation of some of a feeding; 47% of all infants under 2 months of age display normal physiologic gastroesophageal reflux without associated symptoms at least two times daily and outgrow by 10 months to 1 year
- May cause damage to esophageal mucosa with or without failure to thrive, occult blood loss, anemia, and possibly aspiration pneumonia with or without wheezing

Etiology

- Inappropriate lower esophageal sphincter (LES) relaxation allows for gastric contents to be refluxed into esophagus. The turgor of the LES is influenced by age, intra-abdominal pressure, length of esophagus below diaphragm, hormones, food, and neurologic innervations.

Incidence and Demographics

- Affects up to 10% to 20% of the U.S. adult population; 65% of adults have had heartburn, 15% with weekly symptoms
- 47% of all infants younger than 2 months display physiologic reflux, outgrown by 18 months in 90% of cases

Risk Factors

- Smoking, obesity, alcohol use, caffeine use, position of acid pocket above diaphragm in patients with hiatal hernia

Prevention and Screening

- Avoid spicy foods, caffeine, smoking, mints.

Assessment

History

- Typical symptoms: heartburn (pyrosis) is described as a burning retrosternal discomfort radiating upward toward the neck that occurs 30 to 60 minutes after meals.

- Symptoms are exacerbated by lying supine or bending over and improve with sitting up or taking antacids.
- Excessive salivation, regurgitation, halitosis, sour or bitter taste into the mouth are common.
- In children, inquire about type, amount, and frequency of feedings and regurgitation; choking during feedings; any bile or blood in regurgitation; any fevers, diarrhea; upper respiratory infection symptoms, history of respiratory illnesses, otitis media; and any developmental delays.
- Atypical symptoms: dysphagia, odynophagia (painful swallowing), chest pain, hoarseness, cough, sore throat, nausea, and asthma

Physical Exam

- Exam often normal; assess hydration status
- Adults: weight; children: plot height/weight on growth curve
- Respiratory and cardiac exam; abdominal exam to check for tenderness and masses; stool for occult blood
- Mental status, irritability, lethargy
- Assess developmental milestones in infants; neurologic exam if presents as unexplained vomiting

Diagnostic Studies

- Diagnosis can be made without further diagnostic tests in children if typical symptoms of heartburn and regurgitation are present, history and physical exam are normal, and child is developmentally on track and growing appropriately.
- Diagnostic studies are recommended when the diagnosis of GERD is uncertain, when symptoms are not resolved with 4 weeks of empiric treatment, or if complications are suspected as indicated by atypical symptoms (dysphagia, odynophagia (painful swallowing), chest pain, hoarseness, cough, sore throat, nausea, and asthma); symptoms that indicate a more serious etiology such as a cardiac cause for chest pain; evidence of bleeding (guaiac-positive stools or hematemesis); anemia; weight loss; symptoms that persist despite treatment, or daily symptoms.
- Barium swallow/upper GI study is usually the first test ordered, but it is the least sensitive for diagnosing GERD; its main value is to assess anatomy and rule out malrotation and obstruction. It is useful as a screening test to exclude complications of GERD (mucosal irregularities and ulcer) and evaluate dysphagia (caused by stricture).

- Fluoroscopy can demonstrate presence of reflux, as well as rule out other causes of vomiting, such as gastric outlet obstruction.
- Esophageal pH monitoring can measure the number of acid reflux events, as well as the duration of each event in a given period of time. A pH probe is indicated to tailor medical management but not necessary in those infants who present with pathologic reflux that has caused a life-threatening event.
- Esophagogastroduodenoscopy (EGD) aids in the evaluation of the degree of esophagitis from reflux. Biopsies are obtained to assess mucosal integrity. Evaluation of other disorders such as Crohn's disease, eosinophilic or infectious esophagitis, peptic ulcers, stricture or webs, and bleeding points can also be made.
- Stool for occult blood; CBC to rule out anemia

Differential Diagnosis

Infants

- Overfeeding
- UTI
- Pyloric stenosis
- Partial upper intestinal obstruction
- Otitis media
- Pneumonia

Older Ages

- Cardiac spasm or myocardial infarction (MI)
- Peptic ulcer disease
- Esophageal tumor/stricture
- Esophagitis, infectious, chemical
- Esophageal motility disorders
- Esophageal structural disorders
- Hiatal hernia

All Ages

- Gastroenteritis
- Milk/soy intolerance
- Celiac disease
- Infections
- Hepatitis
- Drug-induced

Drugs Affecting the LES

- Nitrates
- Nicotine
- Narcotics
- Theophylline
- Anticholinergics
- Estrogen
- Somatostatin
- Prostaglandins

Management

- Goals are to relieve symptoms, heal esophagitis, and prevent complications.

Nonpharmacologic Treatment

- Lifestyle modification is Step 1 therapy and the key component to management.
- In adults, elevate head of bed on 6-inch blocks or use wedge under mattress.
- Avoid eating 2 to 3 hours before lying down and eat smaller, more frequent meals.
- In infants, hold infant upright for 15 to 30 minutes after feeding; prop upright in infant seat/car seat.

- In infants, also recommend smaller and more frequent feedings.
- Lose weight if overweight; avoid tight-fitting clothing.
- Avoid substances that cause symptoms, including foods high in fat, citrus and spicy foods, mint, chocolate, caffeine, and alcohol; patients with GERD and breastfeeding mothers of infants with GERD should stop smoking.
- If taking medications that decrease LES tone, seek appropriate alternatives.

Pharmacologic Treatment

- Pharmacological treatment in children under the age of 2 years is discouraged.
- Acid-neutralizing drugs may be initiated if nonpharmacologic treatment is not effective.
  - In mild symptoms, use over-the-counter antacids (also used for breakthrough symptoms of protein pump inhibitors [PPIs] and histamine-2 [H2] receptor antagonists).
  - Liquid more effective than tablet form
  - Antacids can decrease absorption of other medications (e.g., fluoroquinolones, tetracycline, ferrous sulfate); separate dosing by 2 hours.
  - Aluminum or magnesium hydroxide: adults: 10–30 mL orally four times a day; children: 0.5–2 mL/kg/dose three to six times/day
- Step 2 therapy involves adding H2 receptor antagonists if symptoms not relieved by lifestyle modification or antacids within 2 to 3 weeks.
- H2 receptor antagonists suppress gastric acid secretion; symptomatic improvement occurs in approximately 80% within 6 weeks.
  - Cimetidine (Tagamet): adults: 400 mg four times a day, maximum 800 mg twice a day; children: 10 mg/kg/dose four times a day
  - Potential drug interactions with theophylline, warfarin, nifedipine, propranolol, and phenytoin
  - Ranitidine (Zantac): 150 mg twice a day; famotidine (Pepcid) 20 mg twice a day; nizatidine (Axid) 150 mg twice a day
- Reevaluate 2 weeks after starting therapy with H2 receptor antagonists; if effective, continue for 8 to 12 weeks.
- If symptoms do not resolve, go to Step 3 therapy: Add a prokinetic agent, use higher dose H2 receptor antagonist for an additional 8 to 12 weeks, or change from H2 antagonist to a PPI for 4 to 8 weeks.

- Prokinetic agents increase LES tone and promote gastric emptying; used for mild to moderate symptoms, typically in combination with H2 receptor antagonists or PPIs
  - Metoclopramide (Reglan): adults: 5–10 mg four times a day; children: 0.1 mg/kg/dose 20 to 30 min before meals and at bedtime
  - Used less frequently because of its potential for dopamine blocking. Side effects such as drowsiness, confusion, depression, and extrapyramidal reactions of dystonia and tardive dyskinesia can occur.
- PPIs suppress gastric acid secretion to a greater degree than H2 blockers and are the initial treatment in patients with erosive esophagitis confirmed by endoscopy; take 1 hour before meal—PPIs should ideally be administered 15 to 30 minutes before the first meal of the day.
  - Omeprazole (Prilosec): adults: 20 mg every a.m.; children: 0.7–3.3 mg/kg/day in one to two doses
  - Lansoprazole (Prevacid): 30 mg once a day; esomeprazole (Nexium) 40 mg once a day; or rabeprazole (Aciphex) 20 mg once a day (1 to 11 years, under 30 kg, 15 mg daily; 30 kg and above, 30 mg daily)
  - Reports of blood dyscrasias with PPIs and H2 blockers. H2 blockers need to be renally dosed. B12 levels should be checked in people taking PPIs. B12, iron, and calcium absorption compromised with PPIs.
  - PPIs and H2 receptor antagonists: multiple cytochrome P450 (CYP) interactions with drugs such as warfarin, phenytoin, and antifungals

How Long to Treat

- Reconsider diagnosis if there is no response to PPIs after 8 weeks.
- Treat erosive esophagitis with PPIs for 8 to 12 weeks—more effective than H2 receptor antagonists.
- 85% of infants with GERD improve with age as they begin to stand and maintain a more erect, upright position, and advance to a more solid diet.
- If patient has a good response to therapy, gradually withdraw medication while continuing lifestyle modifications.
- Maintenance therapy with H2 receptor antagonists (continue usual treatment dosage) or PPIs (omeprazole 20 mg or lansoprazole 30 mg daily) should be considered to prevent relapse that occurs in 80% within 6 months; lifestyle modification should continue throughout treatment and indefinitely to prevent relapse.

Special Considerations

- Pregnancy: predisposition due to elevated hormone levels and increased intraabdominal pressure from pregnant uterus; antacids generally safe
- Lactation: antacids generally safe
- Patients with GERD showed higher incidence of dementia, and older adult patients had the highest risk of developing dementia.
- Consult with, or refer to, a physician or gastroenterologist when the patient does not respond to treatment or has symptoms of dysphagia, evidence of blood loss, iron-deficiency anemia, or significant weight loss, or for pediatric patients with anatomic abnormalities suspected, or if there is poor weight gain or developmental delay.
- Refer for surgery (gastric fundoplication; Step 4 therapy) when all other approaches have failed.

Follow-Up

- 2-Week intervals until improvement noted, then monthly

Expected Course

- In infants, 85% will have resolution when able to sit/stand and have begun on solids
- Often a chronic, relapsing condition in adults; however, the majority of patients with GERD respond well to medical therapy without developing complications or requiring surgery
- Annual endoscopy with biopsy indicated in patients with Barrett's esophagus

PEPTIC ULCER DISEASE (PUD)

Definition

- Ulceration in the gastric or duodenal mucosa caused when the normal protective coating of the stomach is penetrated and irritated by acid secretion, causing pain

Etiology

- NSAIDs
- *Helicobacter pylori* infection associated with 95% of duodenal ulcers
- Acid hypersecretory states (e.g., Zollinger-Ellison syndrome, caused by a gastrin-secreting tumor)
- Ulceration extends through the muscularis mucosa, usually 5 mm or greater in diameter.

Incidence and Demographics

- In the United States, approximately 500,000 new cases and 4 million occurrences per year
- Duodenal ulcers are five times more common than gastric ulcers; more than 95% occur in the duodenal bulb or pyloric channel; occur more often between the ages of 25 and 64
- Benign gastric ulcers commonly occur in the antrum on the lesser curvature and occur more often between the ages of 55 and 70.
- Older adults: increased mortality with initial attack at age 60 years and older

Risk Factors

- Aging (decrease in gastric mucosal protective mechanisms)
- Corticosteroid use, stress; aspirin (ASA) and chronic NSAID use increased risk of gastric ulcers
- Smoking and alcohol use do not appear to be causes

Prevention and Screening

- Consider using cyclooxygenase 2 (COX-2) inhibitor type of NSAIDs (e.g., celecoxib [Celebrex]) to reduce incidence of ulcer, spare gastric mucosal prostaglandin synthesis
- Misoprostol (prostaglandin analog) 100–200 μm three or four times a day or PPI twice a day, given prophylactically in combination with NSAIDs, to prevent NSAID-induced ulcers, for increased risk with age 70 years and over, use of anticoagulants or corticosteroids, and previous history of peptic ulcer and/or complications

- Smoking cessation; stress management
- NSAIDs with food, only when needed; avoid chronic use

Assessment

History (Diagnosis Often Made by Clinical Presentation)

- Classic symptom is epigastric pain (dyspepsia) described as a gnawing or dull ache that fluctuates throughout the day.
- With duodenal ulcer, discomfort occurs 1 to 3 hours after meals and may awaken patient at night. Pain is relieved by eating, antacids, or vomiting.
- With gastric ulcers, symptoms are more variable; food may increase or decrease symptoms; and anorexia, nausea, vomiting, and weight loss are more common.
- Melanotic stools: In older adults and NSAID-induced ulcers, there may be no symptoms until bleeding or perforation occurs.

Physical Exam

- Abdominal exam may reveal mild, localized epigastric tenderness to deep palpation.
- Stool may be positive for occult blood.

Diagnostic Studies

- *H. pylori* detection by serum antibodies or endoscopic biopsy (see below) should be evaluated in all patients with diagnosed PUD.
- CBC to exclude anemia from GI blood loss and leukocytosis because of ulcer perforation; stool occult blood
- Amylase in patients with significant epigastric pain to exclude pancreatic disease
- Fasting serum gastrin level to screen for Zollinger-Ellison syndrome; consider in patients with multiple recurrent ulcers, and in those with ulcer and no *H. pylori* or NSAID use (hold H2 receptor antagonists for 24 hours and PPI for 1 week because they may falsely elevate levels.)
- Upper endoscopy is best test to diagnose peptic ulcer disease; allows for biopsy to detect malignancy (more than 5% of gastric ulcers are malignant at time of presentation) and *H. pylori* infection (through rapid urease test or histology).

Recommended in patients who test positive for *H. pylori* infection (serum antibody) under age 45 and for all patients 45 years and over .

- Barium upper GI series may be used to screen uncomplicated symptoms of dyspepsia; however, they cannot distinguish between benign and malignant gastric ulcers
- Urea breath test (*H. pylori* generates urease) diagnoses active *H. pylori* infection; useful in evaluating symptomatic patients who have been treated previously for *H. pylori* (if breath test positive, indicates unsuccessful eradication). The serum *H. pylori* antibody may persist for up to 18 months after treatment, even in those patients who have been successfully treated. PPIs should be held for 7 days before test to avoid a false-negative result.

Differential Diagnosis

- GERD
- Cholecystitis
- Pancreatitis
- Diverticulitis
- Biliary tract disease
- Gastric carcinoma
- Cardiovascular disease
- Angina/MI
- Gastritis
- Functional dyspepsia

Management

Goal: Eradicate bacteria, provide environment for ulcer healing.

Nonpharmacologic Treatment

- Stop NSAIDs.
- Maintain well-balanced diet.
- Smoking should be discouraged as it slows ulcer healing and increases risk for reoccurrence.

- Stress management
- Surgery for refractory ulcers is rarely performed.

Pharmacologic Treatment

(see Table 9–3)

- In patients who do not need an endoscopy, have normal CBC, and test negative for H. pylori:
  - ◇ PPIs (omeprazole and lansoprazole) suppress gastric acid secretion to a greater degree than H2 receptor antagonists. Give 1 hour before meals.
    - H2 receptor antagonists suppress basal and nocturnal gastric acid secretion; less effective inhibition of meal-stimulated acid production
- Cimetidine (Tagamet), ranitidine (Zantac), famotidine (Pepcid), or nizatidine (Axid)
- Cimetidine has potential drug interactions with theophylline, warfarin, nifedipine, propranolol, and phenytoin
  - ◇ Sucralfate (Carafate) enhances mucosal defenses; efficacy is equal to H2 receptor antagonists in treating duodenal ulcers. Inhibits the absorption of certain medications (i.e., digoxin), and dosing should be separated by 2 hours and taken 1 hour before meals.

NSAID-induced Ulcer Disease

- Antibiotic therapy not necessary
- Discontinue NSAID if possible.

TABLE 9–3.
DRUG DOSAGES IN ACTIVE PEPTIC ULCER DISEASE

DRUG	PPIS	H2 RECEPTOR ANTAGONISTS
Omeprazole (Prilosec)	20 mg q.d.	Ranitidine 150 mg b.i.d., 300 mg HS
Lansoprazole (Prevacid)	30 mg q.d.	Nizatidine 150 mg b.i.d., 300 mg HS
Rabeprazole (AcipHex)	20 mg q.d.	Cimetidine 400 mg b.i.d., 800 mg HS
Esomeprazole (Nexium)	40 mg q.d.	Famotidine 20 mg b.i.d., 40 mg HS
Pantoprazole (Protonix)	40 mg q.d.	
All PPIs before breakfast		H2 blockers before meals
Sucralfate (Carafate)	1 g q.i.d.	Used as adjunct

- Substitute COX-2 inhibitor for other NSAIDs when possible.
- Once-daily PPI
- Prostaglandin analog (misoprostol) used if NSAID continued
- PPI for acute ulcer for 4 to 8 weeks, or indefinitely for prophylaxis
- Antacids no longer used as first-line treatment because of newer agents; commonly used to provide symptom relief in addition to other therapies on as-needed basis
- *H. pylori* Ulcer Disease
- Triple therapy with two antibiotics and a PPI for 14 days is recommended to treat
- *H. pylori* infection. Omeprazole 20 mg twice a day, lansoprazole 30 mg twice a day, pantoprazole 40 mg twice a day, rabeprazole 20 mg twice a day, or esomeprazole 40 mg twice a day in combination with clarithromycin 500 mg twice a day + amoxicillin 1 g twice a day or metronidazole 500 mg twice a day (penicillin-allergic patients) is the currently recommended regimen. Studies have not concluded that quadruple therapy is any more effective than triple therapy and adherence is more difficult.
- Either a PPI or a H2 receptor antagonist is required to provide an environment for healing of existing ulcer.
- In patients with complicated ulcers (bleeding, nausea, and significant pain), initiate treatment with PPI first to relieve symptoms, followed by treatment regimen for *H. pylori* infection if test is positive.

How Long to Treat

- Active peptic ulcer: Reevaluate in 2 weeks; if symptoms improving, continue treatment.
- With PPIs, treat uncomplicated duodenal ulcer for 4 weeks, gastric or complicated ulcer for 6 to 8 weeks.
- With H2 receptor antagonists, uncomplicated duodenal ulcer for 6 weeks, gastric ulcer for 8 to 12 weeks.
- With *H. pylori*, give medications for 10 to 14 days minimum; may require retreatment if symptoms recur.

Special Considerations

- Pregnancy: Misoprostol may cause uterine contractions, resulting in abortion.
- Refer to a gastroenterologist for endoscopic evaluation in patients with symptoms of GI bleeding (iron-deficiency anemia, hematemesis, or melena), persistent vomiting,

and weight loss; severe epigastric pain that may suggest ulcer penetration or perforation; patients 50 years of age and over with new onset of dyspepsia; persistent symptoms after several weeks of treatment or for recurrent symptoms after finishing treatment; all gastric ulcers.

Follow-Up

- Evaluate effectiveness of therapy 2 weeks after initiation and again after completion (4 to 12 weeks).
- Using a urea breath test, confirm eradication of *H. pylori* in patients who continue to have symptoms or relapse (may require retreatment with a different antibiotic regimen).
- Successful *H. pylori* eradication decreases peptic ulcer recurrence to 20% per year.
- All gastric ulcers should be reevaluated by endoscopy with cytology after treatment to document resolution and exclude malignancy.
- Use of steroids and NSAIDs and *H. pylori* infection were risk factors for recurrence of PUD *Complications*
- Hemorrhage, ulcer perforation or penetration, gastric outlet obstruction

IRRITABLE BOWEL SYNDROME (IBS)

Definition

- American Gastroenterological Association (AGA): combination of chronic and recurrent GI symptoms not explained by structural or biochemical abnormalities
- Rome III criteria for diagnosis: 12 or more weeks in the last 12 months of abdominal pain or discomfort that has 2 of 3 features: relieved by defecation, onset associated in change of frequency of stool, onset associated with change in form of stool

Etiology

- Pathophysiology is unknown but may be related to an increase in serotonin (5-hydroxytryptamine [5-HT]), a neurotransmitter controlling intestinal motility and visceral afferent responses. This increase may be caused by normal or noxious stimuli.
- Specific food intolerance (lactose; high fat; citrus or spicy foods; dietetic sweeteners; and gas-producing foods such as beans, cabbage, and raw onions)

- Malabsorption of bile acids
- Heightened visceral pain perception, especially with stress or around menses
- May have history of abuse or depression

Incidence and Demographics

- Common, occurs in 15% of the population, but only 15% seek treatment; median age 35; also occurs in children and older adults

Risk Factors

- Familial history
- Presence of other functional disorders, history of childhood sexual abuse
- Emotional and physical stress (e.g., anxiety, excessive worry, major loss, improper diet, overwork, decreased sleep, and poor physical fitness) can exacerbate symptoms.

Prevention and Screening

- Stress reduction
- Maintain healthy lifestyle by eating a well-balanced, high-fiber, low-fat diet; taking regular exercise; and getting adequate sleep.
- Avoid foods or other substances that exacerbate symptoms (see specific foods listed above under Etiology).
- Avoid caffeine, tobacco, and alcohol.

Assessment

History

- IBS can present as predominantly constipation, predominantly diarrhea, or mixed.
  - ◊ Constipation is described as small, infrequent, hard stools or straining to defecate.
  - ◊ Diarrhea (usually four to six stools a day) is described as watery, ribbon-like, with clear mucus in the stool.

- Blood in stool and waking at night to defecate is more likely inflammatory bowel disease (IBD).
- Often alternates between both constipation and diarrhea. Increased flatulence and bloating may be present. Symptoms are exacerbated by meals and stress and are usually relieved by defecation.
- History of increased emotional or physical stress, depression, or preoccupation with bowel habits
- Weight loss—none with IBS
- Diet, eating patterns, medications, treatments tried, family history (colon cancer)
- In women, obtain menstrual history and any association of symptoms with menstruation.
- Abdominal pain relieved by defecation; preoccupation with bowel symptoms

Physical Exam

- Usually normal; no weight loss
- Lower abdominal tenderness or distension may be present but not pronounced; a tender cord may be palpated over the sigmoid colon (left lower quadrant), which indicates the presence of stool; abdominal tympany if air trapping is present; mildly hyperactive bowel sounds may be present.
- Digital rectal exam is normal, although patient may have discomfort on exam

Diagnostic Studies

- CBC with differential, erythrocyte sedimentation rate (ESR), and thyroid function tests are normal, tissue transglutaminase, stool test for occult blood negative
- In patients with diarrhea, stool studies are negative (culture, ova and parasite, and *C. difficile*, WBCs, and fat)
- Flexible sigmoidoscopy, colonoscopy, barium enema when symptoms are severe or prolonged, to exclude inflammatory or malignant disease; indicated for patients 40 years of age and older
- Small bowel series to rule out Crohn's disease when diarrhea predominates
- Abdominal plain radiograph during acute episode of abdominal pain to exclude bowel obstruction

Differential Diagnosis

- IBD
- Thyroid disease
- Celiac
- Diverticulitis
- Giardiasis
- Celiac disease
- Endometriosis
- Cystic fibrosis
- Lactose intolerance
- Colon cancer
- Malabsorption

Management

Nonpharmacologic Treatment

- Patients should keep a diary in which foods, symptoms, and daily events are recorded to identify possible exacerbating factors.
- Dietary changes: Avoid foods and other agents that worsen symptoms.
- A lactose-free diet should be tried for 2 weeks in all patients to exclude lactose intolerance.
- A high-fiber diet (20–30 g/day) is recommended; may cause bloating and flatulence initially, but usually resolves in few weeks (increase gradually). Add 1 teaspoon bran powder two to three times/day to food or in 8 oz liquid.
- A diet with low fermentable oligosaccharides, disaccharides, monosaccharides, and polyols (FODMAPs) is recommended to improve the global symptoms associated with IBS-D, such as pain and bloating.
- The efficacy of probiotics in IBS has also been tested, and symptoms of bloating, abdominal pain, and flatulence showed significant improvements
- Management of stress through relaxation techniques and behavior modification, emotional support, addressing patient fears

Pharmacologic Treatment

- Medications required only in severe cases
  - Bulk-forming agents may be better tolerated than bran, used in mixed IBS
- Psyllium (Metamucil) 1 tbsp in 8 oz of fluid up to three times a day
- Methylcellulose (Citrucel) 1 tbsp in 8 oz of fluid up to three times a day
  - Anticholinergic agents: relieve spasm and abdominal pain.
- Dicyclomine hydrochloride (Bentyl) 10–20 mg four times a day as needed.
- Hyoscyamine sulfate (Levsin) 0.125 mg one to two (tabs or tsp.) q.4.h. orally or sublingually prn
  - Antidiarrheal agents: used on an as-needed basis
- Loperamide hydrochloride (Imodium) 4 mg initially, then 2 mg after each loose stool as needed. (max 8 mg/day); diphenoxylate with atropine (Lomotil) one to two tablets four times a day as needed.
  - If constipation is the primary problem, may use lactulose 15–30 mL/dose, max 60 mL/day if increased fiber not effective, or lubiprostone (Amitiza) 8–24 mg twice a day
  - Treatment for flatulence
- Simethicone (Phazyme, Gas-X) 125 mg four times a day as needed. with meals and q.h.s.
  - Antidepressants are controversial but may be effective for some patients with chronic, unremitting abdominal pain.
- Tricyclic: amitriptyline (Elavil) 25–50 mg q.h.s.
- Selective serotonin reuptake inhibitors (SSRIs): citalopram 10–20 mg, initially and increase up to 40 mg daily or fluoxetine (Prozac) 20–40 mg, if depression coexists

How Long to Treat

- High-fiber diet and avoidance of exacerbating agents should be continued indefinitely.
- Use other agents as needed for symptomatic management.

Special Considerations

- Symptoms usually decrease with age.
- Pregnancy: Check safety profile of all medications.

- Refer to or consult with a physician or gastroenterologist for severe symptoms; symptoms of nocturnal diarrhea, hematochezia, fever, and weight loss; new onset of symptoms in patients 40 years of age and older; and patients who have persistent symptoms despite treatment with diet, bulking agents, and antispasmodics.
- Refer to a psychologist for counseling and stress management if appropriate.

Follow-Up

- Every 2 weeks until symptoms improve; then every month for 6 months if continued improvement

Expected Course

- Most respond well to treatment during the initial 12-month period; however, IBS is a chronic relapsing condition that may require prolonged therapy.

ULCERATIVE COLITIS

Definition

- A chronic, relapsing inflammatory disease of the colon and rectal mucosa
- May be limited to the rectum (ulcerative proctitis) or involve the entire colon
- Characterized by acute exacerbations and remissions

Etiology

- Unknown but possibly autoimmune or genetic predisposition
- Inflammatory process causes diffuse friability and erosions that result in bleeding.
- Abuse of laxatives can weaken the colon wall.

Incidence and Demographics

- Usually manifests between ages of 15 and 35, with a second smaller peak in seventh decade of life; can occur as early as 5 years of age

- In the United States, occurs in 5 to 12 per 100,000, females more common than males
- Geriatric patients: increased mortality with initial attack if 60 years old and older

Risk Factors

- Tenfold increased risk of disease if first-degree relatives affected
- Jewish and Middle Eastern descent

Assessment

History

- Classic symptom is bloody diarrhea; other symptoms include crampy lower abdominal pain (commonly left lower quadrant, relieved by defecation), fecal urgency, tenesmus, nocturnal diarrhea.
- More severe cases have fever, anemia, anorexia, weight loss, and arthralgias.
- Extraintestinal manifestations such as oligoarticular arthritis, ankylosing spondylitis, uveitis, oral aphthous ulcers, pyoderma gangrenosum, and erythema nodosum occur in about 25% of cases as in Crohn's disease.
- In children, growth retardation, delayed puberty

Physical Exam

- Orthostatic blood pressure and heart rate measurements are done to determine volume status.
- Abdominal exam may reveal tenderness or signs of peritonitis; digital rectal exam may reveal red blood and mucus.
- Signs of extraintestinal manifestations such as arthritis, skin rashes, and eye manifestations

Diagnostic Studies

- CBC to evaluate anemia from bleeding; may show leukocytosis
- ESR and C-reactive protein (CRP) level are increased in active inflammation.
- Albumin may be low; electrolytes may be distorted.

- Stool studies to exclude infection (culture, ova and parasites, *C. difficile* toxin)
- Sigmoidoscopy is diagnostic; mucosa appears friable and inflamed; purulent exudates and ulcers may also be present; biopsy can differentiate ulcerative colitis from specific types of infectious colitis.
- Colonoscopy should not be performed in severe active disease because of the risk of perforation; may be performed when symptoms improve on therapy to determine the extent of disease.
- Plain abdominal radiographs are obtained in severe colitis to exclude toxic megacolon (colon becomes atonic and dilated more than 6 cm and is associated with symptoms of toxicity).
- Barium enemas are not useful during acute disease and may precipitate toxic megacolon.

Differential Diagnosis

- Crohn's disease
- Trauma
- Enterocolitis
- Infectious colitis
- Juvenile polyps
- IBS
- Ischemic colitis
- Neoplasms
- Diverticulitis
- Radiation-induced proctitis
- Hemorrhoids

Management

Nonpharmacologic Treatment

- Maintain well-balanced, high-fiber diet; avoid caffeine and gas-producing foods.
- Surgical intervention: curative with total colectomy; indications include severe colitis that does not respond to steroid treatment, patients with toxic megacolon that fail to improve after 48 to 72 hours (before perforation occurs), and high-grade dysplasia

Pharmacologic Treatment

- Fiber supplements or bulk-forming agents if not achieved through diet
  - Bran powder 1 to 2 tbsp twice a day, or psyllium (Metamucil) 1 tbsp in 8 oz of fluid up to 3 times day, *or*
  - Methylcellulose (Citrucel) 1 tbsp in 8 oz of fluid up to three times day
- Anti-inflammatory agent in mild to moderate disease, effective in inducing remission
  - Sulfasalazine (Azulfidine) and prednisone tablets or liquid for children over 2 years and adults; mesalamine (Rowasa) suppository for rectal involvement, enema for left-sided colitis; hydrocortisone suppository/enema. Treatment is moving from anti-(tumor necrosis factor (TNF)-α drugs to biologicals such as infliximab. Antidiarrheal agents should not be used during the acute phase as they may precipitate toxic megacolon but are safe and beneficial in mild chronic symptoms.
  - Loperamide (Imodium) 4 mg initially, then 2 mg after each loose stool prn (max 8 mg/day)
  - Diphenoxylate with atropine (Lomotil) one to two tablets four times a day as needed.
  - Immunomodulators for more severe disease

How Long to Treat

- Treatment is dictated by symptoms; exacerbations treated several weeks to 2 to 3 months
- Establish good working relationship with patient and gastroenterologist as you manage the primary care problems of the patient.

Special Considerations

- Pregnancy: Acute exacerbations typically occur in the first trimester; advise to postpone becoming pregnant until after 1 year of remission; continue sulfasalazine with folic acid supplementation during pregnancy to maintain remission. Prednisone is safe in pregnancy; immunosuppressants are unsafe and should be avoided.

When to Consult, Refer, Hospitalize

- Refer to a gastroenterologist for initial diagnostic studies and management and when acute exacerbation does not respond to usual therapy.

- Refer to a surgeon for surgical intervention when severe disease is unresponsive to treatment.
- Hospitalization is indicated for patients who present with fulminant colitis with symptoms of high fever, sepsis, profuse bloody diarrhea, abdominal pain, and severe dehydration.

Follow-Up

- Colon cancer screening with colonoscopy and biopsy every 1 to 2 years, beginning 7 to 8 years after disease onset (colon cancer incidence triple in patients with ulcerative colitis for over 10 years)

Expected Course

- Acute exacerbations are usually well controlled with medication and patients do not require surgery.
- Most never require hospitalization.
- Patients who have more severe disease that is resistant to therapy require surgery (up to 20% of patients), which results in complete cure of the disease.

Complications

- Toxic megacolon, perforation, strictures, anemia, colorectal cancer

CROHN'S DISEASE (REGIONAL ENTERITIS)

Definition

- A chronic, relapsing disease characterized by patchy inflammation that occurs anywhere in the gastrointestinal tract, but most commonly the terminal ileum and proximal colon

Etiology

- Pathogenesis unknown
- Often causes ulcerations, strictures, fistulas, and abscesses because inflammatory process involves all layers (transmural) of intestinal wall

- One-third of patients have small bowel involvement only, often of terminal ileum (ileitis); one-half of patients have small bowel and colon involvement, commonly terminal ileum and proximal ascending colon (ileocolitis); 20% of patients have only colon involvement.
- Possible genetic predisposition
- Possible environmental factors, bacteria, viral, dietary

Incidence and Demographics

- Onset usually occurs at 15 to 25 years with a second, smaller peak at 55 to 65 years
- More common in women than men
- Incidence 20 to 100/100,000 in the United States
- 25% present in childhood with an average age at onset 7.5 years
- More common in White people and those of Ashkenazi Jewish descent

Risk Factors

- First-degree relative has disease.
- Anxiety may exacerbate symptoms.

Assessment

History

- Findings variable; depend on location and extent of disease
- Delayed growth and development in children
- Common presentation includes non-bloody diarrhea, abdominal pain (often right lower quadrant or periumbilical), nausea, vomiting, weight loss; low-grade fever and malaise may be present.
- More serious disease may present with bowel obstruction, fistulas complicated by infection, and perianal disease (anal fissure, perianal abscess, or fistula).
- Patients may have high fever, dehydration, severe abdominal pain, significant weight loss, malnutrition, and postprandial bloating.

- Extraintestinal manifestations occur in 25% and include oligoarticular arthritis, ankylosing spondylitis, uveitis, oral aphthous ulcers, pyoderma gangrenosum, and erythema nodosum.
- If disease is confined to the colon, may present with rectal bleeding and diarrhea.

Physical Exam

- Abdominal exam may reveal a tender mass, which represents thickened or inflamed intestine; commonly found in the right lower quadrant.
- Rectal exam to evaluate for perianal disease (fissures, skin tags, fistulas, abscesses, and "blind" sinus tracts)
- Exam for extraintestinal findings

Diagnostic Studies

- CBC may reflect leukocytosis from inflammation or abscess, iron-deficiency anemia due to mucosal blood loss, megaloblastic anemia from B12 deficiency due to terminal ileum disease and malabsorption, or anemia of chronic disease.
- ESR or CRP elevated during active inflammation
- Decreased albumin levels because of malabsorption, intestinal protein loss, or chronic disease
- Stool culture, ova and parasites, and *C. difficile* toxin to exclude infectious cause for diarrhea
- Upper gastrointestinal series with small bowel follow-through
- Colonoscopy is superior to barium enema in evaluating the colon, as it allows for biopsy.
- Serologic testing to distinguish between Crohn's disease and ulcerative colitis
  - Antineutrophil cytoplasmic antibodies (pANCA) present in only 5% to 10% patients with Crohn's disease—much higher in ulcerative colitis
  - Antibodies to yeast *Saccharomyces cerevisiae* (anti-*Saccharomyces cerevisiae* antibodies [ASCA]) present in 60% to 70% patients with Crohn's disease (much lower in ulcerative colitis).
  - The combination of negative pANCA and positive ASCA is 50% sensitive and 97% specific for Crohn's disease.

Differential Diagnosis

- Ulcerative colitis
- Gastroenteritis
- Hemolytic uremic syndrome
- Acute appendicitis
- PUD
- Henoch-Schönlein purpura
- IBS
- Constipation
- Psychosocial problems
- Lactose intolerance
- Infectious diarrhea
- Lymphoma
- Ischemic colitis
- Carcinoma

Management

- Goals are to treat symptoms and control the disease process.

Nonpharmacologic Treatment

- Maintain a well-balanced diet high in protein and vitamins, particularly B12 and iron.
- Avoid dairy products that contain lactose if they exacerbate symptoms.
- A low-roughage diet (no raw fruits or vegetables, nuts, seeds, etc.) may be beneficial during acute exacerbations.
- Stress management; relaxation techniques
- Psychosocial support is very important in these patients, given the chronicity of this disease.
- Surgical intervention: not curative; one-half of patients require at least one surgery

Pharmacologic Treatment

- Parenteral vitamin B12 and medium-chain triglyceride (MCT) supplementation are given if malabsorption results (common in patients with extensive terminal ileum disease or resection).
- Iron supplements are needed in patients with chronic blood loss.
- Drug of choice: 5-ASA (aminosalicylic acids) and prednisone for acute exacerbations: 40–60 mg/day for 2 to 3 weeks; taper to 5 - 20 mg/day; taper to 2.5 mg per week to a maintenance dose required for some persons.
- Azathioprine (Imuran) and 6-MP are used to sustain remission.
- Anti-TNF-α are used first-line in rapidly progressive disease. Treatment is moving from anti-TNFα drugs to biologicals such as infliximab
- Loperamide (Imodium) as needed
- Enteral therapy (tube feedings) or total parental nutrition (TPN) is indicated when patients are unable to tolerate an oral diet for 5 days.

How Long to Treat

- Acute exacerbation: Treatment with sulfasalazine (Sulfazine) or mesalamine (Asacol) for 3 weeks usually improves symptoms; however, some may require 2 to 3 months.
- Patients who fail to improve after 3 weeks of mesalamine should have systemic corticoids added.
- Work closely with the specialist while providing primary care to this patient.

Special Considerations

- Pregnancy: Sulfasalazine and steroids are safe in pregnancy.
- Refer to gastroenterologist for treatment of diarrhea with bile acid sequestrants, antidiarrheal medications, sulfasalazine, corticosteroids, some antibiotics, and immunomodulators.
- Refer to or consult with a gastroenterologist for initial diagnostic studies and management and for acute exacerbations.
- Hospitalization is required in acute exacerbations when symptoms persist.
- Surgical intervention may be required to remove severely affected bowel or to provide bowel rest.

Follow-Up

- Provide patient education about disease process, medication, diet; colonoscopy screening after 10 years of disease because of increased incidence of colon cancer.
- Follow-up according to specialist recommendations and for exacerbation of symptoms.
- All patients will require emotional support.

Expected Course

- Chronic, with acute exacerbations and periods of remission; progression of disease is common, with the average patient having surgery every 7 years.

Complications

- Toxic megacolon fistula, abscess, perforation, bowel obstruction, perianal disease, malabsorption, and colon cancer (increased risk, but not as high as with ulcerative colitis)
- From chronic steroid use: aseptic necrosis of the hip, cataracts, osteoporosis, diabetes, and hypertension
- Depression in 30% to 50% of patients with severe disease

Conditions that May Warrant Surgery

APPENDICITIS

Definition

- Inflammation of the vermiform appendix (small, blind pouch projecting from the cecum), causing obstruction of the lumen of the appendix. Early diagnosis is key to decreasing both morbidity and mortality associated with rupture.

Etiology

- Obstruction is the cause in 30% to 40% of cases and is commonly caused by a fecalith (a hard concentration of fecal matter and calcium salts), foreign body, inflammation, or neoplasm.

- Other causes include hypertrophy of the lymphoid tissue associated with a viral infection (e.g., measles), trapped barium after an imaging study, foreign body (e.g., seeds), intestinal worms (e.g., pin worms), tumor, or adhesions that cause obstruction.
- Obstruction leads to a build-up of mucosal secretions that cause the appendix to become inflamed and may lead to gangrene or perforation.

Incidence and Demographics

- Most common in people ages 10 to 30, with peak incidence at ages 15 to 24
- In patients 50 years and older and younger than 5 years, classic symptoms are less frequent, although perforation is more common, with a higher mortality and morbidity.
- A ruptured appendix occurs in one-half of children under 6 years of age with appendicitis.
- Most common cause of abdominal pain requiring surgery in childhood and adolescence

Risk Factors

- Family history, intra-abdominal tumors, recent gastrointestinal illness—especially viral or worm infestation

Assessment

History

- Classic presentation
  - Pain begins gradually; usually starts as vague, colicky, cramping, and poorly localized to the periumbilical or epigastric area, often associated with the urge to defecate or pass flatus, which helps to reduce the pain. Pain can vary depending on the location of appendix. Migration of periumbilical pain to right lower quadrant (RLQ) is one of the most predictive features of appendicitis.
  - Lasts approximately 4 to 6 hours, followed by increased, steady pain that is more localized, generally to the RLQ (although site can vary because appendix is not always located in RLQ)
  - Usually aggravated by motion or coughing; pain during car ride is suspicious for rebound tenderness
  - Anorexia is a frequent cause; nausea and vomiting can also occur.
  - May have constipation or diarrhea; fever usually low grade or absent

- Atypical presentation in children
  - Initial symptom is vomiting
  - May have GI and genitourinary (GU) complaints
  - Upper respiratory infection symptoms, fever (temperature over 101°F)
  - Less likely to exhibit abdominal tenderness, rebound tenderness, anorexia, and altered bowel sounds
- Atypical presentation in older adults
  - Mental confusion, no fever, less abdominal tenderness

Physical Exam

- Normal or mild elevation in temperature; if febrile, may also have tachycardia
- Patient may be lying with knees flexed, guarding abdomen.
- Abdominal exam: RLQ tenderness with rebound and guarding usually present at McBurney's point; positive Rovsing's sign (pain referred to the right when direct pressure applied to the left lower quadrant [LLQ]), positive psoas sign (pain when raises right leg against resistance), and positive obturator sign (pain when the right hip and knee are flexed and thigh is rotated inward)
- In neonates, a palpable abdominal mass and abdominal wall cellulitis may be evident.
- In children under 2 years, fever and diffuse abdominal tenderness are the primary presentation.
- In children 2 to 12 years, fever and RLQ tenderness are paramount.
- Abdominal tenderness may be absent if appendix is located in pelvis or behind cecum.
- Involuntary guarding and rebound tenderness are indicative of a ruptured appendix.
- May present with tender flank, rectum, or pelvis; therefore, a rectal and pelvic exam plus assessing for CVA tenderness are essential.
- Mass from abscess may be palpable if perforation occurred several days before exam.
- Serial exams are important until diagnosis is made or ruled out.

Diagnostic Studies

- CBC frequently shows a moderate leukocytosis with polymorph nuclear predominance of shift to left (more than 90%).

- CRP, a nonspecific inflammatory marker, if elevated and combined with leukocytosis, increases likelihood of appendicitis.
- Antibiotics and steroids may alter lab results.
- Urinalysis to exclude hematuria and infection
- Urine beta-HCG should be performed in post-menarchal women.
- Flat-plate and upright abdominal X-ray to exclude intestinal obstruction, bowel perforation, or ureteral calculus; identification of a fecalith
- Abdominal CT preferred over X-ray to detect appendiceal inflammation, free fluid, abscess, or other causes of abdominal pain.

Differential Diagnosis

Life-Threatening

- Ectopic pregnancy
- Intestinal obstruction
- Torsion or perforation of viscus
- Abdominal aneurysm
- Atypical presentation of MI

Other Possible Differential Diagnoses

- Acute gastroenteritis
- Ruptured ovarian cyst or follicle
- Twisted ovarian cyst and endometriosis
- Perforated ulcer
- Acute diverticulitis
- Pelvic inflammatory disease
- Acute pancreatitis
- Cholecystitis
- Ureteral calculus
- Pyelonephritis constipation

- Hemolytic uremic syndrome
- Henoch-Schönlein purpura
- IBD
- UTI
- Mesenteric adenitis
- Meckel's diverticulum
- Pneumonia
- Sickle cell
- Pharmacologic disease
- Pelvic inflammatory disease
- Intussusception

Management

Nonpharmacologic Treatment

- Surgery (appendectomy) required, may have an interval appendectomy.
- Nonoperative management of uncomplicated appendectomy is increasing.
- Avoid use of cathartics or enemas because of risk of perforation.
- Push fluids before appendectomy.
- Antibiotics should not be given if the diagnosis of appendicitis is in question, because they can mask the presence or development of perforation.
- If perforation or abscess does occur, IV antibiotics are given perioperatively.

Special Considerations

- Pregnancy: may present with atypical pain due to displacement of the appendix by the uterus
- Acute appendicitis may be the first manifestation of Crohn's disease.

When to Consult, Refer, Hospitalize

- Immediate referral to a surgeon for appendectomy

Follow-Up

Expected Course

- Recovery from an uncomplicated appendectomy is approximately 1 week

Complications

- Abscess and/or perforation of the bowel with subsequent peritonitis—either requires drainage and IV antibiotics

HERNIAS

Description

- A defect in the wall of the abdomen and groin that allows intra-abdominal contents to protrude from the normal location
- Can develop at sites of previous surgical incisions (incisional hernia)
- Clinically, all hernias can be described as reducible (contents can be pushed back into the abdominal cavity), nonreducible (contents cannot be pushed back into the abdominal cavity), incarcerated (a nonreducible hernia in which the flow of intestinal contents is obstructed), or strangulated (an incarcerated hernia in which the blood supply of the hernia contents is compromised).

Etiology

- Congenital or acquired defect in the abdominal wall
- Situations or conditions that raise intra-abdominal pressure increase occurrence (e.g., Valsalva, ascites, pregnancy).
- Incomplete or poor healing of a surgical incision that can predispose to the development of an incisional hernia

Incidence and Demographics

- Umbilical: common in infants; more common in Black children, higher incidence in low-birth-weight infants. In adults, occur in middle-age multiparous women, patients with ascites, and older adults

- Epigastric: common in men 20 to 50 years of age
- Incisional: common in peritoneal dialysis patients
- Inguinal: herniation into the inguinal canal; direct hernias are acquired, indirect are congenital—most common hernia
- Femoral: second-most common in both men and women, rare in children; incidence increases with age

Risk Factors

- Congenital defect in abdominal wall
- Activities and conditions that increase intra-abdominal pressure, such as constipation, straining during micturition, chronic cough, weight-lifting, ascites, pregnancy, obesity
- Postoperative wound infection, dehiscence

Prevention and Screening

- Avoid excessive straining and lose weight if overweight; use good body mechanics
- Screen on physical exams

Assessment

History

- Umbilical hernia: in infants, asymptomatic; adults may have vague, intermittent pain and tenderness
- Epigastric hernias: present with a small painless mass
- Incisional or ventral hernia: recent surgery, smoker, post-operative wound infection
- Peristomal hernia: patients with ostomy
- Strangulated hernias present with severe pain, fever, nausea and vomiting, abdominal distension, and constipation.

Physical Exam

- Inspection and palpation in both the supine and standing positions, while the patient performs a Valsalva maneuver; abdominal exam to evaluate tenderness, masses, hepatomegaly, and ascites; digital rectal exam to exclude enlarged prostate
- Inguinal hernia may be palpable in scrotal sac; inguinal canal can best be palpated with patient standing and exam performed through the scrotal sac.
- Umbilical or ventral: Palpate the umbilical region in the supine position while the patient raises head and performs a Valsalva maneuver.
- Epigastric: usually a small mass located midline between the umbilicus and xiphoid cartilage
- Incisional: presents as a bulge through a surgical incision

Diagnostic Studies

- Diagnosed by history and physical examination
- CBC may show leukocytosis if strangulation is present
- Ultrasound may be helpful to diagnose a hernia in patients who report symptoms but have no palpable mass; can differentiate an incarcerated hernia from an enlarged lymph node or other cause.

Differential Diagnosis

- Muscle strain
- Arthritis
- Lipoma
- Lymphadenopathy
- Hydrocele, varicocele

Management

Nonpharmacologic Treatment

- A patient with a symptomatic, reducible inguinal hernia who has relative contraindications to surgery may wear a truss (keeps hernia reduced); however, this is not always effective.

- Elective herniorrhaphy (hernia repair) is indicated for all abdominal hernias before incarceration and strangulation occur. Patients with evidence indicating a strangulated hernia must undergo emergency surgery.
- Uncomplicated hernia repair is often done under local or spinal anesthesia on an outpatient basis.

Pharmacologic Treatment

- None indicated
- Significant pain, if present, is suggestive of a more serious complication such as incarceration or strangulation and should not be masked by narcotics.

Special Considerations

- Geriatric patients: inguinal and umbilical more common with increasing age
- Diastasis recti is a separation of the two rectus abdominis muscles, causing a ridge of abdominal contents to bulge slightly; it has no clinical consequence.
- Pregnancy: increases risk for developing a hernia because of increased abdominal pressure.
- Patients with portal hypertension and ascites are at increased risk for umbilical hernias.

When to Consult, Refer, Hospitalize

- Refer to a surgeon for evaluation.

Follow-Up

Expected Course

- Risk of reoccurrence after hernia repair: epigastric up to 10%; non-mesh incisional hernias recur 30% to 50%; mesh-repaired hernias recur 20%.

Complications

- Ischemic bowel with a strangulated hernia; bowel obstruction

CHOLECYSTITIS

Description

- Acute or chronic inflammation of the gallbladder

Etiology

- Over 90% of cases are because of cystic duct obstruction by an impacted stone.
- Formation of gallstones is from supersaturation of products in bile exceeding their maximum solubilities.
- Gallstones consist predominantly of either cholesterol or calcium.
- Other causes include gallbladder stasis that can occur from prolonged acute illness, fasting and hyperalimentation, gallbladder infection; vasculitis; carcinoma of the gallbladder and/or bile ducts; other tumors that compress the gallbladder and/or bile ducts; or infectious agents in clients with AIDS.
- Pain arises from the gallbladder contracting against an obstruction.

Incidence and Demographics

- Occurs in 16 to 20 million people in the United States, with 1 million new cases each year
- Less common in Black people except for those with sickle cell anemia
- Geriatric patients: atypical presentation; at higher risk for developing complications, most common indication for abdominal surgery

Risk Factors

- Mnemonic: fat, fair, forty, flatulent, female
- Increases with age, body habitus, obesity, or rapid weight loss
- Childbearing, pregnancy, being female; family, maternal history of gallstones
- Drugs: contraceptive hormones, hormone replacement therapy, ceftriaxone
- Ethnicity: Pima Indian, Scandinavian

- Hyperalimentation; ileal and other metabolic diseases such as diabetes mellitus, Crohn's disease
- Rapid weight loss following bariatric surgery

Prevention and Screening

- Low-fat, low-carbohydrate, high-fiber diet, and physical activity

Assessment

History

- Acute
  - ◊ Epigastric or right upper quadrant pain, nausea, vomiting, and fever
  - ◊ Pain may radiate to right shoulder, scapula, or between shoulder blades if there is irritation of the phrenic nerve (Kehr's sign)
  - ◊ Pain usually precipitated by a large or fatty meal
  - ◊ Past medical history of biliary colic
- Chronic
  - ◊ Less-severe abdominal pain
  - ◊ Episodes shorter in duration (less than 3 hours) and recurrent

Physical Exam

- Jaundice may be present if there is biliary obstruction (15% of acute cases).
- Positive Murphy's sign (sudden intake of breath, inspiratory arrest on palpation of the RUQ due to pain)
- Guarding and rebound tenderness may be present.
- Geriatric patients: Localized tenderness may be the only presenting symptom, no fever or pain.

Diagnostic Studies

- Leukocytosis; elevated ALT (over 300 ***IU/L), ***AST, GGT; and alkaline phosphatase usually present
- Elevated bilirubin may be seen with or without obstruction.
- Serum amylase may also be elevated, especially if a biliary duct obstruction has occurred at or near the pancreatic duct, causing a concomitant pancreatitis.
- Ultrasound: 95% sensitivity and specificity for diagnosis of gallstones

Differential Diagnosis

- Pneumonia
- Thoracic disease
- Angina
- Appendicitis
- Bowel obstruction/IBD
- Pancreatitis
- Hepatitis
- Peptic ulcer disease
- GERD
- Cancer of gallbladder or bile ducts
- Right kidney disease

Management

Nonpharmacologic Treatment

- For chronic cholecystitis, decrease fat in diet.
- Laparoscopic cholecystectomy is standard treatment
- Percutaneous cholecystolithotomy is a safe and effective technique for the patients who cannot undergo laparoscopic cholecystectomy due to their comorbid conditions. (Latif, et al., 2022)

Pharmacologic Treatment

- For chronic cholecystitis, consider using ursodiol (Actigall) 8–10 mg/kg/day divided two or three times a day (may also be used prophylactically in patients undergoing bariatric surgery).
- For acute cholecystitis, refer to surgeon.

Special Considerations

- In obese, diabetic, older adults, or immunosuppressed patients, severe inflammation of the gallbladder with gangrene; necrosis may occur without obvious signs and symptoms.
- High risk for gallbladder carcinoma: Pima Indian descent, calcified gallbladder, gallbladder polyps more than 10 mm, gallstones more than 2.5 cm, anomalous pancreaticobiliary duct junction
- Refer all to surgeon for evaluation; those with acute cholecystitis require hospitalization.

Follow-Up

- Provide patient education about diet, medications

Expected Course

- Uncomplicated cholecystectomy usually followed by complete resolution of symptoms

Complications

- Gangrene, necrosis, cholangitis, other complications of surgery
- Mortality rate markedly increased for older adults who have cholecystectomy for acute cholecystitis

COLORECTAL CANCER

Definition

- Malignancy of the large intestine including the rectum

Etiology

- Most colon cancers are adenocarcinomas that begin as adenomatous polyps (benign epithelial growths).

Incidence and Demographics

- Third leading cause of death because of malignancy in the United States, with 50,000 deaths occurring annually
- Increased prevalence in developed countries, urban areas, and advantaged socioeconomic groups
- Higher incidence in people of German, Irish, Czechoslovakian, and French descent

Risk Factors

- Incidence increases after age 40, with 90% of new cases occurring in patients over age 50.
- Previous history or family history of adenomatous polyps
- Family history of colorectal cancer, especially in a first-degree relative diagnosed before age 55
- Familial polyposis
- IBD
- History of breast or gynecological cancer
- Barrett's esophagus
- Obesity
- Cigarette smoking

Prevention and Screening

- Current American Cancer Society screening recommendations include completing one of the following:
    - Fecal occult blood testing annually
    - Fecal immunochemical test annually
    - Stool DNA test, interval not determined

- ◇ Flexible sigmoidoscopy every 5 years
- ◇ Double-contrast barium enema every 5 years
- ◇ Colonoscopy every 10 years
- ◇ CT colonography every 5 years; colonoscopy completed if positive

- Colonoscopy is the recommended screening test for colorectal cancer for the average risk patient beginning at age 45.
- High-risk patients with first-degree relative with colon cancer should have a colonoscopy, recommended beginning at 40 (or 10 years before cancer diagnosis in relative, whichever is earlier). Patients with negative screening colonoscopies need future screenings every 3 to 5 years.
- Direct effect of diet remains unproven; however, a diet high in fiber, fruits, and vegetables and low in red and processed meats shows promise in decreasing colorectal cancer. Calcium supplementation and a daily aspirin have also been shown to be beneficial.

Assessment

History

- Often colorectal cancer reaches advanced stages without symptoms.
- Symptoms may include rectal bleeding and altered bowel habits (constipation, occasional diarrhea, pencil-thin stools).
- Signs and symptoms of anemia

Physical Exam

- A mass may be palpated in the abdomen.
- Rectal mass may be palpated on digital exam.
- The liver should be evaluated for enlargement suggesting metastatic disease.
- Enlarged inguinal lymph nodes

Diagnostic Studies

- Stool for occult blood: False positives can be caused by ingestion of red meat, iron, or aspirin, and from upper GI bleeding; false negatives can occur from vitamin C ingestion and intermittent bleeding.

- CBC to evaluate for iron-deficiency anemia
- Elevated LFTs raise concern for possible liver metastasis.
- Carcinoembryonic antigen (CEA) has not been shown to be efficacious for colorectal cancer screening; however, it is useful as a marker for treatment response in patients who have been diagnosed with colorectal cancer; if treatment response occurs, the CEA level should decrease.
- Colonoscopy with biopsy confirms diagnosis.
- Abdominal CT to evaluate for metastatic disease in patients with colorectal cancer
- Chest X-ray to look for metastasis to chest
- Endoscopic ultrasound to evaluate the extent of rectal cancers
- Intraoperative ultrasound may be used to evaluate solid organ (liver) involvement after colorectal tumor is resected

Differential Diagnosis

- Rectal polyps
- Hemorrhoids
- Rectal fissures
- Colorectal strictures
- Diverticulosis
- Colorectal infections
- Inflammatory lesions
- Other neoplasms
- IBD
- Masses outside bowel wall

Management

- Depends on cancer stage (tumor size and extent of bowel wall invasion, lymph node involvement, presence of metastasis) and type of tumor
- Surgery is the treatment of choice.

Nonpharmacologic Treatment

- Referral to surgeon for surgery and/or radiation.

Pharmacologic Treatment

- Chemotherapy

Special Considerations

- None

When to Consult, Refer, Hospitalize

- If colon cancer is suspected or diagnosed, refer to a surgeon.
- Patients with a family history of colon cancer or a history of adenomatous polyps should be followed regularly by a gastroenterologist.

Follow-Up

Expected Course

- Depends on stage of the cancer and type of tumor

Complications

- Complications associated with chemotherapy, radiation, surgery, and/or metastasis

ACUTE PANCREATITIS

Description

- Inflammation of the pancreas causing release of pancreatic enzymes into the surrounding tissue. With acute pancreatitis, there is usually complete restoration of pancreatic function; when recovery is incomplete, the patient develops chronic pancreatitis.

Etiology

- Most cases are related to biliary tract disease from a large gallstone causing a blockage of the pancreatic duct or from excessive alcohol consumption.
- This causes the release of pancreatic enzymes that cause local and systemic symptoms.
- Other causes include hypercalcemia, hyperlipidemia, viral infections (e.g., mumps), renal failure, certain medications, and abdominal trauma.

Incidence and Demographics

- Estimated 15 per 100,000
- Equal distribution between genders
- Acute, no predominant age
- Chronic, usually related to alcohol intake, ages 35 to 45

Risk Factors

- Alcohol abuse
- Gallstones, hyperlipidemia, hyperparathyroidism, hypercalcemia
- Abdominal trauma, renal failure, certain viral infections
- Certain medications (diuretics, valproic acid, didanosine [ddI], sulfonamides, azathioprine)
- Noncompliance with diabetes and hyperlipidemia treatment

Prevention and Screening

- Decrease alcohol consumption; a low-fat, low-cholesterol diet

Assessment

History

- Abrupt onset of epigastric or left upper quadrant abdominal pain, often radiating to the back, described as steady and severe

- Pain worsens with movement or lying supine and improves when sitting or leaning forward.
- Nausea and vomiting are generally present.
- There may be a history of alcohol intake or a heavy meal before the onset of pain.

Physical Exam

- Low-grade fever, epigastric or left upper abdominal tenderness, and distension are usually present.
- Occasionally an upper abdominal mass can be palpated because of pancreatic inflammation or presence of a pseudocyst (a sac of pancreatic enzymes surrounding the pancreas).
- Absent bowel sounds may occur if a paralytic ileus is present.
- Mild jaundice, tachycardia, hypotension, pallor, and sweating can be seen.

Diagnostic Studies

- Serum amylase and lipase will be significantly elevated.
- Urinalysis may show proteinuria, increased osmolality, glycosuria, and casts.
- CBC may show leukocytosis (10,000–25,000 cells/μL).
- ALP, ALT, and ALT may be mildly elevated; elevated bilirubin is more associated with biliary disease.
- Serum calcium may be decreased in severe acute disease.
- In chronic disease, labs may be normal.
- Flat-plate and upright abdominal film rule out perforated ulcer or intestinal obstruction.
- Chest X-ray may be needed to rule out chest pathology.
- Abdominal CT scan may be used to demonstrate an enlarged pancreas or pseudocyst.

Differential Diagnosis

- Acute cholecystitis
- Acute intestinal obstruction

- Perforated duodenal ulcer
- Leaking aortic aneurysm
- Renal stone
- Acute mesenteric ischemia
- Gastroenteritis

Management

Nonpharmacologic Treatment

- Referral for hospitalization and treatment of underlying cause, unless mild case and tolerating fluids

Pharmacologic Treatment

- Hydromorphone (Dilaudid) is the analgesic of choice in acute pancreatitis. 0.5–1 mg IV every 1 to 2 hours provides adequate pain relief.
- Morphine causes increased sphincter of Oddi pressure, which can worsen pancreatitis and increase ductal pressure.
- Meperidine (Demerol) causes potential occurrence of toxic metabolites, which can worsen pancreatitis.
- NSAIDS are an effective opiate-sparing alternative in the first 24 hours as well as the use of epidural pain management.
- Carbapenems are used for prophylaxis in necrotizing pancreatitis if there is more than 30% necrosis on the CT scan. Use of prophylactic antibiotics is still considered controversial.
- Zosyn or fluoroquinolones are used if cholangitis is present.
- Be vigilant for monilial superinfection with prophylactic antibiotic use.

Special Considerations

- Can occur in children secondary to trauma (should increase suspicion of child abuse).

When to Consult, Refer, Hospitalize

- Hospitalization required for IV hydration while patient has nothing by mouth, nil per os (NPO), pain management is initiated, and patient is monitored for response to treatment
- Surgical consultation is required in all cases of acute pancreatitis with evidence of abscess formation or infected pancreatic tissue.

Follow-Up

- For recurrent episodes of pancreatitis

Expected Course

- Most uncomplicated cases subside in 3 to 7 days.

Complications

- Pancreatic pseudocysts, abscesses, necrosis, stricture of the common bile duct, diabetes mellitus, chronic pancreatitis, and occasionally pancreatic cancer

DIVERTICULAR DISEASE

Description

- Presence of a diverticulum (herniation of mucosa through muscular wall of the colon)
- Inflammation of a diverticulum, usually caused when undigested food and bacteria remain in the diverticular outpouching and serve as an area where localized abscess and peritonitis begin
  - Infection can vary from a small abscess to peritonitis.
  - Size of the inflamed diverticula varies from small to large, and the number can be one to several dozen.
  - Diverticula are more common in the sigmoid colon (left colon) than in the right colon.

Etiology

- Diverticula develop from increased intraluminal pressure that results from insufficient intake of fiber.
- Subsequently, infection and inflammation result from mechanical obstruction from retention of undigested food residues and bacteria in the diverticula.
- Thought to be a result of poor dietary fiber intake over many years that results in hypertrophy, thickening, and fibrosis of bowel wall from movement of hard stool under increased intraluminal pressures

Incidence and Demographics

- Common in Western countries; uncommon in developing countries
- More common in women

Risk Factors

- Low-fiber diet, increased age, sedentary lifestyle

Prevention and Screening

- High-fiber diet; avoid foods with small seeds that can become trapped in the diverticula

Assessment

History

- Complaints vary with severity of the inflammation and infection; diverticulosis is asymptomatic.
- Crampy left lower or mid-abdominal pain may radiate to the back, or acute pain is localized to the left lower quadrant.
- Fever, constipation, loose stool, and/or nausea and vomiting may be present.

Physical Exam

- There may be left lower quadrant tenderness with a palpable mass and hypoactive bowel sounds.
- Rebound tenderness may also be present and may be suggestive of a perforated diverticulum.
- Rectal exam may reveal a palpable mass (indicating a pelvic abscess) and heme-positive stool.

Diagnostic Studies

- CBC shows a mild to moderate leukocytosis; ESR is elevated in diverticulitis; CBC may be normal in diverticulosis; hemoglobin may be low if bleeding is present and causing anemia.
- Flat-plate and upright abdominal film to look for free air (sign of perforation), ileus, and small or large bowel obstruction
- Abdominal scan CT with IV and oral contrast to delineate pericolic abscesses
- Barium enema should not be obtained in the acute phase, because of risk of perforation; perform after patient has responded to medical management to exclude other problems, such as a mass.
- If a mass or stricture is seen, a colonoscopy should be performed to rule out malignancy after acute episode resolves.

Differential Diagnosis

- Appendicitis
- Ruptured ovarian cyst or follicle
- Twisted ovarian cyst
- Endometriosis
- Ruptured ectopic pregnancy
- Pelvic inflammatory disease
- Crohn's disease
- Colon cancer
- Ischemic bowel
- Intestinal obstruction

Management

Nonpharmacologic Treatment

- Outpatient for the majority of cases with only mild abdominal tenderness, tolerating fluids, low-grade fever, and leukocytosis less than 12,000; initial liquid diet followed by low-residue diet
- Gradually increase dietary fiber after acute phase; avoid eating seeds, nuts, and corn.
- If condition worsens or lacks improvement in 48 to 72 hours, or if peritoneal signs or septicemia, then hospitalize.
- Surgical management is required for signs of abscess or perforation.

Pharmacologic Treatment

- Mild symptoms: metronidazole (Flagyl) 250–500 mg orally q.8.h. plus either trimethoprim-sulfamethoxazole 160/180 (Bactrim DS) orally q.12.h. or other antibiotic (Cipro, Augmentin) for 7 to 10 days; however, antibiotic therapy may be omitted for uncomplicated diverticulitis.
- May treat pain with antispasmodics, opiates (not meperidine—increases intraluminal pressure)
- Stool softeners until dietary fiber can be increased
- Moderate to severe symptoms require hospitalization, IV antibiotics, and nasogastric intubation.

How Long to Treat

- Mild symptoms: 14 days
- Moderate to severe symptoms: Length of treatment may vary.

Special Considerations

- Older adults less likely to have classic symptoms; pursue evaluation despite mild presentation
- No alcohol if metronidazole ordered—will provoke severe vomiting

When to Consult, Refer, Hospitalize

- Hospitalization with surgical consultation should be obtained in all patients with severe diverticulitis (fever, elevated WBC count, rebound tenderness, vomiting, rectal pain) and for those who fail to improve after 48 to 72 hours of medical management.
- Hospitalization is often required for older adults with acute diverticulitis and multiple medical problems.

Follow-Up

- Within 3 days, sooner if worsens; response to antibiotics should occur in 3 days

Expected Course

- Diverticulitis recurs in one-third of patients who receive medical management. Recurrent attacks are an indication for elective surgical resection.

Complications

- Perforation, peritonitis, hemorrhage, and bowel obstruction

Conditions of the Rectum and Anus

HEMORRHOIDS

Description

- Varicosities of the hemorrhoidal venous plexus that are classified as either internal (above pectinate line) or external (below pectinate line); both may coexist.
- Varicosities may be dilated, prolapsed, or thrombosed, often causing painful swelling at the anus.
- Forms when vascular anal cushion prolapses through the anal canal and becomes entrapped by the anal sphincter and a hemorrhoid

Incidence and Demographics

- Occurs in 50% of adults 50 years of age.
- Uncommon under age 25 except in pregnancy

Risk Factors

- Constipation, prolonged sitting or standing
- Weightlifting
- Pregnancy, obesity
- Congestive heart failure, portal hypertension
- Rectal surgery, loss of muscle tone
- Anal intercourse
- Portal hypertension
- Pelvic-occupying lesions

Prevention and Screening

- High-fiber diet
- Avoid constipation and straining to defecate.
- Proper body mechanics when lifting
- Avoid prolonged periods of sitting or standing; change position frequently.
- Weight loss if overweight

Assessment

History

- Rectal bleeding (usually painless and bright red); rectal discomfort, itching, burning
- Inquire about possible risk factors.
- Constipation or straining

Physical Exam

- External hemorrhoids are a soft and painless mass exterior to the anal verge.
- Internal hemorrhoids may be palpated by digital rectal exam or visualized by anoscopy.
- If thrombosed, hemorrhoids are bluish in color, firm, and tender to palpation.

Diagnostic Studies

- Diagnosed by physical exam; if normal exam but has bleeding, colonoscopy in persons age 40 and older.
- CBC to rule out anemia

Differential Diagnosis

- Anal skin tags
- Crohn's disease
- Anal fissure
- Prolapse of rectal mucosa (common in older adults)
- Abscess
- Rectal polyps
- Rectal or anal carcinoma
- Condyloma

Management

Nonpharmacologic Treatment

- Eliminate risk factors when possible.
- Avoid direct pressure on hemorrhoid while sitting.
- Warm sitz baths two to three times daily for 20 minutes, witch-hazel compresses (Tucks) three or four times a day as needed.
- High-fiber diet (20–30 g/day) and increased fluid intake (eight 8 oz glasses/day)

Pharmacologic Treatment

- Bulk-forming laxatives to soften stool and prevent constipation
  - Psyllium (Metamucil) 1 tbsp in 8 oz of fluid up to three times day
  - Methylcellulose (Citrucel) 1 tbsp in 8 oz of fluid up to three times day
- Stool softeners to reduce straining during defecation
  - Docusate sodium (Colace) 50–200 mg/day
- Topical hydrocortisone preparations to relieve pain, itching, and inflammation; cream, foam, and suppositories are available
  - Anusol-HC, ProctoFoam-HC, hydrocortisone cream 1% to 2.5% as needed.
- Local analgesic spray, suppository, or cream provides pain relief
  - Benzocaine (Hurricane), pramoxine (Anusol), or dibucaine (Nupercainal) as needed.

How Long to Treat

- Use topical hydrocortisone preparations for a maximum of 2 to 3 weeks; stool softeners and bulk-forming laxatives may be used indefinitely to prevent reoccurrence.

Special Considerations

- Pregnancy: common, usually resolve spontaneously after delivery

When to Consult, Refer, Hospitalize

- Refer to a colorectal surgeon when symptoms do not respond to conservative treatment within 3 to 4 weeks; when patients present with severe pain, thrombosis, strangulation, ulceration, perianal infection, rectal prolapse, or recurrent symptomatic hemorrhoids.
- Refer patients age 40 and older with rectal bleeding, despite hemorrhoids, to a gastroenterologist for sigmoidoscopy and/or colonoscopy to evaluate for other causes of GI bleeding and to exclude cancer.

Complications

- Bleeding, thrombosis, strangulation, secondary infection, ulceration, and anemia

Follow-Up

- Further evaluation if there is no improvement in symptoms within 2 weeks of initiating treatment, rectal bleeding is excessive or persists, or constipation continues

ANAL FISSURE

Description

- A tear in the lining of the anal canal distal to the dentate line
- Most seen in posterior midline (men); anterior midline may occur in women
- Once occur, become cyclical in nature

Etiology

- Usually associated with the passage of a large, hard stool; can occur with anal stenosis.
- Trauma to anal wall causing pain and inflammation, but usually no infection due to local defenses

Incidence and Demographics

- Incidence unknown, although very common
- Typically occurs in first 3 to 4 years of life
- Can occur in all age groups

Risk Factors

- Sexual abuse should be considered in a child with any abnormal findings
- Constipation
- Trauma

Prevention and Screening

- Avoid constipation.
- Increase fluids and fiber.

Assessment

History

- Passage of a large or hard, dry stool
- Crying during defecation, severe pain
- Bright-red blood evident on toilet paper
- Streaks of blood around stool

Physical Exam

- Fissure can often be seen with careful inspection of the anal area.

Diagnostic Studies

- Not indicated unless the source of the bleeding cannot be identified; may require anesthesia.

Differential Diagnosis

- Juvenile polyp
- Intussusception
- IBD
- Gastroenteritis
- Necrotizing enterocolitis

Management

Nonpharmacologic Treatment

- Anal dilatation is necessary if anal stenosis is present, requires referral
- High-fiber diet or fiber supplements
- Warm sitz baths

Pharmacologic Treatment

- Stool softener to facilitate easy passage and prevent stool withholding
- Topical antibiotic ointment twice a day
- Hydrocortisone cream two or three times a day.
- Topical anesthetics
- Topical nitroglycerin increases local blood flow and reduces pressure in anal sphincter to facilitate healing.
- Botulin toxin may be used and has fewer side effects than nitroglycerin therapy.

How Long to Treat

- Until soft stool is produced, and the fissure is healed

Special Considerations

- Suspect sexual abuse when more than one fissure is present or if the patient is a child

When to Consult, Refer, Hospitalize

- Consult or refer to surgeon or colorectal specialist if symptoms persist after 90 days of treatment.
- Report to child protective authorities if sexual abuse is suspected.

Follow-Up

- 1 to 2 weeks

Expected Course

- Uncomplicated; resolves when fissure is healed, and constipation resolved

Complications

- Recurrence, skin ulceration
- Fecal incontinence

Conditions of the Liver

VIRAL HEPATITIS

Description

- Inflammation of the liver caused by a viral infection that may be acute (less than 6 months duration) or chronic (over 6 months duration) that produces liver dysfunction with a broad range of severity
- Six types of viral hepatitis have been identified: A, B, C, D, E, and G. (Hepatitis A, B, and C are discussed in this chapter.)
- Hepatitis B virus (HBV) and hepatitis C virus (HCV) account for 60% to 80% of chronic hepatitis.

Etiology

- Hepatitis A virus (HAV): an RNA hepatovirus
- Hepatitis B virus (HBV): a DNA hepadnavirus with an inner core protein and outer surface coat component
- Hepatitis C virus (HCV): an RNA togavirus
- Hepatitis D virus (HDV): a defective RNA virus that occurs only in persons with HBV infection

- Hepatitis E virus (HEV): an RNA virus like calicivirus
- Hepatitis G virus (HGV): a flavivirus

Incidence and Demographics

- HAV: 25,000 infections per year since the development of hepatitis A (Hep A) vaccine; 70% are symptomatic, 33% have serologic evidence for past HAV infection
- HBV: 140,000 to 320,000 infections per year, 2 million with chronic infection; more than 500,000 carriers; post-transfusion infection in less than 1%
- HCV: 40,000 new infections per year; chronic infection will develop in more than 85% of those infected; approximately 4 million HCV carriers; 10% have no known source of infection

Risk Factors

See Table 9–4.

TABLE 9–4.
COMPARISON OF VIRAL HEPATITIS TRANSMISSION

VIRUS	TRANSMISSION	RISK FACTORS	INCUBATION	CHRONICITY
Hepatitis A	Fecal–oral	Contaminated food and water Common in overcrowded, poor sanitation areas; also close contacts	15–50 days	No
Hepatitis B	Blood, body fluids	Transfusion Needle sharing Exposure to infected body fluids Sexual activity Perinatal transmission	45–160 days	Yes
Hepatitis C	Blood, body fluids	Transfusion Needle-sharing High-risk sexual behavior Cocaine use Low risk of perinatal transmission	14–180 days	Yes

Prevention and Screening

- Health care providers need a high index of suspicion.
- Universal precautions should be practiced by all health care and day care workers when in contact with blood, blood products, or body fluids.
- Safe sex practices
- Avoid intravenous drug use and sharing of needles.
- Screen all blood products for HBV and HCV infection.
- Proper hygiene and handwashing by food handlers
- Screen all pregnant women for HBV infection.
- Vaccinate against hepatitis A and B (see Table 9–5).
- Immune globulin to all close personal contacts of persons with hepatitis A; traveling to endemic areas; with chronic liver disease or clotting disorders; sewage workers and food handlers, day care workers

Assessment

- Symptoms of viral hepatitis are similar, but the severity of symptoms may vary among types, ranging from asymptomatic infection without jaundice to fulminant hepatitis (severe form of acute hepatitis indicated by encephalopathy, hypoglycemia, bleeding, and prolonged prothrombin time).

History

- Symptoms vary according to phase of disease:
  - Pre-icteric: fatigue, malaise, anorexia, nausea, vomiting, headache, aversion to smoking and alcohol
- May remain asymptomatic
- Icteric: weight loss, pruritus, RUQ pain, clay-colored stool; frequently, pronounced jaundice and may appear mildly toxic to acutely ill (see Table 9–6).

Physical Exam

- General toxicity varies with disease severity.
- Jaundice of the skin, sclera, and mucous membranes

TABLE 9–5.
HEPATITIS VACCINES

VIRUS	VACCINE	TARGET POPULATION	DOSING REGIMEN	DOSE
Hepatitis A	Havrix, Vaqta Twinrix (A and B)	International travelers Children older than 2 years living in endemic areas Chronic liver disease Men who have sex with men IV drug users Occupational risk	*Age 2–18 years:* Havrix, either 2-or 3-dose schedule; Vaqta, 2-dose schedule *Age older than 18 years:* 2-dose schedule of Havrix; 3–4 dose schedule of Twinrix Second dose given 6–12 months after the first Havrix	*2–18 years:* 0.5 mL *older than 18 year:* 1 mL IM anterolateral thigh in children, deltoid in adults
Hepatitis B	Recombivax or Engerix-B Pediarix (combination DPT, Hep B, and polio) Comvax (combination Haemophilus influenzae type b (HIb)and Hep B)	All infants All children not previously vaccinated Health care workers People with high-risk behaviors	Three doses given at 0, 1, and 6 months Many are given in combination with routine pediatric doses in single injection	*0–19 years:* 0.5 mL *older than 19 years:* 1.0 mL IM in anterolateral thigh for children; deltoid for adults
Hepatitis C, D, E, G	None available			

- Lymphadenopathy usually present in cervical and epitrochlear areas
- Abdominal exam: liver tenderness with hepatomegaly present in more than 50%; splenomegaly present in 15%
- Dark urine or clay-colored stools

TABLE 9–6.
VIRAL HEPATITIS DIAGNOSTIC CRITERIA

VIRUS	SYMPTOMS	CONTAGIOUS INTERVAL	DIAGNOSIS POSITIVE LABS
HAV	Children either asymptomatic or very mild nonspecific symptoms Adults usually symptomatic with 1–2 week prodrome of anorexia, nausea, malaise, fever, then jaundice	1–3 weeks before illness lasting through first week of illness	*Acute:* Anti-HAV IgM Anti-HAV IgG develops later in disease and stays for life
HBV	In young children usually asymptomatic Adult symptoms range from asymptomatic seroconversion to acute illness with anorexia, nausea, malaise, jaundice, arthralgias, arthritis, macular skin rash, to fatal hepatitis	All persons with surface antigen of hepatitis B virus (HBsAg) are infectious.	*Acute:* HBsAg Hepatitis B core antigen (HBcAg) IgM anti-HBc If (hepatitis B e antigen (HBeAg) positive, indication of more serious disease *Recovery:* HBsAg Anti-HBs Anti-HBc *Chronic:* HBsAg Anti-HBc
HCV	Asymptomatic in children Adults often mild disease, difficult to distinguish from Hepatitis A and hepatitis B Jaundice in only 25%	All people with HCV antibody or HCV-RNA are considered contagious. Recombinant ImmunoBlot Assay (RIBA) *Chronic:* Serum anti-HCV antibody	*Acute:* Enzyme-linked immunosorbent assay (ELISA) II

Diagnostic Studies

- ALT and AST levels may be elevated; levels peak (400 to several thousand IU/L) during the icteric phase, and then decrease progressively during the convalescent phase.
- Serum bilirubin normal to markedly elevated; clinical jaundice evident at levels higher than 2.5.
- ALP may be normal or mildly elevated.
- Prothrombin time; if prolonged, may indicate serious disease of the liver
- CBC may reveal an increased number of atypical-appearing lymphocytes.
- Urinalysis may be positive for protein and bilirubin.
- Above tests in Table 9-6 may be normal in patients with chronic hepatitis C.
- Serologic tests for viral hepatitis (see Table 9–6)
- Liver biopsy if diagnosis is uncertain, gold standard for severity and activity of chronic hepatitis

Differential Diagnosis

- CMV, herpes simplex virus
- Coxsackievirus
- Toxoplasmosis
- *Candida, Mycobacteria*
- *Pneumocystis*
- *Leptospira*
- Use of hepatotoxic agents
- Alcoholic hepatitis
- Ischemic hepatitis
- Acute cholecystitis
- Common bile duct stone
- Ascending cholangitis
- Cirrhosis

Management

Nonpharmacologic Treatment

- Activity as tolerated; high-calorie, small, palatable meals; hydration to 4,000 mL daily
- Avoid hepatotoxic agents (i.e., acetaminophen and alcohol)
- Colloid baths and lotions to decrease pruritus if present

Pharmacologic Treatment

- For acute, uncomplicated hepatitis A and B, no pharmacologic treatment is indicated.
- Acute hepatitis C, medications are curative
- Antiemetic medications for nausea and vomiting if needed
- Use oxazepam if a benzodiazepine is indicated; avoid morphine sulfate.
- Chronic hepatitis B is treated with pegylated interferon (PegIFN) or nucleoside analogs (lamivudine, tenofovir, and ribavirin) if there is evidence of liver impairment.
- Direct-acting antivirals (DAAs) are the most common treatment for hepatitis C, with curative rates up to 97%
- There are three types of DAAs used for hepatitis C:
  - NS3/4 protease inhibitors, which target an enzyme
  - NS5A inhibitors, which target a protein
  - NS5B polymerase inhibitors, which target an enzyme
- Postexposure hepatitis B
  - Unvaccinated people: hepatitis B immune globulin (HBIG) 0.06 mL/kg IM given as soon as possible (within 7 days of exposure), followed by initiation of HBV vaccination series (see table 9-5), prevents illness in approximately 75%
  - Recommended after direct transmucosal or parental exposure with HBsAg-infected blood or body fluids. HBIG (0.5 mL IM) is given to all newborns of HBsAg-positive mothers within 12 hours of birth.
- Postexposure hepatitis A
  - All household and sexual contacts, give 0.02 mL/kg of immune globulin as soon as possible (within 2 weeks) and begin HAV vaccine.

How Long to Treat

- In chronic hepatitis B, treatment is continued until loss of HBeAg, loss of HBV-DNA, loss of HBsAg, and normal ALT level achieved.
- In chronic hepatitis C, treatment is continued until viral replication is inhibited, normal ALT levels, loss of HCV-RNA, reduction of hepatic inflammation, and improvement in liver histology.

Special Considerations

- HBV: transmitted vertically (mother to infant) in less than 10% HEV: high mortality rate in pregnancy (10% to 20%)
- Lactation: HBV transmission uncertain; HCV transmission unlikely
- Management strategies may differ in patients with cirrhosis and coinfections of HBV and HCV

When to Consult, Refer, Hospitalize

- Consult with physician or specialist for all cases of hepatitis B, C, or D because of high incidence of chronic hepatitis development.
- Refer to a gastroenterologist/hepatologist and/or an infectious disease specialist for uncertain diagnosis, symptoms of fulminant hepatitis, and chronic hepatitis.

Follow-Up

- Hepatitis A patients in 2 weeks to reevaluate condition
- Hepatitis B, C, and D require frequent follow-up during acute stage, then 4- to 8-week intervals if chronic illness develops.

Expected Course

- Acute hepatitis usually resolves over 4 to 8 weeks.

Complications

- Hepatic necrosis, chronic active or chronic hepatitis, cirrhosis, hepatic failure, hepatocellular carcinoma (HBV and HCV)
- Fatal fulminant hepatitis (HAV)
- Chronic hepatitis B and C increase risk for the development of cirrhosis.

GI Conditions Found in Infants and Children

PHYSIOLOGIC JAUNDICE IN THE HEALTHY TERM NEWBORN

Description

- Increased levels of unconjugated serum bilirubin (more than 2.0 mg/dL) that occur 3 to 5 days after birth and cause jaundice
- Pathologic jaundice occurs when there is erythrocyte destruction because of ABO or Rh incompatibility, glucose-6-phosphate hydrogenase (G6PD) deficiency, or other pathologic conditions.
- Overproduction of bilirubin and delayed conjugation of bilirubin caused by increased rate of hemolysis and inefficient hepatic breakdown of bilirubin
- About 60% of infants will have clinical physiologic jaundice with a peak bilirubin level 5–6 mg/dL.
- Approximately 3% of newborns will have more severe jaundice with serum bilirubin levels in the range of 13–15 mg/dL; 2% of breastfed infants will have a 2- to 8-week course of detectable physiological jaundice with an unconjugated bilirubin level in the range of 10–15 mg/dL.
- Parents must be aware that normal physiologic bilirubin levels will not peak until 72 to 96 hours of age for a full-term infant.
- Teach parents how to assess for the presence of jaundice.
- Observe skin color, noting how far down the trunk jaundice has progressed (begins in face and moves downward as bilirubin levels rise).
- Blanch the skin to observe jaundice.
- Abdominal exam: should have normal liver

Diagnostic Studies

- Total bilirubin level, including conjugated bilirubin which is necessary for severe and rapid-onset jaundice in the newborn
- Direct Coombs test, G6PD enzyme assay done if pathologic jaundice or rapidly advancing physiologic jaundice is suspected
- Hematocrit
- Blood type (ABO) and Rh factor

Differential Diagnosis

- Sepsis
- Galactosemia
- Hemolytic disease

Management

- Phototherapy may be necessary: Light enhances bile excretion; home phototherapy can occur in uncomplicated cases.
- Guidelines for initiation vary with age of infant, presence of risk factors (i.e., breastfed infants are expected to reach higher levels), hydration status, and gestational age.
- Generally, consider in full-term infants with total serum bilirubin levels 12–15 mg/dL at 24 to 48 hours old, 15–18 mg/dL at 48 to 72 hours old, or 17–20 mg/dL over 72 hours old
- Breastfeeding can continue and supplementation with water is not necessary, but more-frequent feeding should occur.
- Monitor total bilirubin levels daily; continue treatment until levels stabilize or begin to fall. When phototherapy is instituted, the infant's eyes must be protected from the light, temperature should be monitored, and extra fluid should be given to replace that lost from evaporation.
- Consult with physician or refer to neonatal specialist if pathologic jaundice suspected or feeding difficulty, behavior changes, apnea, fever, or temperature instability.
- Suspect pathologic jaundice if it occurs in first 24 hours of life: total bilirubin rises more than 5 mg/dL per day; total bilirubin exceeds 15 mg/dL in full-term infants (10 mg/dL in premature infants); jaundice lasts longer than 10 days in full-term infants (21 days in premature infants); or direct bilirubin exceeds 1.5 mg/dL.
- Physiologic jaundice resolves approximately 1 week after birth.

COLIC

Description

- Excessive crying in an infant who is otherwise well. Crying lasts longer than 3 hours per day, at least 3 days/week, for at least 3 weeks in an infant under 3 months old. Symptoms often peak at 6 weeks.
- Exact pathophysiology unknown; historically believed to be problem with interaction between infant and environment, although many researchers question this assumption.
- Several possible etiologies: normal variant, maternal/child interaction, family tensions, immaturity of GI tract, stimulus sensitivity, infant temperament, food allergy or intolerance
- May be associated with excessive gas, cow's milk, or other food intolerance
- Occurs in one-third of all infants
- Occurs equally in breastfed and bottle-fed, boys and girls
- Discuss crying history, feeding history, elimination patterns, and interventions tried with parents.
- Measure growth parameters and developmental milestones.
- Careful abdominal examination to assess for masses, tenderness
- Observe parent–child interaction.
- Diagnostic studies are not necessary if there is adequate weight gain, infant meets developmental milestones, and physical exam is normal.
- Reassure parents that no physical problem is present; educate regarding normal infant crying
- Soothe infant by providing motion (swing, rocker, car seat), papoose carrier, snug bundling
- Ensure adequate burping during feeding.
- Encourage and provide support for the mother.
- Switching to hypoallergenic formula (hydrolyzed casein whey) may be helpful.
- Avoiding cow's milk in diet of breastfeeding mothers may also help.
- Colic is a self-limiting condition, which gradually improves.
- Virtually gone by the age of 4 months

PYLORIC STENOSIS

Description

- Presents as projectile vomiting in infants between 2 weeks and 5 months of age because of hypertrophy of the pylorus, which causes increasing duodenal obstruction
  - Infant is hungry, willing to eat after vomiting, but becomes progressively dehydrated.
  - Fretfulness is common.
  - There may be visible gastric peristaltic waves from left to right across the abdomen.
  - Palpable pyloric mass, like an olive, best palpable during feeding or immediately after vomiting
  - The infant should be referred to a pediatric surgeon immediately for pyloromyotomy.
- Following surgery, nothing by mouth until 12 to 24 hours, then advance to full feeds by 36 to 48 hours
- Discharge when tolerating full-strength feeds
- Surgery is considered curative.
- Gastric spasms cause continued spitting of feeds after surgery. Encourage parents to feed small volumes slowly and frequently reassure the family.
- Overfeeding a ravenous baby can lead to regurgitation.

FAILURE TO THRIVE (FTT)

Description

- General sign characterized by failure of physical growth, malnutrition, and potential retardation of development in children. It is described as a child with any of the following growth abnormalities:
  - Weight for age less than 5th percentile on more than one occasion
  - Weight that drops 2 or more percentile lines on standard growth charts
  - Weight less than 80% ideal body weight based on National Center for Health Statistics growth charts
  - Weight for height less than 10th percentile
  - Height for age less than 10th percentile
- Children with various syndromes, premature infants, and intrauterine growth restriction follow different growth patterns.

Risk Factors

- Poverty is the leading risk factor.
- Other risk factors include parents with mental health disorders or cognitive impairment; poor parenting skills; hypervigilant parents; history of physical, emotional, or substance abuse; and social isolation.

Assessment

- Labs should be ordered based on history and physical exam findings and age of patient. May include CBC, electrolytes, lead level, LFTs, TSH.
- In addition to growth parameters, children should be evaluated for signs of abuse, genetic disorders, hypothyroidism, cystic fibrosis, chronic diarrhea, lactose intolerance, GERD, HIV, and TB.

Management

- Treat any underlying conditions that may be identified in the workup.
- Parents should be involved in all aspects of the workup and diagnosis, with a focus on building a trusting relationship for future discussions.
- More-frequent visits for weight monitoring, weekly until significant weight gain
- A multidisciplinary approach to therapy is ideal; parent education and mealtime coaching are paramount.
- Provide home resources to evaluate other problems and provide support and teaching.
- High-calorie, high-protein diet calculated to provide 1½–2 times daily caloric needs. Children on this diet should gain significant weight in the first week of therapy.
- Vitamin supplementation is warranted.
- Close monitoring is warranted for months.
- Children who do not respond within 2 to 3 months in the primary care setting should be referred to a pediatric growth specialist or program.
- Children who present as severely malnourished, septic, or abused may need to be hospitalized.
- Failure to identify at-risk children may result in impaired cognitive and developmental delays, short stature, and chronic medical problems.

CYSTIC FIBROSIS (CF)

Description

- Most common lethal genetic disease in the United States
- Caused by defect on chromosome 7, autosomal recessive inheritance pattern
- Classic diagnostic triad is elevated sweat chloride concentration; production of abnormally tenacious mucous secretion in the gut, pancreas, and hepatobiliary system, resulting in obstruction and chronic pulmonary disease
- CF should be considered in any infant with chronic diarrhea and FTT. There is a possible association between GERD and CF. Although CF affects the GI system, long-term progressive pulmonary disease leads to mortality.
- 1:2,500 White births
- Median survival rate is 47 years.
- Characterized by poor growth, wheezing, dyspnea and cough, digital clubbing, cyanosis, increased flatulence and foul-smelling, greasy stools, and abdominal distention and pain
- Diagnosis is made with a positive sweat test: sweat chloride more than 60 mmol/L; may be unreliable in infants under 1 month old; therefore confirmation through genetic testing is recommended.
- Differential diagnosis includes FTT, celiac disease, bronchiectasis, reactive airway disease, and chronic sinusitis

Management

- High-caloric nutritional support, 100–150 kcal/day
- Multidisciplinary team approach
- Nighttime nasogastric/gastrostomy/jejunostomy supplementation as necessary
- Chest physiotherapy before meals
- Pancreatic enzyme supplementation (lipase) 2,500 units/kg/meal or less
- Vitamin replacement, particularly A, E, D, and K, as these are poorly absorbed secondary to steatorrhea
- May need aerosolized bronchodilator therapy
- Hospitalization is frequently necessary to treat infection and for pulmonary symptom management.

- The average life span is 47 years; with current improved treatment regimens including potential benefits of cystic fibrosis transmembrane conductance regulator (CFTR) modulators and lung transplant, life expectancy is increasing.

INTUSSUSCEPTION

Description

- Telescoping of part of the bowel into another; results in decreased blood flow. Ischemia and infarction of intestine may occur if not treated. Ileocolic intussusception is most common, accounting for 80% of cases.
- Idiopathic: most commonly, cause is unknown.
- Pathologic: lead point found, occurs secondary to an abnormality in the bowel such as Meckel's diverticulum, polyps, intestinal duplication, hematoma, intestinal parasites, or, in older children, a malignancy
- Recent history of viral illness postulated to cause an increase in lymph tissue called Peyer's patches, thought to be a lead point for the intussusception
- Peak incidence is 3 to 36 months of age; ratio of boys to girls is 2:1
- Presents with cramping, intermittent colicky pain
- Screaming, pulling legs upward during episode, followed by period of lethargy
- Pallor
- Bloody stool after the onset of symptoms
- "Currant jelly" stool is a late finding.
- Sausage-shaped mass may be palpable across the midline.
- Bowel sounds may be normal early, hyperactive during painful episodes. Absent bowel sounds are a late finding.

Diagnostic Studies

- CBC to rule out infection
- Abdominal X-ray reveals staircase pattern due to invagination of intestine.
- Ultrasound is diagnostic.
- Contrast enema is both diagnostic and therapeutic.

Differential Diagnosis

- Gastroenteritis
- Tumor
- Constipation/impaction
- Meckel's diverticulum
- Incarcerated inguinal hernia
- Malrotation/volvulus
- Hirschsprung's disease

Management

- Placement of a nasogastric tube and contrast enema reduction done by experienced radiologist is both diagnostic and curative.
- Surgery is indicated if signs of peritonitis, shock, or incomplete radiologic reduction. Resection of the affected bowel may be indicated.
- If reduction complete, restart feedings. Discharge from the hospital takes place after the child has tolerated a full liquid diet.
- Radiologic reduction should not be attempted if symptoms present longer than 5 days, in infants under 3 months of age, or in any child with peritonitis or shock, in whom perforation is suspected.
- Urgent surgical consultation recommended before radiologic reduction undertaken.
- Children are usually discharged from the hospital 24 hours after reduction.

ENCOPRESIS

Description

- Fecal soiling or staining underwear after 4 years of age because of constipation (retentive) or other factors such as resistance to toilet training or reluctance to leave activities to use toilet
- Most common cause is functional, including poor dietary intake of fiber and fluids, behavioral habits such as change in environment with travel or schedule, sedentary

lifestyle. Occurs in children, most often when cereal is first introduced to diet, during toilet training, or entry to school.

- Psychogenic; chronic constipation can begin in the first year of life

Management

Nonpharmacologic Treatment

- Infants under 6 months old
  - If exclusively on formula or breast milk, continue with same; review formula preparation and fluid intake of breastfeeding mother
- Infants 6 to 12 months old
  - Continue present formula or breastfeeding.
  - Offer water between feedings.
  - Add high-fiber food such as prunes, apricots, plums, peas, and beans.
  - May add apple juice or Karo syrup to diet.
- Toddlers and preschoolers
  - Increase water intake and decrease juice intake.
  - Offer whole fruits instead of juice.
  - Increase fiber in diet so child is receiving child's age plus 5 as grams of fiber per day.
- All 5 years of age and older
  - Increase fiber; age 5 to 15: age plus 5 equals g of fiber/day; adults: 20–35 g/day
  - Increase fiber gradually, over a 2-week period.
  - Increase fluid intake, particularly water; for adults, 1.5–2 liters/day
  - Physical exercise; bowel training program/behavior modification
- Non-retentive encopresis
  - Increase child's responsibility, provide incentives.
  - Counsel parents to stop any pressures on child regarding defecation, accidents.
  - No punishment for defecating in pants
- If the nonpharmacological methods are not effective after a month, resort to pharmacologic therapy.

Pharmacologic Treatment

- Lactulose, sorbitol, and Miralax are generally well tolerated in children.
- Mineral oil orally 1–3 mL/kg/day (should not be used under a year of age because of risk of aspiration). This must be disguised to get children to swallow it. Is usually second-line treatment.
- Initiation phase: Home colonic clean-out (goal: yellow, liquid stools), often achieved using high doses of Miralax (two to three capfuls for 2 or more days, with dosing more dependent on findings on physical exam than age and weight dosing or using repeated doses of magnesium citrate [use age-and-weight dosing and repeat two or three times a day for 2 or more days]). Fleet enemas often needed in this phase. Because this is more invasive and often difficult for parents and children, this decision needs to be made in the context of a physical examination.
- Surfactants: used to soften stools; docusate sodium (Colace) for children 3 to 6 years, 20–60 mg/day; 6 to 12 years, 40–150 mg/day; short-term up to 2 weeks; may be used longer and do not induce dependency.

CASE STUDIES

CASE 1

A 6-week-old infant presents to the clinic for a well-baby exam. The mother tells you the baby is spitting up with every feeding. She has decreased the amount per feeding and increased the frequency, but the child still spits up a large portion of the feeding. He is on Isomil, and Mom is feeding 1–2 oz every 1 to 2 hours around the clock. There is no weight loss; he has gained 6 oz since his 2-week visit. Mother denies projectile vomiting.

Past Medical History: He is the product of an uncomplicated pregnancy and term birth. Currently the infant is on no medications.

1. What other history would you ask for?

   Exam: Vital signs, growth parameters stable. Head, eyes, ears, nose, and throat, normal; lungs clear; heart RRR, no murmur; abdomen: normal bowel sounds, soft, no masses, organomegaly.

2. What laboratory tests would you order?
3. What other studies would you order?
4. What is the most probable diagnosis, and what treatment would you provide?

CASE 2

An 18-year-old woman presents with abdominal pain. She has had some vague lower abdominal cramping off and on for the last 2 months, but today the pain intensified, and she was unable to attend school. She has had episodes of loose stools and that has seemed to ease the pain until today; otherwise, her bowel habits have been normal.

1. What other history questions would you ask this patient?

   Exam: Alert and oriented woman lying in a fetal position. Vital signs are stable . Abdomen: increased bowel sounds, softly distended, no masses, organomegaly, diffuse tenderness in right lower quadrant and left lower quadrant, no rebound or guarding. Rectal: no masses or tenderness. Hemoccult: negative.

Pelvic: normal.

2. What laboratory tests would you order?
3. What other studies would you consider?
4. What is the likely diagnosis if laboratory tests are normal, and what treatment would you provide?

CASE 3

A family of three presents to you complaining of vomiting and diarrhea for 2 days. It started with the 3-year-old son, then the mother, and now the father. They are most concerned about their son because he has not had anything to eat or drink since yesterday and has had a fever with temperature of 101°F. He is otherwise healthy and has had no past medical illness other than an occasional cold.

1. What other questions would you ask this family?

   Exam: 3-year-old male child appears lethargic. Temperature 101.4°, pulse 120, respirations 22.

   Head, eyes, ears, nose, and throat: Normal heart: RRR, no murmur. Lungs: clear.

   Abdomen: Increased bowel sounds, soft, no masses or tenderness, organomegaly.

2. What laboratory tests would you order?
3. Are any other diagnostic studies warranted at this time?
4. What is the likely diagnosis, and what treatment would you provide?

CASE STUDIES DISCUSSION

CASE 1

1. What other history would you ask for?

   Ask if there is any choking during feeding (if so, consider congenital anomalies), any bile or blood in regurgitation (obstruction), fevers, upper respiratory infection symptoms (infection), other illnesses? Are developmental milestones appropriate (smiling, lifting head when prone)? Neurological disorders, stooling pattern, irritability, consolability (intussusception, Hirschsprung's disease), any projectile vomiting (pyloric stenosis), feeding position and post-feeding position? Family history of food allergies (food intolerances/allergies), sleeping pattern.

2. What laboratory tests would you order?

   CBC, to look for infection, anemia; electrolytes, to evaluate hydration status; urinalysis (U/A), to look for UTI, hydration status

3. What other studies would you order?

   Chest X-ray, to look for congenital anomalies, lung status, cardiac enlargement

4. What is the most probable diagnosis, and what treatment would you provide?

   If all studies are normal, would consider change in formula to Nutramigen for possible allergy. Upright with feeding and post-feeding. Review burping techniques and frequency during feedings. Close follow-up and if not resolving referral to pediatric gastroenterologist.

CASE 2

1. What other history questions would you ask this patient?

   Stool pattern more than three per day or less than three per week, straining or feeling of incomplete evacuation, mucus in stools, feeling abdominal distention (IBS), any blood in stools, nocturnal diarrhea (ulcerative colitis (UC)), fever, anorexia, weight loss (UC), last menstrual period, birth control, history of STDs (pelvic inflammatory disease), ectopic pregnancy), any association with certain foods (lactose intolerance), UTI symptoms, family history of bowel disease, nausea, vomiting, low-fiber diet (diverticulosis)

2. What laboratory tests would you order?

   CBC: infection, anemia, blood loss; ESR: inflammatory process; beta-HCG: pregnancy; stool for WBCs, culture; ova and parasites: infectious etiology; albumin: malabsorption, chronic disease

3. What other studies would you consider?

   Abdominal ultrasound: ectopic, ovarian abscess; sigmoidoscopy: UC; colonoscopy: Crohn's disease

4. What is the likely diagnosis if laboratory tests are normal, and what treatment would you provide?

   If all laboratory tests are normal, the most likely diagnosis is IBS. Have patient keep a diary of food intake and symptoms, avoid foods that increase symptoms, trial for 2 weeks on a lactose-free diet, increase fiber. Antidiarrheal or anticholinergic as needed. Close follow-up, if unresponsive refer for further evaluation.

CASE 3

1. What other questions would you ask this family?
   - Frequency of vomiting, color of vomitus, waking at night to vomit
   - Frequency of diarrhea, description of stools, blood, mucus
   - Fever, lethargy, urine output, crying with tears
   - Recent travel, camping, day care
   - Any common food source that all members have eaten
2. What laboratory tests would you order?
   - CBC with differential to evaluate for infection, parasites
   - U/A: hydration status
   - Stool for WBC, culture, ova and parasites
3. Are any other diagnostic studies warranted at this time? No
4. What is the likely diagnosis, and what treatment would you provide? Acute gastroenteritis

   While awaiting lab results, maintain and improve hydration status. Give oral replacement therapy (ORT) at 50 mL/kg over a 4-hour period, start with sips and gradually increase if no vomiting occurs. If vomiting occurs, either wait an hour and retry or give an antiemetic, and then try to rehydrate again with ORT. Once child is rehydrated (crying with tears, alert, good urine output, thirsty), resume regular diet.

REFERENCES

Agency for Healthcare Research & Quality. *Comparing effectiveness of management strategies for gastroesophageal reflux disease: An update of the 2005 report.* http://effectivehealthcare.ahrq.gov

Alsinnari, Y. M., Alqarni, M. S., Attar, M., Bukhari, Z. M., Almutairi, M., Baabbad, F. M., & Hasosah, M. (2022). Risk factors for recurrence of peptic ulcer disease: A retrospective study in tertiary care referral center. *Cureus, 14*(2), e22001. doi: 10.7759/cureus.22001. PMID: 35282517; PMCID: PMC8907029

American Cancer Society (2023). *Guidelines for the early detection of cancer.* https://www.cancer.org/cancer/screening/american-cancer-society-guidelines-for-the-early-detection-of-cancer.html

American College of Gastroenterology. (2005). Chronic Constipation Task Force: An evidence-based approach to the management of chronic constipation in North America. *American Journal of Gastroenterology, 100*(Suppl. 1), 51–54.

American Gastroenterological Association. (2002). Medical position statement: Irritable bowel syndrome. *Gastroenterology, 123*(6), 2108–2131.

American Gastroenterological Association. (2005). Guidelines: Elevation of liver chemistry tests. *Gastroenterology, 126,* 1364.

Gau, S. Y., Lai, J. N., Yip, H. T., Wu, M. C., & Wei, J. C. (2022). Higher Dementia Risk in People with Gastroesophageal Reflux Disease: A Real-World Evidence. *Frontiers in Aging Neuroscience, 14,* 830729. doi: 10.3389/fnagi.2022.830729. PMID: 35444524; PMCID: PMC9014245.

Gilbert, D. N., Moellering, R. C., & Eliopoulos, G. M. (2012). *The Sanford guide to antimicrobial therapy 2012.* Hyde Park, VT: Antimicrobial Therapy, Inc.

Katz, P. O., Dunbar, K. B., Schnoll-Sussman, F. H., Greer, K. B., Yadlapati, R., & Spechler, S. J. (2022). ACG Clinical Guideline for the Diagnosis and Management of Gastroesophageal Reflux Disease. *The American Journal of Gastroenterology, 117*(1), 27–56. https://doi.org/10.14309/ajg.0000000000001538

Kornbluth, A., & Sachar, D. B. (2010). Ulcerative colitis practice guidelines in adults (update): American College of Gastroenterology, Practice Partners Committee. *American Journal of Gastroenterology, 105,* 501–523.

Latif, E. A., Inam-U-Llah, Mahdi, H., Zarour, A., Aftab, Z., & Aboumarzouk, O. M., (2022) Is percutaneous extraction of gallstones safe and effective in high-risk patients? Evidence from a systematic review. *Surgeon, 20,* 99–107. doi: 10.1016/j.surge.2022.04.007.. PMID: 35606261.

Lipsett, S. C., Monuteaux, M. C., Shanahan, K. H., & Bachur, R. G. (2022). Nonoperative management of uncomplicated appendicitis. *Pediatrics, 149*(5), e2021054693. doi: 10.1542/peds.2021-054693. PMID: 35434736.

Mijač, D., Krstić, M. N., Marković, A. P., Popović, D. D., Krstić, J. M., & Milosavljević, T. (2022). Abnormal liver blood tests: Primary care approach. *Digestive Diseases, 40*(2), 215–222. doi: 10.1159/000517016. Epub 2021 May 5. PMID: 33951646.

Mora-Capín, A., López-López, R., Guibert-Zafra, B., de Ceano-Vivas La Calle, M., Porto-Abad, R., Molina-Cabañero, J. C., Gilabert-Iriondo, N., Ferrero-García-Loygorri, C., Montero-Valladares, C., García-Herrero, M. Á.; Grupo de Trabajo de Hidratación y Trastornos electrolíticos de la Sociedad Española de Urgencias Pediátricas. (2022). Recommendation document on rapid intravenous rehydration in acute gastroenteritis. *Annals of Pediatrics* (Engl ed), *24,* S2341-2879(22)00124-7. doi: 10.1016/j.anpede.2021.04.011. Epub ahead of print. PMID: 35624005.

Morrow, L., & Greenwald, B. (2022). The American College of Gastroenterology's 2021 Colorectal Cancer Screening Guidelines: A Summary for Gastroenterology Nurses & Associates. Gastroenterology Nursing *45*(3), 184–187. doi: 10.1097/SGA.0000000000000638. Epub 2022 Feb 28. PMID: 35657357

Najeeb, H., Yasmin, F., & Surani, S. (2022). Emerging role of biosimilars in the clinical care of inflammatory bowel disease patients. *World Journal of Clinical Cases, 10*(14):4327–4333. doi: 10.12998/wjcc.v10.i14.4327. PMID: 35663066; PMCID: PMC9125297.

Satish Kumar, L., Pugalenthi, L. S., Ahmad, M., Reddy, S., Barkhane, Z., & Elmadi, J. (2022). Probiotics in irritable bowel syndrome: A review of their therapeutic role. *Cureus, 14*(4), e24240.https://doi.org/10.7759/cureus.24240

Sawayama, H., Miyamoto, Y., Yoshida, N., & Baba, H. Essential updates 2020/2021: Colorectal diseases (benign)-Current topics in the surgical and medical treatment of benign colorectal diseases. *Annals Gastroenterology Surgery, 6*(3), 321–335. doi: 10.1002/ags3.12548. PMID: 35634190; PMCID: PMC9130914.

Sokic-Milutinovic, A., Pavlovic-Markovic, A., Tomasevic, R. S., & Lukic, S. (2022). Diarrhea as a clinical challenge: General practitioner approach. *Digestive Diseases, 40,* 282–289

Thavanesan, N., White, S., Lee, S., Ratnayake, B., Oppong, K. W., Nayar, M. K., Sharp, L., Drewes, A. M., Capurso, G., De-Madaria, E., Siriwardena, A. K., Windsor, J. A., & Pandanaboyana, S. (2022). Analgesia in the initial management of acute pancreatitis: A systematic review and meta-analysis of randomised controlled trials. *World Journal of Surgery, 46*(4), 878–890. doi: 10.1007/s00268-021-06420-w. Epub 2022 Jan 7. PMID: 34994837.

Triggs, J., & Pandolfino, J. (2019). Recent advances in dysphagia management. *F1000Research, 8,* F1000 Faculty Rev-1527. https://doi.org/10.12688/f1000research.18900.1

Wu, B. U., & Conwell, D. L. (2010a). Acute pancreatitis part I: Approach to early management. *Clinical Gastroenterology and Hepatology, 8*(5), 410–416.

Wu, B. U., & Conwell, D. L. (2010b). Acute pancreatitis part II: Approach to follow-up. *Clinical Gastroenterology and Hepatology, 8*(5), 417–422.

